INTRODUCTION TO RADIOLOGICAL PHYSICS AND RADIATION DOSIMETRY

INTRODUCTION TO RADIOLOGICAL PHYSICS AND RADIATION DOSIMETRY

FRANK HERBERT ATTIX
Professor of Medical Physics
University of Wisconsin Medical School
Madison, Wisconsin

A Wiley-Interscience Publication
JOHN WILEY & SONS
New York Chichester Brisbane Toronto Singapore

Attix, Frank H.
     Introduction to radiological physics and radiation dosimetry.

     "A Wiley-Interscience publication."
     Bibliography: p.
     Includes index.
     1. Medical physics. 2. Radiation dosimetry.
I. Title.
R895.A84 1986   612'.01448   86-13222
ISBN 0-471-01146-0

Printed in the United States of America

10 9 8 7 6 5

This book is dedicated to my parents
Ulysses Sheldon Attix and Alma Katherine Attix (nee Michelsen),
my wife Shirley Adeline Attix (nee Lohr),
my children Shelley Anne and Richard Haven,
and to radiological physics students everywhere

Preface

This book is intended as a text for an introductory course at the graduate or senior undergraduate level. At the University of Wisconsin this is a three-credit course: Medical Physics 501—Radiological Physics and Dosimetry, consisting of about 45 lectures and 15 problem discussion sessions, each 50 minutes in length. By moving along briskly and by scheduling the exams at other times, the material in the book can be adequately covered in one semester. The chapters are designed to be taught in sequence from 1 through 16.

The book is written on the assumption that the student has previously studied integral calculus and atomic or modern physics. Thus integrals are used without apology wherever necessary, and no introductory chapter to review atomic structure and elementary particles is provided. Chapter 1 in Johns and Cunningham's book *The Physics of Radiology*, 3rd or 4th edition, for example, can be used for remedial review if needed.

The present text is pragmatic and classical in approach, not necessarily developing equations from first principles, as is more often done by Anderson (1984) in his admirable book *Absorption of Ionizing Radiation*. Missing details and derivations that are relevant to interaction processes may be found there, or in the incomparable classic *The Atomic Nucleus* by Robley Evans, recently republished by Krieger.

A challenging problem in writing this book was how to limit its scope so that it would fit a coherent course that could be taught in one semester and would not reach an impractical and unpublishable length. It had to be in a single volume for convenient use as a text, as it was not intended to be a comprehensive reference like the three-volume second edition of *Radiation Dosimetry*, edited by Attix, Roesch, and Tochilin. Although that treatise has been used for textbook purposes in some courses, it was never intended to be other than a reference. In limiting the scope of this text the following topic areas were largely omitted and are taught as separate courses in the University of Wisconsin Department of Medical Physics: radiotherapy physics, nuclear medicine, diagnostic radiological physics, health physics (radiation protection), and radiobiology. Other texts are used for those courses. Radiation-generating equipment is described in the courses on radiotherapy and diagnostic physics, as the design of such equipment is specific to its use.

What is included is a logical, rather than historical, development of radiological physics, leading into radiation dosimetry in its broadest sense. There is no such thing as a *perfect* sequence—one that always builds on material that has gone before and never has to reach ahead for some as yet untaught fact. However, the present order of chapters has evolved from several years of trial-and-error classroom testing and works quite well.

A few specifics deserve mentioning:

Extensive, but not exclusive, use is made of SI units. The older units in some instances offer advantages in convenience, and in any case they are not going to vanish down a ''memory hole'' into oblivion. The rad, rem, roentgen, curie, and erg will remain in the existing literature forever, and we should all be familiar with them. There is, moreover, no reason to restrain ourselves from using centimeters or grams when nature provides objects for which convenient-sized numbers will result. I believe that units should be working for us, not the other way around.

The recommendations of the International Commission on Radiation Units and Measurements (ICRU) are used as the primary basis for the radiological units in this book, as far as they go. However, additional quantities (e.g., collision kerma, energy transferred, net energy transferred) have been defined where they are needed in the logical development of radiological physics.

Several important concepts have been more clearly defined or expanded upon, such as radiation equilibrium, charged-particle equilibrium, transient charged-particle equilibrium, broadbeam attenuation, the reciprocity theorem (which has been extended to homogeneous but nonisotropic fields), and a rigorous derivation of the Kramers x-ray spectrum.

Relegating neutron dosimetry to the last chapter is probably the most arbitrary and least logical chapter assignment. Initially it was done when the course was taught in two halves, with the first half alone being prerequisite for radiotherapy physics. Time constraints and priorities dictated deferring all neutron considerations until the second half. Now that the course (and text) has been unified, that reason is gone, but the neutron chapter remains number 16 because it seems to fit in best after all the counting detectors have been discussed. Moreover it provides an appropriate setting for introducing microdosimetry, which finds its main application in characterizing neutron and mixed n-γ fields.

The tables in the appendixes have been made as extensive as one should hope to find in an introductory text. The references for all the chapters have been collected together at the back of the book to avoid redundancy, since some references are repeated in several chapters. Titles of papers have been included. A comprehensive table of contents and index should allow the easy location of material.

For the authors-to-be among this book's readers: This book was begun in 1977 and completed in 1986. It started from classroom notes that were handed out to students to supplement other texts. These notes gradually evolved into chapters that were modified repeatedly, to keep what worked with the students, and change what didn't. This kind of project is not for anyone with a short attention span.

The original illustrations for this book were drawn by F. Orlando Canto. Kathryn A. McSherry and Colleen A. Schutz of the office staff were very helpful. I also thank the University of Wisconsin Department of Medical Physics for allowing me to use their copying equipment.

Finally, it is a pleasure to acknowledge that the preparation of this book could not have been accomplished without the dedicated partnership and enthusiasm of my wife Shirley. Not only did she do all the repetitious typing, during a time before a word processor was available, but she never complained about the seemingly endless hours I spent working on it.

HERB ATTIX

Madison, Wisconsin
August 1986

Contents

INTRODUCTION TO
RADIOLOGICAL PHYSICS
AND
RADIATION DOSIMETRY

CHAPTER 1

Ionizing Radiation

I. INTRODUCTION

Radiological physics is the science of ionizing radiation and its interaction with matter, with special interest in the energy thus absorbed. Radiation dosimetry has to do with the quantitative determination of that energy. It would be awkward to try to discuss these matters without providing at the outset some introduction to the necessary concepts and terminology.

Radiological physics began with the discovery of x-rays by Wilhelm Röntgen, of radioactivity by Henri Becquerel, and of radium by the Curies in the 1890s. Within a very short time both x-rays and radium became useful tools in the practice of medicine. In fact, the first x-ray photograph (of Mrs. Röntgen's hand) was made by Röntgen late in 1895, within about a month of his discovery, and physicians on both sides of the Atlantic were routinely using x-rays in diagnostic radiography within a year, thus setting some kind of record for the rapid adoption of a new technology in practical applications.

The historical development of the science of radiological physics since then is itself interesting, and aids one in understanding the quantities and units used in this field today. However, such an approach would be more confusing than helpful in an introductory course. Historical reviews have been provided by Etter (1965), Parker and Roesch (1962), and by Roesch and Attix (1968).

II. TYPES AND SOURCES OF IONIZING RADIATIONS

Ionizing radiations are generally characterized by their ability to excite and ionize atoms of matter with which they interact. Since the energy needed to cause a valence electron to escape an atom is of the order of 4–25 eV, radiations must carry kinetic or quantum energies in excess of this magnitude to be called "ionizing." As will be seen from Eq. (1.1), this criterion would seem to include electromagnetic radiation with wavelengths up to about 320 nm, which includes most of the ultraviolet (UV) radiation band ($\sim$10–400 nm). However, for practical purposes these marginally ionizing UV radiations are not usually considered in the context of radiological physics, since they are even less capable of penetrating through matter than is visible light, while other ionizing radiations are generally more penetrating.

The personnel hazards presented by optical lasers and by radiofrequency (RF) sources of electromagnetic radiation are often administratively included in the area of a health physicist's responsibilities, together with ionizing radiation hazards. Moreover, the determination of the energy deposition in matter by these radiations is often referred to as "dosimetry". However, the physics governing the interaction of such radiations with matter is totally different from that for *ionizing* radiations, and this book will not deal with them.

The important types of ionizing radiations to be considered are:

1. *γ-rays:* Electromagnetic radiation emitted from a nucleus or in annihilation reactions between matter and antimatter. The quantum energy of any electromagnetic photon is given in keV by

$$E_\gamma = h\nu = \frac{hc}{\lambda} = \frac{12.398 \text{ keV-Å}}{\lambda}$$

$$= \frac{1.2398 \text{ keV-nm}}{\lambda} \tag{1.1}$$

where 1 Å (Angstrom) $= 10^{-10}$ m, Planck's constant is

$$h = 6.626 \times 10^{-34} \text{ J s}$$

$$= 4.136 \times 10^{-18} \text{ keV s}$$

(note that 1.6022×10^{-16} J $= 1$ keV), and the velocity of light *in vacuo* is

$$c = 2.998 \times 10^{8} \text{ m/s}$$

$$= 2.998 \times 10^{18} \text{ Å/s}$$

$$= 2.998 \times 10^{17} \text{ nm/s}$$

Evidently, by Eq. (1.1) the quantum energy of a photon of 0.1-nm wavelength is 12.4 keV, within one part in 6000.

The practical range of photon energies emitted by radioactive atoms extends from 2.6 keV (K_α characteristic x-rays from electron capture in $^{37}_{18}$Ar) to the 6.1- and 7.1-MeV γ-rays from $^{16}_{7}$N.

2. *X-rays:* Electromagnetic radiation emitted by charged particles (usually electrons) in changing atomic energy levels (called *characteristic* or *fluorescence* x-rays) or in slowing down in a Coulomb force field (*continuous* or *bremsstrahlung* x-rays). Note that an x-ray and a γ-ray photon of a given quantum energy have identical properties, differing only in mode of origin. Older texts sometimes referred to all lower-energy photons as x-rays and higher energy photons as γ-rays, but this basis for the distinction is now obsolete. Most commonly, the energy ranges of x-rays are now referred to as follows, in terms of the generating voltage:

0.1–20 kV	Low-energy or "soft" x-rays, or "Grenz rays"
20–120 kV	Diagnostic-range x-rays
120–300 kV	Orthovoltage x-rays
300 kV–1 MV	Intermediate-energy x-rays
1 MV upward	Megavoltage x-rays

3. *Fast Electrons:* If positive in charge, they are called positrons. If they are emitted from a nucleus they are usually referred to as β-rays (positive or negative). If they result from a charged-particle collision they are referred to as "δ-rays". Intense continuous beams of electrons up to 12 MeV are available from Van de Graaff generators, and pulsed electron beams of much higher energies are available from linear accelerators ("linacs"), betatrons, and microtrons. Descriptions of such accelerators, as encountered in medical applications, have been given by Johns and Cunningham (1974) and Hendee (1970).

4. *Heavy Charged Particles:* Usually obtained from acceleration by a Coulomb force field in a Van de Graaff, cyclotron, or heavy-particle linear accelerator. Alpha particles are also emitted by some radioactive nuclei. Types include:

- Proton—the hydrogen nucleus.
- Deuteron—the deuterium nucleus, consisting of a proton and neutron bound together by nuclear force.
- Triton—a proton and two neutrons similarly bound.
- Alpha particle—the helium nucleus, i.e., two protons and two neutrons. ^{3}He particles have one less neutron.
- Other heavy charged particles consisting of the nuclei of heavier atoms, either fully stripped of electrons or in any case having a different number of electrons than necessary to produce a neutral atom.
- Pions—negative π-mesons produced by interaction of fast electrons or protons with target nuclei.

5. *Neutrons:* Neutral particles obtained from nuclear reactions [e.g., (p, n) or fission], since they cannot themselves be accelerated electrostatically.

The range of kinetic or photon energies most frequently encountered in applications of ionizing radiations extends from 10 keV to 10 MeV, and relevant tabulations of data on their interactions with matter tend to emphasize that energy range. Likewise the bulk of the literature dealing with radiological physics focuses its attention primarily on that limited but useful band of energies. Recently, however, clinical radiotherapy has been extended (to obtain better spatial distribution, and/or more direct cell-killing action with less dependence on oxygen) to electrons and x-rays up to about 50 MeV; and neutrons to 70 MeV, pions to 100 MeV, protons to 200 MeV, α-particles to 10^3 MeV, and even heavier charged particles up to 10 GeV are being investigated in this connection. Electrons and photons down to about 1 keV are also proving to be of experimental interest in the context of radiological physics.

The ICRU (International Commision on Radiation Units and Measurements, 1971) has recommended certain terminology in referring to ionizing radiations which emphasizes the gross differences between the interactions of charged and uncharged radiations with matter:

1. *Directly Ionizing Radiation.* Fast charged particles, which deliver their energy to matter directly, through many small Coulomb-force interactions along the particle's track.

2. *Indirectly Ionizing Radiation.* X- or γ-ray photons or neutrons (i.e., uncharged particles), which first transfer their energy to charged particles in the matter through which they pass in a relatively few large interactions. The resulting fast charged particles then in turn deliver the energy to the matter as above.

It will be seen that the deposition of energy in matter by indirectly ionizing radiation is thus a *two-step process*. In developing the concepts of radiological physics the importance of this fact will become evident.

The reason why so much attention is paid to ionizing radiation, and that an extensive science dealing with these radiations and their interactions with matter has evolved, stems from the unique effects that such interactions have upon the irradiated material. Biological systems (e.g., humans) are particularly susceptible to damage by ionizing radiation, so that the expenditure of a relatively trivial amount of energy (~ 4 J/kg) throughout the body is likely to cause death, even though that amount of energy can only raise the gross temperature by about $0.001°C$. Clearly the ability of ionizing radiations to impart their energy to individual atoms, molecules, and biological cells has a profound effect on the outcome. The resulting high local concentrations of absorbed energy can kill a cell either directly or through the formation of highly reactive chemical species such as free radicals* in the water medium that constitutes the bulk of the biological material. Ionizing radiations can also produce gross changes, either desirable or deleterious, in organic compounds by breaking molecular bonds, or in crystalline materials by causing defects in the lattice structure.

---

*A free radical is an atom or compound in which there is an unpaired electron, such as H or CH_3.

Even structural steel will be damaged by large enough numbers of fast neutrons, suffering embrittlement and possible fracture under mechanical stress.

Discussing the details of such radiation effects lies beyond the scope of this book, however. Here we will concentrate on the basic physics of the interactions, and methods for measuring and describing the energy absorbed in terms that are useful in the various applications of ionizing radiation.

III. DESCRIPTION OF IONIZING RADIATION FIELDS

A. Consequences of the Random Nature of Radiation

Suppose we consider a point P in a field of ionizing radiation, and ask: ''How many *rays* (i.e., photons or particles) will strike P per unit time?'' The answer is of course zero, since a point has no cross-sectional area with which the rays can collide. Therefore, the first step in describing the field at P is to associate some nonzero volume with the point. The simplest such volume would be a sphere centered at P, as shown in Fig. 1.1, which has the advantage of presenting the same cross-sectional target area to rays incident from all directions. The next question is how large this imaginary sphere should be. That depends on whether the physical quantities we wish to define with respect to the radiation field are *stochastic* or *nonstochastic*.

A stochastic quantity has the following characteristics:*

    a. Its values occur randomly and hence cannot be predicted. However, the probability of any particular value is determined by a probability distribution.

    b. It is defined for finite (i.e. noninfinitesimal) domains only. Its values vary discontinuously in space and time, and it is meaningless to speak of its gradient or rate of change.

    c. In principle, its values can each be measured with an arbitrarily small error.

    d. The *expectation value N_e* of a stochastic quantity is the mean $\overline{N}$ of its measured values N as the number n of observations approaches ∞. That is, $\overline{N} \rightarrow N_e$ as $n \rightarrow \infty$.

A nonstochastic quantity, on the other hand, has these characterstics:

    a. For given conditions its value can, in principle, be predicted by calculation.

    b. It is, in general, a ''point function'' defined for infinitesimal volumes; hence it is a continuous and differentiable function of space and time, and one may speak of its spatial gradient and time rate of change. In accordance with common usage in physics, the argument of a legitimate differential quotient may always be assumed to be a nonstochastic quantity.

*Further discussion of stochastic vs. nonstochastic physical quantities will be found in ICRU (1971) and ICRU (1980).

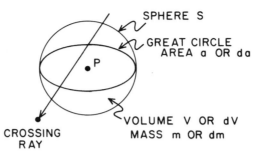

FIGURE 1.1. Characterizing the radiation field at a point *P* in terms of the radiation traversing the spherical surface *S*.

    c.   Its value is equal to, or based upon, the *expectation value* of a related stochastic quantity, if one exists. Although nonstochastic quantities in general need not be related to stochastic quantities, they are so related in the context of ionizing radiation.

It can be seen from these considerations that the volume of the imaginary sphere surrounding point *P* in Fig. 1.1 may be small but must be *finite* if we are dealing with stochastic quantities. It may be infinitesimal (dV) in reference to nonstochastic quantities. Likewise the great-circle area (da) and contained mass (dm) for the sphere, as well as the irradiation time (dt), may be expressed as infinitesimals in dealing with nonstochastic quantities. Since the most common and useful quantities for describing ionizing radiation fields and their interactions with matter are all nonstochastic, we will defer further discussion of stochastic quantities (except when leading to nonstochastic quantities) until a later chapter (16) dealing with *microdosimetry*, that is, the determination of energy spent in small but finite volumes. Microdosimetry is of particular interest in relation to biological-cell damage.

    In general one can assume that a "constant" radiation field is strictly random with respect to how many rays arrive at a given point per unit area and time interval. It can be shown (e.g., see Beers, 1953) that the number of rays observed in repetitions of the measurement (assuming a fixed detection efficiency and time interval, and no systematic change of the field vs. time) will follow a Poisson distribution. For large numbers of events this may be approximated by the normal (Gaussian) distribution. If N_e is the expectation value of the number of rays detected per measurement, the standard deviation of a single random measurement N relative to N_e is equal to

$$\sigma = \sqrt{N_e} \cong \sqrt{N} \qquad (1.2a)$$

and the corresponding percentage standard deviation is

$$S = \frac{100\sigma}{N_e} = \frac{100}{\sqrt{N_e}} \cong \frac{100}{\sqrt{N}} \qquad (1.2b)$$

That is, a single measurement would have a 68.3% chance of lying within $\pm\sigma$

of the expectation value N_e, where σ is given by Eq. (1.2a), if the fluctuations are due to the stochastic nature of the field itself. Likewise N would have a 95.5% chance of lying within $\pm 2\sigma$ of N_e, or a 99.7% chance within $\pm 3\sigma$.

The approximation of N_e by the mean value $\overline{N}$ in Eqs. (1.2a,b) is necessary because N_e is unknown but can be approached as closely as desired by the mean value $\overline{N}$ of n measurements, i.e., $\overline{N} \rightarrow N_e$ as $n \rightarrow \infty$. It is useful to know how closely $\overline{N}$ is likely to approximate N_e for a given number of measurements n. This information is conveyed by the standard deviation of the mean value $\overline{N}$ relative to N_e:

$$\sigma' = \frac{\sigma}{\sqrt{n}} = \sqrt{\frac{N_e}{n}} \cong \sqrt{\frac{\overline{N}}{n}} \tag{1.3a}$$

and the corresponding percentage standard deviation is

$$S' = \frac{100\sigma'}{N_e} = \frac{100}{\sqrt{nN_e}} \cong \frac{100}{\sqrt{n\overline{N}}} = \frac{100}{\sqrt{N_T}} \tag{1.3b}$$

where $N_T = n\overline{N}$ is the total number of rays detected in all n measurements combined. $\overline{N}$ will have a 68.3% chance of lying within $\pm\sigma'$ of N_e. Notice in Eq. (1.3b) that it makes no difference how many measurements (n) are made in acquiring a given total count N_T, and thus a given value of S'.

It is important to emphasize that the foregoing statements of standard deviation in Eqs. (1.2) and (1.3) are based exclusively upon the stochastic nature of radiation fields, not taking account of instrumental or other experimental fluctuations. Thus one should expect to observe experimentally greater standard deviations than these, but never smaller. An estimate of the *precision* (i.e., proximity to N_e) of any single random measurement N made by a radiation detector should be determined from the data of n such measurements by means of the equation:

$$\sigma \cong \left[\frac{1}{n-1} \sum_{i=1}^{n} (N_i - \overline{N})^2 \right]^{1/2} \tag{1.4a}$$

instead of Eq. (1.2a). Here N_i is the value obtained in the ith measurement, and $\overline{N} = (\Sigma N_i)/n$.

An estimate of the precision of the mean value $\overline{N}$ of n measurements should likewise be obtained from the experimental data by

$$\sigma' \cong \left[\frac{1}{n(n-1)} \sum_{i=1}^{n} (N_i - \overline{N})^2 \right]^{1/2} \tag{1.4b}$$

in place of Eq. (1.3a), since $\sigma' = \sigma/\sqrt{n}$.

It should also be pointed out that the expectation value N_e of the measurements is not necessarily the physically *correct* value, and in fact will not be if the measuring instrument is improperly calibrated or is otherwise biased. N_e is merely the value of $\overline{N}$ approached as $n \rightarrow \infty$.

An example will illustrate the meaning of Eq. 1.3a:

Example 1.1. A γ-ray detector having 100% counting efficiency is positioned in a constant field, making 10 measurements of equal duration, $\Delta t = 100$ s (exactly). The average number of rays detected ("counts") per measurement is 1.00×10^5. What is the mean value of the count rate, including a statement of its precision (i.e., standard deviation)?

In Eq. (1.3a) $\overline{N} = 1.00 \times 10^5$ counts, $n = 10$ measurements, and so

$$\sigma' \cong \sqrt{\frac{\overline{N}}{n}} = \sqrt{\frac{1 \times 10^5}{10}} = 10^2 \text{ counts}$$

Thus the count rate is:

$$\frac{\overline{N}}{\Delta t} = \frac{1.00 \times 10^5 \pm 10^2 \text{ counts}}{100 \text{ } s}$$

$$= 1.00 \times 10^3 \pm 1 \text{ c/s} \qquad \text{(S.D.)}$$

This standard deviation is due entirely to the stochastic nature of the field, since the detector counts every incident ray.

B. Simple Description of Radiation Fields by Nonstochastic Quantities

1. FLUENCE

Referring to Fig. 1.1, let N_e be the expectation value of the number of rays striking a finite sphere surrounding point P during a time interval extending from an arbitrary starting time t_0 to a later time t. If the sphere is reduced to an infinitesimal at P with a great-circle area of da, we may define a quantity called the *fluence*, Φ, as the quotient of the differential of N_e by da:

$$\Phi = \frac{dN_e}{da} \tag{1.5}$$

which is usually expressed in units of m^{-2} or cm^{-2}.

2. FLUX DENSITY (OR FLUENCE RATE)

Φ may be defined by (1.5) for all values of t through the interval from $t = t_0$ (for which $\Phi = 0$) to $t = t_{max}$ (for which $\Phi = \Phi_{max}$). Then at any time t within the interval we may define the *flux density* or *fluence rate* at P as

$$\varphi = \frac{d\Phi}{dt} = \frac{d}{dt}\left(\frac{dN_e}{da}\right) \tag{1.6}$$

where $d\Phi$ is the increment of fluence during the infinitesimal time interval dt at time t, and the usual units of flux density are m^{-2} s^{-1} or cm^{-2} s^{-1}.

Since the flux density φ may be defined by means of Eq. (1.6) for all values of t, we may thereby determine the function $\varphi(t)$, and express the fluence at P for the time interval from t_0 to t_1 by the definite integral

$$\Phi(t_0, t_1) = \int_{t_0}^{t_1} \varphi(t)\, dt \tag{1.7}$$

For the case of a time-independent field, $\varphi(t)$ is constant and Eq. (1.7) simplifies to

$$\Phi(t_0, t_1) = \varphi \cdot (t_1 - t_0) = \varphi \, \Delta t \tag{1.8}$$

It should be noted that φ and Φ express the sum of rays incident from all directions, and irrespective of their quantum or kinetic energies, thereby providing a bare minimum of useful information about the field. However, different types of rays are usually not lumped together; that is, photons, neutrons, and different kinds of charged particles are measured and accounted for separately as far as possible, since their interactions with matter are fundamentally different.

3. ENERGY FLUENCE

The simplest field-descriptive quantity which takes into account the energies of the individual rays is the *energy fluence* Ψ, for which the energies of all the rays are summed.

Let R be the expectation value of the total energy (exclusive of rest-mass energy) carried by all the N_e rays striking a finite sphere surrounding point P (see Fig. 1.1) during a time interval extending from an arbitrary starting time t_0 to a later time t^*. If the sphere is reduced to an infinitesimal at P with a great-circle area of da, we may define a quantity called the *energy fluence*, Ψ, as the quotient of the differential of R by da:

$$\Psi = \frac{dR}{da} \tag{1.9}$$

which is usually expressed in units of J m^{-2} or erg cm^{-2}.

For the special case where only a single energy E of rays is present, Eqs. (1.5) and (1.9) are related by

$$R = EN_e \tag{1.9a}$$

and

$$\Psi = E\Phi \tag{1.9b}$$

Individual particle and photon energies are ordinarily given in MeV or keV, which is the kinetic energy acquired by a singly charged particle in falling through a potential difference of one million or one thousand volts, respectively. Energies in MeV

---

*ICRU (1980) calls R the *radiant energy*, and defines it as "the energy of particles (excluding rest energy) emitted, transferred, or received."

can be converted into ergs and joules through the following statements of equivalence:

$$1 \text{ MeV} = 1.602 \times 10^{-6} \text{ erg} = 1.602 \times 10^{-13} \text{ J}$$

$$1 \text{ erg} = 10^{-7} \text{ J} \qquad\qquad = 6.24 \times 10^5 \text{ MeV} \qquad (1.10)$$

$$1 \text{ J} = 6.24 \times 10^{12} \text{ MeV} = 10^7 \text{ erg}$$

4. ENERGY FLUX DENSITY (OR ENERGY FLUENCE RATE)

Ψ may be defined by Eq. (1.9) for all values of t throughout the interval from $t = t_0$ (for which $\Psi = 0$) to $t = t_{max}$ (for which $\Psi = \Psi_{max}$). Then at any time t within the interval we may define the *energy flux density* or *energy fluence rate* at P as:

$$\psi = \frac{d\Psi}{dt} = \frac{d}{dt}\left(\frac{dR}{da}\right) \qquad (1.11)$$

where $d\Psi$ is the increment of energy fluence during the infinitesimal time interval dt at time t, and the usual units of energy flux density are J m^{-2} s^{-1} or erg cm^{-2} s^{-1}.

By identical arguments to those employed in deriving Eqs. (1.7) and (1.8), one may write the following corresponding relations for Ψ:

$$\Psi(t_0, t_1) = \int_{t_0}^{t_1} \psi(t)\, dt \qquad (1.12)$$

and for constant $\psi(t)$,

$$\Psi(t_0, t_1) = \psi \cdot (t_1 - t_0) = \psi\, \Delta t \qquad (1.13)$$

For monoenergetic rays of energy E the energy flux density ψ may be related to the flux density φ by an equation similar to (1.9b):

$$\psi = E\varphi \qquad (1.13a)$$

C. Differential Distributions vs. Energy and Angle of Incidence

The quantities introduced in Section III.B are widely useful in practical applications of ionizing radiation, but for some purposes are lacking in sufficient detail. Most radiation interactions are dependent upon the energy of the ray as well as its type, and the sensitivity of radiation detectors typically depends on the direction of incidence of the rays striking it. Thus one sometimes needs a more complete description of the field.

In principle one could measure the flux density at any time t and point P as a function of the kinetic or quantum energy E and of the polar angles of incidence θ and β (see Fig. 1.2), thus obtaining the *differential flux density*

$$\varphi'(\theta, \beta, E) \qquad (1.14)$$

typically expressed in units of m^{-2} s^{-1} sr^{-1} keV^{-1}.

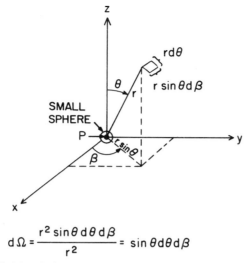

$$d\Omega = \frac{r^2 \sin\theta\, d\theta\, d\beta}{r^2} = \sin\theta\, d\theta\, d\beta$$

FIGURE 1.2.   Polar coordinates. The element of solid angle is $d\Omega$.

Instead of the flux density distribution one could have chosen the distribution of energy flux density, or (for a given time period) the fluence or energy fluence, expressed in the proper units. The following discussion of flux density distributions can be applied to these other quantities as well.

Since the element of solid angle is $d\Omega = \sin\theta\, d\beta\, d\theta$, as shown in Fig. 1.2, it can be seen that the number of rays per unit time having energies between E and $E + dE$ which pass through the element of solid angle $d\Omega$ at the given angles θ and β before striking the small sphere at P, per unit great-circle area of the sphere, is given by

$$\varphi'(\theta,\, \beta,\, E)\, d\Omega\, dE \tag{1.15}$$

typically expressed in $m^{-2}\, s^{-1}$ or $cm^{-2}\, s^{-1}$. Integrating this quantity over all angles and energies will of course give the flux density φ:

$$\varphi = \int_{\theta=0}^{\pi} \int_{\beta=0}^{2\pi} \int_{E=0}^{E_{max}} \varphi'(\theta,\, \beta,\, E)\, \sin\theta\, d\theta\, d\beta\, dE \tag{1.16}$$

also in $m^{-2}\, s^{-1}$ or $cm^{-2}\, s^{-1}$.

1.   ENERGY SPECTRA

Simpler, more useful differential distributions of flux density, fluence, energy flux density, or energy fluence are those which are functions of only one of the variables θ, β, or E. When E is the chosen variable, the resulting differential distribution is called the *energy spectrum* of the quantity. For example the energy spectrum of the flux density summed over all directions is written as $\varphi'(E)$, in typical units of $m^{-2}\, s^{-1}\, keV^{-1}$ or $cm^{-2}\, s^{-1}\, keV^{-1}$:

$$\varphi'(E) = \int_{\theta=0}^{\pi} \int_{\beta=0}^{2\pi} \varphi'(\theta, \beta, E) \sin \theta \, d\theta \, d\beta \qquad (1.17)$$

Integration of $\varphi'(E)$ over all energies of the rays present then gives the flux density:

$$\varphi = \int_0^{E_{max}} \varphi'(E) \, dE \qquad (1.18)$$

To illustrate such a spectrum, Fig. 1.3a shows how a "flat" distribution of photon flux density $\varphi'(E)$ would be plotted as the ordinate vs. the quantum energy as abscissa. Fig. 1.3b shows the corresponding spectrum of energy flux density $\psi'(E)$, where

$$\psi'(E) = E\varphi'(E) \qquad (1.19)$$

That is, the ordinates in Fig. 1.3b are E times those in 1.3a. The unit ordinarily used for the factor E in Eq. (1.19) is the erg or joule, so that $\psi'(E)$ is expressed in J m^{-2} s^{-1} keV^{-1} or erg cm^{-2} s^{-1} keV^{-1}. These units convey the concept intended more clearly than would be the case if the factor E were chosen also be in keV, thus allowing cancellation of the energy units and leaving only m^{-2} s^{-1}. The joule (preferably) and the erg are the units commonly employed in describing gross energy transport in radiological physics [see Eq. (1.10)].

An equation corresponding to (1.18) can also be written for ψ:

$$\psi = \int_{E=0}^{E_{max}} \psi'(E) \, dE = \int_0^{E_{max}} E\varphi'(E) \, dE \qquad (1.20)$$

In carrying out this integration in closed form it will be necessary for E to be in the same units throughout (e.g., keV), contrary to the immediately foregoing comments. The result will then be in keV/(area) (time), which can be converted to other energy units by Eq. (1.10). For numerical integration of (1.20), one may employ $\psi'(E)$ in J m^{-2} s^{-1} keV^{-1} (or erg cm^{-2} s^{-1} keV^{-1}) and still use limits and energy intervals dE expressed in keV.

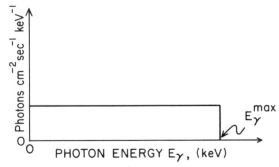

FIGURE 1.3a.   A flat spectrum of photon flux density $\varphi'(E)$.

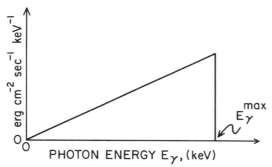

FIGURE 1.3b. Spectrum of energy flux density $\psi'(E)$ corresponding to Fig. 1.3a.

2. ANGULAR DISTRIBUTIONS

If the field is symmetrical with respect to the vertical (z) axis shown in Fig. 1.2, it will be convenient to describe it in terms of the differential distribution of, say, the flux density as a function of the polar angle θ only. This distribution per unit polar angle is given by

$$\varphi'(\theta) = \int_{\beta=0}^{2\pi} \int_{E=0}^{E_{max}} \varphi'(\theta, \beta, E) \sin \theta \; d\beta \; dE \tag{1.21}$$

so that the flux-density component consisting of the particles of all energies arriving at P through the annulus lying between the two polar angles $\theta = \theta_1$ and θ_2 would be

$$\varphi(\theta_1, \theta_2) = \int_{\theta_1}^{\theta_2} \varphi'(\theta) \; d\theta \tag{1.22}$$

where $\varphi'(\theta)$ can be expressed in $m^{-2} \, s^{-1} \, radian^{-1}$, for example. For θ-limits of 0 and π, this integral of course gives φ.

Alternatively one can obtain the differential distribution of flux density per unit *solid angle*, for particles of all energies, as

$$\varphi'(\theta, \beta) = \int_{E=0}^{E_{max}} \varphi'(\theta, \beta, E) \; dE \tag{1.23}$$

in typical units of $m^{-2} \, s^{-1} \, sr^{-1}$. This may be integrated over all directions to again obtain the total flux density:

$$\varphi = \int_{\theta=0}^{\pi} \int_{\beta=0}^{2\pi} \varphi'(\theta, \beta) \sin \theta \; d\theta \; d\beta \tag{1.24}$$

For a field that is symmetrical about the z-axis, $\varphi'(\theta, \beta)$ is independent of β; hence Eq. (1.24) can be integrated over all β-values to obtain

$$\varphi = 2\pi \int_{\theta=0}^{\pi} \varphi'(\theta, \beta) \sin \theta \, d\theta \qquad (1.25)$$

Comparing this equation with Eq. (1.22) over the limits $\theta = 0$ to π reveals that, for the case of z-axis symmetry, $\varphi'(\theta)$ is related to $\varphi'(\theta, \beta)$ by

$$\varphi'(\theta) = (2\pi \sin \theta) \, \varphi'(\theta, \beta), \qquad (1.26)$$

where $\varphi'(\theta)$ has the units $m^{-2} s^{-1}$ radian^{-1} and $\varphi'(\theta, \beta)$ is given in $m^{-2} s^{-1} sr^{-1}$. Figure 1.4 illustrates this relationship for the case of a completely isotropic field (solid curves), and for the case where $\varphi'(\theta, \beta)$ is still β-independent but varies as some function of θ(dashed curves). $\varphi'(\theta, \beta)$ is arbitrarily taken as $(1 - \theta/\pi)$ in the latter case shown.

Sometimes one is interested in expressing the flux density of particles of all energies as a function only of the azimuthal angle β. Then $\varphi'(\theta, \beta)$ from Eq. (1.23) may be used, where one usually sets $\theta = \pi/2$.

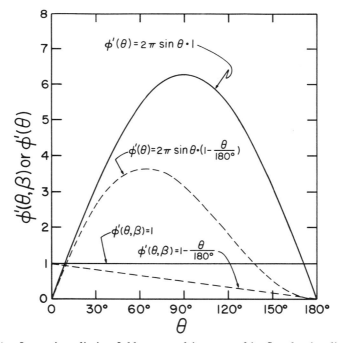

FIGURE 1.4. Isotropic radiation field expressed in terms of its flux-density distribution per unit solid angle, $\varphi'(\theta, \beta) = $ constant $\equiv 1 \ m^{-2} s^{-1} sr^{-1}$ (lower solid curve). The same field is also shown in terms of its distribution per unit polar angle, $\varphi'(\theta)$, in $m^{-2} s^{-1}$ radian^{-1} (upper solid curve). These two curves are related by the factor $2\pi \sin \theta$, which is also true if $\varphi'(\theta, \beta)$ is a function of θ only [e.g., see dashed curves for $\varphi'(\theta, \beta) = 1 - (\theta/180°)$].

D. An Alternative Definition of Fluence

Chilton (1978, 1979) has proven the validity of an alternative definition of fluence, namely:

> The fluence at a point P is numerically equal to the expectation value of the sum of the particle track lengths (assumed to be straight) that occur in an infinitesimal volume dV at P, divided by dV.

This statement was shown to be true for nonisotropic as well as isotropic fields, irrespective of the shape of the volume. Thus one need not require a spherical volume to define fluence in this way. Moreover this definition lends itself to dosimetry calculations by the Monte Carlo method.

E. Planar Fluence

Planar fluence is the number of particles crossing a fixed plane in either direction (i.e., summed by scalar addition) per unit area of the plane. The name "planar fluence" was given to it by Roesch and Attix (1968), who also defined a vector-sum quantity corresponding to the planar flux density that they called the *net flow*, that is, the number of particles per unit time passing through unit area of the plane in one sense (say side A to side B) *minus* those going the other way ($B \rightarrow A$). This quantity is of little dosimetric relevance, however. Although vectorial methods are convenient for field calculations, as shown by Rossi and Roesch (1962) and Brahme (1981), radiation dosimetry finally requires scalar, not vector, addition of the effects of individual particles.

The concept of net flow was first put forward in the context of radiological physics by Whyte (1959). He dealt with the flow of energy carried by particles, and applied the name "plane intensity" to the vector sum of the energy flowing through a fixed plane. Whyte's illustrative diagram is reproduced in Fig. 1.5, which will be used here to discuss fluence vs. planar fluence.

A plane homogeneous beam of radiation is shown perpendicularly incident upon a flat scattering (but not absorbing) foil. All particles are shown for simplicity being scattered through the same angle θ, at any azimuthal angle β. A spherical and a flat detector of equal cross-sectional area are shown positioned above and below the foil. The flat detector is oriented parallel to the foil, and thus is perpendicular to the beam of incident radiation. The number of incident particles striking each detector above the foil is clearly the same, and the planar fluence with respect to the plane of the flat detector is identical to the fluence in the same field. This can only be true in a plane-parallel beam, orthogonal to the flat detector, as shown.

The number of scattered particles striking the spherical detector below the foil is $|1/\cos \theta|$ times the number striking the flat detector, which in turn is the same as the number it received above the foil. Thus the fluence is $|1/\cos \theta|$ times the planar fluence. This increase in fluence contributes to an effect sometimes seen in broad-beam geometry, in which the fluence behind an attenuating layer can be greater than that incident (see Chapter 3, Section V).

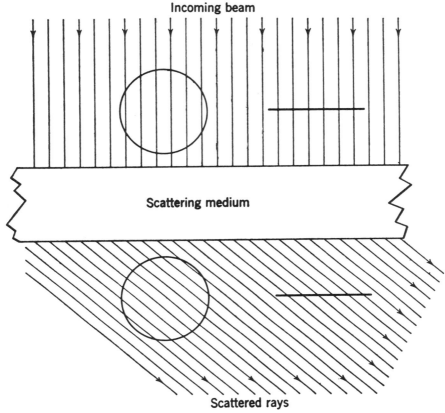

FIGURE 1.5. Particles scattered through an angle θ in a nonabsorbing foil, illustrating effect on fluence vs. planar fluence. (After Whyte, 1959.)

The effect of radiation striking a detector depends on the penetrating power of the radiation. Consider the two limiting cases in which: (a) the radiation penetrates straight through both detectors shown in Fig. 1.5, and (b) the radiation is stopped and absorbed in both detectors. For both cases we will take the response of the detector to be proportional to the energy imparted in it.

For case (a) we will also assume that the energy imparted is approximately proportional to the total track length of the rays crossing the detector, or to the fluence according to the Chilton definition. This assumption is by no means proven at this point, but it is reasonably good for homogeneous radiation crossing a small, easily penetrated detector. The spherical detector in Fig. 1.5 will read more below the foil in proportion to the number of rays striking it, which is $|1/\cos\theta|$ times the number striking it above the foil. The average length of the paths in the sphere is obviously the same above and below. The number of rays striking the flat detector is the same above and below the foil, but the length of each track within the detector is $|1/\cos$

$\theta|$ times as long below as it is above the foil. Thus the total track length in the flat detector is also $|1/\cos \theta|$ times as great below the foil as above. Evidently, then, both of the detectors read more by the factor $|1/\cos \theta|$ below the foil for the case of penetrating radiation.

Now consider the easily stopped radiation in case (b). The sphere again reads more below the foil than above by the factor $|1/\cos \theta|$, since that is the factor by which the number of striking rays increases, and each ray deposits all its energy. The flat detector, however, responds *the same* below as above the foil, since the number of rays striking it does not change, and track length is now irrelevant.

In other words, for the case of *nonpenetrating* rays striking a flat detector or other absorber, the energy deposited is related to the planar fluence with respect to the detector plane, instead of the fluence. Only in this case does planar fluence arise as a practical concept in dosimetry.

To quantify planar fluence for multidirectional radiation fields, we consider a particular great circle of the small sphere at P in Fig. 1.2: the one that is fixed in the x–y plane. The number of particles per unit time, having energies between E and $E + dE$, that pass through the element of solid angle $d\Omega = \sin \theta\, d\beta\, d\theta$ at the given angles θ and β before passing through the fixed great circle, per unit area of the circle, can be expressed [from Eq. (1.15)] as

$$\varphi'(\theta,\, \beta,\, E)|\cos \theta|\, d\Omega\, dE \tag{1.27}$$

The absolute value of $\cos \theta$ means that the particles are counted positively, regardless of the direction from which they come.

Inserting the factor $|\cos \theta|$ into Eq. (1.16) gives an equation for the planar flux density φ_p with respect to the x–y plane in Fig. 1.2:

$$\varphi_p = \int_{\theta=0}^{\pi} \int_{\beta=0}^{2\pi} \int_{E=0}^{E_{max}} \varphi'(\theta,\, \beta,\, E)|\cos \theta|\, \sin \theta\, d\theta\, d\beta\, dE \tag{1.28}$$

and the planar fluence Φ_p is simply the time integral of φ_p over any desired time interval, as in Eq. (1.7).

In an isotropic field of radiation we have $\varphi_p = \frac{1}{2}\varphi$; hence $\Phi_p = \frac{1}{2}\Phi$ for a given time interval. The factor $\frac{1}{2}$ is obtained as the ratio of Eq. (1.28) to Eq. (1.16), which can be simplified in steps, as in Eqs. (1.23)–(1.25) to give

$$\frac{\varphi_p}{\varphi} = \frac{\displaystyle\int_{\theta=0}^{\pi} |\cos \theta|\sin \theta\, d\theta}{\displaystyle\int_{\theta=0}^{\pi} \sin \theta\, d\theta} = \frac{\sin^2 \theta\, \big|_0^{\pi/2}}{-\cos \theta\, \big|_0^{\pi}} = \frac{1}{2} \tag{1.29}$$

For the same case the net flow through the x–y plane is zero, since

$$\int_{\theta=0}^{\pi} \cos \theta\, \sin \theta\, d\theta = 0 \tag{1.30}$$

PROBLEMS

1. What is the photon energy range corresponding to the UV radiation band?

2. The following set of count readings was made in a gradient-free γ-ray field, using a suitable detector for repetitive time periods of one minute: 18,500; 18,410; 18,250; 18,760; 18,600; 18,220; 18,540; 18,270; 18,670; 18,540.

   (a) What is the mean value of the number of counts?

   (b) What is its standard deviation (S.D.)?

   (c) What is the theoretical minimum S.D. of the mean?

   (d) What is the actual S.D. of a single reading?

   (e) What is the theoretical minimum S.D. of a single reading?

3. A broad plane-parallel beam of electrons is perpendicularly incident upon a thin foil which scatters the electrons through an average angle of 20°, stopping none of them.

   (a) What is the ratio of the flux density of primary electrons just behind the foil to that with the foil removed?

   (b) What is the ratio of the number of electrons per cm^2 passing through a plane just behind (and parallel to) the foil to that with the foil removed?

4. The flux density decreases with increasing distance from a point source of rays as the inverse square of the distance. The strength of the electric field surrounding a point electric charge does likewise. At a point midway between two identical charges the electric field is zero.

   (a) What is the flux density midway between two identical sources?

   (b) What is the essential difference between the two cases?

5. A point source of ^{60}Co gamma rays emits equal numbers of photons of 1.17 and 1.33 MeV, giving a flux density of 5.7×10^9 photons/cm^2 sec at a specified location. What is the energy flux density there, expressed in erg/cm^2 sec and in J/m^2 min?

6. In problem 5, what is the energy fluence of 1.17-MeV photons during 24 hours, in erg/cm^2 and J/m^2?

7. A point source isotropically emitting 10^8 fast neutrons per second falls out of its shield onto a railroad platform 3 m horizontally from the track. A train goes by at 60 miles per hour. Ignoring scattering and attenuation, what is the fluence of neutrons that would strike a passenger at the same height above the track as the source?

8. An x-ray field at a point P contains 7.5×10^8 photons/m^2-sec-keV, uniformly distributed from 10 to 100 keV.

   (a) What is the photon flux density at P?

   (b) What would be the photon fluence in one hour?

   (c) What is the corresponding energy fluence, in J/m^2 and erg/cm^2?

9. Show that, for a spherical volume, Chilton's definition of fluence gives the same value as the conventional definition in a uniform monoenergetic field. *Hint:* The mean chord length in any convex volume is $4V/S$, where V is the volume and S is the surface area.

SOLUTIONS TO PROBLEMS

1. 10–400 nm corresponds to 124–3.1 eV.
2. (a) $\overline{N} = 18476$ counts.
   (b) $\sigma' = 58$.
   (c) $\sigma'_{min} = 43$.
   (d) $\sigma = 184$.
   (e) $\sigma_{min} = 136$.
3. (a) 1.06
   (b) Unity.
4. (a) Twice that due to one of the sources.
   (b) Flux density is a *scalar* quantity; electric field strength is a *vector*. Vector addition depends on orientation; scalar addition does not.
5. 1.14×10^4 erg/cm^2-s, 685 J/m^2-min.
6. 4.62×10^8 erg/cm^2, 4.62×10^5 J/m^2.
7. 3.11×10^5 n/m^2.
8. (a) 6.75×10^{10} photons/m^2 s,
   (b) 2.43×10^{14} photons/m^2,
   (c) 2.14 J/m^2 or 2.14×10^3 erg/cm^2.
9. From Eq. (1.5), for a finite sphere of radius r,

$$\Phi = \frac{N}{\pi r^2}$$

Chilton's formulation:

$$\Phi = \frac{N \cdot 4V/S}{V} = \frac{4N}{S} = \frac{N}{\pi r^2}$$

CHAPTER 2

Quantities for Describing the Interaction of Ionizing Radiation with Matter

I. INTRODUCTION

In Chapter 1 we discussed how a field of ionizing radiation could be described non-stochastically in terms of the expectation value of the number of rays, or of the energy they carry, striking an infinitesimal sphere around the point of interest. In this chapter we will define three nonstochastic quantities that are useful for describing the interactions of the radiation field with matter, also in terms of expectation values for the infinitesimal sphere at the point of interest. These quantities are (a) the *kerma* K, describing the first step in energy dissipation by indirectly ionizing radiation, that is, energy transfer to charged particles; (b) the *absorbed dose D*, describing the energy imparted to matter by all kinds of ionizing radiations, but delivered by the charged particles; and (c) the *exposure*, X, which describes x- and γ-ray fields in terms of their ability to ionize air. The mean energy expended per ion pair produced in a gas, $\overline{W}$, will also be briefly introduced in this chapter in its connection with exposure. A more detailed discussion of $\overline{W}$ will be delayed until Chapter 12. Finally, some additional quantities relevant to radiation protection will be briefly discussed.

A word about neutrinos is required with respect to the following definitions, to avoid confusion in Chapter 4 when we deal with equilibria. Neutrinos are elementary particles having no electric charge and practically zero mass, hence they have an exceedingly small cross section for interacting with matter. For this reason the *energy given to, or carried by, neutrinos may be (and always is) totally ignored in the context of radiological physics and dosimetry*. Terms in the following definitions that refer to indirectly ionizing radiation could include neutrinos, since they are uncharged, *but they will be arbitrarily* *excluded. The rest mass conversion term ΣQ likewise will ignore mass-energy transactions with neutrinos.*

Actually the definitions in the present chapter are valid whether or not one excludes neutrinos, but consideration of equilibria in Chapter 4 will be much simpler and more practical if the neutrinos are ignored; hence we will do so from now on. No error results from this.

II. KERMA

This nonstochastic quantity is relevant only for fields of indirectly ionizing radiations (photons or neutrons) or for any ionizing radiation source distributed within the absorbing medium.

A. Definition

The kerma K can be defined in terms of the related stochastic quantity *energy transferred*, ϵ_{tr} (Attix, 1979, 1983) and the *radiant energy R* (ICRU, 1980). The energy transferred in a volume V is:

$$\epsilon_{tr} = (R_{in})_u - (R_{out})_u^{nonr} + \Sigma Q \tag{2.1}$$

where $(R_{in})_u$ = radiant energy of uncharged particles entering V,

$(R_{out})_u^{nonr}$ = radiant energy of uncharged particles leaving V, *except* that which originated from radiative losses of kinetic energy by charged particles while in V, and

ΣQ = net energy derived from rest mass in V ($m \rightarrow E$ positive, $E \rightarrow m$ negative).

By radiative losses, we mean conversion of charged-particle kinetic energy to photon energy, through either bremsstrahlung x-ray production or in-flight annihilation of positrons. In the latter case only the kinetic energy possessed by the positron at the instant of annihilation (which is carried away by the resulting photons along with 1.022 MeV of rest-mass energy) is classified as radiative energy loss.

Radiant energy R is defined as the energy of particles (excluding rest energy) emitted, transferred, or received (ICRU, 1980).

Upon consideration of Eq. (2.1) it will be seen that energy transferred is just the kinetic energy received by charged particles in the specified finite volume V, regardless of where or how they in turn spend that energy. However any kinetic energy passed from one charged particle to another is not to be counted in ϵ_{tr}, as defined.

We may now define the kerma K at point of interest P in V as

$$K = \frac{d(\epsilon_{tr})_e}{dm} \equiv \frac{d\epsilon_{tr}}{dm} \tag{2.2}$$

where $(\epsilon_{tr})_e$ is the expectation value of the energy transferred in the finite volume

V during some time interval, $d(\epsilon_{tr})_e$ is that for the infinitesimal volume dv at the internal point P, and dm is the mass in dv. Since the argument of any legitimate differential quotient may always be taken to be nonstochastic, the symbol $d(\epsilon_{tr})_e$ may be simplified to $d\epsilon_{tr}$ as indicated in Eq. (2.2).

Thus *the kerma is the expectation value of the energy transferred to charged particles per unit mass at a point of interest, including radiative-loss energy but excluding energy passed from one charged particle to another.*

The average value of the kerma throughout a volume containing a mass m is simply the expectation value of the energy transferred divided by the mass, or $(\epsilon_{tr})_e/m$.

Kerma can be expressed in units of erg/g, rad, or J/kg. The latter unit is also called the *gray* (Gy) in honor of L. H. Gray, a pioneer in radiological physics. The rad is still commonly employed for kerma and absorbed dose at the time of this writing, but J/kg is to be preferred as part of a general shift to the International System of units. Fortunately all these units are simply related by

$$1 \text{ Gy} = 1 \text{ J/kg} = 10^2 \text{ rad} = 10^4 \text{ erg/g} \qquad (2.3)$$

B. Relation of Kerma to Energy Fluence for Photons

For monoenergetic photons the kerma at a point P is related to the energy fluence there by the *mass energy-transfer coefficient* $(\mu_{tr}/\rho)_{E,Z}$, which is characteristic of the photon energy E and the atomic number Z of the matter at P:

$$K = \Psi \cdot \left(\frac{\mu_{tr}}{\rho}\right)_{E,Z} \qquad (2.4)$$

Here μ_{tr} is called the *linear energy-transfer coefficient* in units of m^{-1} or cm^{-1}, and ρ is the density in kg/m^3 or g/cm^3. Ψ is the energy fluence at P in J/m^2 (preferred) or erg/cm^2. K is the kerma at P, expressed in J/kg (preferred) or in erg/g, respectively, either of which can be converted into rads, if desired, by Eq. (2.3).

If a spectrum of photon energy fluence $\Psi'(E)$ is present at the point of interest P (let's assume for simplicity that $\Psi'(E)$ is constant during the irradiation period) and if $(\mu_{tr}/\rho)_{E,Z}$ is the mass energy-transfer coefficient as a function of photon energy E for material Z, then the kerma at P will be obtained from the appropriate integration:

$$K = \int_{E=0}^{E_{max}} \Psi'(E) \cdot \left(\frac{\mu_{tr}}{\rho}\right)_{E,Z} dE \qquad (2.5)$$

where $\Psi'(E)$ is the differential distribution of photon energy fluence, in units of $\text{J m}^{-2} \text{ keV}^{-1}$ or $\text{erg cm}^{-2} \text{ keV}^{-1}$ (sometimes MeV is used in place of keV). Note that $(\mu_{tr}/\rho)_{E,Z}$ does not have the dimensions of a differential distribution; it is a set of numerical values tabulated at convenient photon energies for a selection of materials. The tables of J. H. Hubbell are widely employed for this purpose. They will be found in a chapter by Evans (1968), and have been excerpted in Appendix D.3 of the present text.

Since dE is usually expressed in keV, K is obtained from Eq. (2.5) in J/kg or erg/g for the units shown.

An average value of (μ_{tr}/ρ) for the spectrum $\Psi'(E)$ is given by

$$\left(\overline{\frac{\mu_{tr}}{\rho}}\right)_{\Psi'(E), Z} = \frac{K}{\Psi} = \frac{\int_E \Psi'(E) \cdot \left(\frac{\mu_{tr}}{\rho}\right)_{E, Z} dE}{\int_E \Psi'(E) \, dE} \tag{2.5a}$$

C. Relation of Kerma to Fluence for Neutrons

Equations (2.4) and (2.5) could be applied to neutrons as well as x- and γ-ray photons, but this is not customary. Usually neutron fields are described in terms of flux density and fluence, instead of *energy* flux density and *energy* fluence as is usually the case with photons. Thus for consistency a quantity called the *kerma factor* F_n is tabulated for neutrons instead of the mass energy-transfer coefficient:

$$(F_n)_{E, Z} = \left(\frac{\mu_{tr}}{\rho}\right)_{E, Z} \cdot E \tag{2.6}$$

If $(\mu_{tr}/\rho)_{E, Z}$ is given in units of cm^2/g, the neutron energy E in this relation is commonly expressed in g-rad/neutron in place of MeV/neutron, through the following unit conversion:

$$E\left(\frac{MeV}{neutron}\right) \times 1.602 \times 10^{-6} \frac{erg}{MeV} \times 10^{-2} \frac{g \text{ rad}}{erg} = E\left(\frac{g \text{ rad}}{neutron}\right) \tag{2.7}$$

so that the energy of a 1-MeV neutron is also 1.602×10^{-8} g-rad.

Thus, instead of Eq. (2.4), for monoenergetic neutrons one uses the following relation:

$$K = \Phi \cdot (F_n)_{E, Z} \qquad \text{(rad)} \tag{2.8}$$

where Φ is the fluence of monoenergetic neutrons of energy E in neutrons/cm^2 and $(F_n)_{E, Z}$ is the kerma factor for those neutrons in the irradiated material Z, so that K is given directly in rads or centiGrays (cGy).

Likewise, for neutrons having an energy spectrum $\Phi'(E)$ of particle fluence, Eq. (2.5) can be replaced by

$$K = \int_{E=0}^{E_{max}} \Phi'(E) \cdot (F_n)_{E, Z} \, dE \qquad \text{(rad)} \tag{2.9}$$

where $\Phi'(E)$ is commonly in units of neutrons/cm^2 MeV, $(F_n)_{E, Z}$ represents tabulated kerma-factor values in rad cm^2/neutron, and dE is expressed in MeV.

Tabulations of $(F_n)_{E, Z}$ for a wide range of neutron energies and materials have been published by Caswell et al. (1980); an extract of those tables is contained in Appendix F. Future tables may be expressed in Gy m^2/n.

An average value of F_n for the spectrum $\Phi'(E)$ is given by

$$\overline{(F_n)}_{\Phi'(E),Z} = \frac{K}{\Phi} = \frac{\int_E \Phi'(E) \cdot (F_n)_{E,Z} \, dE}{\int_E \Phi'(E) \, dE} \tag{2.9a}$$

D. Components of Kerma

The kerma for x- or γ-rays consists of the energy transferred to electrons and positrons per unit mass of medium. The kinetic energy of a fast electron may be spent in two ways:

1. Coulomb-force interactions with atomic electrons of the absorbing material, resulting in the local dissipation of the energy as ionization and excitation in or near the electron track. These are called *collision* interactions.

2. Radiative interactions with the Coulomb force field of atomic nuclei, in which x-ray photons (bremsstrahlung, or "braking radiation") are emitted as the electron decelerates. These x-ray photons are relatively penetrating compared to electrons and they carry their quantum energy far away from the charged-particle track.

In addition, a *positron* can lose an appreciable fraction of its kinetic energy through in-flight annihilation, in which the kinetic energy possessed by the particle at the instant of annihilation appears as extra quantum energy in the resulting photons. Hence this is also a type of radiative loss of kinetic energy, in which the resulting photons can carry kinetic energy away from the charged-particle track.

Since the kerma includes kinetic energy received by the charged particles whether it is destined to be spent by the electrons in collision or radiative-type interactions, we can subdivide K into two parts according to whether the energy is spent nearby in creating excitation and ionization (K_c) or is carried away by photons (K_r):

$$K = K_c + K_r \tag{2.10}$$

where the subscripts refer to "collision" and "radiative" interactions, respectively.

For the case of neutrons as the indirectly ionizing radiation, the resulting charged particles are protons and heavier recoiling nuclei, for which K_r is vanishingly small. Thus $K = K_c$ for neutrons, and we need not consider the partition of K in that case.

It will be convenient in discussing the concept of charged-particle equilibrium (CPE) in Chapter 4 if we now define the *collision kerma* (K_c) in a manner corresponding to that employed for K in Eqs. (2.1) and (2.2).

Let ϵ_{tr}^n be the related stochastic quantity called the *net energy transferred*, which can be defined for a volume V as

$$\epsilon_{tr}^n = (R_{in})_u - (R_{out})_u^{nonr} - R_u^r + \Sigma Q = \epsilon_{tr} - R_u^r \tag{2.11}$$

where R_u^r is the radiant energy emitted as radiative losses by the charged particles which themselves originated in V, regardless of where the radiative loss events occur. This equation is identical to Eq. (2.1) except for the inclusion here of the term R_u^r; the remaining terms are defined as in Eq. (2.1). Thus ϵ_{tr} and K include energy that goes to radiative losses, while ϵ_{tr}^n and K_c do not.

Now we can define K_c at a point of interest P as

$$K_c = \frac{d\epsilon_{tr}^n}{dm} \tag{2.12}$$

where ϵ_{tr}^n is now the expectation value of the net energy transferred in the finite volume V during some time interval, $d\epsilon_{tr}^n$ is that for the infinitesimal volume dv at point P, and dm is the mass in dv.

Thus *the collision kerma is the expectation value of the net energy transferred to charged particles per unit mass at the point of interest, excluding both the radiative-loss energy and energy passed from one charged particle to another.* The average value of K_c throughout a volume containing mass m is given by $(\epsilon_{tr}^n)_e/m$.

The radiative kerma K_r need not be defined further than simply as the difference between K and K_c, as in Eq. (2.10). However it can be written as $K_r = dR_u^r/dm$, having the same form as Eqs. (2.2) and (2.12).

For monoenergetic photons K_c is related to the energy fluence Ψ by another energy- and material-dependent coefficient $(\mu_{en}/\rho)_{E,Z}$ called the *mass energy-absorption coefficient*, so that the equation corresponding to Eq. (2.4) becomes

$$K_c = \Psi\left(\frac{\mu_{en}}{\rho}\right)_{E,Z} \tag{2.13}$$

where the units are as given for Eq. (2.4). Likewise, for an energy spectrum $\Psi'(E)$, equations corresponding to (2.5) and (2.5a) can also be written for K_c and $(\mu_{en}/\rho)_{\Psi'(E),Z}$, respectively.

The value of $(\mu_{en}/\rho)_{E,Z}$ at a point P is not only characteristic of the atomic number Z of the material present there [as is the case for $(\mu_{tr}/\rho)_{E,Z}$], but is also dependent to some degree upon the material present along the tracks of the electrons which originate at P. This is because radiative energy losses by electrons are greater in higher-Z materials, for which K_r is larger and K_c correspondingly less. All tabulations of $(\mu_{en}/\rho)_{E,Z}$, including those of Hubbell given in Appendix D.3, are based on the assumption that the electrons spend their entire range in the same material in which they started, i.e., that the point P is not near a boundary with another medium. Also, (μ_{en}/ρ) for compounds usually has been calculated on the basis of weight fractions of the elements present. Although this is correct for μ_{tr}/ρ, it is not strictly so for μ_{en}/ρ, as will be discussed in Chapter 7.

$(\mu_{en}/\rho)_{E,Z}$ is close to $(\mu_{tr}/\rho)_{E,Z}$ in value for low Z and E where radiative losses are small; Table 2.1 lists the percentage by which $(\mu_{en}/\rho)_{E,Z}$ is less than $(\mu_{tr}/\rho)_{E,Z}$ (and K_c less than K) for a few sample cases.

The relationship of $(\mu_{tr}/\rho)_{E,Z}$ and $(\mu_{en}/\rho)_{E,Z}$ to the basic interactions of photons will be discussed in Chapter 7.

TABLE 2.1

γ-ray Energy (MeV)	100 $(\mu_{tr} - \mu_{en})/\mu_{tr}$		
	$Z = 6$	29	82
0.1	0	0	0
1.0	0	1.1	4.8
10	3.5	13.3	26

E. Kerma Rate

The kerma rate at a point P and time t [referring to Eq. (2.2)] is given by

$$\dot{K} = \frac{dK}{dt} = \frac{d}{dt}\left(\frac{d\epsilon_{tr}}{dm}\right) \tag{2.14}$$

in units of J/kg s preferred, erg/g s, or rad/s, with other time units often substituted.

Equation (2.14) can be used to define $\dot{K}$ for all times within some extended period of irradiation, thus providing the kerma rate as a function of t, $\dot{K}(t)$. The kerma occurring between selected time limits t_0 and t_1 will then be

$$K(t_0, t_1) = \int_{t_0}^{t_1} \dot{K}(t) \, dt \tag{2.15}$$

or, for a constant kerma rate,

$$K(t_0, t_1) = \dot{K} \, (t_1 - t_0) \tag{2.16}$$

In this equation $\dot{K}$ may be replaced by $\overline{\dot{K}}$, thereby defining that quantity as the average value of $\dot{K}$ during the time interval $t_1 - t_0$.

III. ABSORBED DOSE

The absorbed dose is relevant to all types of ionizing radiation fields, whether directly or indirectly ionizing, as well as to any ionizing radiation source distributed within the absorbing medium.

A. Definition

The absorbed dose D can best be defined in terms of the related stochastic quantity *energy imparted* ϵ (ICRU, 1980). The energy imparted by ionizing radiation to matter of mass m in a finite volume V is defined as

$$\epsilon = (R_{in})_u - (R_{out})_u + (R_{in})_c - (R_{out})_c + \Sigma Q \tag{2.17}$$

where $(R_{in})_u$ and ΣQ are defined the same as for Eq. (2.1), $(R_{out})_u$ is the radiant energy of all the uncharged radiation leaving V, $(R_{in})_c$ is the radiant energy of the charged particles entering V, and $(R_{out})_c$ is the radiant energy of the charged particles leaving V. We can now define the absorbed dose D at any point P in V as

$$D = \frac{d\epsilon}{dm} \qquad (2.18)$$

where ϵ is now the expectation value of the energy imparted in the finite volume V during some time interval, $d\epsilon$ is that for an infinitesimal volume dv at point P, and dm is the mass in dv.

Thus the absorbed dose D is the expectation value of the energy imparted to matter per unit mass at a point. The dimensions and units of absorbed dose are the same as those used for K. The average value $\overline{D}$ of the absorbed dose throughout a volume containing mass m is $(\epsilon)_e/m$. $(\epsilon)_e = \overline{D}m$ is also called the *integral dose*, expressed in units of g rad or joules.

It should be recognized that D represents the energy per unit mass which remains in the matter at P to produce any effects attributable to the radiation. Some kinds of effects are proportional to D, while others depend on D in a more complicated way. Nevertheless, if $D = 0$ there can be no radiation effect. Consequently, the absorbed dose is the most important quantity in radiological physics.

It is not possible to write an equation relating the absorbed dose directly to the fluence or energy fluence of a field of indirectly ionizing radiation, as was done for the kerma in Eqs. (2.4) and (2.8) and for collision kerma in Eq. (2.13). The absorbed dose is not directly related to such a field, being deposited by the resulting secondary charged-particles. The relation of absorbed dose to the fluence of charged particles will be discussed in Chapter 8.

B. Absorbed Dose Rate

The absorbed dose rate at a point P and time t is given by

$$\dot{D} = \frac{dD}{dt} = \frac{d}{dt}\left(\frac{d\epsilon}{dm}\right) \qquad (2.19)$$

Equations corresponding to Eqs. (2.15) and (2.16) may also be written for the absorbed dose, substituting D for K and $\dot{D}$ for $\dot{K}$. The time-averaged value of the absorbed dose rate $\dot{D}$ may likewise be defined by an equation corresponding to (2.16).

IV. COMPARATIVE EXAMPLES OF ENERGY IMPARTED, ENERGY TRANSFERRED, AND NET ENERGY TRANSFERRED

To see how these quantities can be applied, first consider Fig. 2.1a. Photon $h\nu_1$ is shown entering volume V, and undergoing a Compton interaction which produces scattered photon $h\nu_2$ and an electron with kinetic energy T. The electron is assumed to produce one bremsstrahlung x-ray ($h\nu_3$) before leaving V with remaining energy

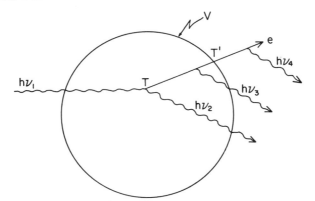

FIGURE 2.1a. Illustration of the concepts of energy imparted, energy transferred, and net energy transferred for the case of a Compton interaction followed by bremsstrahlung emission (Attix, 1983).

T'. It then produces another x-ray ($h\nu_4$). In this example the energy imparted, energy transferred, and net energy transferred in V are, respectively,

$$\epsilon = h\nu_1 - (h\nu_2 + h\nu_3 + T') + 0$$

$$\epsilon_{tr} = h\nu_1 - h\nu_2 + 0 = T$$

$$\epsilon_{tr}^n = h\nu_1 - h\nu_2 - (h\nu_3 + h\nu_4) + 0$$

$$= T - (h\nu_3 + h\nu_4)$$

A second example is shown in Fig. 2.1b, illustrating the significance of the ΣQ term in Eqs. (2.1), (2.11), and (2.17). A γ-ray $h\nu_1$ is emitted by a radioactive atom in V. The photon undergoes pair production, giving kinetic energy T_1 to the electron and T_2 to the positron. Both are assumed to run their course in V. The positron is then annihilated and the resulting two photons (0.511 MeV each) are shown escaping from V. For this case the quantities ϵ, ϵ_{tr}, and ϵ_{tr}^n are all equal, and are given in MeV by

$$\epsilon = \epsilon_{tr} = \epsilon_{tr}^n = 0 - 1.022 \text{ MeV} + \Sigma Q$$

where

$$\Sigma Q = h\nu_1 - 2m_0c^2 + 2m_0c^2 = h\nu_1$$

Hence

$$\epsilon = \epsilon_{tr} = \epsilon_{tr}^n = h\nu_1 - 1.022 \text{ MeV}$$

$$= T_1 + T_2$$

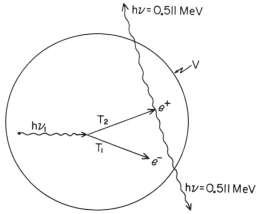

FIGURE 2.1b. Example involving γ-ray emission, pair production, and positron annihilation (Attix, 1983).

Note that there are no radiative losses in this case, since the annihilation photons derive their entire energy from rest mass (the term $+2m_0c^2$), not from kinetic energy.

If the positron in Fig. 2.1b had been annihilated in flight when its remaining kinetic energy was T_3, then the total quantum energy of the annihilation photons would have been 1.022 MeV $+ T_3$. Assuming they escaped from V, the quantities in question become

$$\epsilon = 0 - (1.022 + T_3) + h\nu_1 = T_1 + T_2 - T_3$$
$$\epsilon_{\text{tr}} = 0 - 1.022 + h\nu_1 = T_1 + T_2$$
$$\epsilon_{\text{tr}}^n = 0 - 1.022 - T_3 + h\nu_1 = T_1 + T_2 - T_3$$

Here T_3 was derived from the charged-particle kinetic energy, hence it constitutes radiative loss. ϵ_{tr}^n is less than ϵ_{tr} by that amount. Also, $\epsilon = \epsilon_{\text{tr}}^n$ in this case, the significance of which will be discussed in Chapter 4.

V. EXPOSURE

Exposure is the third of the important fundamental nonstochastic quantities with which we are concerned in radiological physics. It is historically the oldest of the three, and in earlier times (before 1962) was known as "exposure dose"; still earlier (before 1956), it had no name but was merely the quantity that was measured in terms of the roentgen (R) unit, which had been defined by the ICRU in 1928. By convention exposure is defined only for x-ray and γ-ray photons.

A. Definition

Exposure is symbolized by X, and is defined by the ICRU (1980) as "the quotient of dQ by dm, where the value of dQ is the absolute value of the total charge of the ions of one sign produced in air when all the electrons (negatrons and positrons) liberated by photons in air of mass dm are completely stopped in air." Thus

$$X = \frac{dQ}{dm} \tag{2.20}$$

In a note of clarification the ICRU also points out that "the ionization arising from the absorption of bremsstrahlung emitted by the electrons is not to be included in dQ." (Presumably the same can be said for the small radiative losses of kinetic energy that occur through in-flight annihilation of positrons.)

When one puzzles through the foregoing statements to reach a fundamental understanding of their meaning, it will become clear that:

The exposure X is the ionization equivalent of the collision kerma K_c in air, for x- and γ-rays.

B. Definition of $\overline{W}$

We must define precisely what is meant by "ionization equivalent" in the above statement of exposure. Here we must introduce a conversion factor symbolized by $\overline{W}$, *the mean energy expended in a gas per ion pair formed*. We will discuss $\overline{W}$ more generally in Chapter 12; hence the present considerations will be minimal and specific to its relationship with the exposure (see ICRU, 1971).

Let T_i be the initial kinetic energy of the ith electron (or positron) set in motion by x- or γ-rays in the infinitesimal volume of air dV at point P during some specified time interval. Let g_i be the fraction of T_i that is spent by the particle in radiative interactions along its full path in air, so that $1 - g_i$ is the remaining fraction spent in collision interactions. The sum of all the kinetic energy spent by all such electrons in collision interactions can then be written as $\Sigma_i T_i(1-g_i)$.

Now let N_i be the total number of ion pairs that are produced in air by the ith electron or positron of energy T_i, and let g_i' be the fraction of those ion pairs that are generated by the photons resulting from radiative loss interactions (i.e., mostly bremsstrahlung). Thus $1 - g_i'$ is the fraction of the ion pairs that are produced by collision interactions that occur along the particle track, and $N_i(1 - g_i')$ is the number of such ion pairs produced by that particle. Hence the sum of all such ion pairs produced in collision interactions by all the electrons and positrons originating in dV is $\Sigma_i N_i(1-g_i')$.

Assuming that one sums over the energies and ionizations of a large enough number of charged particles to allow $\overline{W}$ to achieve its expectation value for the radiation and gas in question, we can write

$$\overline{W} = \frac{\Sigma T_i(1-g_i)}{\Sigma N_i(1-g_i')} \tag{2.21}$$

Thus by this definition $\overline{W}$ does not count the energy going into radiative losses, nor the ionization produced by the resulting photons, since the exposure also excludes them. $\overline{W}$ is usually expressed in units of eV per ion pair, and the best current value for x and γ rays in dry air is 33.97 eV/i.p. (Boutillon and Perroche, 1985). By dividing $\overline{W}$ by the charge of the electron in coulombs (noting that only the ions of *either* sign, not both, are counted in the definition of exposure) and converting the energy from electron volts to joules, one obtains $\overline{W}$ in a form that is more convenient for relating $(K_c)_{air}$ and X:

$$\frac{\overline{W}_{air}}{e} = \frac{33.97 \text{ eV/i.p. (or electron)}}{1.602 \times 10^{-19}C/\text{electron}} \times 1.602 \times 10^{-19}J/eV$$

$$= 33.97 \text{ J/C} \tag{2.22}$$

We see that the conversion constants cancel each other so as to give $\overline{W}/e$ in J/C the same *numerical* value as $\overline{W}$ has in eV/i.p., which is a convenience. Moreover $\overline{W}$ may be regarded as a *constant* for each gas, independent of photon energy, for x- and γ-ray energies above a few keV.

C. Relation of Exposure to Energy Fluence

It is now possible to describe specifically what is meant by "ionization equivalent" in the statement of exposure at the end of Section III.A. Referring to Eq. (2.13), we can write that the exposure at a point due to an energy fluence Ψ of monoenergetic photons of energy E is given by

$$X = \Psi \cdot \left(\frac{\mu_{en}}{\rho}\right)_{E,\,air} \left(\frac{e}{\overline{W}}\right)_{air} = (K_c)_{air}\left(\frac{e}{\overline{W}}\right)_{air} = (K_c)_{air}/33.97 \tag{2.23}$$

where Ψ is most conveniently expressed in J/m^2,
$(\mu_{en}/\rho)_{E,\,air}$ is in m^2/kg,
K_c is in J/kg,
$(e/\overline{W})_{air} = (1/33.97)$ C/J, and
X is the exposure in C/kg.

The roentgen (R) is the customary and more commonly encountered unit of exposure. It is defined as the exposure that produces, in air, one esu of charge of either sign per 0.001293 g of air (i.e., the mass contained in 1 cm^3 at 760 Torr, 0°C) irradiated by the photons. Thus

$$1 \text{ R} = \frac{1 \text{ esu}}{0.001293\text{g}} \times \frac{1C}{2.998 \times 10^9 \text{ esu}} \times \frac{10^3\text{g}}{1 \text{ kg}}$$

$$= 2.580 \times 10^{-4} \text{ C/kg} \tag{2.24}$$

serves as a conversion factor from R to C/kg. That is

$$X \text{ (C/kg)} = 2.58 \times 10^{-4} X \text{ (R)}$$

$$X \text{ (R)} = 3876 \, X \text{ (C/kg)} \tag{2.25}$$

If a spectrum of photon energy fluence $\Psi'(E)$ (in J/m^2-keV) is present at the point of interest P, and if $(\mu_{en}/\rho)_{E,\,air}$ (in m^2/kg) is the energy-absorption coefficient as a function of photon energy E for air, then the exposure at P will be given by the following integral:

$$X = \int_{E=0}^{E_{max}} (\mu_{en}/\rho)_{E,\,air} \; (e/\overline{W})_{air} \; \Psi'(E) \; dE \qquad (2.26)$$

where $(e/\overline{W})_{air} = (1/33.97)$ C/J,
dE is in keV, and
X is in C/kg;

multiplying the result by 3876 [see Eq. (2.25)] converts it into roentgens.

Likewise the exposure due to any segment of the spectrum lying between two energy limits would be given by Eq. (2.26) with those limits inserted.

One may speak of an "exposure spectrum" of x- or γ-rays, by which is meant

$$X'(E) = (\mu_{en}/\rho)_{E,\,air} \; (e/\overline{W})_{air} \; \Psi'(E) \qquad (2.27)$$

in typical units of R/keV or C/kg keV. Its integral from $E = 0$ to E_{max} gives the exposure, as in Eq. (2.26).

D. Exposure Rate

The exposure rate at a point P and time t is

$$\dot{X} = \frac{dX}{dt} \qquad (2.28)$$

which can be used to define X for all times within some extended period of irradiation, thus providing the exposure rate as a function of t, $\dot{X}(t)$. The exposure occurring between selected time limits t_0 and t will then be

$$X = \int_{t_0}^{t_1} \dot{X}(t) \; dt \qquad (2.29)$$

where $\dot{X}(t)$ has units the same as for $\dot{X}$ at any instant: C/kg-sec or R/sec (or with other time units).

For a constant kerma rate $\dot{X}$ this simplifies to

$$X = \dot{X}(t_1 - t_0) \qquad (2.30)$$

where $\dot{X}$ may be replaced by $\overline{\dot{X}}$ to define the latter as the time-averaged value of the exposure rate.

E. Significance of Exposure

Exposure (and its rate) provides a convenient and useful means of characterizing an x- or γ-ray field, for the following reasons:

1. The energy fluence Ψ is proportional to the exposure X for any given photon energy [see Eq. (2.23)] or spectrum [Eq. (2.26)].
2. The mixture of elements in air is sufficiently similar in "effective atomic num-

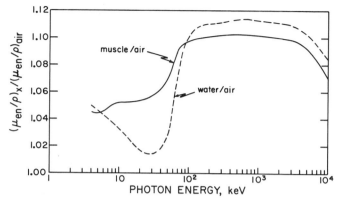

FIGURE 2.2a. Ratio of mass energy-absorption coefficients for muscle and water relative to air. [Based on data of Hubble, as given by Evans (1968) for $hv > 0.15$ MeV, and by Greening, (1972) for $hv \leq 0.15$ MeV.]

ber'' to that in soft biological tissue (i.e., muscle) to make air an approximately ''tissue-equivalent'' material with respect to x- or γ-ray energy absorption. Thus if one is interested in the effects of such radiations in tissue, air may be substituted as a reference medium in a measuring instrument.

3.   Because of the approximate tissue equivalence of air noted in item 2, the value of the collision kerma K_c in muscle, per unit of exposure X, is nearly independent of photon energy. This follows from the fact that for a given energy fluence Ψ of photons of energy E, the exposure X is proportional to $(\mu_{en}/\rho)_{E,\,air}$, while K_c in muscle is proportional to $(\mu_{en}/\rho)_{E,\,musc}$ [see Eqs. (2.13) and (2.23), and $(\mu_{en}/\rho)_{E,\,musc}/(\mu_{en}/\rho)_{E,\,air}$ is nearly constant $(1.07 \pm 3\%$ total spread) vs. E over the range 4 keV–10 MeV, as shown in Fig. 2.2a. That figure also shows corresponding ratios of $(\mu_{en}/\rho)_{E,\,Z}$ for water/air, and Fig. 2.2b shows compact bone and acrylic plastic

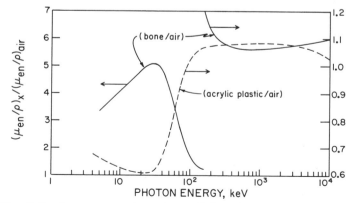

FIGURE 2.2b. Ratio of mass energy-absorption coefficients for acrylic plastic and compact bone relative to air. Acrylic plastic ($C_5H_8O_2$) is variously called Lucite, Plexiglas, and Perspex. Data sources as in Fig. 2.2a.

relative to air. Water/air ($1.07 \pm 5\%$) is nearly as constant as muscle/air, but both acrylic plastic and compact bone show larger differences from air, especially below 0.1 MeV, due to the *photoelectric effect*, which will be discussed in Chapter 7.

4. One can characterize an x-ray field at a point by means of a statement of exposure or exposure rate *regardless of whether there is air actually located at the point in question*. The statement that "the exposure at point P is X" simply means that the photon energy fluence Ψ [or its spectrum $\Psi'(E)$] at the point is such that Eq. (2.23) [or (2.26)] would give the stated value of X. Similar remarks apply also to the kerma K or collision kerma K_c, except that the reference medium is not necessarily air, and must therefore be specified.

VI. QUANTITIES AND UNITS FOR USE IN RADIATION PROTECTION

A. Quality Factor, Q

The *quality factor Q* is a dimensionless variable weighting factor to be applied to the absorbed dose to provide an estimate of the relative human hazard of different types and energies of ionizing radiations. Values of Q are selected from experimental values of the *relative biological effectiveness* (RBE), which is the ratio of x- or γ-ray dose to that of the radiation in question giving the same kind and degree of biological effect. Q is chosen by the International Commission on Radiological Protection (ICRP) to be a smooth function of the *unrestricted linear energy transfer* (L_∞) of the radiation. This latter quantity is defined in Chapter 8, Section III.I. It is also called the collision stopping power. Figure 2.3 shows the currently accepted functional dependence of Q, indicating that higher-density charged particle tracks are generally more biologically damaging per unit dose than low-density tracks.

Information concerning radiobiology has been given by Hall (1973) among others, and will not be discussed here. However, it should be noted that the Q-values in Fig. 2.3 are appropriate only for routine radiation-protection applications, and should not be used in connection with high-level accidental exposures (ICRP, 1971).

B. Dose Equivalent, H

The *dose equivalent H*, is defined as

$$H \equiv DQN \qquad (2.31)$$

where D is the absorbed dose, Q is the quality factor, and N is the product of all other modifying factors (currently assigned the value 1).

If D is given in J/kg, then so is H, since Q is dimensionless. The J/kg has the special name gray (Gy) when applied to absorbed dose, but has the special name sievert (Sv) when applied to dose equivalent. Thus it is apparent that if Q has a value of, say, 5, then a point in the body where the dose is 1 Gy = 1 J/kg would also have a dose equivalent of 5 Sv = 5 J/kg. This has the appearance of a paradox, since 1 J/kg $\neq$

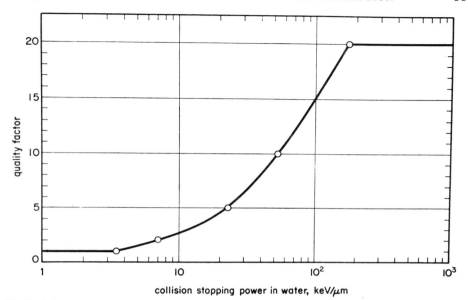

quality factor

collision stopping power in water, keV/μm

FIGURE 2.3. Quality factor Q of charged particles as a function of collision stopping power (L_∞) in water, as recommended by the ICRP (1971). (Reproduced with permission from Pergamon Press, Ltd.)

5 J/kg. However, the situation is one in which *two different quantities* (D and H) are stated in terms of the same units. A similar case would be that of a room having a *width* of 3 meters and *length* of 5 meters. This does not mean that 3 meters = 5 meters.

This kind of argument has been used by the ICRU (1980) as justification for assigning the sievert the value 1 J/kg. However, the argument applies only to physical quantities, and dose equivalent is not strictly a physical quantity. An alternative approach to the problem would have been to assign only the special unit sievert to H, and let Q have the units Sv/Gy instead of making it dimensionless. The present situation is tenable, however, so long as one arbitrarily chooses to treat H as a physical quantity.

If the absorbed dose in Eq. (2.31) is stated in rad ($=10^{-2}$ J/kg), then H is given in terms of the special unit *rem* ($=10^{-2}$ J/kg). These units are no longer recommended by the ICRU, however.

In the common case where the dose is delivered by primary or secondary charged particles having a spectrum of values of L_∞,

$$H = D\overline{Q}N \tag{2.32}$$

and

$$\overline{Q} = \frac{1}{D} \int_0^\infty QD(L_\infty)\,dL_\infty \tag{2.33}$$

and $D(L_\infty)$ is the differential distribution of dose with respect to L_∞, in typical units of Gy μm/keV.

C. Specification of Ambient Radiation Levels

To estimate the absorbed dose or dose equivalent in the presence of the perturbing (scattering and attenuating) influence of the human body in a radiation field, the quantities *absorbed-dose index* (D_I) and *dose-equivalent index* (H_I) were defined (ICRU, 1980).

The absorbed-dose index at a point in a field of ionizing radiation is defined as the maximum absorbed dose occurring within a 30-cm-diameter sphere (simulating the body) centered at the point, and consisting of material equivalent to soft tissue with a density of 1 g/cm^3. The preferred unit is Gy.

The dose-equivalent index at such a point is the maximum dose equivalent occurring within the same sphere, also centered at the point. The preferred unit is the Sv.

For this purpose, soft tissue is taken as 76.2% O, 10.1% H, 11.1% C and 2.6% N, by weight. The outer 70 μm of the sphere's surface is ignored, as it simulates the dead layer of skin, which is biologically irrelevant. Generally the maximum values of D, $\overline{Q}$, and H all occur at different locations in the sphere, although in practice $\overline{Q}_{max} D_I$ will not underestimate H_I.

Singh and Madhvanath (1981) have pointed out that this phantom is too small to adequately represent a human body with respect to the (n, γ) generation of γ-rays, particularly for neutrons incident with energies below 10 keV. They suggest that the sphere should be replaced by a cylindrical phantom 60 cm tall and 30 cm in diameter, centered at the point of interest. This of course would require additional specification of orientation if the field is nonisotropic. Substitution of a 40-cm-diameter sphere should be considered in any future modification of these definitions, as it would retain the advantages of isotropic geometry while providing closer body simulation of n, γ production.

PROBLEMS

1. What is $(K_c)_{air}$ in Gy at a point in air where $X = 47$ roentgens?

2. An electron enters a volume V with a kinetic energy of 4 MeV, and carries 0.5 MeV of that energy out of V when it leaves. While in the volume it produces a bremsstrahlung x-ray of 1.5 MeV which escapes from V. What is the contribution of this event to:

   (a) The energy transferred?

   (b) The net energy transferred?

   (c) The energy imparted?

3. A 10-MeV γ-ray enters a volume V and undergoes pair production, thereby disappearing and giving rise to an electron and positron of equal energies. The

electron spends half its kinetic energy in collision interactions before escaping from V. The positron spends half of its kinetic energy in collisions in V before being annihilated in flight. The resulting photons escape from V. Determine (a), (b), and (c) as in problem 2.

4. The flux density of 6-MeV γ-rays is $3.4 \times 10^6/\text{cm}^2$ s at a point in Pb. What are the values of K and K_c there after one week? (Express in units of erg/g, rad, and gray.) (See Appendix D.3.)

5. A field of 14.5-MeV neutrons deposits a kerma of 1.37 Gy at a point of interest in water. What is the fluence? (See Appendix F).

6. In Chapter 1, problem 8, assuming that the medium at P is aluminum.
   (a) Calculate the collision kerma there for the one-hour irradiation, in Gy.
   (b) Calculate the exposure there, in C/kg. (Note: You may use linear interpolation in Appendix D.3.)

7. Consider two flasks containing 5 and 25 cm^3 of water, respectively. They are identically and homogeneously irradiated with γ-rays, making the average kerma equal to 1 Gy in the smaller flask.
   (a) Neglecting differences in γ-ray attenuation, what is the average kerma in the larger flask?
   (b) What is the energy transferred in each volume of water?

SOLUTIONS TO PROBLEMS

1. 0.412 Gy.
2. (a) 0.
   (b) 0.
   (c) 2 MeV.
3. (a) 8.98 MeV.
   (b) 6.73 MeV.
   (c) 4.49 MeV.
4. $K = 6.54 \times 10^5$ erg/g $= 6.54 \times 10^3$ rad $= 65.4$ Gy,
   $K_c = 5.38 \times 10^5$ erg/g $= 5.38 \times 10^3$ rad $= 53.8$ Gy.
5. 1.93×10^{10} n/cm^2.
6. (a) 0.113 Gy,
   (b) 6.45×10^{-4} C/kg.
7. (a) 1 Gy,
   (b) 0.005 J, 0.025 J

CHAPTER 3

Exponential Attenuation

I. INTRODUCTION

The rational study of radiological physics calls for the introduction of the concept of *exponential attenuation* at this point, as it plays an important role in Chapter 4 and following chapters. This concept is relevant primarily to *uncharged ionizing radiations* (i.e., photons and neutrons), which lose their energy in relatively few large interactions, rather than charged particles (see Chapter 8), which typically undergo many small collisions, losing their kinetic energy gradually.

An individual uncharged particle (photon or neutron) has a significant probability of passing straight through a thick layer of matter without losing any energy, while a charged particle must always lose some or all of its energy. An uncharged particle has no limiting ''range'' through matter, beyond which it cannot go; charged particles all encounter such a range limit as they run out of kinetic energy. For comparable energies, uncharged particles penetrate much farther through matter, on the average, than charged particles, although this difference gradually decreases at energies above 1 MeV.

II. SIMPLE EXPONENTIAL ATTENUATION

Consider a monoenergetic parallel beam consisting of a very large number N_0 of uncharged particles incident perpendicularly on a flat plate of material of thickness L, as shown in Fig. 3.1. We will assume for this ideal case that each particle either is completely absorbed in a single interaction, producing no secondary radiation, or passes straight through the entire plate unchanged in energy or direction.

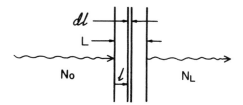

FIGURE 3.1.   Simple exponential attenuation.

Let $(\mu \cdot 1)$ be the probability that an individual particle interacts in a unit thickness of material traversed. Then the probability that it will interact in an infinitesimal thickness dl is μdl. If N particles are incident upon dl, the change dN in the number N due to absorption is given by

$$dN = -\mu N \, dl \qquad (3.1)$$

where μ is typically given in units of cm^{-1} or m^{-1}, and dl is correspondingly in cm or m.

The fractional change in N due to absorption of particles in dl is just

$$\frac{dN}{N} = -\mu \, dl \qquad (3.2)$$

Integrating over the depth l from 0 to L, and corresponding particle populations from N_0 to N_L, gives

$$\int_{N=N_0}^{N_L} \frac{dN}{N} = - \int_{l=0}^{L} \mu \, dl$$

$$\ln N \Big|_{N_0}^{N_L} = -\mu l \Big|_{0}^{L}$$

$$\ln N_L - \ln N_0 = \ln \frac{N_L}{N_0} = -\mu L$$

$$\frac{N_L}{N_0} = e^{-\mu L} \qquad (3.3)$$

This is the law of exponential attenuation, which applies either for the ideal case described above (simple absorption, no scattering or secondary radiation), or where scattered and secondary particles may be produced but are *not counted* in N_L. More will be said about this point later.

The quantity μ is called the *linear attenuation coefficient*, or simply the *attenuation coefficient*. When it is divided by the density ρ of the attenuating medium, the *mass attenuation coefficient* μ/ρ (cm^2/g or m^2/kg) is obtained. μ is sometimes referred to as the "narrow-beam attenuation coefficient," the meaning of which will be discussed in Section IV.

Equation (3.3) can be replaced by the following infinite series:

$$\frac{N_L}{N_0} = e^{-\mu L} = 1 - \mu L + \frac{(\mu L)^2}{2!} - \frac{(\mu L)^3}{3!} + \cdots \qquad (3.4)$$

which may be approximated by its first two terms $(1 - \mu L)$ if μL is sufficiently small compared with unity. As a practical matter, if $\mu L < 0.05$ (i.e., $<5\%$ attenuation), this approximation

$$\frac{N_L}{N_0} = e^{-\mu L} \cong 1 - \mu L \qquad (3.5)$$

is valid within about a tenth of one percent.

The quantity $1/\mu$ (cm or m) is known as the *mean free path* or *relaxation length* of the primary particles. It is the average distance a single particle travels through a given attenuating medium before interacting. It is also the depth to which a fraction $1/e$ ($\cong 37\%$) of a large homogeneous population of particles in a beam can penetrate. A distance of three mean free paths, $3/\mu$, reduces the primary beam intensity to 5%; $5/\mu$ to $<1\%$; and $7/\mu$ to $<0.1\%$.

III. EXPONENTIAL ATTENUATION FOR PLURAL MODES OF ABSORPTION

Suppose that more than one absorption process is present in the preceding case. Again we will assume that each event by each process is totally absorbing, producing no scattered or secondary particles. Then we can write that the total linear attenuation coefficient μ is equal to the sum of its parts:

$$\mu = \mu_1 + \mu_2 + \cdots$$

or

$$1 = \mu_1/\mu + \mu_2/\mu + \cdots \qquad (3.6)$$

where μ_1 is called the *partial linear attenuation coefficient* for process 1, and likewise for the other processes. Substituting Eq. (3.6) into Eq. (3.3) gives

$$\frac{N_L}{N_0} = e^{-(\mu_1 + \mu_2 + \cdots)L}$$

or

$$N_L = N_0(e^{-\mu_1 L})(e^{-\mu_2 L}) \cdots \qquad (3.7)$$

which proves that the number N_L of particles penetrating through the slab L depends on the total effect of all the partial attenuation coefficients.

The total number of interactions by all types of processes is given by

$$\Delta N = N_0 - N_L = N_0 - N_0 e^{-\mu L} \qquad (3.8)$$

and the number of interactions by, say, a single process x alone is

$$\Delta N_x = (N_0 - N_L)\frac{\mu_x}{\mu} = N_0\left(1 - e^{-\mu L}\right)\frac{\mu_x}{\mu} \tag{3.9}$$

where μ_x/μ is the fraction of the interactions that go by process x.

The significance of the preceding equations can be illustrated by the following example:

Example 3.1: Let $\mu_1 = 0.02$ cm^{-1} and $\mu_2 = 0.04$ cm^{-1} be the partial linear attenuation coefficients in the slab shown in Fig. 3.1. Let $L = 5$ cm, and $N_0 = 10^6$ particles. How many particles N_L are transmitted, and how many are absorbed by each process in the slab?

Solution:

$$N_L = N_0 e^{-(\mu_1 + \mu_2)L} = 10^6\, e^{-(0.02 + 0.04)5}$$

$$= 7.408 \times 10^5$$

The total number of particles absorbed is

$$N_0 - N_L = (10^6 - 7.408 \times 10^5) = 2.592 \times 10^5$$

The number absorbed by process 1 is

$$\Delta N_1 = (N_0 - N_L)\frac{\mu_1}{\mu} = 2.592 \times 10^5 \times \frac{0.02}{0.06} = 8.64 \times 10^4$$

and by process 2,

$$\Delta N_2 = (N_0 - N_L)\frac{\mu_2}{\mu} = 2.592 \times 10^5 \times \frac{0.04}{0.06} = 1.728 \times 10^5$$

Notice that in this problem we cannot derive the number of process-1 events on the basis of μ_1 alone, since the number of particles available for interaction at any depth in the slab depends on the total attenuation coefficient μ. Confusion on this point sometimes results from the fact that in an *infinitesimal* layer the number of interactions by each process can be gotten from Eq. (3.1):

$$dN_1 = -\mu_1 N\, dl$$

$$dN_2 = -\mu_2 N\, dl$$

However, for noninfinitesimal layers this formula does not apply. If one attempts to use this equation to solve the foregoing Example 3.1, one obtains

$$\Delta N_1 \neq -0.02 \text{ cm}^{-1} \times 10^6 \times 5 \text{ cm} = 1 \times 10^5 \text{ interactions}$$

by process No. 1 and

$$\Delta N_2 \neq -0.04 \text{ cm}^{-1} \times 10^6 \times 5 \text{ cm} = 2 \times 10^5 \text{ interactions}$$

by process No. 2, which overestimate the correct answers by 16% in this case. The thicker the layer, the greater the error due to assuming it to be infinitesimal.

Another common error in doing Example 3.1 is to try to calculate the number of individual-process interactions from the following incorrect equations:

$$\Delta N_1 \neq N_0 - N_0 e^{-\mu_1 L} = 10^6 - 10^6 e^{-0.02 \times 5} = 9.52 \times 10^4$$

and

$$\Delta N_2 \neq N_0 - N_0 e^{-\mu_2 L} = 10^6 - 10^6 e^{-0.04 \times 5} = 1.813 \times 10^5$$

which overestimate the correct answers by 10% and 5%, respectively. The latter answer is the more nearly correct because μ_2 more closely approximates the value of μ. The closer a partial attenuation coefficient approximates the total coefficient μ, the more nearly the foregoing statements approach the correct Eq. (3.9).

Mathematically the treatment of partial attenuation coefficients will be found very similar to that of partial decay constants in radioactivity (see Chapter 6).

IV. "NARROW-BEAM" ATTENUATION OF UNCHARGED RADIATION

We have seen that exponential attenuation will be observed for a monoenergetic beam of identical uncharged particles that are "ideal" in the sense that they are absorbed without producing scattered or secondary radiation. Real beams of photons or neutrons interact with matter by processes (to be described in later chapters) that may generate either charged or uncharged secondary radiations, as well as scattering primaries either with or without a loss of energy. The total number of particles that exit from the slab shown in Fig. 3.1 is hence greater than just the surviving un-scattered primaries, and one must decide which kinds of particles should be included in N_L in Eq. (3.3). That equation will not be valid in every case, as we shall see.

Secondary charged particles are certainly not to be counted as uncharged particles. This exclusion on logical grounds is further supported by the practical consideration that charged particles are usually much less penetrating, and thus tend to be absorbed in the attenuator. Those that do escape can be prevented from entering the detector by enclosing it in a thick enough shield. Energy given to charged particles is thus regarded as having been absorbed, inasmuch as it does not remain a part of the uncharged radiation beam.

The scattered and secondary uncharged particles can either be counted in N_L, or not. If they are counted, then Eq. (3.3) becomes invalid in describing the variation of N_L vs. L, due to violation of its underlying assumption that only simple absorbing events can occur. Such cases are referred to generally as *broad-beam attenuation*, which will be discussed in the next section.

If scattered or secondary uncharged radiation reaches the detector, *but only the primaries are counted in N_L*, one has broad-beam geometry but narrow-beam attenuation. As a consequence Eq. (3.3) remains valid under these conditions even for real beams of uncharged primary radiation.

The value of the attenuation coefficient μ includes the partial coefficients for all types of interactions by the primary particles [see Eq. (3.6)], since a particle ceases to be primary when it undergoes its first interaction of any kind, even small-angle scattering with no energy loss. Therefore μ must be numerically larger than the value of any corresponding *effective attenuation coefficient μ'* that is observed under broad-beam attenuation conditions. That is, μ is an upper limit for the value of μ', which will be discussed further in the next section. If one gradually reduces the fraction of scattered and secondary radiation measured, broad-beam attenuation gradually approaches narrow-beam attenuation, and μ' increases to approach μ.

There are two general methods of achieving narrow-beam attenuation:

a. *Discrimination* against all scattered and secondary particles that reach the detector, on the basis of particle energy, penetrating ability, direction, coincidence, anticoincidence, time of arrival (for neutrons), etc.

b. *Narrow-beam geometry*, which prevents any scattered or secondary particles from reaching the detector.

Figure 3.2 illustrates the essential features of narrow-beam geometry. The detector is placed far enough from the attenuating layers so that any particle S that is deflected in an interaction will miss the detector. The beam is collimated to be just large enough to cover the detector uniformly, thereby minimizing the number of scattered or secondary particles generated in the attenuator. The radiation beam source is located a large distance from the attenuator so that the particles are almost perpendicularly

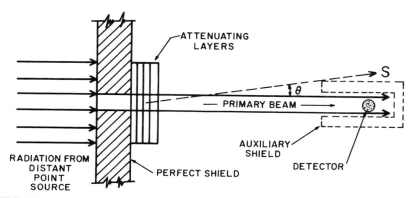

FIGURE 3.2. Narrow-beam geometry. The diameter of the primary photon or neutron beam is made just large enough to cover the detector uniformly. The detector is placed at a large enough distance from the attenuator that the number of scattered or secondary particles (S) that reach the detector is negligible in comparison with the number of primary rays.

incident. Moreover, the intensity of the primary beam at the detector will then be nearly independent of distance from the attenuator, while the intensity of the scattered and secondary particles will decrease as the inverse square of that distance. Thus the relative strength of the primary beam increases with detector distance, allowing reduction of the nonprimary radiation fraction to a negligible level at the detector.

The shield is assumed to stop all radiation incident upon it except that passing through its aperture. If it allows any leakage, it may be necessary to put a supplementary shield around the detector, as shown in Fig. 3.2, that allows entry of radiation only at angles $\theta \cong 0°$. Lead is the usual shielding material for x- or γ-rays, especially where space is limited. Iron and hydrogenous materials are preferable for fast neutrons. Radiation shielding generally is beyond the scope of this book, belonging more properly to the disciplines of radiation protection (NCRP 1976, 1977) and nuclear engineering (e.g., see Schaeffer, 1973). It can be said however that shielding usually involves broad-beam geometry.

It is not difficult in practice to achieve reasonably narrow-beam geometry experimentally, and thus closely to approximate narrow-beam attenuation as required, for example, in specifying x-ray half-value layers (see Chapter 9). Published values of the attenuation coefficients for various materials and energies are based on measurements done under rigorous conditions of narrow-beam geometry, whence the alternative name "narrow-beam attenuation coefficient" for μ. Appendixes D.2 and D.3 contain tabulations of μ/ρ for photons, as discussed in Chapter 7. The corresponding data for fast neutrons are usually given in the form of atomic interaction cross sections $_a\sigma_T = \mu A/\rho N_A$ (cm^2/atom or m^2/atom), where A is the atomic weight, ρ is the density of the attenuating medium, and N_A is Avogadro's constant.

Narrow-beam geometry is sometimes referred to as "good" geometry (e.g., Evans, 1955).

V. BROAD-BEAM ATTENUATION OF UNCHARGED RADIATION

Any attenuation geometry other than narrow-beam geometry—i.e., in which at least some nonprimary rays reach the detector—is called broad-beam geometry. While one can easily understand what is meant by "ideal" narrow-beam geometry (i.e., that in which *no* scattered or secondary particles strike the detector), the corresponding concept of an ideal broad-beam geometry is more difficult to define, and is experimentally less accessible. Nevertheless it will be found useful to establish such a concept for comparison with actual cases. It may be defined as follows:

In ideal broad-beam geometry every scattered or secondary uncharged particle strikes the detector, but only if generated in the attenuator by a primary particle on its way to the detector, or by a secondary charged particle resulting from such a primary.

This requires that the attenuator be thin enough to allow the escape of all the uncharged particles resulting from first interactions by the primaries, plus the x-rays and annihilation γ-rays emitted by secondary charged particles that are generated by primaries in the attenuator. Multiple scattering is excluded from this ideal case.

If, in addition to having (or accurately simulating) ideal broad-beam *geometry*, we require the detector to respond in proportion to the *radiant energy* of all the primary, scattered, and secondary uncharged radiation incident upon it, then we have a case that may be called *ideal broad-beam attenuation*. For this case we can write an exponential equation in the form of Eq. (3.3):

$$\frac{R_L}{R_0} = e^{-\mu_{en}L} \tag{3.10}$$

where R_0 is the primary radiant energy incident on the energy detector when $L = 0$, R_L is the radiant energy of uncharged particles striking the detector when the attenuator is in place, L is the attenuator thickness, which must remain thin enough to allow escape of all scattered and secondary uncharged particles, and μ_{en} is the energy-absorption coefficient, as already defined in Eq. (2.13).

μ_{en} is often used as an approximation to the effective attenuation coefficient μ' for thin absorbing layers in broad-beam attenuation situations, even though they may be less than ideal. This application of μ_{en} is referred to by Goldstein (1957) as the "straight-ahead approximation," to convey the idea that the scattered and secondary particles are supposed to continue straight ahead until they strike the detector. In real broad-beam attenuation experiments the observed μ' may approximate μ_{en} only poorly, even for thin absorbers. Nevertheless μ_{en} is often employed in this connection where better values of effective broad-beam attenuation coefficients are not available. It gives fairly good results, for example, in calculating photon attenuation in the wall of a cavity ionization chamber made of low-Z material.

Practical broad-beam geometries usually fall short of the ideal case because some of the scattered and secondary radiation that is supposed to reach the detector fails to arrive. This loss of radiation can be called *out-scattering*, illustrated by particles labeled S_1 in Fig. 3.3, *b–f* (Section VI below). Similarly, we can define *in-scattering* as the arrival at the detector of scattered and secondary uncharged particles that are generated in the attenuator by primaries that are *not* aimed at the detector (particles S_2 in Fig. 3.3, *b–f*). Ideal broad-beam geometry may be simulated to the extent that in-scattered particles replace those being out-scattered, with respect to both type and energy. For perfect balance an energy detector would then respond in accordance with Eq. (3.10).

Generally, however, out-scattering is not exactly compensated by in-scattering. Usually out-scattering exceeds in-scattering, resulting (for a radiant-energy detector) in a value of μ' that exceeds μ_{en} (i.e., $\mu_{en} < \mu' < \mu$). If in-scattering is the greater, then $\mu' < \mu_{en}$ for a radiant-energy detector. In-scattering may so strongly exceed out-scattering that μ' may be less than zero, i.e., the detector response may initially *increase* with L. This effect is shown in the data in Fig. 3.4*b* and in Fig. 3.5*b*, curve D (Section VI below).

As L is increased to great thicknesses of attenuator, the value of μ' observed in broad-beam attenuation of monoenergetic radiation gradually increases to approach μ. This happens in the following way: For small L, the scattered + secondary $(s+s)$ particles generated in an increment of thickness dL exceed those absorbed + out-scattered in dL. Gradually with increasing L the rate of generation of $s+s$ particles by primaries decreases, while the rate of absorption + out-scattering of $s+s$ particles increases as their population increases, until equilibrium is reached. If a narrower beam is employed, out-scattering is increased so that the equilibrium is reached at a smaller value of L. For a very narrow beam, out-scattering equals generation for all values of L; hence $\mu' = \mu$ and again one has narrow-beam geometry.

The different types of geometries and attenuations can be summarized as follows:

1. *Narrow-beam geometry.*   Only primaries strike the detector; μ is observed for monoenergetic beams.

2. *Narrow-beam attenuation.*   Only primaries are counted in N_L by the detector, regardless of whether secondaries strike it; μ is observed for monoenergetic beams.

3. *Broad-beam geometry.*   Other than narrow-beam geometry; at least some scattered and secondary radiation strikes the detector.

4. *Broad-beam attenuation.*   Scattered and secondary radiation is counted in N_L by the detector. $\mu' < \mu$ is observed. (Note: Narrow-beam attenuation can be obtained in broad-beam geometry if only the primaries are counted in N_L.)

5. *Ideal broad-beam geometry.*   Every scattered or secondary uncharged particle that is generated directly or indirectly by a primary on its way to the detector, strikes the detector. No other scattered or secondary radiation strikes the detector. (Note: Ideal broad-beam geometry can be simulated if each out-scattered particle is replaced by an identical in-scattered particle.)

6. *Ideal broad-beam attenuation.*   Ideal broad-beam geometry exists (or is simulated), and the detector responds in proportion to the radiant energy incident on it. In that case $\mu' = \mu_{\text{en}}$.

In the next section several types of broad-beam geometries will be examined in relation to these concepts.

VI. SOME BROAD-BEAM GEOMETRIES

Figure 3.3 illustrates some arrangements which are characterized in varying degree as broad-beam geometries. The detector in each case is taken to be isotropically sensitive to uncharged radiation, but totally insensitive to incident charged particles (e.g., a thick-walled spherical ionization chamber).

In Fig. 3.3a the radiation beam (which in this case is narrow) enters through a small hole and impinges on the attenuating layers of material inside of a (hypothetical) spherical-shell detector, so that practically all scattered rays (S_1) originating in the attenuator will strike the detector, regardless of their direction (except $\cong 180°$). A deep well-type detector could roughly approximate this geometry. This approaches ideal broad-beam geometry, as defined in the preceding section.

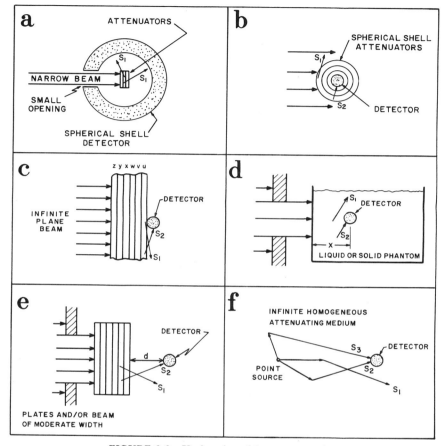

FIGURE 3.3   Various broad-beam geometries.

In Fig. 3.3*b* the situation is reversed: The attenuating material is arranged in spherical shells surrounding the detector. The beam is made large enough to irradiate the attenuators fully. In this case the out-scattered rays such as S_1 generated in the attenuator upstream of the detector, but not striking it, tend to be compensated by in-scattered rays such as S_2 originating elsewhere in the attenuator. This probably simulates ideal broad-beam geometry at least as closely as any arrangement that relies on such compensation, i.e., any geometry other than that in Fig. 3.3*a*.

Figure 3.3*c* shows a plane beam that is infinitely wide compared to the effective maximum range of scattered and secondary radiation, and incident perpendicularly on similarly wide attenuating plates. The detector is kept as close as possible to the attenuator to allow laterally out-scattered rays such as S_1 to be maximally replaced by in-scattered rays such as S_2. In practice this usually means that the detector is kept stationary, and the attenuating slabs are added in sequence of increasing distance forward of the detector ($u \rightarrow z$). For a perfectly plane-parallel beam the same result would be observed by adding the slabs in reverse order ($z \rightarrow u$), so long as the chamber were kept in contact with the rearmost slab, moving back as slabs were added. In a diverging beam this would exaggerate the observed attenuation by a loss of intensity in proportion to the inverse square of the distance from the source. For this reason experimental attenuation measurements are usually made with the detector in a fixed position. Our discussion in this chapter will assume (unless otherwise specified) that the inverse-square effect is absent, either because the detector is fixed, or the radiation beam is plane-parallel.

In the geometry of Fig. 3.3c it is clear that the detector receives no back-scattered radiation, since there is no material behind it. The irradiated attenuator thus subtends a solid angle at the detector of only about 2π radians, as compared to 4π radians for Fig. 3.3b (and effectively also for Fig. 3.3a, where the detector subtends approximately 4π radians at the attenuator). The smaller the subtended solid angle, the poorer the ''coupling'' between the detector and the attenuator, and the less scattered radiation will reach the detector. However, as will be shown in later chapters, scattered rays predominately tend to move in a forward direction (i.e., $\theta < 90°$ relative to the primary particle direction). This is because of conservation of momentum, the effect of which becomes more pronounced for primary particles of higher energies. The result is that the attenuators upstream from the detector generally contribute most of the scattered rays.

Figure 3.3d shows a detector that may be positioned at a variable depth x from the front surface of a large mass of solid or liquid medium, which is designed to simulate the attenuating properties of the human body. Such a mass, called a *phantom*, often consists of a Lucite-walled cubic tank 30 or 40 cm on an edge, filled with water. Uncharged particle (usually photon) beams of various cross-sectional dimensions are directed perpendicularly on the phantom, as shown, and the detector response is measured vs. depth. The resulting function is used in cancer radiotherapy treatment planning, and is usually referred to as the ''central-axis depth–dose'' of the beam, for a specified SSD (source-to-surface distance).

Ordinarily in such measurements the detector is moved to vary the depth, and since the SSD is finite, the observed depth–dose function includes the inverse-square-law effect as well as attenuation in the medium. However, we will assume for our discussion that the detector remains fixed while the tank is moved, or that the source is very distant. In that case, if the beam and tank were very wide, the attenuation function observed would be similar to that in the geometry of Fig. 3.3c. The detector response enhancement due to the presence of the back-scattering material behind the detector in the phantom remains nearly a constant fraction for all depths (including zero depth), until the rear surface is closely approached.

If a smaller beam size is used in the geometries of Fig. 3.3c and d, out-scattered rays such as S_1 are less fully compensated by in-scattered rays (S_2), and the response of the detector to scattered radiation decreases relative to its response to primary radiation. Thus the effective attenuation coefficient μ' observed at a given depth will be closer to μ, as discussed in the preceding section. This trend is even more accentuated by moving the detector a distance **d** away from the attenuators, as in Fig. 3.3*e*. For a given beam width, this results in fewer scattered rays at the detector than for the cases shown in Fig. 3.3*c* and *d*. The larger the ratio **d/w** (for beam width **w** large enough to cover the detector), the closer the situation approaches narrow-beam geometry.

Still another broad-beam geometry is shown in Fig. 3.3*f*, in which a point source and a detector are immersed in an infinite homogeneous attenuating medium (e.g., water) separated by a variable distance. The effect of attenuation can be separated from that of the inverse square law by comparing the detector response in the medium with that in a vacuum for the same distance. Note that out-scattered rays like s_1 are compensated by in-scattered rays like s_2, but additional backscattered rays such as s_3 may also strike the detector, especially when it is close to the source and the primary energy is low.

Examples of attenuation curves obtained with point γ-ray sources of ^{60}Co ($E \cong$ 1.25 MeV) and ^{203}Hg (0.279 MeV) in the geometry of Fig. 3.3*f*, with water for the attenuator, are shown in Fig. 3.4*a* and *b*. Also shown are lines of slope $-\mu$, indicating the attenuation of the primary photons only (i.e., narrow-beam attenuation), and $-\mu_{\mathrm{en}}$, the slope equivalent to the effective attenuation coefficient for ideal broad-beam attenuation. The slope $-\mu'$ of the broad-beam attenuation curve is not a constant,

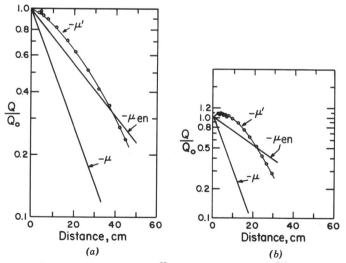

FIGURE 3.4.   Broad-beam attenuation of (*a*) ^{60}Co (1.25 MeV) and (*b*) ^{203}Hg (0.279 MeV) gamma rays as a function of distance from a point source in an infinite water medium. Also shown are lines of slope $-\mu$ and $-\mu_{\mathrm{en}}$. The measured attenuation was gotten as the ratio of the ion chamber response with (Q) to that without (Q_0) the water medium present. (From the thesis of M. A. Van Dilla, as quoted by Evans, 1955.) Figures reproduced with permission of R. D. Evans and the McGraw-Hill Book Company.

but becomes progressively steeper with increasing depth to approach the value $-\mu$, as discussed in Section V. The case of ^{203}Hg is particularly striking because, out to a distance of about 10 cm, more radiation is detected in the presence of the water than when it is removed. In other words, the slope is initially positive in this case. There are two general causes for such an observation in broad-beam geometry:

1. *Excessive in-scattering*, for example caused by backscattering from an attenuating medium located behind the source or the detector, or by crowding of scattered rays in proportion to the cosine of the mean scattering angle θ, so that the particle fluence increases as $1/\cos\theta$ behind a thin plane scatterer in a plane parallel beam (see Fig. 1.5).

2. *Energy-dependence of the detector*, causing it to over-respond to the arriving scattered rays.

Ideal broad-beam geometry, as defined in Section V and illustrated in Fig. 3.3a, could only result in an increase in detector response with attenuator thickness for an energy-dependent detector as in item 2 above. This is because ideal broad-beam geometry does not depend on the compensation of out-scattered by in-scattered rays. Practical simulations of this geometry all rely on such compensation, however, and thus are subject to imbalance of in- vs. out-scattered particles in varying degree.

Some experimental results obtained with narrow- and broad-beam geometries in measuring the attenuation of a fast-neutron beam ($\overline{E} \cong 14$ MeV) are shown in Fig. 3.5. The procedure is described in the legend; other experimental details are given by Attix et al. (1976). The figure inset shows the geometrical arrangement. An ionization chamber was used as the detector.

Curve A is for nearly narrow-beam geometry and is nearly straight (i.e., exponential), with a final slope of $\mu = 0.209$ cm^{-1}. The slight curvature results from the beam being nonmonoenergetic, with the steel filtering out the easiest-to-stop components first. Curve B is for a broader beam, with the attenuator close to the detector. The beam was still broader for curve C, and for curve D equal slabs of attenuator were synchronously added in back and front of the detector. The extra effect of backscattering is evident from the comparison of curves C and D. Curve D shows an initial rise above unity, not shown by C; then they tend to be parallel at greater depths.

VII. SPECTRAL EFFECTS

So far we have ignored the energy response function of the detector, except to require a constant response per unit of radiant energy for ideal broad-beam attenuation. For monoenergetic homogeneous primaries in narrow-beam geometry, there is only one type and energy of particle to be detected. For that simple case the same exponential attenuation vs. depth would be observed irrespective of the physical quantity measured, be it particle fluence, energy fluence, exposure, or other relevant parameter.

Since any broad-beam geometry delivers scattered and secondary particles to the detector, one must consider the relative sensitivity of the detector to those particles vs. primary radiation. In general scattering tends to degrade primaries to lower energies. Moreover neutrons usually also generate secondary γ rays, and conversely, γ rays above a few MeV can generate secondary neutrons in (γ, n) nuclear interactions. Thus the sensitivity of the detector to radiations of differing energies as well as types (n vs. γ) can influence the observed attenuation in broad-beam geometry.

We need not dwell here on the special problem of γ-rays generated by neutron beams and the measurement of such mixed beams. Chapter 16 on neutron physics and dosimetry will discuss this. It is worth mentioning however that the data shown in Fig. 3.5 were gotten with a "tissue-equivalent" ion chamber which measured the beam in terms of the total neutron + γ-ray absorbed dose in muscle. (γ, n) reactions are relatively unimportant contributors to photon-beam attenuation even at high energies, as will be discussed in Chapter 7. Hence we may focus our attention on the influence of the detector's energy dependence on attenuation measurements or calculations. Note, in the latter connection, that one must assign a response function to the detector in a Monte Carlo radiation-transport calculation.

The simple counting of transmitted particles, irrespective of their energies, is generally not a useful measure of the attenuation of radiation except for narrow beams of monoenergetic radiation. In radiological physics and dosimetry our interest is usually directed toward the ability of radiation to deposit energy or produce ionization

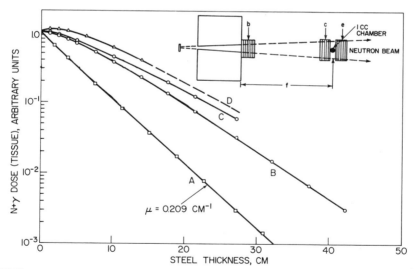

FIGURE 3.5. Narrow vs. broad-beam attenuation of a fast-neutron beam ($\overline{E} \cong 14$ MeV) in steel. (After Attix et al., 1976.) The detector was a 1-cm³ ion chamber, located $f = 161$ cm from the shield. The beam at that distance was 3 cm in diameter for curve A, 13 × 13 cm² for curve B, and 28 × 28 cm² for curves C and D. The attenuators were located at position b for curve A, position c for curves B, C, and D, and also position e for curve D. Curve A is for narrow-beam geometry; curves B, C, and D for progressively broader-beam geometry. Reproduced with permission of *Physics in Medicine and Biology*.

in matter. Thus it is more relevant to weight transmitted particles by the energy they carry, in other words, to measure the energy fluence or the radiant energy arriving at the detector. This can be done by a beam-stopping calorimeter, for example, but such a device may be quite large and massive. Moreover the measurement of absorbed dose in a suitable detector material, or exposure (for photons only) in an air-equivalent detector, is usually even more relevant as a measure of attenuation. In other words, the question "How much is the dose in tissue, or the exposure, diminished as a result of an attenuating layer?" is often of greater interest than "How many photons are counted?" or even "How much energy is measured?" Nevertheless the energy fluence Ψ remains an important fundamental measure of attenuation, since both the exposure and the absorbed dose (which equals the collision kerma under charged-particle-equilibrium conditions; see next chapter) are proportional to Ψ for a given value of μ_{en}/ρ, as discussed in Chapter 2.

While the detector response function can have no influence on the observed narrow-beam attenuation coefficient μ for monoenergetic beams, that is not true for a spectrum consisting of multiple lines or a continuous distribution. Since μ is energy-dependent, different parts of the primary spectrum are attenuated at different rates. Thus, even for narrow-beam attenuation, the observed slope $-\overline{\mu}$ of the attenuation curve changes with depth, generally becoming flatter as the less-penetrating components are removed. Figure 3.5 (curve A) shows a slight curvature due to this effect. Chapter 9, Figs. 9.12 and 9.13 contain examples for x-ray bremsstrahlung spectra.

The narrow-beam attenuation coefficient for a given medium will have a mean value $\overline{\mu}$ that depends on the attenuator thickness L as well as on the detector response function. For the case where the detector responds in proportion to the incident energy fluence (or the radiant energy), the mean narrow-beam attenuation coefficient observed at depth L is given by

$$\overline{\mu}_{\Psi,L} = \frac{\displaystyle\int_{E=0}^{E_{max}} \Psi'_L(E)\,\mu_{E,Z}\,dE}{\displaystyle\int_{E=0}^{E_{max}} \Psi'_L(E)\,dE} \tag{3.11}$$

where $\Psi'_L(E)$ is the differential energy-fluence spectrum (e.g., in J/m^2 keV) reaching the detector through attenuator thickness L, and $\mu_{E,Z}$ is the narrow-beam attenuation coefficient for energy E and atomic number Z.

If the primary beam consists of n spectral lines, Eq. (3.11) is replaced by

$$\overline{\mu}_{\Psi,L} = \frac{\displaystyle\sum_{i=1}^{n} (\Psi_i)_L (\mu_{E,Z})_i}{\displaystyle\sum_{i=1}^{n} (\Psi_i)_L} \tag{3.12}$$

where $(\Psi_i)_L$ is the energy fluence of the ith spectral line at depth L.

Corresponding equations can be written where the detector responds in proportion to other parameters such as particle fluence or exposure.

VIII. THE BUILDUP FACTOR

The concept of *buildup factor B* is very useful in describing broad-beam attenuation quantitatively. It can be applied with respect to any specified geometry, attenuator, or physical quantity in radiological physics (e.g., numbers of particles, energy fluence, exposure, kerma, or dose). The general definition can be written as

$$B = \frac{\text{quantity due to primary} + \text{scattered and secondary radiation}}{\text{quantity due to primary radiation alone}} \qquad (3.13)$$

For narrow-beam geometry it follows that $B = 1$ exactly, and for broad-beam geometry $B > 1$. The value of B is a function of radiation type and energy, attenuating medium and depth, geometry, and the measured quantity.

Restating Eq. (3.3) in terms of, say, energy fluence Ψ, and incorporating the depth-dependent buildup factor B to allow the equation's application in broad-beam geometry, we have

$$\frac{\Psi_L}{\Psi_0} = Be^{-\mu L} \qquad (3.14)$$

in which Ψ_0 is the unattenuated primary energy fluence, Ψ_L is the total energy fluence arriving at the detector behind a medium thickness L, and μ is the narrow-beam attenuation coefficient. Equation (3.14) follows from Eq. (3.13), since $\Psi_0 e^{-\mu L}$ is the attenuated energy fluence due to primaries alone penetrating L.

When L is zero in Eq. (3.14) (i.e., no attenuator thickness between source and detector), B becomes equal to $B_0 \equiv \Psi_L/\Psi_0$, which has the value unity for most broad-beam geometries (e.g., Fig. 3.3a, b, c, e, f). For the case shown in Fig. 3.3d, however, when the detector is at the phantom surface (depth $= x \equiv L = 0$), backscattered rays will still strike it. Hence $\Psi_L > \Psi_0$ in Eq. (3.14), so $B_0 > 1$ even for $L = 0$. In that case B_0 is called the *backscatter factor*. For ^{60}Co γ-rays ($\cong 1.25$ MeV) incident in a very broad beam on a water phantom, $B_0 \cong 1.06$ in terms of the exposure or tissue dose. For lower energy its value is greater (see depth–dose tables, e.g., Johns and Cunningham, 1974).

Some typical calculated buildup factors are given in Fig. 3.6 for the exposure delivered by an infinitely wide plane homogeneous photon beam perpendicularly incident on a semi-infinite water medium. The abscissa is given in terms of μL, the depth of the point of measurement in units of the mean free path, $1/\mu$. The buildup factor B for exposure is seen to increase steadily with depth in all cases. Corresponding buildup factors for other related quantities (energy fluence, dose) generally show similar behavior. Berger (1968) has calculated useful tables of dose buildup factors for γ-ray point sources in water.

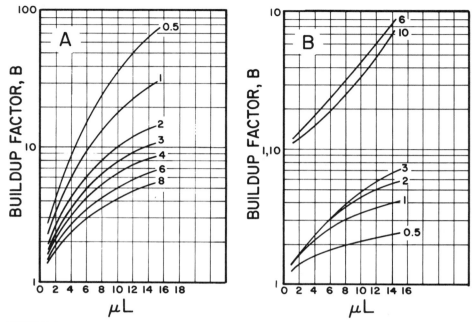

FIGURE 3.6. Exposure buildup factors for a plane, infinitely wide beam of photons perpendicularly incident on semi-infinite media of (A) water and (B) lead. Curves are labeled with photon energies in MeV. Abscissae indicate the depth in units of the mean free path $1/\mu$. (Goldstein, 1957.) Reproduced with the author's permission.

It will also be seen that, for equal depths in terms of mean free paths, B is less in lead than in water for γ-rays below 4 MeV. This results from the much greater photoelectric effect in lead, which absorbs the Compton-scattered photons, preventing their propagation. At higher energies the production of annihilation photons through pair production in lead makes B larger than it is in water. These processes are discussed in Chapter 7.

An alternative concept to the buildup factor is the *mean effective attenuation coefficient*, $\bar{\mu}'$, which can be defined by the following equation:

$$\frac{\Psi_L}{\Psi_0} = Be^{-\mu L} \equiv e^{-\bar{\mu}'L} \tag{3.15}$$

or, solving for $\bar{\mu}'$,

$$\bar{\mu}' \equiv \mu - \frac{\ln B}{L} \tag{3.16}$$

$\bar{\mu}'$ has the computational advantage of being less strongly dependent upon depth L than is the corresponding buildup factor B, as can be seen in Table 3.1.

TABLE 3.1. Comparison of Exposure Buildup Factor B and Mean Effective Attenuation Coefficient $\bar{\mu}'$ for a Plane Beam of 1-MeV γ-Rays in Water[a]

B	μL	X_L/X_o $= Be^{-\mu L}$	L (cm)	$\bar{\mu}'$ (cm^{-1})	$\bar{\mu}'/\mu$	$\bar{\mu}'/\mu_{en}$
3	1.7	0.548	24	0.025	0.35	0.81
6	4.0	0.110	57	0.039	0.55	1.26
10	6.3	1.84×10^{-2}	89	0.045	0.64	1.46
20	10.9	3.69×10^{-4}	154	0.051	0.72	1.65
30	14.6	1.37×10^{-5}	207	0.054	0.76	1.75

[a] $\mu = 0.0706$ cm^{-1}; $\mu_{en} = 0.0309$ cm^{-1}.

The exposure buildup-factor data in the first column were taken from the 1-MeV curve in Fig. 3.6a, varying from $B = 3$ to 30 as μL goes from 1.7 to 14.6. The corresponding $\bar{\mu}'$-values derived from Eq. (3.16) change gradually from 0.025 to 0.054 cm^{-1}.

Figure 3.7 illustrates the data in Table 3.1. The curve is a plot of $Be^{-\mu L}$ vs. μL. Its slope at any depth is $-\mu'$, which gradually gets steeper, approaching $-\mu$ for large values of μL. Also plotted in Fig. 3.7 are the slopes $-\bar{\mu}'$ from Table 3.1, which can be seen as chords joining the curve origin and its values at tabulated depths, so that $\bar{\mu}' < \mu' < \mu$ at each depth.

IX. THE RECIPROCITY THEOREM

In the simplest case, for which it is exact, the *reciprocity theorem* for the attenuation of any kind of radiation is self-evident: *Reversing the positions of a point detector and a point source within an infinite homogeneous medium does not change the amount of radiation detected.* This is shown schematically in Fig. 3.8. If we assume that media P and Q are identical, then clearly it makes no difference whether the rays go from left to right, or vice versa on mirror-image paths.

If P and Q are different with respect to their scattering and/or attenuating properties, *the transmission of primary rays still remains the same*, left or right. However, the generation and/or transmission of a scattered ray such as that shown in Fig. 3.8a vs. b may differ. For example, if the scattered ray is absorbed more strongly in medium Q than in P, all else being equal, it is more likely to reach the detector in case b than in case a, since its path length in medium Q is longer in case a.

Though no longer exact (except for primary rays), the reciprocity theorem remains useful in calculating the attenuation of radiation in dissimilar or nonhomogeneous media, so long as either the primary rays dominate, or the generation and propagation of scattered rays is not strongly dissimilar in the different media. Such is the case, for example, for γ-rays in low-Z media, for which the Compton effect dominates the production and attenuation of scattered rays (see Chapter 7).

Mayneord (1945) extended the reciprocity theorem to the case where the source

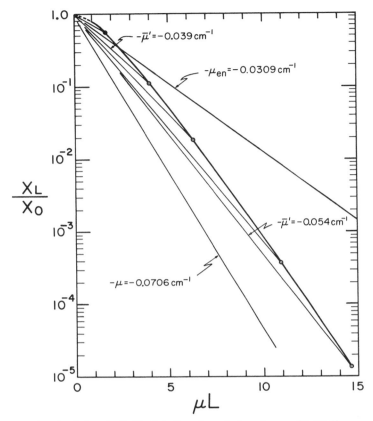

FIGURE 3.7. Graph of data in Table 3.1, for a broad plane beam of 1-MeV γ-rays in water. Note that any slope in this graph is equal to $[\ln(X_L/X_0)/[L(cm)]$, even though the abscissa is labelled μL, that is, the depth L in units of mean free path $1/\mu$.

and detector were both extended volumes such as those shown in Fig. 3.9. He concluded that:

> The integral dose* in a volume V due to a γ-ray source uniformly distributed throughout source volume S is equal to the integral dose that would occur in S if the same activity density per unit mass were distributed throughout V.

Clearly this can be exact with respect to the dose resulting from primary rays only, unless V and S are parts of an infinite homogeneous medium. Furthermore, at the

---

*Assuming charged-particle equilibrium (see Chapter 4), so that D is proportional to Ψ throughout V and S. Note also that integral dose $= (\epsilon)_e$; see Section III.A in Chapter 2.

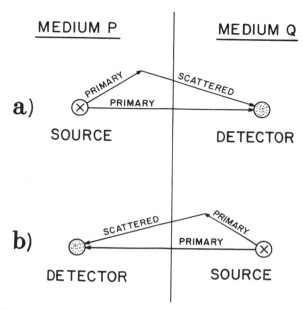

FIGURE 3.8. The reciprocity theorem in radiation transport (see text).

time it was written no distinction was being made between exposure and dose, and Mayneord stated his ''dose'' in roentgens, thus implicitly assuming air as the dosed medium in both S and V. Consequently the theorem as stated is only true if the mass energy-absorption coefficients are the same for the materials in S and V. This can be seen in the following derivation. Although γ-rays are discussed, it is applicable in principle to neutrons as well.

Figure 3.9 shows a source region S containing matter of density ρ_1, and a detector region V of density ρ_2, set at a distance from one another in an infinite medium of density ρ_3 (kg/m^3). Each region is assumed to be homogeneous.

The region S contains a uniformly distributed γ-ray source with specific activity A' (Bq/kg).* Thus the elementary volume ds (m^3) contains an activity $dA = A' \cdot \rho_1 \, ds$ (Bq). We will assume that each atomic decay emits one γ-ray, with the single energy E (MeV). (Note that although we assume a monoenergetic source here for convenience, the theorem works as well for multienergy sources.) The narrow-beam attenuation coefficient for γ-rays of quantum energy E in S is μ_1 (cm^{-1}), in V it is μ_2, and in the matrix medium μ_3.

Consider now a volume element dv in V, at a distance $r_1 + r_2 + r_3 = r$ away from

---

*1 Bq $\equiv$ 1 becquerel $\equiv$ one radioactive disintegration per second, as discussed in Chapter 6, Section III.

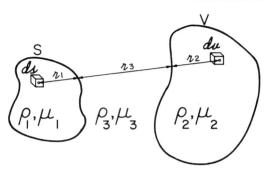

FIGURE 3.9.   Illustration of reciprocity theorem according to Mayneord (1945).

ds. If there were no attenuation, the photon fluence Φ at dv for an irradiation time
of Δt (seconds) would be

$$\Phi = \frac{dA\ \Delta t}{4\pi r^2} \qquad \text{(photons/m}^2\text{)} \tag{3.17}$$

and the energy fluence would be

$$\Psi = 1.602 \times 10^{-13}\ \Phi E \qquad \text{(J/m}^2\text{)} \tag{3.18}$$

giving a collision kerma at dv of

$$K_c = \Psi \left(\frac{\mu_{\text{en}}}{\rho_2}\right)_{E,\,V} \qquad \text{(J/kg)} \tag{3.19}$$

where $(\mu_{\text{en}}/\rho_2)_{E,V}$ is the energy absorption coefficient for γ-ray energy E in medium
V, in m^2/kg [see Eq. (2.13)].

It will be shown in the next chapter that when a condition called "charged-particle
equilibrium" applies, one has $K_c = D$, the absorbed dose. We will assume that to
be the case here, so that the absorbed dose to the material in dv due to the source
in ds is given in J/kg by

$$D = 1.602 \times 10^{-13} \frac{A'\rho_1\ \Delta t\ E(\mu_{\text{en}}/\rho_2)_{E,\,V}\ ds}{4\pi r^2} \tag{3.20}$$

—still assuming no attenuation. To confine ourselves to the attenuation of primary
rays in traveling from ds to dv, Eq. (3.20) must be multiplied by $e^{(-\mu_1 r_1 - \mu_2 r_2 - \mu_3 r_3)}$.

The total absorbed dose at dv due to the entire radioactive source in region S is
gotten by integration of Eq. (3.20) over the volume S:

$$D_{\text{tot}} = \frac{1.602 \times 10^{-13}\ A'\rho_1\ \Delta t\ E(\mu_{\text{en}}/\rho_2)_{E,\,V}}{4\pi} \int_S \frac{e^{-(r_1\mu_1 + r_2\mu_2 + r_3\mu_3)}}{r^2}\ ds \tag{3.21}$$

The element of integral dose in dv is equal to $D_{\text{tot}}\rho_2\ dv$. Thus the integral dose $D(V,
S)$ in the volume V as a result of the source throughout S is gotten in joules from

$$D(V, S) = \frac{1.602 \times 10^{-13} A' \rho_1 \rho_2 \, \Delta t \, E(\mu_{en}/\rho_2)_{E,V}}{4\pi} \int_V \int_S \frac{e^{-(r_1\mu_1 + r_2\mu_2 + r_3\mu_3)}}{r^2} \, dv \, ds$$

$$(3.22)$$

It can be seen from this equation that the corresponding relation for the integral dose in S due to the same source density A in V would be

$$D(S, V) = \frac{1.602 \times 10^{-13} A' \rho_1 \rho_2 \, \Delta t \, E(\mu_{en}/\rho_1)_{E,S}}{4\pi} \int_S \int_V \frac{e^{-(r_1\mu_1 + r_2\mu_2 + r_3\mu_3)}}{r^2} \, ds \, dv$$

$$(3.23)$$

Since the order of integration doesn't matter, Eqs. (3.22) and (3.23) are identical for the case where $(\mu_{en}/\rho_2)_{E,V} = (\mu_{en}/\rho_1)_{E,S}$. Thus Mayneord's statement of the reciprocity theorem is proved for primary rays only, where the two volumes contain media having the same μ_{en}/ρ, and charged-particle equilibrium obtains throughout both. Note that symmetry arguments alone suffice to guarantee reprocity for *all* radiation in an infinite homogeneous medium.

As a corollary to this theorem, one can state that:

If S and V in Fig. 3.9 contain identical, uniformly distributed total activities, they will each deliver to the other the same average absorbed dose.

Furthermore:

If all the activity in S is concentrated at an internal point P, then the dose at P due to the distributed source in V equals the average dose in V resulting from an equal source at P.

This latter statement can be taken a step further to say that:

The dose at any internal point P in S due to a uniformly distributed source throughout S itself is equal to the average absorbed dose in S resulting from the same total source concentrated at P.

This relationship, though exact only in an infinite homogeneous medium, or for primary radiation, is nevertheless practically useful in calculation of internal dose due to distributed sources in the body (see Chapter 5). It is a central feature of the MIRD method for internal dosimetry (Ellett et al., 1964, 1965; Loevinger and Berman, 1968; Brownell et al., 1968; Snyder et al., 1975).

Loevinger et al. (1956) applied the reciprocity theorem to β-rays for sources imbedded in infinite homogeneous media, substituting an empirically derived function to replace the exponential attenuation term in Eqs. (3.22), (3.23). This emphasizes the fact that in an infinite homogeneous medium the reciprocity theorem depends only on symmetry arguments (see Fig. 3.8, with $P = Q$), and therefore is valid for all kinds of radiations, both primary and scattered.

PROBLEMS

1. A plane-parallel monoenergetic beam of 10^{12} uncharged particles per second is incident perpendicularly on a layer of material 0.02 m thick, having a density $\rho = 11.3 \times 10^3$ kg/m^3. For values of the mass attenuation coefficient $\mu/\rho = 1 \times 10^{-3}$, 3×10^{-4}, and 1×10^{-4} m^2/kg, calculate the number of primary particles transmitted in 1 minute. Compare in each case with the approximation in Eq. (3.5); give percentage errors.

2. What is the relaxation length in each case in problem 1?

3. Suppose that the beam in problem 1 is attenuated simultaneously by three different processes having the given attenuation coefficients.
   (a) How many particles are transmitted in 1 minute?
   (b) How many interactions take place by each process?

4. Suppose a beam of uncharged radiation consists one-third of particles of energy 2 MeV, for which $\mu/\rho = 1 \times 10^{-3}$ m^2/kg, one-third of 5-MeV particles, with $\mu/\rho = 3 \times 10^{-4}$ m^2/kg, and one-third of 7-MeV particles, with $\mu/\rho = 1 \times 10^{-4}$ m^2/kg.
   (a) What average value $\overline{(\mu/\rho)_\Phi}$ will be observed by a particle counter when a thin layer of the attenuator is interposed in the beam, with narrow-beam geometry?
   (b) Calculate the average $\overline{(\mu/\rho)_\Psi}$ that will be seen by an energy fluence meter.

5. Let the beam in problem 4 first pass through a layer of the attenuator 250 kg/m^2 thick, in narrow-beam geometry. Then repeat (a) and (b).

6. At a depth of 47 cm in a medium the absorbed dose is found to be 3.95 Gy, while that resulting only from primary radiation is 3.40 Gy. At the front surface of the medium, the dose from primary radiation is 10.0 Gy. Calculate the dose buildup factor B, the linear attenuation coefficient μ, and the mean effective attenuation coefficient $\bar{\mu}'$. Assume CPE and plane, monoenergetic primaries.

SOLUTIONS TO PROBLEMS

1. 4.786×10^{13}, 5.607×10^{13}, 5.866×10^{13}; 4.644×10^{13}, 5.593×10^{13}, 5.864×10^{13}; 3, 0.25, and 0.03% low.

2. 0.0885, 0.295, 0.885 m.

3. (a) 4.373×10^{13}.
   (b) 1.162×10^{13}, 3.49×10^{12}, 1.16×10^{12}.

4. (a) 4.67×10^{-4} m^2/kg;
   (b) 3.00×10^{-4} m^2/kg.

5. (a) 4.31×10^{-4} m^2/kg;
   (b) 2.79×10^{-4} m^2/kg.

6. $B = 1.162$, $\mu = 2.295$ m^{-1}, $\bar{\mu}' = 1.976$ m^{-1}.

CHAPTER 4

Charged-Particle and Radiation Equilibria

I. INTRODUCTION

The concepts of radiation equilibrium (RE) and charged-particle equilibrium (CPE) are useful in radiological physics as a means of relating certain basic quantities. That is, CPE allows the equating of the absorbed dose D to the collision kerma K_c, while radiation equilibrium makes D equal to the net rest mass converted to energy per unit mass at the point of interest.

II. RADIATION EQUILIBRIUM

Consider an extended volume V, as in Fig. 4.1, containing a distributed radioactive source. A smaller internal volume v exists about a point of interest, P. Here V is required to be large enough so that the maximum distance of penetration d of any emitted ray (excluding neutrinos) and its progeny (i.e., scattered and secondary rays) is less than the minimum separation s of the boundaries of V and v. Radioactivity is emitted isotropically on the average.

If the following four conditions exist throughout V, it will be shown that *radiation equilibrium* (RE) exists for the volume v (in the nonstochastic limit):

a.   The atomic composition of the medium is homogeneous.

b.   The density of the medium is homogeneous.*

c.   The radioactive source is uniformly distributed.*

---

*A theorem due to Fano (1954) says that the density of the medium need not be homogeneous if the source strength per unit mass is homogeneous. However, this theorem lacks rigor in the presence of the polarization effect (see Chapter 8). Hence for generality we require condition b.

61

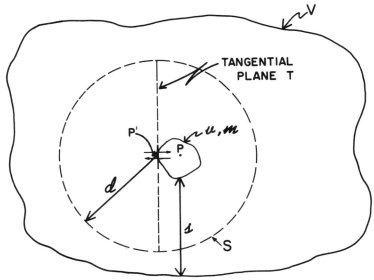

FIGURE 4.1.   Radiation equilibrium. Extended volume *V* contains a homogeneous medium and a homogeneous isotropic source distribution. Radiation equilibrium will exist in the smaller internal volume *v* if the maximum distance of penetration (*d*) of primary rays plus their secondaries is less than the minimum separation (*s*) of *v* from the boundary of **V**. Neutrinos are ignored. (See text.)

    d.   There are no electric or magnetic fields present to perturb the charged-particle paths, except the fields associated with the randomly oriented individual atoms.

The type of radioactive material distributed in the medium need not be specified for purposes of the present argument; radioactivity will be discussed in the next chapter. However, it should be pointed out here that all radioactive sources derive their emitted energy from a reduction in the rest mass of the atoms involved, through Einstein's mass-energy equation $E = mc^2$, where *c* is the velocity of light in vacuum. In the case of positive or negative β-ray emission, a large part of this energy is carried away kinetically by the associated neutrinos. Because of their exceedingly small interaction probability, they can carry their kinetic energy through thousands of kilometers of matter. For this reason the size requirement on the volume *V* above ignores neutrinos; otherwise *V* would have to have unattainable dimensions.

    We have seen in Chapter 3 that the other indirectly ionizing radiations (photons and neutrons) are attenuated in matter more or less exponentially, hence they do not have a true "range" beyond which no particle will penetrate. However, one can (in principle, at least) require *V* to be large enough to achieve any desired reduction in numbers of rays penetrating from its boundaries to reach *v*.

    Imagine now a plane *T* (Fig. 4.1) that is tangent to the volume *v* at a point *P'*, and consider the rays crossing the plane per unit area there. In the nonstochastic limit there will be perfect reciprocity of rays (see arrows in Fig. 4.1) of each type and energy crossing both ways, since the radioactive source distribution within the sphere S of radius d about point P' is perfectly symmetrical with respect to plane T. This will be true for all possible orientations of tangent planes around the volume v; hence one can say that, *in the nonstochastic limit, for each type and energy of ray entering v, another identical ray leaves*. This condition is called *radiation equilibrium* (RE) with respect to v.

Recalling Eq. (2.17), we can write as a consequence of radiation equilibrium that the following equalities of expectation values exist:

$$(\overline{R}_{in})_u = (\overline{R}_{out})_u \tag{4.1a}$$

and

$$(\overline{R}_{in})_c = (\overline{R}_{out})_c \tag{4.1b}$$

—that is, the energy carried in and that carried out of v are balanced for both indirectly and directly ionizing radiation, where the bars signify expectation values.

The energy imparted (Eq. 2.17) can then be simplified to

$$\overline{\epsilon} = \overline{\Sigma Q} \tag{4.2}$$

which means that under RE conditions the expectation value of the energy imparted to the matter in the volume v is equal to that emitted by the radioactive material in v, excluding that given to neutrinos.

Because we are dealing with the nonstochastic case, for which the concept of radiation equilibrium is of practical interest, the volume v may be reduced to an infinitesimal dv about point P, and RE may then be said to exist at that point. The absorbed dose at P will then be given by Eq. (2.18), $D = d\overline{\epsilon}/dm$, where ϵ is equal to $\overline{\Sigma Q}$ in Eq. (4.2). Thus we can make the following statement:

If radiation equilibrium exists at a point in a medium, the absorbed dose is equal to the expectation value of the energy released by the radioactive material per unit mass at that point, ignoring neutrinos.

The concept of radiation equilibrium has practical importance especially in the fields of nuclear medicine and radiobiology, where distributed radioactive sources may be introduced into the human body or other biological systems for diagnostic, therapeutic, or analytical purposes. The resulting absorbed dose at any given point in such circumstances depends on the size of the object relative to the radiation range and on the location of the point within the object. This will be discussed in the next chapter, and references will be given to more detailed treatments.

A few additional comments about the above condition d for the existence of RE are called for. The absence of electric and magnetic fields from V allows the use of the simplest symmetry argument for proving that RE occurs, since radioactive point sources emit radiation isotropically. The presence of a homogeneous, constant magnetic and/or electric field throughout V makes the symmetry argument more difficult to visualize, since the flow of charged particles past a point such as P' will no longer be isotropic. However, isotropicity is not a requirement for RE in the volume v; it is merely necessary that the inward and outward flow of identical particles of the same energy be balanced for all particles present. Even if all the particles flow in one side of v and out the other side, RE will still obtain so long as the in vs out flow is balanced. Any source anisotropy, or distortion of charged-particle tracks, that is homogeneously present everywhere throughout V will have no perturbing effect on the existence of RE in v.

This can be seen with the aid of Fig. 4.2. Consider an elemental volume dv at point of interest P, and two other elemental volumes dv' and dv'' that are symmetrically positioned with respect to dv. We assume dv is located at a distance s from the boundary of volume V that is greater than the maximum range of radiation penetration, d. Throughout V both the medium and the distributed source are homogeneous, as in Fig. 4.1, but now we allow the presence of a homogeneous electric and/or magnetic field, and the source itself need not emit radiation isotropically, so long as the anisotropy is homogeneous everywhere in V.

Assuming that radiation moves preferentially from left to right in Fig. 4.2, homogeneity and symmetry considerations require that the particles (A) traveling from dv' to dv are identical to those (B) traveling from dv to dv'', in the expectation-value limit. Likewise the lesser flow (b) of particles from dv'' to dv is identical to that (a)

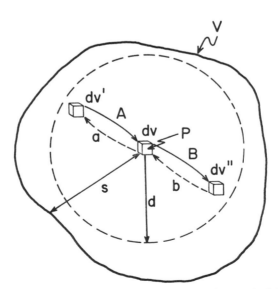

FIGURE 4.2. Radiation equilibrium in homogeneous but anisotropic fields of radiation. (See text.)

from dv to dv'. Consequently $a + B = A + b$, that is, the flow of particles from dv to $dv' + dv''$ is identical to that from $dv' + dv''$ to dv.

The pair of volumes dv' and dv'' can be moved to all possible symmetrical locations within V, and their particle flows can be integrated. Locations outside of the sphere of radius d about point P of course neither receive particles from nor contribute particles to dv. One may conclude from such an argument that each particle flowing out of dv is replaced by an identical particle flowing in. Thus RE exists at P.

This simple proof can also be viewed as an extension of Mayneord's statement of the reciprocity theorem to homogeneous but *anisotropic* sources in infinite homogeneous media: The integral dose (i.e., expectation value of the energy imparted) in dv due to the sources in $dv' + dv''$ equals the integral dose in $dv' + dv''$ resulting from the source in dv. Thus the integral dose throughout V due to the source in dv equals the integral dose in dv resulting from the source throughout V.

Although it is obvious that Eq. (4.1a) would not be perturbed by the presence of a magnetic or electric field, since photons and neutrons are not significantly influenced, the dose resulting from such fields is delivered by secondary charged particles that are affected. For example, Galbraith et al. (1984) have demonstrated that when an electron beam stops in an insulating medium, the resulting nonhomogeneous electric field created by the trapped charge can distort the absorbed dose distribution deposited by a subsequent irradiation, whether x-rays or electrons.

Finally it should not be forgotten that charged particles acquire kinetic energy from motion under the influence of an electric field, or a time-varying magnetic field. This extra energy is spurious with respect to the ionizing radiation field: it does not contribute to the true absorbed dose, even though it may elevate the reading of a dosimeter. Fortunately, such spurious dose contributions are rarely large enough to be significant except for the case of electron multiplication in a gas counter or an ion chamber biased at excessive voltage (see Chapter 12, Section V.A).

III. CHARGED-PARTICLE EQUILIBRIUM

Charged particle equilibrium (CPE) exists for the volume v if each charged particle of a given type and energy leaving v is replaced by an identical particle of the same energy entering, in terms of expectation values (Attix, 1983). If CPE exists, Eq. (4.1b) is of course satisfied. Evidently, where radiation equilibrium exists, so does CPE. In other words, the existence of RE is a *sufficient* condition for CPE to exist. However, the practical importance of CPE stems from the fact that under certain conditions it can be adequately approximated even in the absence of RE. Two important cases will be considered in the following subsections.

A. CPE for Distributed Radioactive Sources

1.

Let us first consider the trivial case where only charged particles are emitted and radiative losses are negligible. Again referring to Fig. 4.1, the dimension s is taken to be greater than the maximum range d of the particles. If the same four conditions (a–d) are satisfied throughout the volume V as required for RE in Section II, then RE and CPE will of course both exist for the volume v, since they are identical in this case. Figure 4.2 applies likewise to CPE.

2.

Consider now the more interesting case where both charged particles and relatively more-penetrating indirectly ionizing radiation are emitted. In Fig. 4.1 let the distance d be the maximum range of the *charged particles only*, and let V be just large enough so the minimum distance s separating V from v exceeds d. If the indirectly ionizing rays are penetrating enough to escape from V without interacting significantly with the medium, then they will produce practically no secondary charged particles. Only the primary charged particles then need be considered in the symmetry argument as before, where again we assume conditions a–d throughout V, as stated for radiation equilibrium. Since the passage of identical charged particles in and out of v is thus seen to be balanced, CPE exists with respect to the primary charged particles, and Eq. (4.1b) is satisfied.

However, RE is not attained, and consequently Eq. (4.1a) is not satisfied, since $(\overline{R}_{out})_u > (\overline{R}_{in})_u$ for the volume v. This is evident from the fact that the indirectly ionizing rays that originate in v and escape from V are not replaced, because there is no source outside of V. The equation for the expectation value of the energy imparted in this case becomes [from Eq. (2.17)]

$$\overline{\epsilon} = (\overline{R}_{in})_u - (\overline{R}_{out})_u + \overline{\Sigma Q} \tag{4.3}$$

Since we are assuming that the indirectly ionizing rays are so penetrating that they do not interact significantly in v, $\overline{\epsilon}$ is equal to the kinetic energy given only to charged-particles by the radioactive source in v, less any radiative losses by those particles while in v. The average absorbed dose in v is thus equal to Eq. (4.3) divided by the mass in v, for CPE conditions.

Suppose now that the size of the volume V occupied by the source is expanded so that distance s in Fig. 4.1 gradually increases from being merely equal to the charged-particle range to being greater than the effective range of the indirectly ionizing rays and their secondaries. That transition will cause the $(\overline{R}_{in})_u$ term in Eq. (4.3) to increase until it equals $(\overline{R}_{out})_u$ in value. Thus RE will be restored, according to the symmetry argument applied to all rays in Section II. The energy imparted, as expressed by Eq. (4.3) for the CPE case, would thence be transformed into Eq. (4.2) for RE.

The calculation of the absorbed dose is evidently straightforward for either of these limiting cases (CPE or RE), but intermediate situations are more difficult to deal with, i.e., when the volume V is larger than necessary to achieve CPE in v, but not large enough for RE. In that case some fraction of the energy of the indirectly ionizing radiation component will be absorbed, and it is relatively difficult to determine what that fraction is. This problem will be discussed in the next chapter.

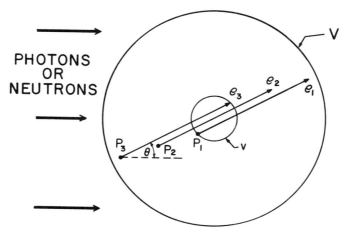

FIGURE 4.3. Charged-particle equilibrium conditions for an external source. The volume V contains a homogeneous medium, uniformly irradiated throughout by indirectly ionizing radiation (i.e., attenuation of the latter is assumed to be negligible). Secondary charged particles are thus produced uniformly throughout V, not necessarily isotropically, but with the same directional and energy distribution everywhere. If the minimum distance separating the boundaries of V and smaller internal volume v is greater than the maximum range of charged particles present, CPE exists in v. (Also see text.)

3.

Achieving CPE for the case of a distributed source of only indirectly ionizing radiation requires that RE also be obtained; hence the discussion in Section II applies.

B. CPE for Indirectly Ionizing Radiations from External Sources

In Fig. 4.3 a volume V is shown, again containing a smaller volume v. The boundaries of v and V are required in this case to be separated by at least the maximum distance of penetration of any secondary charged particle present. If the following conditions are satisfied throughout V, CPE will exist for the volume v (in the nonstochastic limit):

- **a.** The atomic composition of the medium is homogeneous.
- **b.** The density of the medium is homogeneous.*
- **c.** There exists a uniform *field* of indirectly ionizing radiation (i.e., the rays must be only negligibly attenuated by passage through the medium).
- **d.** No inhomogeneous electric or magnetic fields are present.

It is possible for CPE to exist in a volume without satisfying all the above conditions under certain geometrical conditions. The ion-collecting region of a free-air chamber represents such a situation, to be discussed in Chapter 12. Another example is the

---

*The remarks about the Fano theorem in the footnote in Section II also apply here, replacing "source strength" by "number and type of interactions."

trivial case of a point source within a volume large enough so the radiation cannot reach the boundary surface, hence no replacement particles are required.

It will be evident that the above assumed conditions are similar to those listed for radiation equilibrium in Section II, except that a uniform *field* of indirectly ionizing radiation throughout V replaces the uniform radioactive *source* in condition c, and the separation of the boundary of V from that of v now only has to exceed the secondary charged particle range rather than having to be larger than the range of the most penetrating radiation, which is usually the indirectly ionizing radiation present. Condition d was demonstrated by means of Fig. 4.2 to be a sufficient substitute for requiring the absence of electric or magnetic fields.

Because of the uniformity of the indirectly ionizing radiation field and of the medium throughout V, one can say that the number of charged particles produced per unit volume in each energy interval and element of solid angle will be uniform everywhere in V (for the nonstochastic limit). However the particles are not emitted isotropically as in the case of radioactive point sources. Neutron and photon interactions generally result in anisotropic angular distributions of secondary and scattered radiations, as will be seen in later chapters dealing with such interactions. However this anisotropy will be homogeneous throughout V. This condition, together with a uniform medium in which the charged particles can slow down throughout V (as guaranteed by conditions a and b) is sufficient to produce CPE for the volume v, as shown by the reciprocity argument illustrated in Fig. 4.2.

This is further demonstrated in Fig. 4.3 for the simplified case of straight charged-particle tracks, all emitted at angle θ with respect to the monodirectional primary rays. Consider first the track of charged particle e_1, generated by the total absorption of an indirectly ionizing ray at a point P_1 just inside the boundary of v. Particle e_1 crosses v and carries out of that volume a kinetic energy of, say $\frac{2}{3}$ of its original energy. A second identical interaction occurring at point P_2 generates charged particle e_2, which enters v with $\frac{2}{3}$ of its original energy, and leaves with $\frac{1}{3}$ of that energy. Likewise a third identical interaction at P_3 generates charged particle e_3, which enters v with $\frac{1}{3}$ of its original energy, and expends all of that energy in v. Thus CPE exists for the nonstochastic limit, and the total kinetic energy spent in v by the three particles equals that which e_1 alone would have spent if its entire track had remained inside of v.

Substituting Eq. (4.3) into Eq. (2.11) assuming the non-stochastic limit for the latter, we see that for CPE conditions,

$$\overline{\epsilon}_{tr}^n = \overline{\epsilon} + (\overline{R}_{\text{out}})_u - (\overline{R}_{\text{out}})_u^{\text{non-}r} - \overline{R}_u^r \tag{4.4a}$$

However, under those same conditions we may also assume that any radiative interaction by a charged particle after it leaves v will be replaced by an identical interaction inside of v, as shown in Fig. 4.4. Thus

$$(\overline{R}_{\text{out}})_u = (\overline{R}_{\text{out}})_u^{\text{non-}r} + \overline{R}_u^r \tag{4.4b}$$

provided that the volume v is small enough to allow radiative-loss photons to escape,

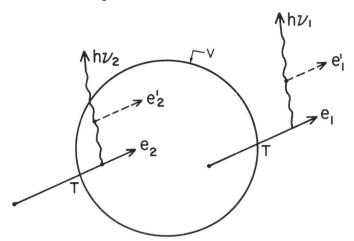

FIGURE 4.4. Illustrating Eqs. (4.4b) and (4.4c). CPE exists (in the nonstochastic limit) because electron e_2 enters the volume v with a kinetic energy T equal to that carried out by electron e_1. If e_1 then emits an x-ray hv_1, e_2 will also emit an identical x-ray hv_2 (on the average). If hv_2 escapes from v, then $(\overline{R}_{out})_u = hv_2 = hv_1 = \overline{R}''_u$, and since $\overline{R}_{out})_u^{non-r} = 0$, Eq. (4.4b) is satisfied. However, if hv_2 is absorbed within v, producing secondary electron e'_2, then $(\overline{R}_{out})_u = 0$ but $\overline{R}''_u$ still equals hv_1 and $(\overline{R}_{out})_u^{non-r} = 0$ as before, so Eq. (4.4b) is no longer satisfied. Therefore Eq. (4.4c) also is only valid for small enough volumes to allow the escape of radiative losses. Equations (4.5) and (4.6) are surely valid because the relevant volume is infinitesimal.

as shown in the same figure. For that case Eqs. (4.4a) and (4.4b) can be simplified to the equality

$$\bar{\epsilon} = \bar{\epsilon}''_{tr} \tag{4.4c}$$

Reducing v to the infinitesimal volume dv, containing mass dm about a point of interest P, we can write

$$\frac{d\bar{\epsilon}}{dm} = \frac{d\bar{\epsilon}''_{tr}}{dm} \tag{4.5}$$

and hence

$$\boxed{\begin{array}{c} \text{CPE} \\ D = K_c \end{array}} \tag{4.6}$$

where the CPE above the equality sign emphasizes its dependence upon that condition. Notice that since Eqs. (4.5) and (4.6) apply to an infinitesimal volume, the required equality of Eq. (4.4b) is assured, since radiative-loss photons will certainly escape in that case.

The derivation of Eq. (4.6) proves that under CPE conditions at a point in a medium, the absorbed dose is equal to the collision kerma there. That is true irrespective of radiative losses. This is a very important relationship, as it equates the measurable quantity D with the calculable quantity K_c $(= \Psi \cdot \mu_{en}/\rho)$.

Moreover, if the same photon energy fluence Ψ is present in media A and B having two different average energy absorption coefficients $\overline{(\mu_{en}/\rho)}_A$ and $\overline{(\mu_{en}/\rho)}_B$, the ratio of absorbed doses under CPE conditions in the two media will be given by

$$\boxed{\frac{D_A}{D_B} \overset{\text{CPE}}{=} \frac{(K_c)_A}{(K_c)_B} = \frac{\overline{(\mu_{en}/\rho)}_A}{\overline{(\mu_{en}/\rho)}_B}} \qquad (4.7a)$$

where $\overline{(\mu_{en}/\rho)}_{A,B}$ can be calculated for the photon fluence spectrum $\Psi'(E)$ from a formula corresponding to Eq. (2.5a). Likewise for the same neutron fluence $\Phi'(E)$ present in the two media,

$$\boxed{\frac{D_A}{D_B} \overset{\text{CPE}}{=} \frac{K_A}{K_B} = \frac{(\overline{F_n})_A}{(\overline{F_n})_B}} \qquad (4.7b)$$

where the average kerma factors $(\overline{F_n})_{A,B}$ can be calculated from Eq. (2.9a).

Note that D_A can differ from D_B in Eqs. (4.7a, b) either because the atomic compositions of A and B are different, or because the radiation spectra present are not identical.

Equation (4.6) is evidently a necessary condition for the existence of CPE at a point in a field of indirectly ionizing radiation, on the basis of Eq. (2.11), (2.12), (2.17), (2.18), and (4.1b). It may also be regarded as a sufficient condition for CPE in terms of *energy* carried by the charged particles, but in the strictest sense CPE must be defined to require not only energy balance but also equal *numbers* of the same types of charged particles passing in and out of the volume in question. Otherwise, to the limited extent that the value of $\overline{W}$ [see Eqs. (2.21)–(2.23)] depends on particle type and energy, the ionization produced within the volume might not be the same as that produced everywhere by the charged particles originating in that volume.

IV. CPE IN THE MEASUREMENT OF EXPOSURE

It was pointed out in Eq. (2.23) that exposure X (which is only defined for x and γ rays) is equal to the product of K_c and $e/\overline{W}$ for air. This poses a practical difficulty in the measurement of X, since collision kerma (K_c) cannot be readily measured by any direct means. The attainment of CPE in an ionization chamber, however, allows the measurement of the ionization collected within a defined volume and mass of air, in place of the ionization produced everywhere by all the secondary electrons that start within the defined volume, as called for by the exposure definition. With

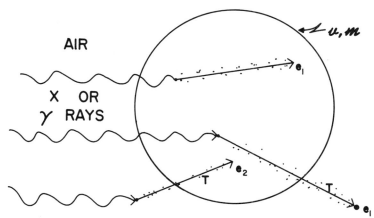

FIGURE 4.5. The role of CPE in the measurement of exposure X. The average exposure in the finite air volume v equals the total charge of either sign released in air by all electrons (e_1) that originate in v, divided by the air mass m in v. If CPE exists, each electron carrying an energy (say, T) out of v is compensated by another electron (e_2) carrying the same energy in. Thus the same ionization occurs in v as if all electrons e_1 remained there. The measurement of that charge divided by m is thus equivalent to a measurement of the average exposure in v. Radiative losses are assumed to escape from v, and any ionization they produce is not to be included in X.

one exception discussed in Chapter 12, all types of standard free-air chambers and cavity ion chambers depend in this way on CPE for measuring exposure.

Figure 4.5 illustrates how such ion chambers operate, in principle. All involve a finite defined volume v (and mass m) of air, hence they actually measure an *average* exposure for that mass. v must be small enough to allow the escape of radiative losses, as noted in Fig. 4.4, and as required by the definition of exposure. Corrections must be made for larger volumes, as discussed in Chapter 12, Section III.A.4.

V. RELATING ABSORBED DOSE TO EXPOSURE FOR x- AND γ-RAYS

It is sometimes useful to know how much absorbed dose would be deposited at some point in air as a result of an exposure X. The relationship is indeterminate in the absence of CPE,* since

$$D_{air} \underset{\substack{\uparrow \\ \text{J/kg}}}{\overset{\text{CPE}}{=}} (K_c)_{air} \underset{\substack{\uparrow \\ \text{J/kg}}}{=} X \underset{\substack{\uparrow \\ \text{C/kg}}}{\cdot} \left(\frac{\overline{W}}{e}\right)_{air} \qquad (4.8)$$

$$\underset{\text{33.97 J/C}}{\uparrow}$$

where the first equality is valid only if CPE exists at the point in question.

*Or TCPE in the case of megavolt photons, see Section VII.C.

If D_{air} is expressed in rads and X in roentgens, Eqs. (2.3) and (2.24) can be used for converting units to rewrite Eq. (4.8) as

$$\overset{\text{CPE}}{0.01 D_{air} = 0.01 (K_c)_{air}} = 2.58 \times 10^{-4} \times 33.97 X \qquad (4.9)$$

or

$$\overset{\text{CPE}}{D_{air} = (K_c)_{air}} = 0.876 X \qquad (4.10)$$

where $(K_c)_{air}$ and D_{air} are in rads, and X in roentgens. It should be emphasized that Eq. (4.10) is valid only where X is the exposure at the point of interest in air, under CPE conditions.

VI. CAUSES OF CPE FAILURE IN A FIELD OF INDIRECTLY IONIZING RADIATION

There are four basic causes for CPE failure in an indirectly ionizing field, which can be identified from the list of CPE conditions given in Section III, referring to Fig. 4.3:

a. Inhomogeneity of atomic composition within volume V.

b. Inhomogeneity of density in V.

c. Non-uniformity of the field of indirectly ionizing radiation in V.

d. Presence of a non-homogeneous electric or magnetic field in V.

Some practical situations where CPE failure occurs are the following:

A. Proximity to a Source

If the volume V in Fig. 4.3 is too close to the source of the indirectly ionizing radiation, then the energy fluence will be significantly nonuniform within V, being larger on the side nearest the source, say on the left. Thus there will be more particles (e_3) produced at points like P_3 than particles e_1 at P_1, and more particles will enter v than leave it. CPE consequently fails for v.

B. Proximity to a Boundary of Inhomogeneity in the Medium

If the volume V in Fig. 4.3 is divided by a boundary between dissimilar media, loss of CPE may result at v, since the number of charged particles then arriving at v will generally be different than would be the case for a homogeneous medium. This difference may be due to a change in charged-particle production, or a change in the range or geometry for scattering of those particles, or a combination of these effects.

A case of special interest is illustrated in Fig. 4.6: that of a beam of megavolt photons incident on a solid unit-density phantom, simulating the body for radiotherapy beam calibration purposes. We will assume for simplicity that the phantom has the atomic composition of air, but with density $\rho = 1$ g/cm^3, and that the photon

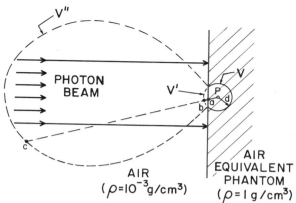

FIGURE 4.6. Dose buildup inside the surface of a phantom irradiated by a beam of megavolt photons. (See text for discussion.)

beam is not contaminated by secondary electrons from the photon source or associated hardware. The absorbed dose D in the phantom increases steeply (roughly as shown in Figure 4.7 below) from a relatively low value at the surface to a maximum; then it decreases more gradually in a condition called *transient charged-particle equilibrium*, (TCPE), which will be described in the next section. For present purposes we may temporarily consider TCPE as being approximately the same as CPE, with D only slightly greater than K_c.

The question to be answered is this: Why is the dose strongly perturbed (i.e., why is it much less than K_c) in the vicinity of the phantom surface, when only the density is discontinuous at that boundary? To simplify even further we may assume that the polarization effect (see first footnote in this chapter) is also negligible. Still the buildup of dose in the phantom will appear more or less as shown in Fig. 4.7. The reason for this is shown in Fig. 4.6. We see there that the spherical volume V, having radius d equal to the maximum range of secondary electrons, must contain a uniformly irradiated homogeneous medium throughout if TCPE is to be produced at point P. If P is too close to the surface, as shown, the portion V' of V will project out of the phantom surface. To replace the solid missing from that lenticular volume, a thousandfold larger volume V'' of air is required (assuming its density to be 10^{-3} g/cm^3). Considering only straight electron paths, an electron which would have started at b and just reached P if V' were filled with solid, now must start at c in gaseous air. (Distance $ac = 1000\ ab$.) However the photon beam is not wide enough to irradiate point c in air, although it does irradiate b.

Thus the replacement of the solid volume V' with the gaseous volume V'' fails to provide as many secondary electrons or as much dose at P, because V'' is not homogeneously (nor even completely) irradiated. Each millimeter of solid air-equivalent medium missing from V' must be replaced by 1 meter of gaseous air, so V''

may be many meters in extent. Clearly it will not be uniformly irradiated in practice. Indeed, the source itself is usually 1 m or less from the phantom surface, and the beam width rarely exceeds 40 cm.

To further complicate the situation, even if the volume V'' were uniformly irradiated, electron out-scattering in air would make it less likely that an electron starting at point c would reach the vicinity of P than an electron starting at b if V' were filled with the solid. An electron scattered at a small angle near point c several meters away might miss the phantom altogether.

Thus we see that the dose-buildup effect observed in phantoms irradiated by high-energy photon beams results from the combination of the density change at the interface and geometric factors involving both photon-beam dimensions and electron scattering. The Fano theorem is not applicable in such cases, even if the polarization effect is negligible.

C. High Energy Radiation

As the energy of indirectly ionizing radiation increases, the penetrating power of the secondary charged particles increases more rapidly than the penetrating power of the primary radiation. Table 4.1 expresses this for both γ-rays and neutrons, and shows that, for example, a 7% attenuation of γ-rays would occur in a water layer equal in thickness ($\cong 5$ cm) to the maximum range of secondary electrons produced by 10-MeV γ-rays. The neutron effect is much smaller (1%) at that energy, assuming hydrogen-recoil proton secondaries.

As a result of this phenomenon, the same type of CPE failure occurs as described in Section VI.A above. That is, in Fig. 4.3, the number of charged particles generated at point P_3 is greater than at P_1, because of the attenuation of the indirectly ionizing radiation in penetrating from the depth of P_3 to that of P_1 in the medium. The degree of CPE failure becomes progressively larger for higher energies, as the table indicates.

Because of this kind of CPE failure, and the usual dependence of x- and γ-ray exposure measurements on the existence of CPE as noted in Section IV, exposure

TABLE 4.1.   **Approximate Attenuation[a] of Gamma Rays and Neutrons within a Layer of Water Equal to the Maximum Range of Secondary Charged Particles**

Primary Radiation Energy (MeV)	Gamma-Ray Attenuation (%) in Maximum Electron Range	Neutron Attenuation (%) in Maximum Proton Range
0.1	0	0
1.0	1	0
10	7	1
30	15	4

[a] For "broad-beam" geometry, see Chapter 3, employing μ_{en} as an effective attenuation coefficient.

measurements have been conventionally assumed to be infeasible for photon energies above about 3 MeV. This limitation is sometimes erroneously interpreted as a failure of the definition of exposure itself; hence the exposure would simply not be defined for high-energy photons, or indeed for any other situation where CPE cannot be achieved. This is not the case however; only the *measurement* of exposure usually depends upon CPE. Moreover, even that constraint has a "loophole": If some other known relationship between D_{air} and $(K_c)_{air}$ can be attained under achievable conditions, and substituted for the simple equality that exists for CPE, exposure can still be measured, at least in principle (Attix, 1979). Such a relationship does exist for a situation known as TCPE, which will be considered in the next section.

VII. TRANSIENT CHARGED-PARTICLE EQUILIBRIUM (TCPE)

TCPE is said to exist at all points within a region in which D is proportional to K_c, the constant of proportionality being greater than unity. This relationship is illustrated in Figs. 4.7a and b. In both cases a broad* "clean" beam of indirectly ionizing radiation (i.e., unaccompanied by charged particles) is shown falling perpendicularly on a slab of material whose surface is supposed to be coincident with the ordinate axis of the figure. In Fig. 4.7a the kerma at the surface is shown as K_0, attenuating exponentially with depth as indicated by the K-curve. We assume in this case that radiative losses by the secondary charged particles are nil ($K_r \cong 0$), which would be strictly true only for incident neutrons. However, in carbon, water, air, and other low-Z media $K_r = K - K_c$ remains less than 1% of K for photons up to 3 MeV. Figure 4.7b shows the corresponding situation where K_r is significant and the radiative-loss photons are allowed to escape from the phantom.

The absorbed-dose curve is shown rising with increasing depth near the surface as the population of charged particles flowing toward the right is augmented by more and more interactions of indirectly ionizing rays. The dose curve reaches a maximum

---

*The beam diameter must be at least twice the maximum range of secondary charged particles, and points of interest must be distant from the edge of the beam by at least that range.

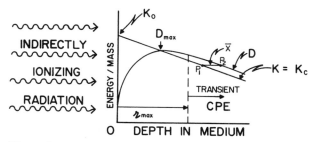

FIGURE 4.7a.   **Illustrating transient CPE for high-energy indirectly ionizing radiation incident from the left on a slab of material. Radiative losses (e.g., bremsstrahlung) are assumed to be absent, so $K_r = 0$ and $K = K_c$.**

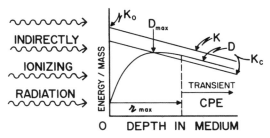

FIGURE 4.7b.   Same as Fig. 4.7*a*, except that radiative losses are significant, so $K = K_c + K_r$ $= K_c (\mu_{tr}/\mu_{en})$, and the resulting photons are assumed to escape from the phantom.

(D_{max}) at the depth where the rising slope due to buildup of charged particles is balanced by the descending slope due to attenuation of the indirectly ionizing radiation. For a "clean" beam of indirectly ionizing radiation D_{max} occurs at approximately the same depth as where the D-curve crosses the K_c-curve.* However, the presence of charged-particle "contamination" in the beam is often observed to shift the depth of D_{max} closer to the surface, where it no longer approximates the depth at which $D = K_c$ (Biggs and Ling, 1979). Thus one should not assume that $D = K_c$ at D_{max}.

At a somewhat greater depth r_{max}, equal to the maximum distance the secondary charged particles starting at the surface can penetrate in the direction of the incident rays, the D-curve becomes parallel to the K_c- and K-curves, although all may gradually change slope together with depth. D therefore becomes proportional to K_c, and we say that TCPE exists. Roesch (1958) suggested a relationship between the D- and K-curves for TCPE conditions, but he assumed that no radiative interactions occurred, and ignored scattered photons. In terms of present terminology we can write that:

$$
\begin{aligned}
D &\overset{\text{TCPE}}{=} K_c e^{\mu' \bar{x}} \\
&\overset{\text{TCPE}}{=} K_c \left(1 + \mu' \bar{x} + \frac{(\mu' \bar{x})^2}{2!} + \ldots \right) \\
&\overset{\text{TCPE}}{=} K_c (1 + \mu' \bar{x})
\end{aligned}
\tag{4.11}
$$

where D and K_c are for the same given depth, at which TCPE is required; μ' is the common slope of the D, K, and K_c curves at that depth; and $\bar{x}$ is the mean distance the secondary charged particles carry their kinetic energy in the direction of the pri-

---

*The situation is mathematically similar to that of a radioactive material and its shorter-lived daughter product, as will be seen in Chapter 6. The K_c-curve corresponds to the parent activity decaying with time, while the D-curve is like the daughter-product activity. This similarity accounts for the adoption of the term "transient equilibrium" (which originated for radioactivity) in the present case. The correspondence between the two situations is only approximate, however, since the initial activity of the daughter product is ordinarily taken to be zero, while the "initial" dose (i.e., that at the surface) is always >0 because of incident and/or backscattered charged particles.

mary rays while depositing it as dose. $\bar{x}$ is shown in Fig. 4.7a as the distance separating the depths of the points P_1 and P_2 where K_c and D have equal values. μ' and $\bar{x}$ of course must be expressed in consistent reciprocal units so their product is dimensionless.

The "TCPE" above the equal signs in Eq. (4.11) indicates that these equalities are valid only where transient CPE exists. The final relation in Eq. (4.11) should actually be an approximation, since only the first two terms of the series are employed. However, the higher-order terms are truly negligible in practical cases.

The above discussion applies equally well to Fig. 4.7a and b, where radiative losses are or are not negligible, respectively. The D-curve continues to bear the same relationship to the K_c-curve, but where $K_r \neq 0$ the K_c-curve moves down below the K-curve by the amount $K_r = [(\mu_{tr} - \mu_{en})/\mu_{tr}]K$. (We assume here that the radiative-loss photons escape from the medium.)

It is instructive to do a "*Gedankenexperiment*" with respect to Figs. 4.7a and b. Imagine a strong constant magnetic field being applied to the phantom with lines of force parallel to its surface plane. All charged particles would then be forced to remain near the depth plane of their origin, following helical paths with the helix axis lying in the plane of origin of the particle. For a sufficiently strong magnetic field the particles hypothetically could be forced to remain arbitrarily close to their depth of origin.

What happens to the D-curve under these conditions? *It would align itself with the K_c-curve, coinciding with it at all depths, and CPE likewise would exist at all depths.* * Since the magnetic field will not affect the bremsstrahlung losses in Figure 4.7b, the K_c-curve remains below the K-curve by the same amount as before. It seems clear from this that the integral of the D-curve from depth 0 to ∞, with or without the magnetic field and regardless of radiative losses, should equal the corresponding integrated value of K_c (neglecting losses of charged particles scattering out the front surface of the medium when the magnetic field is absent).

In conclusion, with respect to Eq. (4.11), this relationship in principle allows the relating of D and K_c where transient CPE conditions exist for high-energy indirectly ionizing radiations. However, a knowledge of $\bar{x}$ and the effective attenuation coefficient μ' is required for each case, so Eq. (4.11) is not as readily applicable as the simple equality of D and K_c that exists under CPE conditions.

PROBLEMS

1. Approximately what diameter for a sphere of water would be required to approach radiation equilibrium within 1% at its center, assuming it contains a uniform, dilute solution of ^{60}Co (1.25-MeV γ-rays)? Use μ_{en} and μ as ap-

---

*Limited of course to the volume within the radiation beam, and remote from the beam edges by a distance at least equal to the range of the charged particles, which are still allowed to move with a velocity component aligned in either direction along the magnetic lines of force.

proximations to the effective γ-ray attenuation coefficient; this will over- and under-estimate the size, respectively.

2. How large a diameter would be required in problem 1 if one wanted to achieve RE for the neutrinos as well? Assume the neutrinos' interaction cross section to be 10^{-31} cm^2/electron (it is probably smaller). (Note: The number of electrons in a gram of water is $6.02 \times 10^{23} \times 10/18$.)

3. A radioactive source is distributed homogeneously throughout a medium, producing RE at a point of interest. What is the absorbed dose there if 10^{-16} of the total mass present is converted to energy, 60% of which is given to neutrinos?

4. A point P in an x-ray beam receives an exposure of 275 R.

    (a) If there is air at the point, what is the value of $(K_c)_{air}$?

    (b) What is the absorbed dose in air at P?

    (c) What condition must exist at P for (b) to be answerable?

5. Suppose the x-rays in problem 4 have an energy of 200 keV, and that the air at P is replaced by copper. For CPE conditions, what is the absorbed dose in the copper assuming that the exposure remains unchanged?

6. Consider a beam of 3-MeV γ-rays perpendicularly incident on an Fe foil that is very thin in comparison with the range of the secondary electrons.

    (a) What are the values of K, K_c, and K_r in the foil for a fluence of 5.6×10^{15} photons/m^2? (Assume $\mu_{tr}/\rho = 0.00212$ and $\mu_{en}/\rho = 0.00204$ m^2/kg).

    (b) Approximately what is the absorbed dose in the foil, assuming no charged particles are incident from elsewhere?

    (c) What would happen to K, K_c, K_r, and D if a strong magnetic field were applied with the lines of force lying in the foil?

7. A broad beam of low-energy x-rays with $\psi = 3.7 \times 10^{-4}$ J/cm^2 s irradiates a plate of Al perpendicularly, and is completely absorbed.

    (a) What is the energy absorbed per cm^2 in 5 min?

    (b) If the slab is 2 cm thick and has a density of 2.7 g/cm^3, what is the average value of $(K_c)_{Al}$ throughout the medium?

    (c) Assuming no electrons enter or leave the plate, what is the average absorbed dose?

    (d) What would be the average dose if the slab were 4 cm thick?

SOLUTIONS TO PROBLEMS

1. 312 cm, 144 cm.

2. 2760 km.

3. 3.60 Gy.

4. (a) 2.41 Gy.
    (b) 2.41 Gy.
    (c) CPE.
5. 5.37 Gy.
6. (a) $K = 5.70$ Gy; $K_c = 5.49$ Gy; $K_r = 0.22$ Gy.
    (b) D indeterminate, but $\to 0$ as foil thickness $\to 0$, because all electrons leaving and none entering; $\therefore$ CPE fails.
    (c) K, K_c, and K_r unchanged. $D \to K_c$ as magnetic field strength increases, trapping the electrons in the foil, thus approaching CPE.
7. (a) 0.111 J/cm^2.
    (b) 20.6 Gy.
    (c) 20.6 Gy.
    (d) 10.3 Gy.

CHAPTER **5**

Absorbed Dose in Radioactive Media

I. INTRODUCTION

In this chapter we will consider radioactive processes and the deposition of absorbed dose in radioactive media. It was said in Chapter 4 that the computation of the absorbed dose is straightforward for either CPE or RE conditions, but is more difficult for intermediate situations. If the radiation emitted consists of charged particles plus much longer-range γ-rays, as is often the case, one can determine if CPE or RE is present, depending on the size of the radioactive object. Assuming the satisfaction of conditions a through d in Chapter 4, Section II.A, and referring to Fig. 4.1, we may consider these two limiting cases:

    1. In a *small* radioactive object V (i.e., having a mean radius not much greater than the maximum charged-particle range d), CPE is well approximated at any internal point P that is at least a distance d from the boundary of V. Then, if $d \ll 1/\mu$ for the γ-rays, the absorbed dose D at P approximately equals the energy per unit mass of medium that is given to the charged particles in radioactive decay (less their radiative losses),* since the photons practically all escape from the object and are assumed not to be scattered back by its surroundings.

    2. In a *large* radioactive object (i.e., with mean radius $\gg 1/\mu$ for the most penetrating γ-rays), RE is well approximated at any internal point P that is far enough from the boundary of V so γ-ray penetration through that distance is negligible.

---

*In low-Z media radiative losses are $\approx 1\%$ or less for β-rays, and nil for α's, so they are ordinarily ignored.

80

The dose at P will then equal the sum of the energy per unit mass of medium that is given to charged particles plus γ-rays in radioactive decay.

Deciding upon a maximum γ-ray "range" for case 2 requires some kind of quantitative criterion. Less than 1% of primary γ-rays penetrate through a layer 5 mean free paths in thickness, and less than 0.1% through 7 mean free paths. (The mean free path is defined as the reciprocal of the attenuation coefficient μ, see Chapter 3). However, one must take at least crude account of the propagation of the scattered photons, since we are dealing with a type of broad-beam geometry.

Referring to the example in Fig. 3.7 (1-MeV γ-rays, broad plane beam in water), we see that at a depth of 7 mean free paths the true attenuation is closer to 10^{-2} than 10^{-3}. Roughly 10 mean free paths are evidently necessary to reduce beam penetration to $<0.1\%$ in this case. Assuming the "straight-ahead" approximation (i.e., substituting μ_{en} for $\overline{\mu}'$ as an effective attenuation coefficient; see Chapter 3) would evidently require about 16 mean free paths ($L \cong 16/\mu \cong 7/\mu_{en}$) to reach 0.1% penetration in Fig. 3.7. One concludes that if the relevant data for buildup factors or effective attenuation coefficients $\overline{\mu}'$ are not available for a particular situation, the use of the straight-ahead approximation ($\overline{\mu}' = \mu_{en}$) will overestimate the size of a radioactive object necessary to approximate RE at its center within desired limits. Assuming $\overline{\mu}' = \mu$ will underestimate that size by ignoring scattered rays.

To estimate the γ-ray dose at an internal point in an intermediate-sized radioactive object, it will be helpful to define a quantity called the *absorbed fraction* (Ellett et al., 1964, 1965):

$$AF = \frac{\gamma\text{-ray radiant energy absorbed in target volume}}{\gamma\text{-ray radiant energy emitted by source}} \qquad (5.1)$$

(Ellett et al. use the symbol φ, but we use AF to avoid confusion with the symbol for flux density).

Figure 5.1 illustrates the situation to be considered. The volume V, representing

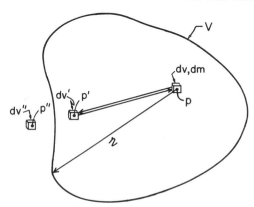

FIGURE 5.1. Illustration of the reciprocity theorem as applied to estimate the γ-ray dose at point P within a homogeneous, uniformly radioactive object V. (See text.)

the radioactive object, is filled by a homogeneous medium and a uniformly distributed γ-ray source. It may be surrounded either by (1) an infinite homogeneous medium identical to that in V, but *non*radioactive, or (2) an infinite vacuum. In the first case a γ-ray escaping from V may be scattered back in; in the second case it will be irrevocably lost. The first case simulates more closely an organ in the body; the second an object surrounded by air.

First let us consider case (1). The energy spent* in the volume element dv, at an internal point of interest P, by γ-rays from the source in dv' at any other internal point P', is equal to the energy spent in dv' by the source in dv. (Outside volume elements such as dv'' have no source, hence do not expend energy in dv.) The reciprocity theorem is exact in this case, because of the infinite homogeneous medium. Since this equality holds for all points P' throughout V, we may conclude that the energy spent in dv by the source throughout V is equal to the energy spent throughout V by the source in dv. If $\overline{R}_{dv}$ is the expectation value of the γ-ray radiant energy emitted by the source in dv and $\overline{\epsilon}_{dv,V}$ the part of that energy that is spent in V, then the absorbed fraction with respect to source dv and target V is

$$\mathrm{AF}_{dv,V} = \frac{\overline{\epsilon}_{dv,V}}{\overline{R}_{dv}} \tag{5.2}$$

For very small radioactive objects ($V \rightarrow dv$) this absorbed fraction approaches zero; for an infinite radioactive medium it equals unity.

It has already been shown that $\overline{\epsilon}_{dv,V} = \overline{\epsilon}_{V,dv}$, where $\overline{\epsilon}_{V,dv}$ is the energy spent in dv by gamma rays from the source throughout V. Thus we can make a substitution in Eq. (5.2), obtaining

$$\mathrm{AF}_{dv,V} = \frac{\overline{\epsilon}_{V,dv}}{\overline{R}_{dv}} \tag{5.3}$$

Evidently then, if one can calculate the absorbed fraction in Eq. (5.2), its value is equal to the ratio of photon energy spent in dv by the source throughout V to the energy emitted by the source in dv. This equals the ratio of the photon absorbed dose at P to that under RE conditions. Thus if, say, 10% of the γ-ray energy from the source in dv escapes from V, this results in a 10% reduction in γ-ray dose at P below its RE value, and $\mathrm{AF}_{dv,V} = 0.90$.

Assuming $\overline{\mu}'$ to be the mean effective attenuation coefficient for γ-ray energy fluence transmission through a distance r of the medium in Fig. 5.1, the fraction escaping from V in the direction of r from point P is $e^{-\overline{\mu}'r}$. In terms of the polar coordinates in Fig. 1.2, with point P at the origin, the value of the absorbed fraction in Eq. (5.2) is given by

$$\mathrm{AF}_{dv,V} = \frac{1}{4\pi} \int_{\theta=0}^{\pi} \int_{\beta=0}^{2\pi} (1 - e^{-\overline{\mu}'r}) \sin\theta \, d\theta \, d\beta \tag{5.4}$$

*For brevity we substitute "energy spent" for "expectation value of the energy imparted".

Carrying out this integration is complicated by the fact that $\bar{\mu}'$ [or the buildup factor B; see Eq. (3.15)] is a function of r as well as $h\nu$; moreover some radionuclides emit γ-rays of many different energies. An average value of $\overline{AF}_{dv, V}$ for n different γ-ray energy lines can be gotten by

$$\overline{AF}_{dv, V} = \frac{\displaystyle\sum_{i=1}^{n} (AF_{dv}, V)_i (\overline{R}_{dv})_i}{\displaystyle\sum_{i=1}^{n} (\overline{R}_{dv})_i} = \frac{\displaystyle\sum_{i=1}^{n} (AF_{dv}, V)_i (\overline{R}_{dv})_i}{\overline{R}_{dv}} \tag{5.4a}$$

Calculations by Monte Carlo or moments methods have been reported by Ellett (1968), Berger (1968), Brownell et al. (1968), Ellett and Humes (1971), and Snyder et al. (1975). All but the first of these references were published as reports of the MIRD (Medical Internal Radiation Dose) Committee of the Society of Nuclear Medicine.

A simple example of these results is shown in Fig. 5.2 (Brownell et al., 1968), which gives the radius of a unit-density tissue sphere required to produce absorbed fractions of 0.5 and 0.9, as a function of the photon quantum energy of a point source at the center. This example applies to case (1), in which the sphere is part of an infinite homogeneous medium. The equality of Eq. (5.3) to Eq. (5.2) means that Fig. 5.2 also gives the γ-dose at the center of the sphere if it were uniformly radioactive, as a fraction of the RE γ-dose there.

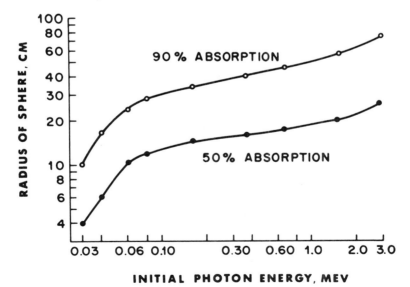

INITIAL PHOTON ENERGY, MEV

FIGURE 5.2. Radius of unit-density tissue sphere needed to absorb 50% and 90% of the emitted photon energy from a central point source in an infinite homogeneous medium. (After Brownell et al., 1968.) Reproduced with permission of the authors and The Society of Nuclear Medicine.

The dose decreases gradually as the point of interest is moved from the center of a γ-active object toward its boundaries. In a radioactive volume V large enough to have RE at its center, imbedded in an infinite homogeneous medium, the γ-ray dose is reduced by approximately half in moving to the boundary of V. At the interface between a semi-infinite homogeneous radioactive medium and another semi-infinite volume of the same medium without radioactivity, the dose would of course be exactly $\frac{1}{2}$ of its RE value.

For purposes of internal dosimetry, one may be interested in the *average* γ-ray dose within a radioactive organ, rather than the dose at some specific point. For this purpose one wants the value of $AF_{V,V}$, which is just the average of $AF_{dv,V}$ for all points P throughout the source volume V. The MIRD literature already cited is mostly focused on such average-dose calculations, and Snyder et al. (1975) also give average doses deposited in one organ by γ-rays emitted from another radioactive organ.

Case (2) mentioned in connection with Fig. 5.1, for which the volume V is surrounded by a void, is more difficult to calculate. The reciprocity theorem is only approximate in that case because of the lack of backscattering. Ellett (1968) has calculated the average absorbed dose in a uniformly radioactive tissue sphere of 780 g (5.7-cm radius) and 2.3 kg (8.2-cm radius), with and without a surrounding tissue scattering medium. The results are given in Fig. 5.3. A maximum 30% dose increase is seen at 80 keV. This decreases at lower energies because of the increasing influence of photoelectric absorption, and at higher energies because scattered rays are more forward directed. These effects will be described in Chapter 7.

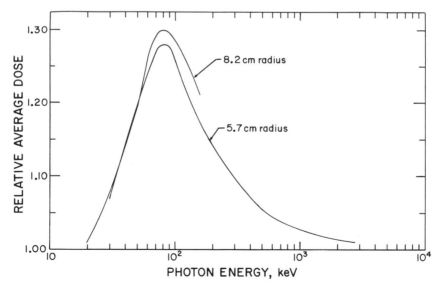

FIGURE 5.3. Ratio of average absorbed doses in uniformly radioactive tissue spheres with/without surrounding non-radioactive tissue medium. Lower curve: 780-g (5.7-cm-radius) sphere; upper curve: 2.3-kg (8.2-cm-radius) sphere. (Data from Ellett, 1968.)

To obtain a crude estimate of the dose at some point P within a uniformly γ-active homogeneous object, it may suffice to obtain the average distance $\bar{r}$ from the point to the surface of the object, either by inspection or using

$$\bar{r} = \frac{1}{4\pi} \int_{\theta=0}^{\pi} \int_{\beta=0}^{2\pi} r \sin\theta \; d\theta \; d\beta \tag{5.5}$$

Then one may employ $\mu_{en} \cong \bar{\mu}'$ in the straight-ahead approximation to obtain

$$\mathrm{AF}_{dv, V} \cong 1 - e^{-\mu_{en}\bar{r}} \tag{5.6}$$

which roughly approximates the ratio of γ-ray dose at P to that present if RE conditions existed.

Example 5.1. An object contains a uniformly distributed β- and γ-ray source. The rest-mass loss is spent half in 1-MeV γ-ray production and half in β^--decay, for which $E_{max} = 5$ MeV and $E_{avg} = 2$ MeV. The point of interest P is located > 5 cm inside the boundary of the object, and at an average distance $\bar{r} = 20$ cm from the boundary. $\mu_{en} = 0.0306$ cm^{-1} and $\mu = 0.0699$ cm^{-1} for the γ-rays. For a total energy of 10^{-2} J converted from rest mass in each kilogram of the object, estimate the absorbed dose at P.

Solution: $1/\mu$ is much larger than the maximum β-ray range (see Appendix E), which in turn is less than the distance of P from the boundary of the object. Thus CPE may be assumed to exist at P for the β-rays, and they contribute $\frac{2}{5} \times 5 \times 10^{-3}$ J/kg $= 2 \times 10^{-3}$ J/kg to the dose there. (This will be explained in Section II.B.)

For the γ-rays, $e^{-\mu_{en}\bar{r}} = 0.54$; hence $\mathrm{AF}_{dv, V} \cong 1 - e^{-\mu_{en}\bar{r}} = 0.46$ is the approximate fraction of the γ-ray energy that contributes to the dose at P. Now $0.46 \times 5 \times 10^{-3}$ J/kg $= 2.3 \times 10^{-3}$ J/kg, so the total dose $\cong 4.3 \times 10^{-3}$ J/kg $= 4.3 \times 10^{-3}$ Gy. For a very large object the RE dose at P (including β-rays) would be 7.0×10^{-3} J/kg, the other 3.0×10^{-3} J/kg being carried away by the neutrinos.

If we had assumed the object to be a 40-cm-diameter sphere of unit density tissue with P at its center, we could compare our result with the Monte Carlo calculation of Brownell et al. shown in Fig. 5.2. It can be seen there that about 50% absorption of 1-MeV γ-rays occurs; therefore the γ-ray dose at the center is roughly half of its RE value of 5×10^{-3} J/kg, or 2.5×10^{-3} J/kg. This is fortuitously close to our estimate of 2.3×10^{-3} J/kg. Furthermore, the central point is far enough from the boundary so that the effect of backscattering is negligible, whether the object is surrounded by inert tissue, or a void. According to Ellett (1968) the influence of γ-ray backscatter affects the dose very little at points more than one mean free path from a boundary, and in this case $1/\mu \cong 14$ cm.

The present chapter ignores temporal variations in source strength. Chapter 6 will consider radioactive decay. Biological uptake, transfer, and elimination of radioactive sources are beyond the scope of this book and are left to other references.

II. RADIOACTIVE DISINTEGRATION PROCESSES

Radioactive nuclei, either natural or artificially produced by nuclear reactions, are unstable and tend to seek more stable configurations through expulsion of energetic particles, including one or more of the following,* where corresponding changes in the atomic number (Z) and number of nucleons (A) are indicated:

	ΔZ	ΔA
α-particle	-2	-4
β^--particle†	$+1$	0
β^+-particle†	-1	0
γ-ray	0	0

The total energy (mass, quantum, and kinetic) of the photons and other particles released by the disintegration process is equal to the net decrease in the rest mass of the *neutral atom*, from parent to daughter. Energy, momentum, and electric charge are each conserved in the process.

In this connection it should be noted that, according to Einstein's mass-energy equation $E = mc^2$, the energy equivalent of rest mass is as follows:

$$1 \text{ atomic mass unit (amu)} = \tfrac{1}{12} \text{ of the mass of the } {}^{12}_{6}\text{C nucleus}$$

$$= 931.50 \text{ MeV}$$

$$1 \text{ electron mass } (+ \text{ or } -) = 0.51100 \text{ MeV}$$

A. Alpha Disintegration

Alpha disintegration occurs mainly in heavy nuclei. An important example is the decay of radium to radon, represented by the following mass-energy balance equation:

$$\underset{\tau_{1/2} = 1602\,y}{{}^{226}_{88}\text{Ra} \xrightarrow{\hspace{2cm}}} {}^{222}_{86}\text{Rn} + {}^{4}_{2}\text{He} + 4.78 \text{ MeV} \qquad (5.7)$$

where $\tau_{1/2}$ symbolizes the *half-life*, or the time needed for $\tfrac{1}{2}$ of the original number of "parent" atoms of ${}^{226}_{88}$Ra to decay to the "daughter product", ${}^{222}_{86}$Rn. *Each of the elemental terms in Eq. (5.7) (and in other mass-energy balance equations to follow) represents the rest mass of a neutral atom of that element.* Notice that when the α-particle (He nucleus) is emitted by the ${}^{226}_{88}$Ra atom, its atomic number decreases by 2 and it consequently sheds two atomic electrons from its outermost shell, to become a neutral atom of ${}^{222}_{86}$Rn. After the α-particle slows down it captures two electrons from its surround-

---

*Other more complex decay modes, including spontaneous fission, are also possible; see the introduction to Lederer and Shirley, (1979).
†Accompanied by neutrino emission.

ings, thereby becoming a neutral $_2^4$He atom. The 4.78 MeV shown in the above equation is the energy equivalent of the rest mass decrease in transforming a neutral $_{88}^{226}$Ra atom into neutral atoms of $_{86}^{222}$Rn + $_2^4$He. It nearly all appears as particle kinetic energy, except for a small part that is given to 0.18-MeV photons, as discussed below.

The corresponding mass-energy-level diagram for this disintegration is shown in Fig. 5.4, where the vertical scale is given in terms of relative values of neutral atomic masses or their energy equivalents, as it will in later diagrams for other types of disintegrations. Two branches are available for the disintegration of $_{88}^{226}$Ra. 94.6% of these nuclei decay directly to $_{86}^{222}$Rn, making available 4.78 MeV, which is shared as kinetic energy between the α-particle (4.70 MeV) and the recoiling $_{86}^{222}$Rn atom (85 keV), the shares being proportional to the reciprocal of their masses to conserve momentum.

The alternative branch for the decay of $_{86}^{226}$Ra occurs in only 5.4% of the nuclei, which release 4.60 MeV of kinetic energy and give rise to a nuclear excited state of $_{86}^{222}$Rn. This promptly relaxes to the ground state through the emission of a 0.18-MeV γ-ray. The same total kinetic + quantum energy is released by either route, and the net reduction in atomic rest mass is identical for each.

In Fig. 5.4 the rest masses of the $_{86}^{222}$Rn and $_2^4$He atoms have been combined into the lower mass-energy levels to allow the diagram to emphasize the details of the kinetic and quantum energies released. The kinetic + quantum energy (4.78 MeV) comprises only about $[4.78/(4 \times 931)]100 \cong 0.1\%$ of the energy equivalent to the total rest-mass decrease of the neutral atoms of $_{88}^{226}$Ra $\rightarrow$ $_{86}^{222}$Rn, since the rest mass of the α-particle is so large.

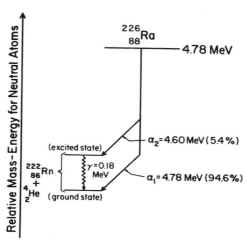

FIGURE 5.4. Atomic energy level diagram for $_{88}^{226}$Ra $\rightarrow$ $_{86}^{222}$Rn, showing branching in the modes of disintegration. Note that the rest-mass energy of the $_{86}^{222}$Rn atom has been augmented by that of the $_2^4$He atom so that the vertical scale need not be expanded to include the loss of energy equivalent to the α-particle mass ($\cong 4 \times 938$ MeV).

1. Absorbed Dose from α-Disintegration

In computing the absorbed dose in a medium from radioactive disintegration processes the calculation is always made under the assumption of the nonstochastic limit, and therefore the *average* branching ratios are used. Again considering our example of radium decaying to radon, the average kinetic energy given to charged particles per disintegration is equal to

$$E_\alpha = 0.946 \ (4.78 \ \text{MeV}) + 0.054 \ (4.60 \ \text{MeV})$$

$$= 4.77 \ \text{MeV} \tag{5.8}$$

Under CPE conditions in a small (1-cm-radius) radium-activated object, if n such disintegrations occurred in each gram of the matter, the resulting absorbed dose would be given by $4.77n$ MeV/g, convertible into more conventional dose units through Eqs. (1.10) and (2.3).

Under RE conditions, on the other hand, the dose for the same concentration of radium would be simply $4.78n$ MeV/g, since the small additional γ-ray energy would then be included.

The foregoing considerations deal exclusively with the energy released by the decay of radium to radon. Any further dose that may be deposited by the radon or its daughter products would have to be calculated separately.

B. Beta Disintegration

Nuclei having an excess of neutrons tend to emit an electron (β^--particle), thus leaving the nucleus with one less neutron and one more proton, i.e., the atomic number Z is increased by 1. Conversely, nuclei with excess of protons usually emit a positron (β^+), effectively decreasing Z by 1 while increasing the neutron count by 1. In either case the total number of nucleons (protons + neutrons) remains constant, so that the daughter product is an *isobar* of its parent.* β-ray emission leaves many kinds of nuclei in an excited state, and one or more γ-rays are then emitted to reach the ground state.

The β-rays emitted in a given mode of disintegration (averaged over many such disintegrations) have a spectrum of kinetic energies extending from zero to a fixed maximum $E_{\max}$, with a skewed bell-shaped differential distribution exemplified by the spectrum of β^--rays from $^{32}_{15}\text{P}$ shown in Fig. 5.5. The maximum β^- kinetic energy ($E_{\max} = 1.71$ MeV in this case) represents the net decrease in the rest mass of the neutral $^{32}_{15}\text{P}$ atom in becoming a neutral $^{32}_{16}\text{S}$ atom, since the ground state of the $^{32}_{16}\text{S}$ is reached directly without γ-ray emission. The atomic mass-energy balance equation is

$$^{32}_{15}\text{P} + e^- \xrightarrow[\tau_{1/2} = 14.3 \text{d}]{} {}^{32}_{16}\text{S} + \beta^- + {}^0_0\nu + 1.71 \ \text{MeV (k.e.)} \tag{5.9}$$

*Nuclei with odd Z and an even number of nucleons, and having stable neighboring isobars at both Z + 1 and Z − 1, can decay either by β^-, β^+, or electron-capture processes, as for example in the case of $^{84}_{37}\text{Rb}$, (see Evans, 1955).

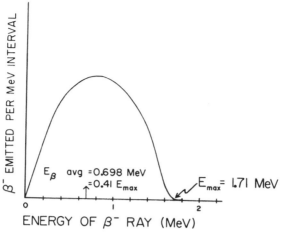

FIGURE 5.5. β^--ray spectrum emitted from $^{32}_{15}$P. The average energy of the particles is 0.694 MeV. The abscissa may be alternatively labeled "1.71 − neutrino energy (MeV)" to make the curve indicate the neutrino spectrum.

where the atomic mass decrease $^{32}_{15}$P − $^{32}_{16}$S = 1.71 MeV, which appears as kinetic energy shared between the β^- and the neutrino.

The electron on the left of the equation is required to balance the charge and rest mass of the β^- on the right. Physically, when the $^{32}_{15}$P nucleus emits the β^-, a positively charged ion ($^{32}_{16}$S$^+$) results, which promptly captures a bystanding electron to become a neutral $^{32}_{16}$S atom.

The symbol $^0_0\nu$ in Eq. (5.9) represents a neutrino, which is a nearly zero-mass,[*] zero-charge particle that is emitted along with each β-particle, thus conserving energy and momentum in the disintegration process. The difference between the β^--ray kinetic energy and E_{max} = 1.71 MeV in each disintegration is carried away by the associated neutrino, and the differential distribution of the neutrino kinetic energy is therefore complementary to that of the β^--particles, as also shown in Fig. 5.5. Figure 5.6 shows the corresponding atomic energy-level diagram.

The average kinetic energy of the β^-- or β^+-particles in a β-ray spectrum is found to be roughly 0.3–0.4 times E_{max}, depending on the individual spectral shape, which is determined by the "forbiddenness" classification of the β-ray transition. This matter is discussed by Evans (1955), and an excellent summary of the relation between the average and maximum β-ray energy has been written by Dillman and Von der Lage (1975). Often, for purposes of roughly estimating the absorbed dose deposited by charged particles, $E_{avg} \cong \frac{1}{3} E_{max}$ is assumed for β-rays, if more accurate information is not available.

Since the neutrino is radiologically irrelevant, the energy spent in the material

---

[*]The actual neutrino mass is probably $\simeq 1/17,000$ of that of an electron (Lubkin, 1981).

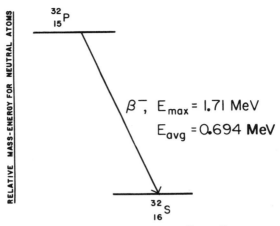

FIGURE 5.6.   Atomic energy-level diagram for $^{32}_{15}P \rightarrow ^{32}_{16}S$ β^--disintegration.

in which the β-ray emitter is located is just the product of the number of β-rays by their *average* energy, not their maximum energy. It is important not to confuse E_{avg} with E_{max}. Extensive tables of such data for 122 radionuclides have been provided by Dillman and Von der Lage (1975); some E_{avg} data are given in Appendix C.

An excellent general reference on decay schemes, maximum β-ray energies, and other relevant isotopic data has been prepared by Lederer and Shirley (1979).

A simple example of β^+-disintegration is that of $^{15}_8O \rightarrow ^{15}_7N$, for which the atomic mass-energy balance equation is

$$^{15}_8O \xrightarrow[\tau_{1/2} = 122 \text{ s}]{} {}^{15}_7N + \overbrace{e^- + \beta^+}^{2m_0 = 1.022 \text{ MeV}} + {}^0_0\nu + 1.73 \text{ MeV (k.e.)} \quad (5.10)$$

where the atomic-mass decrease from $^{15}_8O$ to $^{15}_7N = 1.022$ MeV $+ 1.73$ MeV $= 2.75$ MeV, as illustrated in Fig. 5.7, and the 1.73 MeV kinetic energy is shared between the β^+ and the neutrino.

During β^+-emission a valence electron is simultaneously released by the $^{15}_8O$ atom. Thus both the β^+ and the electron are lost by the parent atom and appear as free particles on the right of Eq. (5.10). The decrease in atomic mass is equal to the sum of the released kinetic energy (1.73 MeV) and the rest masses (0.511 MeV each) of the e^- and the β^+. When the β^+ stops, it combines in an annihilation interaction with a nearby electron, emitting 1.022 MeV in the form of two 0.511-MeV oppositely directed γ-rays. Sometimes the positron is annihilated "in flight" before it stops, in which case the photons also carry away the remaining kinetic energy.

1.   Absorbed Dose from Beta Disintegration

For present purposes we will ignore any radiative losses (bremsstrahlung and in-flight positron annihilation) by the β-rays, and simply assume that their kinetic energy

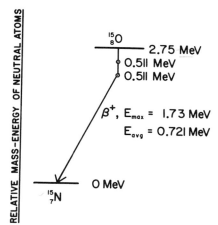

RELATIVE MASS-ENERGY OF NEUTRAL ATOMS

$^{15}_{8}O$

2.75 MeV
0.511 MeV
0.511 MeV

β^+, E_{max} = 1.73 MeV

E_{avg} = 0.721 MeV

0 MeV

$^{15}_{7}N$

FIGURE 5.7. Atomic energy-level diagram for β^+-emission by $^{15}_{8}O$. The vertical line segments below the $^{15}_{8}O$ energy level indicate the loss of the rest-mass energy of the β^+ and the corresponding valence electron released by the atom during disintegration.

is all spent in collision interactions resulting in absorbed-dose deposition. Such radiative-loss corrections are relatively unimportant in low-Z media (e.g., water and tissue).

Under CPE conditions the absorbed dose due to n β-disintegrations per gram of medium is nE_{avg} (MeV/g). Additional absorbed-dose contributions due to any γ-rays resulting from a particular radionuclide must be treated as described in Section I.

Example 5.2. What is the absorbed dose rate (Gy/h) at the center of a sphere of water 1 cm in radius, homogeneously radioactivated by $^{32}_{15}P$, with 6 × 10⁵ disintegrations per second occurring per gram of water? (Assume time constancy.)

Solution: The maximum energy of β^+-rays from $^{32}_{15}P$ is 1.71 MeV, and the corresponding maximum range of these electrons is ≈ 8 mm of water (see Appendix E). Thus CPE will be produced at the center of the 1-cm-radius sphere. The absorbed dose rate there will be

$$\dot{D} = 3600 \frac{s}{hr} \times 6 \times 10^5 \frac{dis}{g\ sec} \times 0.694 \frac{MeV}{dis}$$

$$\times 1.602 \times 10^{-10} \frac{Gy}{MeV/g}$$

$$= 0.24\ Gy/h$$

Example 5.3. A sphere of water with a radius of 5 cm contains a uniform distribution of $^{15}_{8}O$, with a level of activity of 10^6 dis/g s.
(a) What is the approximate absorbed dose rate (Gy/s) at the center of the sphere, estimated by the mean-radius $(\bar{r})$ method [see Eqs. (5.5) and (5.6)]?

(b) What would the answer to (a) become if the radioactive water sphere were increased to a radius of 150 cm?

Solution: (a) CPE exists at the center, since the maximum β^+-range is only about 8 mm of water. The absorbed dose rate contributed by the β^+-rays is

$$\dot{D}_{\beta^+} = 10^6 \frac{\text{dis}}{\text{g s}} \times 0.721 \frac{\text{MeV}}{\text{dis}} \times 1.602 \times 10^{-10} \frac{\text{Gy}}{\text{MeV/g}}$$

$$= 1.155 \times 10^{-4} \text{ Gy/s}$$

For each disintegration producing one β^+-particle, two 0.511-MeV γ-rays are produced when the particle stops. For these γ-rays $\mu_{en} = 0.0330 \text{ cm}^{-1}$ (Appendix D.3) for unit-density water. The absorbed fraction of the energy per unit mass emitted as γ-rays that contributes to the dose is $\text{AF} \cong (1 - e^{-\mu_{en}\bar{r}}) = (1 - e^{-0.0330 \times 5}) = 0.15$. Thus the dose rate contributed by γ-rays is

$$\dot{D}_\gamma = 10^6 \frac{\text{dis}}{\text{g s}} \times 1.022 \frac{\gamma\text{-ray MeV produced}}{\text{dis}}$$

$$\times 0.15 \frac{\gamma\text{-energy absorbed}}{\gamma\text{-energy produced}}$$

$$\times 1.602 \times 10^{-10} \frac{\text{Gy}}{\text{MeV/g}}$$

$$= 2.46 \times 10^{-5} \text{ Gy/s}$$

Therefore the total absorbed dose rate at the center, including the β^+-contribution, is

$$\dot{D}_{tot} = 1.155 \times 10^{-4} + 2.46 \times 10^{-5} = 1.40 \times 10^{-4} \text{ Gy/s}$$

(b) Increasing $\bar{r}$ to 150 cm increases the absorbed fraction to 0.993; hence the γ-ray dose rate contribution at the center becomes

$$\dot{D}_\gamma = 2.46 \times 10^{-5} \times \frac{1 - e^{-0.0330 \times 150}}{0.15}$$

$$= 1.625 \times 10^{-4} \text{ Gy/s}$$

So the total dose rate is

$$\dot{D}_{tot} = 1.155 \times 10^{-4} + 1.625 \times 10^{-4} = 2.78 \times 10^{-4} \text{ Gy/s}$$

Note that since the sphere radius in (b) is so large ($\simeq 14/\mu$), RE should be closely approximated at the center. This means that the atomic rest-mass decrease should nearly all appear as dose except for what escapes with neutrinos. From Fig. 5.7 it can be seen that the total energy derived from rest mass per disintegration of $^{15}_{8}\text{O}$

→ $^{15}_{7}$N is 2.75 MeV, while the amount carried away by neutrinos is 1.73 − 0.721 = 1.01 MeV. Thus the energy going into dose under RE conditions is simply 2.75 MeV − 1.01 MeV = 1.74 MeV per disintegration (which approximates E_{max} only by coincidence in this case).

Therefore the dose rate assuming RE is

$$\dot{D}_{tot} = 10^6 \frac{dis}{g\ s} \times 1.74 \frac{MeV}{dis} \times 1.602 \times 10^{-10} \frac{Gy}{MeV/g}$$

$$= 2.79 \times 10^{-4}\ Gy/s$$

This figure is nearly the same as that obtained above, as it should be.

C. Electron-Capture (EC) Transitions

Radioactive disintegrations through electron capture (EC) are competitive with those by β^+-disintegration. In the EC process the parent nucleus, instead of emitting a β^+-particle, captures one of its own atomic electrons and emits a monoenergetic neutrino. The electrons most likely to be captured in the EC process are K-shell electrons ($\cong 90\%$), with L-shell electrons supplying practically all of the remainder ($\cong 10\%$; see Evans, 1955). Resulting shell vacancies are promptly filled by an electron from a higher orbit, with the release of a fluorescence x-ray (see Fig. 7.15). The probability that a fluorescence photon will escape from its native atom is called the *fluorescence yield*, Y_K or Y_L (see Fig. 7.14).

The parallel atomic mass-energy equations for the case of $^{22}_{11}$Na → $^{22}_{10}$Ne are given below in Eq. (5.11) for β^+-decay and Eq. (5.12) for the EC process. The half-life for decay by both branches together is 2.60 y. The corresponding atomic energy-level diagram is shown in Fig. 5.8.

1. β^+-*Branch:*

$$2m_0 = 1.022\ MeV$$

$$^{22}_{11}\text{Na} \rightarrow\ ^{22}_{10}\text{Ne} + \overbrace{e^- + \beta^+} +\ ^{0}_{0}\nu + 0.546\ MeV\ (k.e.)$$
$$+ 1.275\ MeV\ (E_\gamma) \tag{5.11}$$

where the atomic mass decrease is equal to

$$^{22}_{11}\text{Na} -\ ^{22}_{10}\text{Ne} = 1.022\ MeV + 0.546\ MeV + 1.275\ MeV$$

$$= 2.843\ MeV$$

2. *EC Branch:*

$$^{22}_{11}\text{Na} \rightarrow\ ^{22}_{10}\text{Ne} +\ ^{0}_{0}\nu + \underbrace{E_b + 1.275\ MeV\ (E_\gamma)}_{1.568\ MeV} \tag{5.12}$$

where the atomic mass decrease is equal to

$$^{22}_{11}\text{Na} -\ ^{22}_{10}\text{Ne} = 1.568\ MeV + 1.275\ MeV = 2.843\ MeV$$

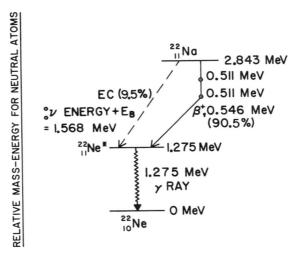

FIGURE 5.8. Atomic energy-level diagram for β^+ and EC disintegration of $^{22}_{11}\text{Na} \xrightarrow{\tau_{1/2} = 2.60 \text{ y}} {}^{22}_{10}\text{Ne}$. $(E_\beta)_{\text{max}} = 0.546$ MeV; $\overline{E}_\beta = 0.216$ MeV.

It will be seen from Fig. 5.8 that for β^+-disintegration to take place in any radionuclide requires a minimum mass difference between the parent neutral atom and its daughter atom of $2m_0$ ($= 1.022$ MeV). Otherwise only EC can occur, since no kinetic energy would be available for a β^+-particle, and in that case the dose deposited in EC events becomes relatively important.

In Eq. (5.12) the E_b-term indicates the electron binding energy in the K- or L-shell. The kinetic energy of the emitted neutrino equals the difference in atomic rest mass between $^{22}_{11}\text{Na}$ and the excited state of $^{22}_{10}\text{Ne}$ ($=1.568$ MeV), less the electron binding energy E_b ($\cong 1$ keV for the K shell).

1. Absorbed Dose for the EC Process

When a β^+ is emitted, it contributes its average kinetic energy to the production of absorbed dose, and then its annihilation γ-rays may contribute more dose, depending upon the size and shape of the radioactive mass of material. If an EC event occurs instead of β^+-emission, neither of these dose components is present, and virtually all of the energy they represent is carried away by the neutrino. The only remaining energy available for absorbed dose in an EC event (if there is no subsequent γ-ray emission from an excited state) is contained in the electron-binding term E_b, which is very small compared to the energy that is removed by the neutrino. An example based on $^{22}_{11}\text{Na}$ will illustrate this.

Example 5.4. A water sphere of 2-cm radius contains a uniformly distributed source of $^{22}_{11}\text{Na}$ which undergoes 10^5 disintegrations per g-s. Estimate the absorbed dose deposited at the center in one week, using the mean-radius method [Eqs. (5.5) and (5.6)].

Solution: CPE exists for the β^+ particles. Thus the dose they deposit is

$$D_{\beta^+} = 10^5 \frac{dis}{g\ s} \times 0.905 \frac{\beta^+}{dis} \times 0.216 \frac{MeV}{\beta^+}$$

$$\times 1.602 \times 10^{-10} \frac{Gy}{MeV/g} \times 6.048 \times 10^5\ s$$

$$= 1.89\ Gy$$

The very small additional dose due to the E_b-term for EC events may be calculated as follows, although here, as in most cases, it will be found to be negligible unless the competing β^+-transitions are forbidden by energy considerations.

All of the binding energy of the electrons captured in the parent nuclei of ^{22}Na is given either to Auger electrons or to fluorescence photons. Figure 7.15 shows that K-fluorescence photons from Ne (the daughter atom) have a very low energy (actually 0.85 keV). Moreover the fluorescence yield $Y_K = Y_L \cong 0$ for Ne (see Fig. 7.14), which means that the E_b of the parent-atom electrons is entirely absorbed in the immediate vicinity of the atom in question. E_b for the K-shell of sodium is $(E_b)_K = 1.07$ keV, while $(E_b)_{L1} = 0.06$ keV (from Appendix B).

The dose contributed through EC events is

$$D_{EC} = 10^5 \frac{dis}{g\ s} \times 0.095 \frac{EC\ events}{dis} \times 1.602 \times 10^{-10} \frac{Gy}{MeV/g}$$

$$\times 6.048 \times 10^5\ s \times f_{EC} \frac{MeV}{EC\ event}$$

The last term, containing the energy spent on the dose per EC event, can be approximated by

$$f_{EC} \cong 0.9(E_b)_K + 0.1(E_b)_L = 9.7 \times 10^{-4} \frac{MeV}{EC\ event} \qquad (5.13)$$

Thus $D_{EC} \cong 8.9 \times 10^{-4}$ Gy, which is of course negligible.

Next we must calculate the γ-ray contribution to the dose at the center of the sphere, for which $\bar{r} = 2$ cm. For each disintegration, 0.905 β^+-particles are emitted on the average; consequently $2 \times 0.905 = 1.81$ photons of 0.511 MeV each are emitted, for which $\mu_{en} = 0.0330$ cm^{-1}. The resulting dose is estimated by the straight-ahead approximation to be

$$D_{0.511} = 10^5 \frac{dis}{g\ s} \times 1.81 \frac{photons}{dis} \times 0.511 \frac{MeV}{photon}$$

$$\times 1.602 \times 10^{-10} \frac{Gy}{MeV/g} \times 6.048 \times 10^5\ s \times AF$$

$$= 0.572\ Gy$$

where $AF \cong 1 - e^{-0.0330 \times 2}$. For the final relaxation γ-ray from $^{22}_{10}Ne^* \rightarrow ^{22}_{10}Ne$, which occurs for every disintegration, the energy-absorption coefficient μ_{en} is 0.0289 cm^{-1} in water, and the dose is

$$D_{1.275} = 10^5 \frac{dis}{g \ s} \times 1 \frac{photon}{dis} \times 1.275 \frac{MeV}{photon}$$

$$\times 1.602 \times 10^{-10} \frac{Gy}{MeV/g} \times 6.048 \times 10^5 \ s \times AF$$

$$= 0.694 \ Gy$$

where $AF \cong 1 - e^{-0.0289 \times 2}$. Hence the total dose is

$$D_{tot} = D_{\beta^+} + D_{EC} + D_{0.511} + D_{1.275}$$
$$= 1.89 + 8.9 \times 10^{-4} + 0.572 + 0.694$$
$$= 3.16 \ Gy$$

or 67% more than for β^+ alone.

EC contributes a more significant fraction of the dose when β^+-emission is prohibited and only EC can occur. An example is $^{55}_{26}Fe \rightarrow ^{55}_{25}Mn$, which emits Mn fluorescence x-rays of 5.9 keV and no other radiation (besides monoenergetic neutrinos). These photons are so easily attenuated that radiation equilibrium exists at the center of a 1-cm-radius water sphere. Thus the energy contributing to the dose there per EC event is equal to the electron binding energy E_b in each case, whether a fluorescence x-ray is emitted or not. Since approximately 88% of these EC events involve the K-shell, and the other 12% can be assumed to be with the L, the energy spent on the dose per EC event [Eq. (5.13)] is

$$f_{EC} = 0.88(6.54 \ keV) + 0.12(0.7 \ keV)$$

$$= 5.84 \ keV$$

where the binding energies are those for the daughter product, Mn (see Appendix B).

D. Internal Conversion vs. γ-Ray Emission

An excited nucleus, instead of emitting a γ-ray of energy $h\nu$, can impart the same amount of energy *directly* to one of its own atomic electrons, which then escapes the atom with a net kinetic energy of $h\nu - E_b$, where E_b is the binding energy of the electron's original shell. This process, called *internal conversion* (IC), has nothing to do with the photoelectric effect (see Chapter 7), since the nucleus emits no photon in this case. The ratio of the number N_e of conversion electrons emitted to the number N_γ of γ-rays emitted by a given species of excited nucleus is called the *internal-conversion coefficient*.

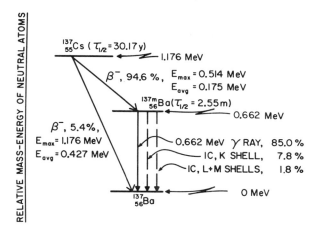

FIGURE 5.9. Atomic energy-level diagram for $^{137}_{55}$Cs $\xrightarrow[\tau_{1/2} = 30.17y]{}$ $^{137}_{56}$Ba, illustrating competition between γ-ray emission and internal conversion. Percentages all refer to disintegrations of parent atoms of $^{137}_{55}$Cs. $(e_K/\gamma) = 0.0916$, $K/(L + M + \ldots) = 4.41$.

An example of internal conversion is shown in Fig. 5.9 for

$$^{137}_{55}\text{Cs} \xrightarrow[\tau_{1/2} = 30.17\,y]{} {}^{137}_{56}\text{Ba}.$$

It will be seen that 94.6% of the $^{137}_{55}$Cs atoms decay to an excited state of $^{137}_{56}$Ba, indicated as $^{137m}_{56}$Ba, where the m indicates a *metastable* or *long-lived isomeric state* with a half-life of 2.55 minutes. (Isomers are nuclei having the same Z and the same number A of nucleons, but differing energy states.) These excited nuclei then decay in the following proportions: 89.9% γ-ray emission (0.662 MeV), 8.2% conversion of K-shell electrons, and 1.9% other-shell conversion.

This branching information is listed under the metastable $^{137m}_{56}$Ba by Lederer and Shirley (1979), in the following format: γ 89.9%, e_K/γ 0.0916; $K/L + M + \cdots$ 4.41. Normally IC branching is not shown on energy-level diagrams, but Fig. 5.9 includes it for clarity. Note that the percentages shown there have been normalized to a total of 94.6%, so that, for example, there are 85.0 γ-rays emitted per 100 disintegrations of $^{137}_{55}$Cs.

Internal conversion is always possible in place of γ-ray emission by an excited nucleus. However, in many cases the probability of IC is negligibly small and can be ignored.

1. Absorbed Dose for Internal Conversion

When IC occurs in competition with γ-ray emission, it generally results in a net *increase* in absorbed dose in small objects, since the penetrating γ-radiation is thus replaced by a relatively short-range electron of nearly the same energy. That is, the energy of the conversion electron is

$$E_{IC} = h\nu - E_b \tag{5.14}$$

which will all be spent on absorbed dose under CPE conditions, neglecting radiative losses. In addition, the binding energy E_b also will be entirely contributed to the dose, provided that no part of it escapes from the radioactive body in the form of fluorescence x-rays. If the fraction $p = 1 - AF$ of these x-rays can escape from the radioactive body, then the energy contributed per IC event to dose under CPE conditions becomes

$$f_{IC} = h\nu - p_K Y_K h\bar{\nu}_K - p_L Y_L h\bar{\nu}_L \tag{5.15}$$

where

$$p \cong e^{-\mu_{en}\bar{r}} \tag{5.16}$$

with μ_{en} and $\bar{r}$ defined as before.

Example 5.5.   A sphere of water 10 cm in diameter contains a uniform source of ^{137}Cs undergoing 10^3 disintegrations per g s. What is the absorbed dose at the center, in grays, for a 10-day period, due only to the decay of $^{137m}_{56}$Ba? Use the mean-radius, straight-ahead approximation.

Solution: For the γ-rays of 0.662 MeV, $\mu_{en} = 0.0327$ cm^{-1}, and the dose in 10 days is

$$D_\gamma = 10^3 \, \frac{\text{dis}}{\text{g s}} \times 0.85 \, \frac{\gamma\text{-rays}}{\text{dis}} \times 0.662 \, \frac{\text{MeV}}{\gamma\text{-ray}}$$

$$\times 1.602 \times 10^{-10} \, \frac{\text{Gy}}{\text{MeV/g}} \times 8.64 \times 10^5 \, \text{s} \times AF$$

$$= 1.17 \times 10^{-2} \, \text{Gy}$$

where $AF \cong 1 - e^{-0.0327 \times 5}$.

For the K-shell conversion process, making use of Eq. (5.15), the dose contribution will be

$$D_{IC}^K = 10^3 \, \frac{\text{dis}}{\text{g s}} \times 0.078 \, \frac{IC(K) \text{ events}}{\text{dis}} \times (h\nu - p Y_K h\bar{\nu}_K) \, \frac{\text{MeV}}{IC(K)}$$

$$\times 1.602 \times 10^{-10} \, \frac{\text{Gy}}{\text{MeV/g}} \times 8.64 \times 10^5 \, \text{s}$$

$$= 1.080(0.662 - p_K Y_K h\bar{\nu}_K) \times 10^{-2} \, \text{Gy}$$

From Fig. 7.15, $h\bar{\nu}_K = 0.032$ MeV, and from Fig. 7.14, $Y_K = 0.90$. Appendix D.3 gives $\mu_{en} \cong 0.13$ cm^{-1} for 0.032 MeV, by interpolation. Hence Eq. (5.16) becomes

$$p_K = e^{-0.13 \times 5} = 0.52$$

and

$$D_{IC}^K = 6.99 \times 10^{-3} \text{ Gy}$$

Likewise, for the IC process in the $L + M + \cdots$ shells, which we may assume to be all L_1 shell, $h\bar{\nu}_L = E_b^L = 6$ keV, for which $\mu_{en} = 24 \text{ cm}^{-1}$ water. Thus $p_L \cong 0$, and

$$D_{IC}^L = 10^3 \frac{\text{dis}}{\text{g s}} \times 0.018 \frac{\text{IC}(L)}{\text{dis}} \times (0.662 - 0) \frac{\text{MeV}}{\text{IC}(L)}$$

$$\times 1.602 \times 10^{-10} \frac{\text{Gy}}{\text{MeV/g}} \times 8.64 \times 10^5 \text{ s}$$

$$= 1.65 \times 10^{-3} \text{ Gy}$$

Hence the total absorbed dose in 10 days due to the disintegration of $^{137m}_{56}\text{Ba}$ atoms is

$$D_{tot} = D_\gamma + D_{IC}^K + D_{IC}^L = 1.17 \times 10^{-2} + 6.99 \times 10^{-3} + 1.65 \times 10^{-3}$$

$$= 2.03 \times 10^{-2} \text{ Gy}$$

E. Tables for Dose Estimation in Appendix C

Appendix C contains data excerpted from the tables of Dillman and Von der Lage (1975), providing abbreviated dose information about a selection of radionuclides. For each source the table gives the types of radiations emitted, the number of particles (or photons) of each type emitted per parent disintegration, the *mean* energy per particle, and the corresponding "equilibrium dose constant" in g rad/μCi h. The latter quantity can be converted into J/Bq h by multiplying by 2.703×10^{-10}. It represents the energy contributed to the absorbed dose, per unit activity and time, under RE conditions (or CPE conditions for β-rays).

The use of these tables can be demonstrated by reference to Example 5.4, in which a source of ^{22}Na distributed in a 2-cm-radius water sphere undergoes 10^5 dis/g s. That is equivalent to 10^8 Bq/kg. The table in Appendix C shows that the main β^+-disintegration has an equilibrium dose constant of 0.4163 g rad/μCi h, which converts to 1.125×10^{-10} J/Bq h. The β^+-dose under CPE conditions is then given by

$$D_{\beta^+} = 10^8 \frac{\text{Bq}}{\text{kg}} \times 1.125 \times 10^{-10} \frac{\text{J}}{\text{Bq h}} \times 168 \text{ h}$$

$$= 1.89 \text{ Gy}$$

For obtaining the dose due to the 1.2746-MeV γ-rays under RE conditions one uses the equilibrium dose constant of 2.7148 g rad/μCi h, which converts to 7.338×10^{-10} J/Bq h. Thus the dose is

$$D_{\gamma,RE} = 10^8 \frac{\text{Bq}}{\text{kg}} \times 7.338 \times 10^{-10} \frac{\text{J}}{\text{Bq h}} \times 168 \text{ h}$$

$$= 12.33 \text{ Gy}$$

The absorbed fraction may be estimated as in Example 5.4, obtaining the value AF = 0.0562. Thus at the center of the water sphere D_γ from these γ-rays is 12.33 × 0.0562 = 0.693 Gy, in good agreement with the value obtained before.

PROBLEMS

1. What is the mean radius $\bar{r}$ from the midpoint of a cylinder of radius a and height h to its boundary surface? Evaluate $\bar{r}$ for $a = h/2 = 10$ cm.

2. A $^{137}_{55}$Cs source is homogeneously distributed throughout a right cylindrical bucket of water having diameter = height = 30 cm. What is the approximate absorbed dose rate in Gy per day in water at the center of the bucket if 160 atoms of $^{137}_{55}$Cs disintegrate per g s? Use the straight-ahead approximation and the mean-radius method of calculating the photon dose. Give the answers for each component of the dose.

3. Repeat problem 2 for a mouse-sized cylindrical mass of water 3 cm in diameter by 3 cm long.

4. Redo Examples 5.2 through 5.5 in this chapter by application of Appendix C.

SOLUTIONS TO PROBLEMS

1. 11.32 cm.

2. $\dot{D}_{\beta-(0.427)} = 5.1 \times 10^{-5}$ Gy/d,
$\dot{D}_{\beta-(0.175)} = 3.67 \times 10^{-4}$ Gy/d,
$\dot{D}_\gamma = 5.31 \times 10^{-4}$ Gy/d,
$\dot{D}^K_{IC} = 1.14 \times 10^{-4}$ Gy/d,
$\dot{D}^L_{IC} = 2.6 \times 10^{-5}$ Gy/d,
$\dot{D}_{tot} = 1.09 \times 10^{-3}$ Gy/d.

3. $\dot{D}_{\beta-(0.427)} = 5.1 \times 10^{-5}$ Gy/d,
$\dot{D}_{\beta-(0.175)} = 3.67 \times 10^{-4}$ Gy/d,
$\dot{D}_\gamma = 6.7 \times 10^{-5}$ Gy/d,
$\dot{D}^K_{IC} = 1.10 \times 10^{-4}$ Gy/d,
$\dot{D}^L_{IC} = 2.6 \times 10^{-5}$ Gy/d,
$\dot{D}_{tot} = 6.22 \times 10^{-4}$ Gy/d.

CHAPTER 6

Radioactive Decay

I. TOTAL DECAY CONSTANTS

Consider a large number N of identical radioactive atoms. We define λ as the *total radioactive decay* (or transformation) *constant*, which has the dimensions reciprocal time, usually expressed in inverse seconds (s^{-1}). The product of λ by a time in consistent units (e.g., seconds), and that is $\ll 1/\lambda$, is the probability that an individual atom will decay during that time interval.

We make the (well-established) assumption that λ is independent of the age of the atom (and of all physical and chemical conditions such as temperature, pressure, concentration, etc.).

The expectation value of the total number of atoms in the group that disintegrate per unit of time very short in comparison to $1/\lambda$ is called the *activity* of the group, λN. This is also expressed in units of reciprocal time, since N is a dimensionless number.

So long as the original group is not replenished by a source of more nuclei, the rate of change in N at any time t is equal to the activity:

$$-\frac{dN}{dt} = \lambda N \qquad (6.1)$$

Separating variables and integrating from $t = 0$ (when $N = N_0$) to time t, we have

$$\int_{N_0}^{N} \frac{dN}{N} = -\int_{0}^{t} \lambda \, dt \qquad (6.2)$$

whence

$$\ln N - \ln N_0 = -(\lambda t - 0)$$

$$\ln \left(\frac{N}{N_0}\right) = -\lambda t$$

$$\frac{N}{N_0} = e^{-\lambda t} \tag{6.3}$$

So we can write for the ratio of activities at time t to that at $t_0 = 0$

$$\frac{\lambda N}{\lambda N_0} = e^{-\lambda t} \tag{6.4}$$

which is found to agree with the experimentally observed law of radioactive decay.

II. PARTIAL DECAY CONSTANTS

If a nucleus has more than one possible mode of disintegration (i.e., to different *daughter products*), the total decay constant can be written as the sum of the partial decay constants λ_i:

$$\lambda = \lambda_A + \lambda_B + \cdots \tag{6.5}$$

and the total activity is

$$N\lambda = N\lambda_A + N\lambda_B + \cdots \tag{6.6}$$

The *partial activity* of the group of N nuclei with respect to the ith mode of disintegration can be written

$$\lambda_i N = \lambda_i N_0 e^{-\lambda t} \tag{6.7}$$

where N has been expressed in terms of N_0 according to Eq. (6.3). Note that each partial activity $\lambda_i N$ in Eq. (6.7) decays at the rate determined by the total decay constant λ, rather than λ_i itself, since the stock of nuclei (N) available at time t for each type of disintegration is the same for all types, and its depletion is the result of their combined action.* Also note that the partial activities $\lambda_i N$ are always proportional to the total activity λN, independent of time, since each λ_i is constant. That is, the $\lambda_i N/\lambda N$ are constant fractions, and their sum for all i modes of disintegration is unity, from Eq. (6.6).

III. UNITS OF ACTIVITY

The old unit of activity was the curie (Ci), originally defined as the number of disintegrations per second occurring in a mass of 1 g of $^{226}_{88}$Ra. Later the definition of

---

*Note the mathematical similarity of decay constants to attenuation coefficients in Chapter 3, Sections I–III.

the curie was divorced from the mass of radium, and was simply set equal to 3.7 $\times 10^{10}$ s^{-1}. Subsequent measurements of the activity of radium have determined that 1 g of $^{226}_{88}$Ra has an activity of 3.655×10^{10} s^{-1}, or 0.988 Ci (Martin and Tuck, 1959).

More recently it was decided by an international standards body to establish a new special unit for activity, the *becquerel* (Bq), equal to 1 s^{-1}. Thus

$$1 \text{ Ci} = 3.7 \times 10^{10} \text{ Bq,}$$

$$1 \text{ mCi} = 3.7 \times 10^{7} \text{ Bq,} \qquad (6.8)$$

$$1 \text{ } \mu\text{Ci} = 3.7 \times 10^{4} \text{ Bq}$$

It will be recognized that the *becquerel* and the *hertz* have identical dimensions, both having units of 1 s^{-1}. The only difference between them is in their application, the hertz being intended for expressing the frequency of periodic motion, while the becquerel is used solely for radioactivity. In other fields of application requiring s^{-1} as a unit, no special name has been assigned.

It is difficult to predict how soon the becquerel might replace the curie in common usage; certainly there will be a period of coexistence between the two units. It is of the greatest importance that errors must not result from confusion arising from unit conversion, especially in clinical nuclear medicine.

In addition to the curie and becquerel as defined above a third option exists for expressing activity, but *only* for *radium* sources. Such a source can be said to have an "activity" equal to the *mass* of $^{226}_{88}$Ra that it contains, typically in milligrams. For historical reasons this usage is very common in spite of its irregularity and lack of consistency with the proper dimensions of activity (s^{-1}). However, it causes no difficulty, so long as one remembers that 1 mg of $^{226}_{88}$Ra has a true activity of 0.988 mCi. The latter value should be used, for example, in calculating production of the daughter product radon.

IV. MEAN LIFE AND HALF LIFE

The expectation value of the time needed for an initial population of N_0 radioactive nuclei to decay to $1/e$ of their original number is called the *mean life* τ. Thus

$$\frac{N}{N_0} = \frac{1}{e} = 0.3679 = e^{-\lambda\tau}$$

$$\ln e^{-1} = -1 = -\lambda\tau \qquad (6.9)$$

$$\therefore \quad \text{mean life } \tau = \frac{1}{\lambda}$$

The mean life τ has interesting and useful properties. As its name implies, it represents the average lifetime of an individual nucleus from an arbitrary starting time t_0 until it disintegrates at a later time t. Here $t - t_0$ may have any value from 0 to ∞.

τ is also the time that would be needed for all the nuclei to disintegrate if the initial activity of the group, λN_0, were maintained constant instead of decreasing exponentially. This can be easily seen from the following argument: Suppose that the initial number of nuclei present is N_0. The initial rate at which they disintegrate is the initial activity, λN_0. Multiplying this rate (now assumed constant) by any period of time would give the total number of nuclei disintegrating during that time. If that time is the mean life τ, then

$$\lambda N_0 \tau = \frac{\lambda N_0}{\lambda} = N_0 \tag{6.10}$$

indicating that all of the nuclei would disintegrate. This can also be seen from Fig. 6.1. The slope of the decay curve of activity may be obtained by differentiation:

$$\frac{d(\lambda N)}{dt} = \frac{d(\lambda N_0 e^{-\lambda t})}{dt} = -\lambda^2 N_0 e^{-\lambda t} = -\lambda^2 N \tag{6.11}$$

Thus the initial slope is $-\lambda^2 N_0$. The time it takes for the straight line along that direction to reach 0 activity can be obtained from:

$$\lambda N_0 - \lambda^2 N_0 t = 0$$

$$\therefore \quad t = \frac{\lambda N_0}{\lambda^2 N_0} = \frac{1}{\lambda} = \tau \tag{6.12}$$

Thus the initial slope intersects the zero-activity axis at the mean life τ, as expected.

A second important characteristic time period associated with exponential decay is the *half-life* $\tau_{1/2}$, which is the expectation value of the time required for one-half

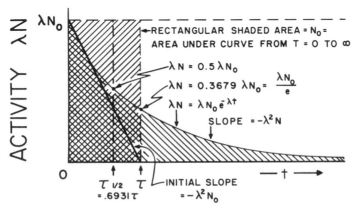

FIGURE 6.1.   Illustrating exponential decay, and the concepts of mean life τ and half-life $\tau_{1/2}$.

of the initial number of nuclei to disintegrate, and hence for the activity to decrease by half:

$$\frac{\lambda N}{\lambda N_0} = 0.5 = e^{-\lambda \tau_{1/2}}$$

$$\ln 0.5 = -0.6931 = -\lambda \tau_{1/2} \tag{6.13}$$

$$\tau_{1/2} = \frac{0.6931}{\lambda} = 0.6931 \, \tau$$

V. RADIOACTIVE PARENT-DAUGHTER RELATIONSHIPS

Consider an initially pure large population $(N_1)_0$ of parent nuclei, which start disintegrating with total decay constant λ_1 at time $t = 0$. The number of parent nuclei remaining at time t is $N_1 = (N_1)_0 e^{-\lambda_1 t}$.

Let λ_1 be composed of partial decay constants λ_{1A}, λ_{1B}, and so on. We focus our interest solely on the daughter product resulting from disintegrations of the A type, which occur with decay constant λ_{1A}. The rate of production of these daughter nuclei at time t is given by $\lambda_{1A}N_1 = \lambda_{1A}(N_1)_0 e^{-\lambda_1 t}$. Simultaneously they in turn will disintegrate with a total decay constant of λ_{2A}, where the 2 refers to the generation doing the decaying (i.e., daughter, or 2nd generation) and the A identifies the type of parental disintegration that gave rise to the daughter in question. Since we will not be concerned here with the fate of any other daughter products, we can simplify terminology by dropping the A from the λ_{2A}. The rate of removal of the N_2 daughter nuclei which exist at time t_0 will be equal to the negative of their total activity, $-\lambda_2 N_2$. Thus the net rate of accumulation of the daughter nuclei at time t is

$$\frac{dN_2}{dt} = \lambda_{1A}N_1 - \lambda_2 N_2$$

$$= \lambda_{1A}(N_1)_0 e^{-\lambda_1 t} - \lambda_2 N_2 \tag{6.14}$$

The general solution of this differential equation for N_2 at time t will be of the form

$$N_2 = (N_1)_0 \, (x_1 e^{-\lambda_1 t} + x_2 e^{-\lambda_2 t}) \tag{6.15}$$

where x_1 and x_2 are constants to be determined. Differentiating with respect to time gives

$$\frac{dN_2}{dt} = (N_1)_0 [\, x_1(-\lambda_1 e^{-\lambda_1 t}) + x_2(-\lambda_2 e^{-\lambda_2 t})] \tag{6.16}$$

Now substituting Eqs. (6.15) and (6.16) into Eq. (6.14), we get

$$-(N_1)_0 [\, x_1 \lambda_1 \, e^{-\lambda_1 t} + x_2 \lambda_2 e^{-\lambda_2 t}] = \lambda_{1A}(N_1)_0 e^{-\lambda_1 t} - \lambda_2 (N_1)_0 (x_1 e^{-\lambda_1 t} + x_2 e^{-\lambda_2 t})$$

$$\tag{6.17}$$

which becomes, upon canceling and collecting terms,

$$x_1[(N_1)_0 \, e^{-\lambda_1 t}(\lambda_2 - \lambda_1)] + x_2[0] - (N_1)_0 \lambda_{1A} e^{-\lambda_1 t} = 0$$

or

$$e^{-\lambda_1 t}[x_1(N_1)_0(\lambda_2 - \lambda_1) - \lambda_{1A}(N_1)_0] = 0$$

The factor in brackets must equal zero to satisfy the equation for all t-values, so

$$x_1(N_1)_0(\lambda_2 - \lambda_1) = \lambda_{1A}(N_1)_0 \qquad (6.18)$$

whence

$$x_1 = \frac{\lambda_{1A}}{\lambda_2 - \lambda_1}$$

Assuming now that the population N_2 of daughter nuclei is zero at $t = 0$, we can solve Eq. (6.15) for x_2:

$$N_2 = 0 = (N_1)_0 \, (x_1 e^{-\lambda_1 t} + x_2 e^{-\lambda_2 t})$$

$$= (N_1)_0 \, (x_1 + x_2) \qquad (6.19)$$

$$\therefore \quad x_2 = -x_1 = \frac{-\lambda_{1A}}{\lambda_2 - \lambda_1}$$

Substituting Eq. (6.19) into (6.15), we have

$$N_2 = (N_1)_0 \left[\frac{\lambda_{1A}}{\lambda_2 - \lambda_1} \, e^{-\lambda_1 t} - \frac{\lambda_{1A}}{\lambda_2 - \lambda_1} \, e^{-\lambda_2 t} \right] = (N_1)_0 \frac{\lambda_{1A}}{\lambda_2 - \lambda_1} \, (e^{-\lambda_1 t} - e^{-\lambda_2 t})$$

Then the activity of the daughter product at any time t, assuming $N_2 = 0$ at $t = 0$, is

$$\lambda_2 N_2 = \lambda_{1A}(N_1)_0 \frac{\lambda_2}{\lambda_2 - \lambda_1} \, (e^{-\lambda_1 t} - e^{-\lambda_2 t}) \qquad (6.20)$$

Remembering that the activity of the parent at time t is $\lambda_1 N_1 = \lambda_1(N_1)_0 e^{-\lambda_1 t}$, we can divide Eq. (6.20) by this equation to obtain the ratio of daughter to parent activities vs. time:

$$\frac{\lambda_2 N_2}{\lambda_1 N_1} = \frac{\lambda_{1A}}{\lambda_1} \cdot \frac{\lambda_2}{\lambda_2 - \lambda_1} \, (1 - e^{-(\lambda_2 - \lambda_1)t}) \qquad (6.21)$$

It is evident from Eq. (6.21) that if the partial decay constant λ_{1A} of the parent were equal to its total decay constant λ_1 (i.e., only *one* daughter were produced by the parent), then

$$\frac{\lambda_2 N_2}{\lambda_1 N_1} = \frac{\lambda_2}{\lambda_2 - \lambda_1} \, (1 - e^{-(\lambda_2 - \lambda_1)t}) \qquad (6.22)$$

Thus the only difference between Eqs. (6.22) and (6.21) is that (6.21) gives, for all

t-values, an activity for the daughter (relative to that of the parent) that is smaller by the factor λ_{1A}/λ_1, which is just the fractional decay constant of the parent for the type of disintegration that produces the daughter. We may therefore ignore the influence of branching in the modes of parent disintegration until the final step when the activity of the daughter has been determined as a function of t on the basis of Eq. (6.22), and then simply multiply by the ratio λ_{1A}/λ_1 to decrease the daughter's activity by the proper factor.

In each of the following equilibrium cases to be considered, we will assume the initial activity of daughter product to be zero ($N_2 = 0$ at $t = 0$).

VI. EQUILIBRIA IN PARENT–DAUGHTER ACTIVITIES

It can be seen from Eq. (6.20) that the activity of a daughter resulting from an initially pure population of parent nuclei will have the value zero both at $t = 0$ and ∞. Evidently $\lambda_2 N_2$ reaches a maximum at some intermediate time t_m when

$$\frac{d(\lambda_2 N_2)}{dt} = 0 = (-\lambda_1 e^{-\lambda_1 t_m} + \lambda_2 e^{-\lambda_2 t_m})$$

and therefore

$$\lambda_1 e^{-\lambda_1 t_m} = \lambda_2 e^{-\lambda_2 t_m}$$

$$\frac{\lambda_2}{\lambda_1} = e^{(\lambda_2 - \lambda_1)t_m}$$

and

$$\ln \frac{\lambda_2}{\lambda_1} = (\lambda_2 - \lambda_1)\, t_m$$

$$t_m = \frac{\ln (\lambda_2/\lambda_1)}{\lambda_2 - \lambda_1} \tag{6.23}$$

This maximum occurs at the same time $t = t_m$ that the activities of the parent and daughter are equal if, and only if, $\lambda_{1A} = \lambda_1$ (i.e., the parent has only one daughter). This can be seen from the following considerations. From Eq. (6.22) we have

$$\frac{\lambda_2 N_2}{\lambda_1 N_1} = 1 = \frac{\lambda_2}{\lambda_2 - \lambda_1}(1 - e^{-(\lambda_2 - \lambda_1)t})$$

$$\frac{\lambda_2 - \lambda_1}{\lambda_2} = 1 - e^{-(\lambda_2 - \lambda_1)t}$$

$$e^{-(\lambda_2 - \lambda_1)t} = 1 - \frac{\lambda_2 - \lambda_1}{\lambda_2} = \frac{\lambda_1}{\lambda_2}$$

$$(\lambda_2 - \lambda_1)t = \ln \frac{\lambda_2}{\lambda_1}$$

Therefore

$$t = \frac{\ln (\lambda_2/\lambda_1)}{\lambda_2 - \lambda_1} = t_m \tag{6.24}$$

which is the same as Eq. (6.23), proving that the maximum of the sole daughter's activity does occur at the same time as the parent's and daughter's activity curves cross, assuming N_2 is initially zero. If, however, $\lambda_{1A} < \lambda_1$, then Eq. (6.21) must be used in place of Eq. (6.22), and the time for equal parent and daughter activities will be shifted from $t = t_m$ to a later time, or to infinite time if the curves no longer cross at all.

The specific relationship of the daughter's activity to that of the parent depends upon the relative magnitudes of the total decay constants of parent (λ_1) and daughter (λ_2).

A. Daughter Longer-Lived than Parent, $\lambda_2 < \lambda_1$

Equation (6.21) can be altered by changing signs to obtain the following for the ratio of daughter to parent activities:

$$\frac{\lambda_2 N_2}{\lambda_1 N_1} = \frac{\lambda_{1A}}{\lambda_1} \cdot \frac{\lambda_2}{\lambda_1 - \lambda_2} (e^{(\lambda_1 - \lambda_2)t} - 1) \tag{6.25}$$

or, where only one daughter is produced,

$$\frac{\lambda_2 N_2}{\lambda_1 N_1} = \frac{\lambda_2}{\lambda_1 - \lambda_2} (e^{(\lambda_1 - \lambda_2)t} - 1) \tag{6.26}$$

This activity ratio is thus seen to increase continuously with t for all times. Remembering that the parent activity at time t is

$$\lambda_1 N_1 = \lambda_1 (N_1)_0 \, e^{-\lambda_1 t}$$

one can construct the activity curves vs. time for the representative case of metastable tellurium-131 decaying to its only daughter iodine-131; and thence to xenon-131:

$$^{131m}_{52}\text{Te} \xrightarrow[\tau_{1/2}=30\,\text{h}]{\beta^-} {}^{131}_{53}\text{I} \xrightarrow[\tau_{1/2}=193\,\text{h}]{\beta^-} {}^{131}_{54}\text{Xe}$$

$$\lambda_1 = 2.31 \times 10^{-2} \, \text{h}^{-1}, \qquad \lambda_2 = 3.59 \times 10^{-3} \, \text{h}^{-1}$$

$$\therefore \ \lambda_1 > \lambda_2$$

The resulting curves are shown in Fig. 6.2.

B. Daughter Shorter-Lived than Parent, $\lambda_2 > \lambda_1$

For $t \gg t_m$ the value of the daughter/parent activity ratio in Eq. (6.21) becomes a constant, assuming as usual that $N_2 = 0$ at $t = 0$:

$$\frac{\lambda_2 N_2}{\lambda_1 N_1} = \frac{\lambda_{1A}}{\lambda_1} \cdot \frac{\lambda_2}{\lambda_2 - \lambda_1} \tag{6.27}$$

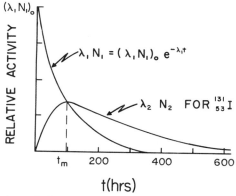

FIGURE 6.2. Qualitative relationship of activity vs. time for $^{131m}_{52}$Te as parent and $^{131}_{53}$I as daughter. $\lambda_1 = 2.31 \times 10^{-2}\,\mathrm{h}^{-1}$, $\lambda_2 = 3.59 \times 10^{-3}\,\mathrm{h}^{-1}$, and hence $\lambda_2 < \lambda_1$. At $t = 0$ the activity of $^{131m}_{52}$Te is equal to $(\lambda_1 N_1)_0$ and that of $^{131}_{53}I$ equals zero.

or, where only a single daughter is produced (i.e., $\lambda_{1A} = \lambda_1$),

$$\frac{\lambda_2 N_2}{\lambda_1 N_1} = \frac{\lambda_2}{\lambda_2 - \lambda_1} \qquad (6.28)$$

The existence of such a constant ratio of activities as in Eq. (6.27) or (6.28) is called *transient equilibrium*, in which the daughter activity decreases at the same rate as that of the parent.

For $\lambda_{1A} = \lambda_1$, the daughter activity is always greater than that of the parent during transient equilibrium, and the two activities are equal at the time $t = t_m$ [see Eqs. (6.23) and (6.24)], at which time $\lambda_2 N_2$ is also a maximum. For $\lambda_{1A} < \lambda_1$, $\lambda_2 N_2$ still maximizes at t_m, but the crossover of $\lambda_1 N_1$ occurs later, if it occurs at all. Obviously if

$$\frac{\lambda_1}{\lambda_{1A}} > \frac{\lambda_2}{\lambda_2 - \lambda_1}$$

then Eq. (6.27) will give $\lambda_2 N_2 / \lambda_1 N_1 < 1$, and no crossover will occur. The daughter's activity will still follow that of the parent during transient equilibrium, but always remain the lower of the two.

For the special case where

$$\frac{\lambda_1}{\lambda_{1A}} = \frac{\lambda_2}{\lambda_2 - \lambda_1} \qquad (6.29)$$

in Eq. (6.27), the activity of the Ath daughter in transient equilibrium equals that of the parent. Equality of daughter and parent during transient equilibrium is referred to as *secular equilibrium*, which will be discussed in the next section.

It is convenient to know how closely a daughter has approached a transient-equilibrium relationship with its parent at a given time. The time t_m when the daughter's activity reaches a maximum is given by Eq. (6.23), which may be substituted into Eq. (6.21) to obtain the daughter-to-parent activity ratio at time t_m:

$$\left(\frac{\lambda_2 N_2}{\lambda_1 N_1}\right)_{t_m} = \frac{\lambda_{1A}}{\lambda_1} \cdot \frac{\lambda_2}{\lambda_2 - \lambda_1} \left[1 - \exp\left(-(\lambda_2 - \lambda_1)\frac{\ln(\lambda_2/\lambda_1)}{\lambda_2 - \lambda_1}\right)\right]$$

$$= \frac{\lambda_{1A}}{\lambda_1} \cdot \frac{\lambda_2}{\lambda_2 - \lambda_1} (1 - e^{-\ln \lambda_2/\lambda_1})$$

$$= \frac{\lambda_{1A}}{\lambda_1} \cdot \frac{\lambda_2}{\lambda_2 - \lambda_1} \cdot \frac{\lambda_2 - \lambda_1}{\lambda_2} = \frac{\lambda_{1A}}{\lambda_1} \tag{6.30}$$

which of course equals unity for $\lambda_{1A} = \lambda_1$.

When transient equilibrium is reached, from Eq. (6.27) we have for the daughter-to-parent activity ratio

$$\left(\frac{\lambda_2 N_2}{\lambda_1 N_1}\right)_{t_e} = \frac{\lambda_{1A}}{\lambda_1} \cdot \frac{\lambda_2}{\lambda_2 - \lambda_1} \tag{6.31}$$

Thus at time t_m the ratio of $\lambda_2 N_2/\lambda_1 N_1$ to its transient-equilibrium value is

$$\frac{\left(\dfrac{\lambda_2 N_2}{\lambda_1 N_1}\right)_{t_m}}{\left(\dfrac{\lambda_2 N_2}{\lambda_1 N_1}\right)_{t_e}} = \frac{\lambda_{1A}/\lambda_1}{\dfrac{\lambda_{1A}}{\lambda_1} \cdot \dfrac{\lambda_2}{\lambda_2 - \lambda_1}} = \frac{\lambda_2 - \lambda_1}{\lambda_2} \tag{6.32}$$

By similar algebra it can be shown that at any time nt_m (i.e., at a time expressed in units of t_m), the ratio of $(\lambda_2 N_2/\lambda_1 N_1)$ to its transient-equilibrium value will be given by

$$\frac{\left(\dfrac{\lambda_2 N_2}{\lambda_1 N_1}\right)_{nt_m}}{\left(\dfrac{\lambda_2 N_2}{\lambda_1 N_1}\right)_{t_e}} = \frac{\dfrac{\lambda_{1A}}{\lambda_1} \cdot \dfrac{\lambda_2}{\lambda_2 - \lambda_1}(1 - e^{-n \ln(\lambda_2/\lambda_1)})}{\dfrac{\lambda_{1A}}{\lambda_1} \cdot \dfrac{\lambda_2}{\lambda_2 - \lambda_1}}$$

$$= 1 - e^{-n \ln(\lambda_2/\lambda_1)} \tag{6.33}$$

which approaches unity for large n.

An interesting example of transient equilibrium, which also exhibits branching of the decay to more than one daughter, is provided by $^{99}_{42}\text{Mo}$ ($\tau_{1/2} = 66.7$ h). The total parent decay constant $\lambda_1 = 0.693/(66.7 \text{ h}) = 0.0104 \text{ h}^{-1}$. In 86% of its β^--disintegrations, $^{99}_{42}\text{Mo}$ decays to $^{99m}_{43}\text{Tc}$, a metastable daughter having a 6.03-h half-life in decaying to its ground-state isomer $^{99}_{43}\text{Tc}$ by γ-ray emission. The other 14% of the $^{99}_{42}\text{Mo}$ nuclei decay by β^--emission to other excited states of $^{99}_{43}\text{Tc}$, which then promptly decay by γ-ray emission to the ground state. Thus we can regard $^{99}_{43}\text{Tc}$ as a second daughter of $^{99}_{42}\text{Mo}$, to which that parent decays in 14% of its disintegrations.

We have a special interest in the first daughter $^{99m}_{43}\text{Tc}$ for clinical diagnostic applications, because its intermediate half-life (6.03 h) and γ-ray energy of 140 keV make it useful for injection into the body for tissue scanning in nuclear medical procedures. This daughter can be periodically "milked" from a $^{99}_{42}\text{Mo}$-containing generator, or "cow", enclosed in a lead-shielded container kept in the hospital. The milking process withdraws both $^{99m}_{43}\text{Tc}$ and $^{99}_{43}\text{Tc}$ together, but the latter has a long $(2 \times 10^5$ y) half-life and emits no γ-rays. The γ-rays emitted during the decay of the short-lived excited states of $^{99}_{43}\text{Tc}$ occur in the generator and are absorbed in its lead container. Consequently only $^{99m}_{43}\text{Tc}$ still emits γ-rays after withdrawal from the generator, and that is the only daughter that concerns us.

The partial decay constant λ_{14} for $^{99}_{42}\text{Mo}$ disintegrating to $^{99m}_{43}\text{Tc}$ is 0.86 times the total decay constant for $^{99}_{42}\text{Mo}$, or 0.00894 h^{-1}. $^{99m}_{43}\text{Tc}$ itself decays to $^{99}_{43}\text{Tc}$, exhibiting a half-life of 6.03 h, so $\lambda_2 = 0.115$ h^{-1}. The time t_m at which the activity of $^{99m}_{43}\text{Tc}$ reaches a maximum is given by Eq. (6.23):

$$t_m = \frac{\ln(\lambda_2/\lambda_1)}{\lambda_2 - \lambda_1} = \frac{\ln(0.115/0.0104)}{0.115 - 0.0104} = 23.0 \text{ h}$$

The ratio of daughter to parent activity at transient equilibrium in this case is given by Eq. (6.27) as

$$\frac{\lambda_2 N_2}{\lambda_1 N_1} = \frac{0.00894}{0.0104} \cdot \frac{0.115}{0.115 - 0.0104} = 0.945$$

If, *hypothetically*, $^{99m}_{43}\text{Tc}$ had been the *only* daughter of $^{99}_{42}\text{Mo}$, then Eq. (6.28) would have described $\lambda_2 N_2/\lambda_1 N_1$ at transient equilibrium, and its value would have been

$$\frac{\lambda_2 N_2}{\lambda_1 N_1} = \frac{0.115}{0.115 - 0.0104} = 1.099$$

Both the real and hypothetical $^{99m}_{43}\text{Tc}$ activity curves are shown in Fig. 6.3, where the latter is shown dashed.

The approach to transient equilibrium of $^{99m}_{43}\text{Tc}$ can be calculated from Eq. (6.33) as a function of t in units of $t_m = 23$ h:

t	Eq. (6.33)	$(\lambda_2 N_2/\lambda_1 N_1)_{n t_m}$
t_m	0.910	0.860
$2t_m$	0.992	0.937
$3t_m$	0.999	0.944
$4t_m$	0.9999	0.945

It will be seen that in this example transient equilibrium is approached within 0.1% at a time equal to $3t_m$. In general, it can be seen from Eq. (6.33) that the ratio of daughter to parent activity will reach 90% of its transient-equilibrium value

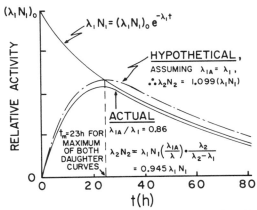

FIGURE 6.3. Example of transient equlibrium: Activity vs. time for $^{99}_{42}$Mo as parent and $^{99m}_{43}$Tc as daughter. $\lambda_1 = 0.0104 \text{ h}^{-1}$; $\lambda_2 = 0.115 \text{ h}^{-1}$, hence $\lambda_2 > \lambda_1$. The activity of $^{99}_{42}$Mo is equal to $(\lambda_1 N_1)_0$ at $t = 0$, and $(\lambda_2 N_2)_0 = 0$ also. Both *actual* $(\lambda_{1A}/\lambda_1 = 0.86)$ and *hypothetical* (assuming $\lambda_{1A}/\lambda_1 = 1$) curves of daughter activity are shown, the latter dashed.

$$\frac{\lambda_{1A}}{\lambda_1} \cdot \frac{\lambda_2}{\lambda_2 - \lambda_1}$$

when $n \ln (\lambda_2/\lambda_1) = 2.3$, 99% when $n \ln (\lambda_2/\lambda_1) = 4.6$, and 99.9% when $n \ln (\lambda_2/\lambda_1) = 6.9$. Thus a relatively large value of λ_2/λ_1 produces a given approximation to transient equilibrium at a relatively short time (i.e., small n). For $\lambda_2/\lambda_1 = 10$, Eq. (6.33) gives 0.9 for $t = t_m$, 0.99 for $t = 2t_m$, and 0.999 for $t = 3t_m$.

C. Only Daughter Much Shorter-Lived than Parent, $\lambda_2 \gg \lambda_1$

For long times ($t \gg \tau_2$) in this case Eq. (6.28) reduces to

$$\frac{\lambda_2 N_2}{\lambda_1 N_1} = \frac{\lambda_2}{\lambda_2 - \lambda_1} \cong 1 \qquad (6.34)$$

That is, the activity of the daughter very closely approximates that of its parent, and they decay together at the rate of the parent. Such a special case of transient equilibrium, where the daughter and parent activities are practically equal, is commonly called *secular equilibrium*, because it closely approximates that condition [see Eq. (6.29)]. The practical cases to which this terminology is applied usually include a very long-lived parent, hence the use of the word "secular" in its sense of "lasting through the ages".

An example of this is the relationship of $^{226}_{88}$Ra as parent, decaying to $^{222}_{86}$Rn as daughter, thence to $^{218}_{84}$Po:

$$^{226}_{88}\text{Ra} \xrightarrow[\substack{\tau_{1/2} = 1602\text{y} \\ \lambda_1 = 1.1845 \times 10^{-6}\text{d}^{-1}}]{\alpha, \gamma} {}^{222}_{86}\text{Rn} \xrightarrow[\substack{\tau_{1/2} = 3.824\text{d} \\ \lambda_2 = 0.18125\text{d}^{-1}}]{\alpha} {}^{218}_{84}\text{Po}$$

In this case Eq. (6.33) gives

$$\frac{\lambda_2 N_2}{\lambda_1 N_1} = \frac{0.18125}{0.18125 - 1.1845 \times 10^{-6}} = 1.000007 \cong 1$$

where both activities must be stated in the same units (e.g., Bq).

Since $^{222}_{86}\text{Rn}$ is the only daughter of $^{226}_{88}\text{Ra}$, its activity exactly equals that of its parent at $t_m = 66$ days [from Eq. (6.24), assuming $(\lambda_2 N_2)_0 = 0$], and thereafter the equality is approximated within 7 parts per million, as shown in the preceding equation. The proximity to transient equilibrium for this case is given by Eq. (6.33): within 1% at $t = 26$ days; within 0.1% at $t = 39$ days.

Thus 1 Ci of $^{226}_{88}\text{Ra}$ sealed in a closed container at time t_o will, any time after 39 days later, be accompanied by 1 Ci (within 0.1%) of $^{222}_{86}\text{Rn}$, which is a noble gas. The granddaughter product, $^{218}_{84}\text{Po}$, in turn decays to $^{214}_{82}\text{Pb}$, and so on through six additional series decay steps to reach stable $^{206}_{82}\text{Pb}$, as shown in Fig. 6.4, which gives the entire uranium series beginning with $^{238}_{92}\text{U}$. It can be shown (e.g., see Evans, 1955) that in such a case all the progeny atoms will eventually be nearly in secular equilibrium with a relatively long-lived ancestor (e.g., $^{226}_{88}\text{Ra}$), and will therefore all have practically the same activity (where the activities of RaC′ and RaC″ must be combined, since they are branching sisters).

Where $\lambda_2 \gg \lambda_1$ with decay branching present, giving rise to more than one

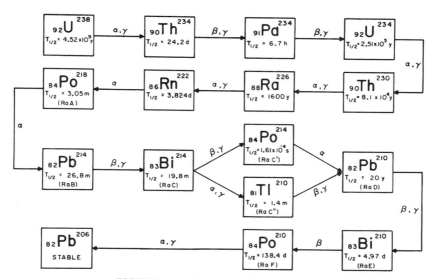

FIGURE 6.4. Uranium-238 decay series.

daughter, the ratio of the activity of the Ath daughter to that of its parent at long times can be gotten from Eq. (6.27):

$$\frac{\lambda_2 N_2}{\lambda_1 N_1} = \frac{\lambda_{1A}}{\lambda_1} \cdot \frac{\lambda_2}{\lambda_2 - \lambda_1} \cong \frac{\lambda_{1A}}{\lambda_1} \tag{6.35}$$

VII. REMOVAL OF DAUGHTER PRODUCTS

In some cases, especially for diagnostic or therapeutic applications of short-lived radioisotopes, as noted in Section VI.B, it is useful to remove the daughter product from its relatively long-lived parent, which continues producing more daughter atoms for later removal and use. The greatest yield *per milking* will of course be gotten at time t_m since the previous milking, assuming complete removal of the daughter product each time. Waiting longer than t_m is counterproductive, as the activity of the daughter present then begins to decline along with the parent. Frequent (or continuous) milking would give a greater *total* yield of the daughter product, however.

Assuming that the initial parent activity is $\lambda_1(N_1)_0$ and the initial Ath-daughter activity is zero at time $t = 0$, the daughter's activity at any later time t is obtained from Eq. (6.20). It is convenient to observe that this equation tells us how much Ath-daughter activity *exists* at time t as a result of the parent-source disintegrations, regardless of whether or how often the daughter has been separated from its source. Thus the amount of daughter activity available to be removed from the source at time t is that given by Eq. (6.20) minus the daughter activity previously removed and still existing elsewhere at the same time t.

Alternatively, if we let $\lambda_1(N_1)_0$ represent the initial activity of the parent source at time $t = 0$, and if the Ath daughter product is completely removed at a later time t_1 (not necessarily the first milking), then the additional Ath daughter activity that can be removed at a subsequent time t_2 is given by

$$\lambda_2 N_2 = \lambda_{1A}(N_1)_0 \, e^{-\lambda_1 t_1} \frac{\lambda_2}{\lambda_2 - \lambda_1} \left(e^{-\lambda_1(t_2 - t_1)} - e^{-\lambda_2(t_2 - t_1)} \right) \tag{6.36}$$

If only a single daughter is produced ($\lambda_{1A} = \lambda_1$) and if we assume $t_1 = 0$ and $t_2 = t$, then

$$\lambda_2 N_2 = (\lambda_1 N_1)_0 \frac{\lambda_2}{\lambda_2 - \lambda_1} \left(e^{-\lambda_1 t} - e^{-\lambda_2 t} \right)$$

$$= (\lambda_1 N_1)_0 \frac{\lambda_2}{\lambda_2 - \lambda_1} \, e^{-\lambda_1 t} \left(1 - e^{-(\lambda_2 - \lambda_1)t} \right) \tag{6.37}$$

$$= \lambda_1 N_1 \frac{\lambda_2}{\lambda_2 - \lambda_1} \left(1 - e^{-(\lambda_2 - \lambda_1)t} \right)$$

The activity $\lambda_2 N_2$ of the daughter product after removal from its parent may not be directly correlated with the radiation output of the resulting new source as a function of time. An important example is radon gas, which itself emits only α-particles and no γ-radiation. Immediately after removal from its $^{226}_{88}$Ra parent and sealing off into a gold "seed", radon is practically "dead" as a γ-ray emitter; hence the seed can be quickly manipulated with little necessity for γ-ray shielding. However, its γ-ray output soon builds up with the production of its granddaughter Ra B and great-granddaughter Ra C (see Fig. 6.4), both of which are prolific γ-ray emitters (Johns and Cunningham, 1974, Table XIV-1). It takes about 4 h for the Ra B and Ra C to reach their maximum activities, and hence for the γ-ray output rate to maximize. Evans (1955) provides an excellent treatment of the problem of calculating the activities of a chain of radioactive progeny as a function of time.

VIII. RADIOACTIVATION BY NUCLEAR INTERACTIONS

Stable nuclei may be transformed into radioactive species by bombardment with suitable particles, or photons of sufficiently high energy. Thermal neutrons are particularly effective for this purpose, as they are electrically neutral, hence are not repelled from the nucleus by Coulomb forces, and are readily captured by many kinds of nuclei. Tables of isotopes (e.g., Lederer and Shirley, 1979) list typical reactions which give rise to specific radionuclides.

Let N_t be the number of target atoms present in the sample to be activated:

$$N_t = \frac{N_A m}{A}, \tag{6.38}$$

where N_A = Avogadro's constant (atoms/mole),
$\quad\quad A$ = gram-atomic weight (g/mole), and
$\quad\quad m$ = mass (g) of *target atoms only* in the sample. (This is equal to the product of the gross sample mass by the weight fraction of target atoms present in the sample.)

If φ is the particle flux density (s^{-1} cm^{-2}) at the sample, assuming that the sample self-shielding is negligible, and σ is the interaction cross section (cm^2/atom) for the activation process in question, then the initial rate of production (s^{-1}) of activated atoms is

$$\left(\frac{dN_{\text{act}}}{dt}\right)_0 = \varphi N_t \sigma \tag{6.39}$$

assuming as usual that we are dealing with expectation values. Correspondingly the initial rate of production of activity of the radioactive source being thus created is given by

$$\left(\frac{d(\lambda N_{\text{act}})}{dt}\right)_0 = \lambda \varphi N_t \sigma \quad\quad (\text{Bq } s^{-1}) \tag{6.40}$$

where λ is the total radioactive decay constant of the new species.

If we may assume that φ is constant and that N_t is not appreciably depleted as a result of the activation process, then the rates of production given by Eqs. (6.39) and (6.40) are also constant.

As the population of active atoms increases, they decay at the rate λN_{act} (s^{-1}). Thus the net rate at which they accumulate can be expressed as

$$\frac{dN_{\text{act}}}{dt} = \varphi N_t \sigma - \lambda N_{\text{act}} \tag{6.41}$$

After an irradiation time $t \gg \tau$, the rate of decay equals the rate of production, and the net rate of population increase becomes zero; thus the equilibrium activity level is given directly by

$$(\lambda N_{\text{act}})_e = \varphi N_t \sigma \quad (\text{Bq}) \tag{6.42}$$

where the subscript e stands for equilibrium.

At any time t after the start of irradiation, assuming the initial activity to be zero ($\lambda N_{\text{act}} = 0$ at $t = 0$), the activity in becquerels can be shown to be related to the equilibrium activity by

$$\lambda N_{\text{act}} = (\lambda N_{\text{act}})_e (1 - e^{-\lambda t}) = \varphi N_t \sigma (1 - e^{-\lambda t}) \tag{6.43}$$

This equation can be derived from Eq. (6.41) in the same way that Eq. (6.20) was derived from Eq. (6.14). Or, assuming that no decay occurs during the irradiation period t (which will be approximately correct if $t \ll \tau$), the activity at time t may be approximated by

$$\lambda N_{\text{act}} \cong \lambda \varphi N_t \sigma t \tag{6.44}$$

where $\lambda \varphi N_t \sigma$ is the *initial* rate of production of activity (Bq/s) from Eq. (6.40).

Figure 6.5 shows the growth of activity as a function of time, according to Eq. (6.43). Also shown is the linear approximation given by Eq. (6.44). It is clear from the graph that this approximation is adequate only for times very short compared

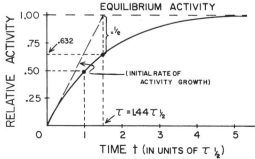

FIGURE 6.5.   Growth of a radionuclide of decay constant λ due to a constant rate of nuclear interaction.

to the mean life τ. At time $t = \tau = 1/\lambda$, Eq. (6.44) predicts that the activity (neglecting decay) would reach $\varphi N_t \sigma$, the equilibrium activity level [Eq. (6.42)].

Sometimes it is necessary to calculate the equilibrium activity level on the basis of the initial rate of growth of activity, without knowing the flux density or cross section for the interaction. An example would be the prediction of the maximum activity level of a particular radionuclide that would be reached ultimately in a neutron shield, knowing only the activity resulting from a short initial irradiation period.

Combining Eqs. (6.40) and (6.42), we have for the equilibrium activity level

$$\lambda(N_{\text{act}})_e = \varphi N_t \sigma = \frac{1}{\lambda}\left(\frac{d(\lambda N_{\text{act}})}{dt}\right)_0$$

$$= \tau \left(\frac{d(\lambda N_{\text{act}})}{dt}\right)_0 \qquad (6.45)$$

Therefore the equilibrium activity level is equal to the initial production rate of activity multiplied by the mean life τ. This method of course requires that the mean life (or the decay constant) be known for the radioactive product of interest.

IX. EXPOSURE-RATE CONSTANT

The *exposure-rate constant* Γ_δ of a radioactive nuclide emitting photons is the quotient of $l^2(dX/dt)_\delta$ by A, where $(dX/dt)_\delta$ is the exposure rate due to photons of energy greater than δ, at a distance l from a point source of this nuclide having an activity A (ICRU, 1971):

$$\Gamma_\delta = \frac{l^2}{A}\left(\frac{dX}{dt}\right)_\delta \qquad (6.46)$$

It is usually stated in units of R m^2 Ci^{-1} h^{-1} or R cm^2 mCi^{-1} h^{-1}.

This quantity was defined by the ICRU to replace the earlier *specific gamma-ray constant* Γ, which only accounts for the exposure rate due to γ-rays, whereas Γ_δ also includes the exposure rate contribution (if any) of characteristic x-rays and internal bremsstrahlung*, and establishes the arbitrary lower energy limit δ (keV) below which all photons are ignored. As of this writing most of the available tabulations of data for γ-ray emitters still list Γ rather than Γ_δ, and the specific γ-ray constant continues to be used in practice where the corresponding exposure-rate constant is not available.

Table 6.1 gives the results of calculations by Dillman, published by the NCRP (1974), quoting Γ- and Γ_δ-values for several γ-emitters with the assumption that δ

---

*Internal bremsstrahlung results from the abrupt change in nuclear charge due to the emission of a β-ray ($+$ or $-$) or the capture of an electron [see Evans (1955) and discussion of bremsstrahlung x-ray production in Chapter 10]. Its contribution to the exposure rate is relatively weak, and usually negligible in strong γ-ray emitters.

TABLE 6.1.   **Data for Selected γ-Ray Sources**[a]

Radionuclide	Half-Life	γ-Photon Energy (MeV)	Specific γ-Ray Constant[b] (R cm^2 mCi^{-1} h^{-1})	Exposure-Rate Constant[b] (R cm^2 mCi^{-1} h^{-1})
^{137}Cs	30.0 y	0.6616	3.200	3.249
^{51}Cr	27.72 d	0.3200	0.1827	0.1827
^{60}Co	5.26 y	1.173–1.322[c]	12.97	12.97
^{198}Au	2.698 d	0.4118–1.088[c]	2.309	2.357
^{125}I	60.25 d	0.03548	0.04194	1.315
^{192}Ir	74.2 d	0.1363–1.062[c]	3.917	3.970
^{226}Ra[d]	1602 y	0.0465–2.440[c]	8.996[e]	10.07
^{182}Ta	115.0 d	0.0427–1.453[c]	7.631	7.753

[a] NCRP (1974).

[b] The specific γ-ray constants and exposure-rate constants were calculated by L. T. Dillman from decay-scheme data, assuming $\overline{W}_{air} = 33.70$ eV/i.p. Values in the present table have been adjusted downward to be consistent with $\overline{W}_{air} = 33.97$ eV/i.p. Contributions to these constants by photons below 11.3 keV were excluded.

[c] Minimum and maximum values included in the calculation of specific γ-ray constant and exposure-rate constant.

[d] With daughters.

[e] This value differs from the currently accepted value of 8.35 R cm^2 mCi^{-1} h^{-1} for radium because the value 8.996 was calculated for no filtration. The value of 8.35 is for a filter of 0.5-mm platinum and includes such secondary radiations as may be generated in the platinum filter; it corresponds to 8.25 R cm^2 mg^{-1} h^{-1}, since 1 mg = 0.988 mCi.

$= 11.3$ keV. It will be seen that Γ_δ is greater than Γ by 2% or less, except for $^{226}_{88}$Ra (12%) and $^{125}_{53}$I (in which case Γ is only about 3% of Γ_δ because K-fluorescence x-rays following electron capture constitute most of the photons emitted). In extreme cases like this, where Γ would be useless if defined literally (i.e., for γ-rays only), x-rays have been sometimes included in Γ even though the definition did not call for it (e.g., Table A8 in Johns and Cunningham, 1974). Moreover, Γ-values derived from experimental measurements of the exposure rate naturally include the effect of any x-rays escaping from the source. Thus the tabulations of Γ available in the literature may be closer to Γ_δ in value than one would expect from the difference in their definitions, and variations in Γ from one table to another constitute a greater practical difficulty at the present time than the lack of Γ_δ data.

The most extensive tables of Γ now available are those of Nachtigall (1969), which were computed in a self-consistent way for 600 radionuclides. Unger and Trubey (1982) have tabulated 500, in terms of tissue CPE dose in place of exposure.

In the following paragraphs we will show how the specific γ-ray constant Γ can be calculated for a given point source. The exposure-rate constant Γ_δ may be calculated in the same way by taking account of the additional x-ray photons (if any) emitted per disintegration.

At a location l meters (in vacuo) from a γ-ray point source having an activity A Ci, the flux density of photons of the single energy E_i is given by

$$\varphi_{E_i} = 3.7 \times 10^{10} \, Ak_i \, \frac{1}{4\pi l^2}$$

$$= 2.944 \times 10^9 \, \frac{Ak_i}{l^2} \quad \text{(photons/s m}^2) \tag{6.47}$$

where k_i is the number of photons of energy E_i emitted per disintegration. This can be converted to energy flux density through Eq. (1.13a) as follows:

$$\psi_{E_i} = E_i \, \varphi_{E_i} = 2.944 \times 10^9 \, \frac{Ak_i E_i}{l^2} \quad \text{(MeV/s m}^2) \tag{6.48}$$

in which E_i is to be expressed in MeV/photon. It will be more convenient to express ψ_{E_i} in units of J/s m^2 (1 MeV $= 1.602 \times 10^{-13}$ J), while still expressing E_i in MeV, in which case the above equation becomes

$$\psi_{E_i} = 4.717 \times 10^{-4} \, \frac{Ak_i E_i}{l^2} \, \text{J/s m}^2 \tag{6.49}$$

We can relate this energy flux density to the exposure rate by recalling Eqs. (1.11), (2.23), and (2.28). For photons of energy E_i the exposure rate is given by

$$\left(\frac{dX}{dt}\right)_{E_i} = \frac{1}{33.97} \left(\frac{\mu_{en}}{\rho}\right)_{E_i, \text{ air}} \left(\frac{d\Psi}{dt}\right)_{E_i} = \frac{1}{33.97} \left(\frac{\mu_{en}}{\rho}\right)_{E_i, \text{ air}} \psi_{E_i} \tag{6.50}$$

and the total exposure rate for all of the γ-ray energies E_i present is

$$\frac{dX}{dt} = \frac{1}{33.97} \sum_{i=1}^{n} \left(\frac{\mu_{en}}{\rho}\right)_{E_i, \text{ air}} \psi_{E_i} \tag{6.51}$$

Substituting Eq. (6.49) into (6.51), we obtain

$$\frac{dX}{dt} = 1.389 \times 10^{-5} \, \frac{A}{l^2} \sum_{i=1}^{n} \left[k_i E_i \left(\frac{\mu_{en}}{\rho}\right)_{E_i, \text{air}} \right] \text{C/kg s} \tag{6.52}$$

This can be converted into R/h, remembering that 1 R $= 2.58 \times 10^{-4}$ C/kg and 3600 s $= 1$ h:

$$\frac{dX}{dt} = 193.8 \, \frac{A}{l^2} \left[\sum_{i=1}^{n} k_i E_i \left(\frac{\mu_{en}}{\rho}\right)_{E_i, \text{air}} \right] \text{R/h} \tag{6.53}$$

The specific γ-ray constant for this source is defined as its exposure rate from all γ-rays *per curie of activity*, normalized to a distance of 1 m by means of an inverse-square-law correction:

$$\Gamma = \frac{dX}{dt} \cdot \frac{l^2}{A} = 193.8 \left[\sum_{i=1}^{n} k_i E_i \left(\frac{\mu_{en}}{\rho} \right)_{E_i, \text{air}} \right] \text{R m}^2/\text{Ci h} \qquad (6.54)$$

where E_i is expressed in MeV and μ_{en}/ρ in m^2/kg. If $(\mu_{en}/\rho)_{E_i, \text{air}}$ is given instead in units of cm^2/g, the constant in this equation is reduced to 19.38. Γ may be obtained in units of R cm^2/mCi h directly with Eq. (6.54) if $(\mu_{en}/\rho)_{E_i, \text{air}}$ is expressed in cm^2/g in place of m^2/kg.

For the special case of $^{226}_{88}Ra$ in equilibrium with its progeny (see Fig. 6.4), Γ is usually expressed in R cm^2/mg h, the activity of the $^{226}_{88}Ra$ is being expressed in terms of its mass (see Section III). Also, the accepted value of 8.25 R cm^2/mg h refers not to a "bare" point source, but rather to one in which the γ-rays are filtered through 0.5 mm of Pt(10% Ir) in escaping. Shalek and Stovall (1969) have provided a table of Γ-values for radium sources in other capsule thicknesses; between 0.5 and 1.0 mm, Γ decreases by approximately 1.3% per 0.1-mm increase in Pt(10% Ir) wall thickness. The specific γ-ray constant for $^{222}_{86}Rn$ in equilibrium with its progeny, with 0.5-mm Pt–Ir filtration, is 8.34 R cm^2/mCi h, nearly the same as that for $^{226}_{88}Ra$ in equilibrium, which is 8.35 R cm^2/mCi h ($= 8.25$ R cm^2 mg^{-1} $h^{-1}/0.988$ mCi mg^{-1}). The tenth-percent difference is due to the weak γ-ray emission in the disintegration of the $^{226}_{88}Ra$ itself. Nearly all of the γ-rays emitted by $^{226}_{88}Ra$ or $^{222}_{86}Rn$ in equilibrium with their decay products result from just two of their progeny: Ra B ($^{214}_{82}Pb$) and Ra C ($^{214}_{83}Bi$), as discussed by Johns and Cunningham (1974).

Applying Eq. (6.54) to an example, ^{60}Co, we note first that each disintegration is accompanied by the emission of two photons, one at 1.17 MeV and the other at 1.33 MeV. Thus the value of k_i is unity at both energies. The mass energy-absorption coefficient values for air at these energies are:

E_i (MeV)	$(\mu_{en}/\rho)_{E_i, \text{air}}$ (m^2/kg)
1.17	0.00270
1.33	0.00262

Hence Eq. (6.54) becomes

$$\Gamma = 193.8(1.17 \times 0.00270 + 1.33 \times 0.00262)$$

$$= 1.29 \text{ R m}^2/\text{Ci h}$$

which is close to the value given in Table 6.1, considering the difference in units.

The exposure rate (R/hr) at a distance l meters from a point source of A curies is given by

$$\frac{dX}{dt} = \frac{\Gamma A}{l^2} \qquad (6.55)$$

where Γ is given for the source in R m^2/Ci h, and attenuation and scattering by the surrounding medium are assumed to be negligible.

A quantity called the *air kerma rate constant* that is related to the exposure rate constant was also defined by the ICRU (1980). The defining equation is identical to Eq. (6.46) except for the replacement of X by K_{air}. The units recommended are $m^2 J kg^{-1}$ or $m^2 Gy Bq^{-1} s^{-1}$. Unfortunately the ICRU chose the same symbol, Γ_δ, for this constant, which may cause confusion. Moreover a more useful quantity would have resulted from the use of *air collision kerma*, as it would then be related to the photon energy fluence through $(\mu_{en}/\rho)_{air}$ instead of $(\mu_{tr}/\rho)_{air}$, and thus would allow the escape of bremsstrahlung losses, as is true of the exposure-rate constant.

PROBLEMS

1. A radium source contains 50 mg of $^{226}_{88}Ra$ in equilibrium with all its progeny. Assuming $\tau_{1/2}$ is 1602 y:

    (a) What is the decay constant for $^{226}_{88}Ra$?

    (b) What is its mean life?

    (c) How many atoms of $^{226}_{88}Ra$ does the source contain, based upon its mass and assuming that 226 g = 1 mole?

    (d) How many atoms of $^{226}_{88}Ra$ does it contain, based upon its activity?

    (e) How many millicuries and how many atoms of $^{222}_{86}Rn$ will be present in secular equilibrium? ($\tau_{1/2} = 3.824$ d.)

2. $^{74}_{33}As$ disintegrates to $^{74}_{32}Ge$ in 68% of the cases, and to $^{74}_{34}Se$ otherwise. $\tau_{1/2}$ for the parent atoms is 17.9 d.

    (a) What is the decay constant for $^{74}_{33}As$?

    (b) What are the partial decay constants for $^{74}_{33}As \rightarrow {}^{74}_{32}Ge$ (λ_{Ge}) and $^{74}_{33}As \rightarrow {}^{74}_{34}Se$ (λ_{Se})?

    (c) What is the activity of a source containing 2.0×10^{17} atoms of $^{74}_{33}As$? Express in becquerels and curies.

    (d) What is the initial rate of production of the $^{74}_{34}Se$ atoms; what is the rate at 47 days?

3. (a) Assuming it to be absent at time $t = 0$, at what time t_m does the activity of $^{131}_{53}I$ reach a maximum as a daughter product of $^{131m}_{52}Te$?

    (b) What are the activities of parent and daughter at time t_m, assuming 5 mCi of the parent at $t = 0$?

    (c) How many atoms of each are present at t_m?

4. (a) Write a formula for the ratio of the numbers of atoms of daughter to parent for a single daughter, initially absent.

    (b) At what time will the numbers of daughter and parent atoms be equal in Problem 3?

    (c) Draw a graph showing the numbers of $^{131m}_{52}Te$ and $^{131}_{53}I$ atoms vs. time.

5. A $^{90}_{38}$Sr source with an initial activity of 20 μCi decays with a half-life of 28.1 y to $^{90}_{39}$Y, which in turn decays with $\tau_{1/2} = 64$ h to stable zirconium. Assuming that the $^{90}_{38}$Sr atoms are initially pure:

(a) When does its daughter maximize?

(b) When does it approach within 1 % of transient equilibrium? Within 0.1 %?

(c) What is the ratio of activities for Y and Sr in transient equilibrium? What kind of equilibrium does this approximate?

(d) How many atoms of Zr have been produced at $t = 120$ d?

6. A generator contains 500 mCi of $^{131}_{56}$Ba ($\tau_{1/2} = 11.6$ d) producing the daughter $^{131}_{55}$Cs ($\tau_{1/2} = 9.7$ d). At $t = 0$ the daughter is completely removed.

(a) When will the ^{131}Cs activity equal that of its parent?

(b) How many becquerels of ^{131}Cs can then be removed (assuming 100 % removal efficiency)?

(c) How much total activity of ^{131}Cs could be obtained if milking were done instead three times, at 122.3-h intervals?

(d) If you saved up the ^{131}Cs obtained in (c), what would be its remaining activity at $t = 367$ h?

7. A gold foil weighing 3.5 mg is irradiated by a thermal-neutron flux density of 10^{13} n cm^{-2} s^{-1}. The interaction cross section is $\sigma = 96 \times 10^{-24}$ cm^2/atom, and $\tau_{1/2} = 2.70$ d for ^{198}Au.

(a) How long will it take for the foil to achieve an activity of 100 mCi of ^{198}Au?

(b) What is the equilibrium level of activity?

(c) How long would it have taken to reach the same activity if the decay of ^{198}Au were negligible during that time?

(d) What is the true activity reached at that time?

8. On the average, for 1000 disintegrations of $^{131}_{53}$I, the following numbers and energies of photons will be emitted:

E_γ (MeV)	No. of Photons/1000 dis
0.723	16
0.637	69
0.503	3
0.364	853
0.326	2
0.284	51
0.177	2
0.164	6
0.080	51
Total	1053

Calculate the specific γ-ray constant, making use of data from Appendix D.3.

SOLUTIONS TO PROBLEMS

1. **(a)** 1.37×10^{-11} s^{-1}.
   (b) 7.29×10^{10} s.
   (c) 1.332×10^{20} atoms.
   (d) 1.333×10^{20} atoms.
   (e) 49.4 mCi, 8.71×10^{14}.
2. **(a)** 4.48×10^{-7} s^{-1}.
   (b) $\lambda_{Ge} = 3.05 \times 10^{-7}$ s^{-1}, $\lambda_{Se} = 1.43 \times 10^{-7}$ s^{-1}.
   (c) 8.96×10^{10} Bq $= 2.42$ Ci.
   (d) 2.87×10^{10} s^{-1}; 4.65×10^{9} s^{-1}.
3. **(a)** 95.4 h.
   (b) Both 2.04×10^{7} Bq.
   (c) 3.18×10^{12} atoms Te, 2.05×10^{13} atoms I.
4. **(a)** —
   (b) 31.4 h.
   (c) —
5. **(a)** 31.8 d.
   (b) 17.7 d, 26.6 d.
   (c) 1.00026. Secular.
   (d) 7.40×10^{12}.
6. **(a)** 367 h
   (b) 7.42×10^{9} Bq.
   (c) 1.10×10^{10} Bq.
   (d) 7.42×10^{9} Bq.
7. **(a)** 1.74 d.
   (b) 278 mCi.
   (c) 1.40 d.
   (d) 84 mCi.
8. $\Gamma = 2.19$ R cm^{2}/mCi h.

CHAPTER **7**

Gamma- and X-Ray
Interactions in Matter

I. INTRODUCTION

There are five types of interactions with matter by x- and γ-ray photons which must be considered in radiological physics:

1. Compton effect
2. Photoelectric effect
3. Pair production
4. Rayleigh (coherent) scattering
5. Photonuclear interactions

The first three of these are the most important, as they result in the transfer of energy to electrons, which then impart that energy to matter in many (usually small) Coulomb-force interactions along their tracks. Rayleigh scattering is elastic; the photon is merely redirected through a small angle with no energy loss. Photonuclear interactions are only significant for photon energies above a few MeV, where they may create radiation-protection problems through the (γ, n) production of neutrons and consequent radioactivation.

The relative importance of Compton effect, photoelectric effect, and pair production depends on both the photon quantum energy $(E_\gamma = h\nu)$ and the atomic number Z of the absorbing medium. Figure 7.1 indicates the regions of Z and E_γ in which each interaction predominates. The curves show where two kinds of interactions are equally probable. It will be seen that the photoelectric effect is dominant at the lower

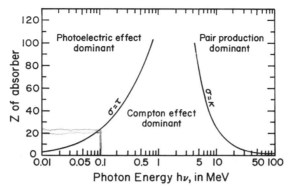

FIGURE 7.1. Relative importance of the three major types of γ-ray interactions. The curves show the values of Z and E_γ for which two types of effects are equal. (Reproduced from Evans (1955) with permission of R.D. Evans and McGraw-Hill Book Company.)

photon energies, the Compton effect takes over at medium energies, and pair production at the higher energies. For low-Z media (e.g., carbon, air, water, human tissue) the region of Compton-effect dominance is very broad, extending from $\cong 20$ keV to $\cong 30$ MeV. This gradually narrows with increasing Z.

In this chapter each of the five kinds of interactions will be discussed, identifying their respective contributions to the coefficients for attenuation (μ/ρ), energy transfer (μ_{tr}/ρ), and energy absorption (μ_{en}/ρ).

II. COMPTON EFFECT

A description of the Compton effect can be conveniently subdivided into two aspects: *kinematics* and *cross section*. The first relates the energies and angles of the participating particles when a Compton event occurs; the second predicts the probability that a Compton interaction will occur. In both respects it is customary to assume that the electron struck by the incoming photon is initially *unbound* and *stationary*. These assumptions are certainly not rigorous, inasmuch as the electrons all occupy various atomic energy levels, thus are in motion and are bound to the nucleus. Nevertheless the resulting errors remain inconsequential in radiological physics applications, because of the dominance of the competing photoelectric effect under the conditions (high Z, low hν) where electron binding effects are the most important in Compton interactions.

In the present chapter the initial motion and binding of the electron will be ignored. The Klein–Nishina treatment of the cross section, to be presented in Section II.B.2, is based on free electrons, and Appendix D.1 tabulates K–N interaction, scattering, and energy-transfer cross sections in units of cm^2/electron, which are applicable to all elements under the zero-binding assumption. Discussion of the influence of electron binding on the Compton effect has been given by Hubbell et al., (1980), Johns and Cunningham (1983), and Anderson (1984).

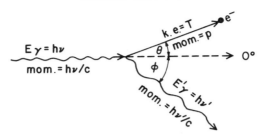

FIGURE 7.2. Kinematics of the Compton effect. A photon of quantum energy $h\nu$ incident from the left strikes an unbound stationary electron, scattering it at angle θ relative to the incident photon's direction, with kinetic energy T. The scattered photon $h\nu'$ departs at angle φ on the opposite side of the original direction, in the same scattering plane. Energy and momentum are each conserved. The assumption of an unbound electron means that the above kinematic relationships are independent of the atomic number of the medium.

A. Kinematics

Figure 7.2 schematically shows a photon of energy $h\nu$ colliding with an electron. The photon's incident forward momentum is $h\nu/c$, where c is the speed of light in vacuum. The stationary target electron has no initial kinetic energy or momentum.

After the collision the electron departs at angle θ, with kinetic energy T and momentum p. The photon scatters at angle φ with a new, lower quantum energy $h\nu'$ and momentum $h\nu'/c$. The solution to the collision kinetics is based upon conservation of both energy and momentum. Energy conservation requires that

$$T = h\nu - h\nu' \tag{7.1}$$

Conservation of momentum along the original photon direction ($0°$) can be expressed as

$$\frac{h\nu}{c} = \frac{h\nu'}{c} \cos \varphi + p \cos \theta$$

or

$$h\nu = h\nu' \cos \varphi + pc \cos \theta \tag{7.2}$$

Conservation of momentum perpendicular to the direction of incidence gives the equation

$$h\nu' \sin \varphi = pc \sin \theta \tag{7.3}$$

pc can be written in terms of T in Eqs. (7.2) and (7.3) by invoking the "law of invariance":

$$pc = \sqrt{T(T + 2 \, m_0 c^2)} \tag{7.4}$$

in which m_0 is the electron's rest mass. This equation can be derived from the following three relativistic relationships:

$$m = \frac{m_0}{\sqrt{1 - (v/c)^2}} \tag{7.5}$$

$$T = mc^2 - m_0c^2 \tag{7.6}$$

$$p = mv \tag{7.7}$$

where v is the electron's velocity, m is its relativistic mass, and p its momentum.

As a result of the substitution for pc, Eqs. (7.1), (7.2), and (7.3) constitute a set of three simultaneous equations in these five parameters: $h\nu$, $h\nu'$, T, θ, and φ. These equations can be solved algebraically to obtain any three of the variables we choose in a single equation. Of the many equations that may be thus derived, the following set of three equations, each in three variables, provides in convenient form a complete solution to the kinematics of Compton interactions:

$$h\nu' = \frac{h\nu}{1 + (h\nu/m_0c^2)(1 - \cos \varphi)} \tag{7.8}$$

$$T = h\nu - h\nu' \tag{7.9}$$

$$\cot \theta = \left(1 + \frac{h\nu}{m_0c^2}\right) \tan\left(\frac{\varphi}{2}\right) \tag{7.10}$$

in which m_0c^2 (the rest energy of the electron) is 0.511 MeV, and $h\nu$, $h\nu'$ and T are also expressed in MeV.

It will be seen from Eq. (7.8) that for a given value of $h\nu$, the energy $h\nu'$ and angle φ of the scattered photon are uniquely correlated to each other. Equation (7.9) then provides the kinetic energy T of the corresponding scattered electron, and Eq. (7.10) gives its scattering angle θ.

Figure 7.3 is a simple graphical representation of the kinematic relationships between $h\nu$, $h\nu'$, and T, as expressed by Eqs. (7.8) and (7.9). It can be seen that for $h\nu$ smaller than about 0.01 MeV, all the curves for different φ-values converge along the diagonal, indicating that $h\nu' = h\nu$ regardless of photon scattering angle. Consequently the electron receives practically no kinetic energy in the interaction. This means that Compton scattering is nearly elastic for low photon energies. An earlier theory of γ-ray scattering by Thomson, based on observations only at low energies, predicted that the scattered photon should always have the same energy as the incident one, regardless of $h\nu$ or φ. That is shown in Fig. 7.3 by the extension of the diagonal line to high energies. This curve also applies to the Compton effect for the trivial case of straight-ahead scattering, $\varphi = 0$.

The failure of the Thomson theory (see next section) to describe high-energy photon scattering necessitated the development of Compton's theory, which provides the other curves in Fig. 7.3 for the representative photon scattering angles φ = 45°, 90°, and 180°. For high-energy incident photons the backscattered photon ($\varphi = 180°$) has an energy $h\nu'$ approaching 0.2555 MeV, while side-scattered photons ($\varphi = 90°$) have $h\nu' \rightarrow 0.511$ MeV.

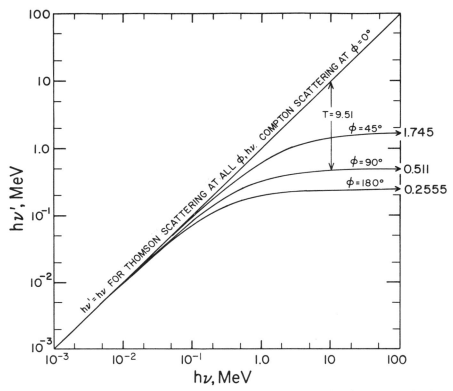

FIGURE 7.3. Graphical representation of the kinematic relationship of $h\nu$, $h\nu'$, and T in the Compton effect, as described by Eqs. (7.8) and (7.9). Curves are shown only for $\varphi = 0$, $45°$, $90°$ and $180°$. Note that T is to be interpreted as the vertical separation of any φ-curve from the $\varphi = 0$ diagonal. In the case shown ($h\nu = 10$ MeV, $\varphi = 90°$), $T = 9.51$ MeV.

The kinetic energy of the recoiling electron is given graphically in Fig. 7.3 as the vertical distance of the curve for the appropriate φ below the diagonal line, in terms of energy on the $h\nu'$ scale. Thus for the example shown by the arrow ($h\nu = 10$ MeV and $\varphi = 90°$), $T = 10 - 0.49 = 9.51$ MeV. For backscattering of photons, the electron is projected forward ($\theta = 0$) with an energy equal to $h\nu - h\nu'$, which approaches $h\nu - 0.2555$ MeV for very large $h\nu$. The photon is evidently able to transfer most of its energy to the electron in that case, but can never give away all of its energy in a Compton collision with a free electron.

Figure 7.4 contains graphs of the relationship between φ, θ, and $h\nu$ as given by Eq. (7.10), for several values of $h\nu$. When $\varphi = 0$, $\theta = 90°$, and when $\varphi = 180°$, $\theta = 0°$, for all photon energies. Obviously the electron can only be scattered in the forward hemisphere by a Compton event. The dependence of θ upon φ is a strong function of $h\nu$ between the angular extremes. For low photon energies $\theta \cong 90° -$

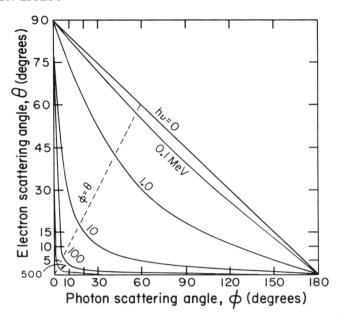

FIGURE 7.4. Relationship of the electron scattering angle θ to the photon scattering angle φ in the Compton effect, from Eq. (7.10). Curves are shown for the incident photon energies 0, 0.1, 1.0, 10, 100, and 500 MeV. The dashed line is the locus where $\theta = \varphi$, when the electron and photon are scattered at equal angles on opposite sides of the incident photon's direction.

$\varphi/2$; the electron scattering angle gradually decreases from 90° to 0° as the photon angle increases from 0° to 180°, and $\theta = \varphi$ at about 60°. At high photon energies the major variation in θ is concentrated at small φ-values, and vice versa. For example, at $h\nu = 500$ MeV, $\theta = \varphi$ at 2.59°. All photons scattered at angles between 2.59° and 180° are kinematically related to the electrons scattered forward at angles $\theta < 2.59°$. All electrons scattered at angles θ between 2.59° and 90° are likewise related to the photons scattered forward between 0 and 2.59°.

It is important to remember that Figs. 7.3 and 7.4 and Eqs. (7.8), (7.9), and (7.10) tell us nothing about the *probability* of a photon or an electron being Compton-scattered in any particular direction; that is a separate matter to be discussed in Section II.B. The foregoing figures and equations only state how the various parameters must be related to each other if a Compton interaction does occur.

B. Interaction Cross Section for the Compton Effect

1. THOMSON SCATTERING

J. J. Thomson provided the earliest theoretical description of the process by which a γ-ray photon can be scattered by an electron (see Evans, 1955). In this theory the electron was assumed to be free to oscillate under the influence of the electric vector

of an incident classical electromagnetic wave, then promptly to reemit a photon of
the same energy. The electron thus retains no kinetic energy as a result of this elastic
scattering event. This agrees with the kinematic predictions of the later relativistic
Compton treatment quite well up to about $h\nu = 0.01$ MeV, for which Eq. (7.8) gives
$h\nu' = 0.0096$ MeV. Figure 7.3 clearly shows this agreement at low photon energies.

   Thomson also deduced that the differential cross section per electron for a photon
scattered at angle φ, per unit solid angle, could be expressed as

$$\frac{d_e\sigma_0}{d\Omega_\varphi} = \frac{r_0^2}{2}(1 + \cos^2 \varphi) \tag{7.11}$$

in typical units of cm^2 sr^{-1} per electron. $r_0 = e^2/m_0c^2 = 2.818 \times 10^{-13}$ cm is called
the "classical electron radius". The value of Eq. (7.11) is 7.94×10^{-26} cm^2 sr^{-1}
e^{-1} at $\varphi = 0$ and $180°$, and half of that at $\varphi = 90°$. Thus the angular distribution
of scattered photons for a large number of events is predicted to be front–back symmetrical, according to Thomson. If the beam of photons is unpolarized, there will
also be cylindrical symmetry around the beam axis. The angular distribution of
Thomson-scattered photons is approximated by the uppermost curve in Fig. 7.5,
which was drawn to show the corresponding distribution of Compton-scattered photons for $h\nu = 0.01$ MeV. When $h\nu$ approaches zero, the two theories converge, as
relativistic considerations become irrelevant.

   The total Thomson scattering cross section per electron, $_e\sigma_0$, can be gotten by
integrating Eq. (7.11) over all directions of scattering. This will be simplified by
assuming cylindrical symmetry and integrating over $0 \le \varphi \le \pi$, noting that the
annular element of solid angle is given in terms of φ by $d\Omega_\varphi = 2\pi \sin \varphi \, d\varphi$:

$$_e\sigma_0 = \int_{\varphi=0}^{\pi} d_e\sigma_0 = \pi r_0^2 \int_{\varphi=0}^{\pi}(1 + \cos^2 \varphi)\sin \varphi \, d\varphi$$

$$= \frac{8\pi r_0^2}{3} = 6.65 \times 10^{-25} \text{ cm}^2/\text{electron} \tag{7.12}$$

   This cross section (which can be thought of as an effective target area) is numerically equal to the probability of a Thomson-scattering event occurring when
a single photon passes through a layer containing one electron per cm^2. It is also the
fraction of a large number of incident photons that scatter in passing through the
same layer, e.g., approximately 665 events for 10^{27} photons. So long as the fraction
of photons interacting in a layer of matter by *all processes combined* remains less than
about 0.05, the fraction may be assumed to be proportional to absorber thickness,
i.e., the linear approximation is adequate. For greater thicknesses the exponential
relation must be used (see Chapter 3).

   More will be said about interaction cross sections for each kind of interaction later
in the present chapter in discussing their contributions to μ_{tr}/ρ, μ_{en}/ρ, and the mass
attenuation coefficient μ/ρ.

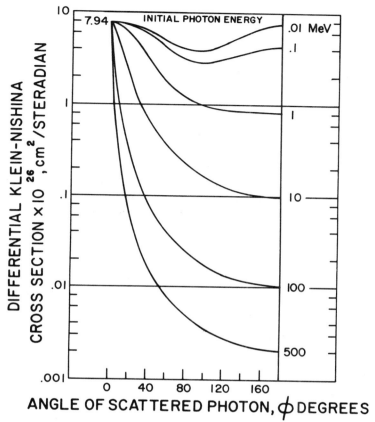

FIGURE 7.5. Differential Klein–Nishina cross section, $d_e\sigma/d\Omega_\varphi$ [see Eq. (7.13)] vs. angle φ of the scattered photon, for $h\nu = 0.01, 0.1, 1.0, 10, 100,$ and 500 MeV. This shows the angular distribution, per unit solid angle, of the scattered photons resulting from the Compton effect. (After Nelms, 1953.)

2. KLEIN–NISHINA CROSS SECTIONS FOR THE COMPTON EFFECT

In 1928 Klein and Nishina (see Evans, 1955) applied Dirac's relativistic theory of the electron to the Compton effect to obtain improved cross sections. Thomson's value of 6.65×10^{-25} cm^2/e, independent of $h\nu$, was known to be too large for $h\nu > 0.01$ MeV. The error reached a factor of 2 at $h\nu = 0.4$ MeV. The Klein–Nishina (K–N) treatment was remarkably successful in predicting the correct experimental value, even though they assumed unbound electrons, initially at rest. The differential cross section for photon scattering at angle φ, per unit solid angle and per electron, corresponding to Eq. (7.11) from Thomson's theory, may be written in the form

$$\frac{d_e\sigma}{d\Omega_\varphi} = \frac{r_0^2}{2} \left(\frac{h\nu'}{h\nu}\right)^2 \left(\frac{h\nu}{h\nu'} + \frac{h\nu'}{h\nu} - \sin^2 \varphi\right) \tag{7.13}$$

in which $h\nu'$ is given by Eq. (7.8). For low energies, as was previously pointed out, $h\nu' \cong h\nu$; hence Eq. (7.13) becomes

$$\frac{d_e\sigma}{d\Omega_\varphi} = \frac{r_0^2}{2} (2 - \sin^2 \varphi) = \frac{r_0^2}{2} (1 + \cos^2 \varphi) \tag{7.14}$$

which is identical to Eq. (7.11), verifying that the K–N differential cross section reduces to that of Thomson for the special case of low photon energies.

Figure 7.5 (Nelms, 1953) is a graphical representation of Eq. (7.13) for six values of $h\nu$. The forward bias of the scattered photons at high energies is apparent. That reference also contains eleven other carefully prepared graphs of $d_e\sigma/d\Omega_\varphi$ vs. φ for many intermediate energies, offering a very convenient display of Compton-effect data for purposes of estimation and hand calculation.*

The total K–N cross section per electron ($_e\sigma$) can be gotten from an integration of Eq. (7.13) over all photon scattering angles φ:

$$_e\sigma = 2\pi \int_{\varphi=0}^{\pi} \frac{d_e\sigma}{d\Omega_\varphi} \sin \varphi \, d\varphi$$

$$= \pi r_0^2 \int_0^\pi \left(\frac{h\nu'}{h\nu}\right)^2 \left(\frac{h\nu}{h\nu'} + \frac{h\nu'}{h\nu} - \sin^2 \varphi\right) \sin \varphi \, d\varphi$$

$$= 2\pi r_0^2 \left\{ \frac{1 + \alpha}{\alpha^2} \left[\frac{2(1 + \alpha)}{1 + 2\alpha} - \frac{\ln(1 + 2\alpha)}{\alpha} \right] + \frac{\ln(1 + 2\alpha)}{2\alpha} - \frac{1 + 3\alpha}{(1 + 2\alpha)^2} \right\} \tag{7.15}$$

where $\alpha = h\nu/m_0c^2$, in which $h\nu$ is to be expressed in MeV and $m_0c^2 = 0.511$ MeV.

Equation (7.15) is shown graphically as the upper curve of Fig. 7.6. As expected, it is almost equal to the Thomson scattering cross section (6.65×10^{-25} cm^2/e) at $h\nu = 0.01$ MeV. It decreases gradually for higher photon energies to approach a $_e\sigma \propto (h\nu)^{-1}$ dependence.

It is important to remember that $_e\sigma$, which is tabulated in Appendix D.1, is independent of the atomic number Z:

$$_e\sigma \propto Z^0 \tag{7.16}$$

since the electron binding energy has been assumed to be zero. Thus the K–N cross section per atom of any Z is given by

$$_a\sigma = Z \cdot {}_e\sigma \quad (\text{cm}^2/\text{atom}) \tag{7.17}$$

The corresponding K–N cross section per unit mass, σ/ρ, which is also called the Compton mass attenuation coefficient, is obtained from

---

*Nelms's report also has extensive families of curves of $h\nu'$ vs. φ, T vs. θ, $d_e\sigma/d\Omega_\theta$ vs. θ, $d_e\sigma/d(h\nu')$ vs. $h\nu'$, and $d\sigma/dT$ vs T. Note that Nelms' symbols differ from the present ones.

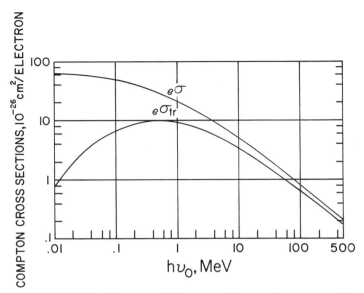

FIGURE 7.6. Klein–Nishina (Compton-effect) cross section per electron ($_e\sigma$) and corresponding energy-transfer cross section per electron ($_e\sigma_{tr}$) as a function of primary photon quantum energy $h\nu$. (After Nelms, 1953.)

$$\frac{\sigma}{\rho} = \frac{N_A Z}{A} \, _e\sigma \qquad (cm^2/g) \tag{7.18}$$

where $N_A = 6.022 \times 10^{23}$ mole^{-1} is Avogadro's constant, the number of atoms in a gram-atomic weight of any element or the number of molecules in a gram-molecular weight of any compound,

Z = number of electrons per atom of an element or per molecule of a compound,

A = number of grams per mole of material (i.e., A is the gram-atomic or molecular-weight),

ρ = density in g/cm^3, and

$N_A Z/A$ = number of electrons per gram of material.

Any interaction coefficient given in units of cm^2/g may of course be divided by 10 to convert it into units of m^2/kg.

Reviewing Eqs. 7.16–7.18 we see that $_e\sigma \propto Z^0$, $_a\sigma \propto Z$, and $\sigma/\rho \stackrel{\sim}{\propto} Z^0$, where the last, approximate proportionality requires some explanation: With the exception of hydrogen, for which $Z/A = 1$, Z/A ranges between 0.5 and 0.4, tending to decrease gradually with increasing Z (see Appendix B). The somewhat crude assumption of constant Z/A means that the Compton mass attenuation coefficient is approximately $Z -$ independent, like the electronic cross section. The atomic cross section (7.17) is proportional to Z, *one power of Z greater than the others*. This latter pattern applies to all interaction cross sections, even though their Z-dependence may differ from that of the Compton effect.

C. Energy-Transfer Cross Section for the Compton Effect

The total K–N cross section, multiplied by a unit thickness of 1 e/cm^2, also may be thought of as the fraction of the incident energy fluence, carried by a beam of many monoenergetic photons, that will be diverted into Compton interactions in passing through that layer of matter. In each interaction the energy of the incident photon ($h\nu$) is shared between the scattered photon ($h\nu'$) and the recoiling electron (T). It is of interest to know the overall fraction of $h\nu$ that is given to the electrons, averaged over all scattering angles, as this energy contributes to the kerma and thence to the dose. That is, we would like to know the value of $\overline{T}/h\nu$, where $\overline{T}$ is the average kinetic energy of the recoiling electrons. This can be obtained through first modifying the differential K–N cross section in Eq. (7.13) to obtain a quantity referred to as the differential K–N energy-transfer cross section, $d_e\sigma_{tr}/d\Omega_\varphi$:

$$\frac{d_e\sigma_{tr}}{d\Omega_\varphi} = \frac{d_e\sigma}{d\Omega_\varphi} \cdot \frac{T}{h\nu} = \frac{d_e\sigma}{d\Omega_\varphi} \cdot \frac{h\nu - h\nu'}{h\nu}$$

$$= \frac{r_0^2}{2}\left(\frac{h\nu'}{h\nu}\right)^2 \left(\frac{h\nu}{h\nu'} + \frac{h\nu'}{h\nu} - \sin^2\varphi\right)\left(\frac{h\nu - h\nu'}{h\nu}\right)$$

$$(cm^2\ sr^{-1}\ e^{-1}) \quad (7.19)$$

Integrating this over all photon scattering angles φ from 0 to 180°, as in Eq. (7.15), yields the following statement of $_e\sigma_{tr}$, the K–N energy-transfer cross section:

$$_e\sigma_{tr} = 2\pi r_0^2\left[\frac{2(1+\alpha)^2}{\alpha^2(1+2\alpha)} - \frac{1+3\alpha}{(1+2\alpha)^2} - \frac{(1+\alpha)(2\alpha^2 - 2\alpha - 1)}{\alpha^2(1+2\alpha)^2}\right.$$

$$\left. - \frac{4\alpha^2}{3(1+2\alpha)^3} - \left(\frac{1+\alpha}{\alpha^3} - \frac{1}{2\alpha} + \frac{1}{2\alpha^3}\right)\ln(1+2\alpha)\right]$$

$$(cm^2/e) \quad (7.20)$$

This cross section, multiplied by the unit thickness 1 e/cm^2, represents the fraction of the energy fluence in a monoenergetic photon beam that is diverted to the recoil electrons by Compton interactions in that layer. The Compton (or K–N) energy-transfer cross section is also plotted in Fig. 7.6 (lower curve). The vertical difference between the two curves represents the K–N cross section for the energy carried by the scattered photons, $_e\sigma_s$. Thus

$$_e\sigma = _e\sigma_{tr} + _e\sigma_s \quad (7.21)$$

The average fraction of the incident photon's energy given to the electron is simply

$$\frac{\overline{T}}{h\nu} = \frac{_e\sigma_{tr}}{_e\sigma} \quad (7.22)$$

and one can obtain the average energy of the Compton recoil electrons generated
by photons of energy $h\nu$ as

$$\overline{T} = h\nu \cdot \frac{_e\sigma_{tr}}{_e\sigma} \tag{7.23}$$

The ratios given in Eq. (7.22) are plotted in Fig. 7.7 on the basis of the data given
in Fig. 7.6. At low energies the average fraction of $h\nu$ given to the electron approaches
zero; for $h\nu = 1.6$ MeV the electrons get half, or $\overline{T} = 0.8$ MeV.

The contribution of the Compton effect to the photon mass attenuation coefficient
μ/ρ is σ/ρ. The corresponding contribution to the mass energy-transfer coefficient
is

$$\frac{\sigma_{tr}}{\rho} = \frac{N_A Z}{A} \cdot {_e\sigma_{tr}} \qquad (\text{cm}^2/\text{g}) \tag{7.24}$$

in reference to Eqs. (7.18) and (7.20).

The contributions of the several kinds of interactions to μ/ρ, μ_{tr}/ρ, and μ_{en}/ρ will
be summarized in a later section.

Before proceeding to discussions of the other types of interactions, it will be helpful
to show and explain two other useful forms of the differential K–N cross section that
were included in the compilation by Nelms (1953). The first is $d_e\sigma/d\Omega_\theta$, the differential
K–N cross section for electron scattering at angle θ, per unit solid angle and per
electron. Note that the solid angle referred to in this case means that through which
the *electron* scatters at angle θ. For $d_e\sigma/d\Omega_\varphi$ the solid angle is that through which the
photon scatters at angle φ. The relationship between these two differential cross sections is

$$\frac{d_e\sigma}{d\Omega_\theta} = \frac{d_e\sigma}{d\Omega_\varphi} \cdot \frac{(1 + \alpha)^2 (1 - \cos\varphi)^2}{\cos^3\theta} \tag{7.25}$$

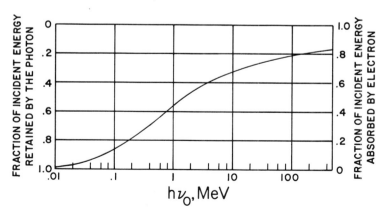

FIGURE 7.7.   Mean fraction $(\overline{T}/h\nu)$ of the incident photon's energy given to the recoiling electron in Compton interactions, averaged over all angles (right ordinate). Also, mean fraction $(h\overline{\nu}'/h\nu)$
$h\nu)$ of energy retained by the scattered photon (left ordinate).

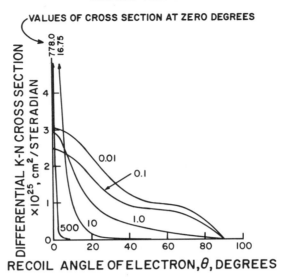

FIGURE 7.8. Differential Klein–Nishina cross section $d_e\sigma/d\,\Omega_\theta$, vs angle θ of the scattered electron for $h\nu = 0.01, 0.1, 1, 10,$ and 500 MeV. This shows the angular distribution, per unit solid angle, of the recoil electrons resulting from the Compton effect. (After Nelms, 1953.)

in which $d_e\sigma/d\Omega_\varphi$ is given by Eq. (7.13), and $\varphi = 2 \tan^{-1} [(\cot \theta)/(1 + \alpha)]$ from Eq. (7.10). Integration over all electron scattering angles from $\theta = 0$ to $90°$ must again give $_e\sigma$, as in Eq. (7.15).

Figure 7.8 displays Eq. (7.25) graphically for several values of $h\nu$, plotting $d_e\sigma/d\Omega_\theta$ vs. θ. The probability of electrons being scattered at $\theta = 90°$ approaches a constant value (zero) for all $h\nu$, while $d_e\sigma/d\Omega_\varphi = 7.94 \times 10^{-26}$ cm^2/sr e for all $h\nu$ at $\varphi = 0°$, as seen in Fig. 7.5. As the cross section decreases to $d_e\sigma/d\Omega_\varphi = 2 \times 10^{-29}$ cm^2/sr e for backscattered photons at $h\nu = 500$ MeV (Fig. 7.5), the corresponding cross section for $0°$-scattered electrons is seen from Fig. 7.8 to reach $d_e\sigma/d\Omega_\theta = 7.78 \times 10^{-23}$. This is an indication of how very strongly forward-directed the electrons become at high incident photon energies, while at the same time it becomes relatively unlikely that photons will be $180°$-backscattered. This seems to be a paradox until one refers again to Fig. 7.4, in which it is evident that high-energy photons scattered at a wide range of angles must be associated with electrons recoiling at nearly $0°$. The high forward momentum in the collision causes most of the electrons and most of the scattered photons to be strongly forward-directed when $h\nu$ is large.

The second additional form of differential K–N cross section that deserves mention here is $d_e\sigma/dT$, typically in cm^2 MeV^{-1} e^{-1}. This is the probability that a single photon will have a Compton interaction in traversing a layer containing one e/cm^2, transferring to that electron a kinetic energy between T and $T + dT$. Thus $d_e\sigma/dT$ is the energy distribution of the electrons, averaged over all scattering angles θ. It is given by the relation:

$$\frac{d_e\sigma}{dT} = \frac{\pi r_0^2 m_0 c^2}{(h\nu')^2}$$

$$\times\left\{\left[\frac{m_0 c^2 T}{(h\nu)^2}\right]^2 + 2\left[\frac{h\nu'}{h\nu}\right]^2 + \frac{h\nu'}{(h\nu)^3}\left[(T - m_0 c^2)^2 - (m_0 c^2)^2\right]\right\} \quad (7.26)$$

Figure 7.9 is a graphical representation of Equation (7.26) for several values of $h\nu$. [Nelms (1953) gives families of curves also for many intermediate energies.] It is evident that the distribution of kinetic energies given to the Compton recoiling electrons tends to be fairly flat from zero almost up to the maximum electron energy, where a higher concentration occurs. As mentioned earlier in discussing Eqs. (7.8) and (7.9), the maximum electron energy T_{max} resulting from a head-on Compton collision ($\theta = 0°$) by a photon of energy $h\nu$ is ($h\nu - h\nu'_{min}$), which is equal to

$$T_{max} = \frac{2(h\nu)^2}{2h\nu + 0.511 \text{ MeV}} \quad (7.27)$$

This approaches $h\nu - 0.2555$ MeV for large hν. The higher concentration of electrons near this energy, as seen in Fig. 7.9, is consistent with the high probability of electron scattering near $\theta = 0°$, shown in Fig. 7.8. Both trends become more pronounced at high energies.

It should be remembered that the energy distributions shown in Fig. 7.9 are those occurring at production. The spectrum of Compton-electron energies present at a point in an extended medium under irradiation is generally degraded by the presence

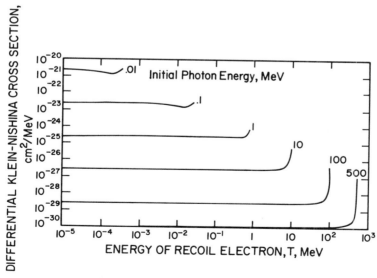

FIGURE 7.9. Differential Klein–Nishina cross section $d_e\sigma/dT$ expressing the initial energy spectrum of Compton recoiling electrons. (After Nelms, 1953.)

of electrons that have lost varying amounts of their energy depending on how far they have traveled through the medium. Under charged-particle equilibrium conditions this degraded electron energy distribution is called an ''equilibrium spectrum.'' Such degraded spectra will be discussed in connection with cavity theory in Chapter 10.

Turner et al. (1980) and Todo et al. (1982) have provided useful spectra of electron starting energies resulting from monoenergetic photon interactions in water, calculated by the Monte Carlo method. They included contributions from the other interaction modes, in addition to Compton recoil-electron spectra.

III. PHOTOELECTRIC EFFECT

The photoelectric effect is the most important interaction of low-energy photons with matter, as indicated in Fig. 7.1. While the Compton effect's interaction cross section approaches a constant value, and its energy-transfer cross section diminishes as $h\nu$ decreases below 0.5 MeV (see Fig. 7.6), the corresponding cross sections for the photoelectric effect both increase strongly, especially for high-Z media. Consequently the photoelectric effect totally predominates over the Compton effect at low photon energies, particularly with respect to the energy transferred to secondary electrons.

A. Kinematics

It was seen in the case of the Compton effect that a photon cannot give up all of its energy in colliding with a free electron. However, it can do so in an encounter with a tightly bound electron, such as those in the inner shells of an atom, especially of high atomic number. This is called the photoelectric effect and is illustrated schematically in Fig. 7.10. An incident photon of quantum energy $h\nu$ is shown interacting with an atomic-shell electron bound by potential energy E_b. The photoelectric effect

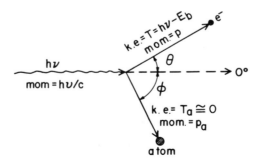

FIGURE 7.10.   Kinematics of the photoelectric effect. A photon of quantum energy $h\nu$ incident from the left strikes an electron bound to an atom with binding energy E_b. The photon vanishes, giving a kinetic energy of $T = h\nu - E_b$ to the electron, which departs at angle θ relative to the incident photon's direction. To conserve momentum the remainder of the atom departs at an angle φ. The atom's kinetic energy T_a is practically zero.

cannot take place with respect to a given electron unless $h\nu > E_b$ for that electron. The smaller $h\nu$ is, the more likely is the occurrence of the photoelectric effect, so long as $h\nu > E_b$. The photon is totally absorbed in the interaction, and ceases to exist. The kinetic energy given to the electron, *independent of its scattering angle θ*, is

$$T = h\nu - E_b - T_a \qquad (7.28)$$

$$= h\nu - E_b \qquad (7.29)$$

The kinetic energy T_a given to the recoiling atom is nearly zero,[*] justifying the conventional use of an equality sign rather than an approximation sign in Eq. (7.29).

The electron departs from the interaction at an angle θ relative to the photon's direction of incidence, carrying momentum p. Since the photon has been totally absorbed, it provides no scattered photon to assist in conserving momentum, as in the Compton effect case. In the photoelectric effect that role is assumed by the atom from which the electron was removed. Although its kinetic energy $T_a \cong 0$, its momentum p_a cannot be negligible. The direction taken by the recoiling atom is of little consequence, since it carries negligible kinetic energy. Suffice it to say that the atom scatters in the direction required to conserve momentum in each photoelectric event, and that $0 < \varphi < 180°$.

B.   Interaction Cross Section for the Photoelectric Effect

Theoretical derivation of the interaction cross section for the photoelectric effect is more difficult than for the Compton effect, because of the complications arising from the binding of the electron. There is no simple equation for the differential photoelectric cross section that corresponds to the K–N formula. However, satisfactory solutions have been reported by different authors for several photon energy regions, as discussed by Evans (1955) and more recently by Hubbell (1969). Published tables of photoelectric interaction coefficients such as those in the latter reference are based on experimental results, supplemented by theoretically assisted interpolations for other energies and absorbing media than those measured.

The directional distribution of photoelectrons per unit solid angle is shown in Fig. 7.11. These are theoretical results from a review by Davisson and Evans (1952). The photoelectrons are seen to be ejected predominately sideways for low photon energies, because they tend to be emitted in the direction of the photon's electric vector. With increasing photon energy this distribution gets pushed more and more toward smaller (but still nonzero) angles. Electron scattering at $0°$ is forbidden because that is perpendicular to the electric vector.

A summary representation of the angular distribution of photoelectrons is conveyed by the bipartition angle shown in Fig. 7.12. One-half of all the photoelectrons are ejected at angles θ less than the bipartition angle. For example, photons of 0.5

---

[*] $T_a/T = m_0/M_0$, where m_0 is the rest mass of the electron and M_0 that of the recoiling atom. For example, an atom of ^{27}Al would carry approximately 0.002 % as much kinetic energy as the photoelectron. Heavier atoms would carry even less.

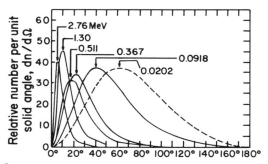

θ= angle photoelectrons make with direction of γ rays

FIGURE 7.11.   Directional distribution of photoelectrons per unit solid angle, for energies as labeled on the curves. The curve areas are not normalized to each other. [After Davisson and Evans (1952). Reproduced with permission of R. D. Evans and the American Physical Society.]

MeV send out half of their photoelectrons within a forward cone of half angle $\cong 30°$, and the remainder at larger angles.

The interaction cross section per atom for photoelectric effect, integrated over all angles of photoelectron emission, can be written as

$$_a\tau \cong k\,\frac{Z^n}{(h\nu)^m} \qquad \text{(cm}^2\text{/atom)} \tag{7.30}$$

where k is a constant,

$n \cong 4$ at $h\nu = 0.1$ MeV, gradually rising to about 4.6 at 3 MeV, and

$m \cong 3$ at $h\nu = 0.1$ MeV, gradually decreasing to about 1 at 5 MeV.

In the energy region $h\nu \cong 0.1$ MeV and below, where the photoelectric effect becomes most important, it is convenient to remember that

$$_a\tau \propto \frac{Z^4}{(h\nu)^3} \qquad \text{(cm}^2\text{/atom)} \tag{7.31}$$

and consequently that the photoelectric mass attenuation coefficient becomes [by employing the conversion factors in Eqs. (7.17) and (7.18)]

$$\frac{\tau}{\rho} \propto \left(\frac{Z}{h\nu}\right)^3 \qquad \text{(cm}^2\text{/g)} \tag{7.32}$$

This approximate relationship may be compared with the curves in Fig. 7.13,

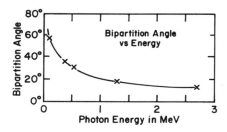

FIGURE 7.12.   Bipartition angle of photoelectrons vs $h\nu$. One-half of all the photoelectrons are ejected within a forward cone of half angle equal to the bipartition angle. [After Davisson and Evans (1952). Reproduced with permission of R. D. Evans and the American Physical Society.]

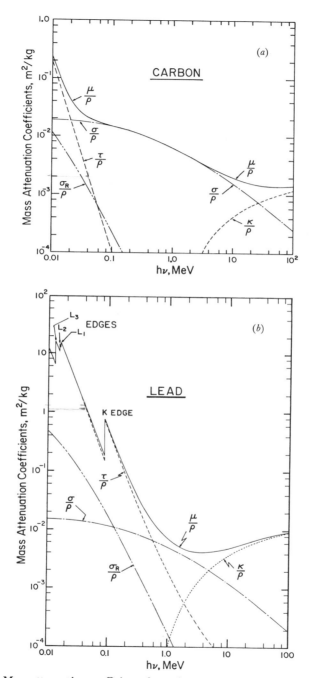

FIGURE 7.13. Mass attenuation coefficients for carbon (*a*) and lead (*b*). τ/ρ indicates the contribution of the photoelectric effect, σ/ρ is that of the Compton effect, κ/ρ that of pair production, and σ_R/ρ that of Rayleigh (coherent) scattering. μ/ρ is their sum, which is closely approximated in Pb by the τ/ρ curve below $h\nu = 0.1$ MeV (From data of Hubbell, 1969).

derived from empirically based tabulated values. The curve labeled τ/ρ in part *a* represents the photoelectric mass attenuation coefficient for carbon, and in part *b* that for lead, plotted vs. $h\nu$. The carbon curve clearly approximates the $(h\nu)^{-3}$ dependence; the lead does likewise except where the breaks occur. Below the so-called ''K-edge'' at 88 keV, the two K-shell electrons cannot participate in the photoelectric effect because their binding energy $(E_b)_K = 88$ keV is too great. Only the L, M, and higher-shell electrons can do so. Just above 88 keV the K-electrons can also participate. Thus the magnitude of the resulting step function (from 7.1 down to 1.7 cm²/g) indicates the importance of the contribution of the two K-shell electrons to the photoelectric cross section, in comparison with the other 80 electrons in the atom. The K-shell contributes over three-fourths, because of the large binding energy of those two electrons and the strong dependence of the photoelectric effect upon binding energy. The L-shell shows a similar effect at the three L edges (L_1 at 15.9, L_2 at 15.2, and L_3 at 13.0 keV) which correspond to the three energy levels in the L shell. The combined L-edge step is smaller than that at the K-edge, because of the lower L-shell binding energies.

Referring again to Fig. 7.13, it can also be seen that the (τ/ρ) curve in lead is roughly three decades higher than that in carbon in the low-energy region, as predicted by Eq. (7.32), since $Z_{Pb} = 82$ is of the order of 10 times greater than $Z_C = 6$.

C. Energy-Transfer Cross Section for the Photoelectric Effect

It is evident from the conservation-of-energy equation (7.29) for the photoelectric effect that the fraction of $h\nu$ that is transferred to the photoelectron is simply

$$\frac{T}{h\nu} = \frac{h\nu - E_b}{h\nu} \tag{7.33}$$

However, this is only a first approximation to the total fraction of $h\nu$ that is transferred to all electrons. The binding energy E_b must be taken into account, and part or all of it is converted into electron kinetic energy through the *Auger effect*, to be considered next.

When an electron is removed from an inner atomic shell by any process, such as the photoelectric effect, internal conversion, electron capture, or charged-particle collision, the resulting vacancy is promptly filled by another electron falling from a less tightly bound shell. For K- and L-shell vacancies this transition is sometimes accompanied by the emission of a fluorescence x-ray of quantum energy $h\nu_K$ or $h\nu_L$, respectively, equal to the difference in potential energy between the donor and recipient levels, as discussed in Chapter 9, Section II.A. The probability of this happening is called the *fluorescence yield*, Y_K or Y_L, respectively; values are plotted in Fig. 7.14 as a function of atomic number. Y_K is seen to rise rapidly for $Z > 10$, gradually approaching unity for high-Z elements, while Y_L is practically zero below copper, rising to only 0.42 at $Z = 90$. The chance of fluorescence x-ray emission during the filling of a vacancy in the M (or higher) shell is negligibly small.

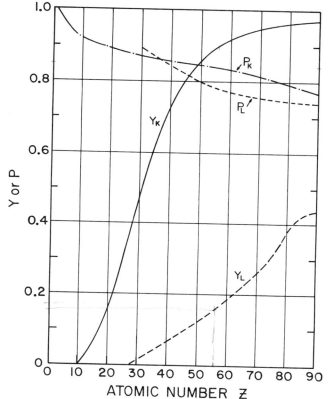

FIGURE 7.14. Fluorescence yield ($Y_{K,L}$) and fractional participation in the photoelectric effect ($P_{K,L}$) by K- and L-shell electrons (see text). P_K and P_L was calculated from tables of Hubbell (1969) and McMaster et al. (1969); Y_K from Lederer and Shirley (1979); and Y_L from Burhop (1952).

The role of the Auger effect is to provide an alternative mechanism by which the atom can dispose of whatever part of the binding energy E_b is not removed by a fluorescence x-ray. If no x-ray is emitted, then all of E_b is disposed of by the Auger process. In the Auger effect the atom ejects one or more of its electrons with sufficient kinetic energy to account collectively for the excess energy. Thus any energy invested in such Auger electrons contributes to the kerma.

An atom may emit a number of Auger electrons more or less simultaneously in a kind of chain reaction. The atom thus exchanges one energetically "deep" inner-shell vacancy for a number of relatively shallow outer-shell vacancies. These vacancies are finally neutralized by conduction-band electrons.

The energy budget in the Auger effect is illustrated in the following example: Suppose a K-shell vacancy appears, with binding energy $(E_b)_K$. Assume that an electron falls in from the L-shell, as is most often the case. Letting the binding energy in that shell be $(E_b)_L$, either the atom will emit an x-ray of energy $h\nu_K = (E_b)_K - (E_b)_L$, or it must dispose of that energy [as well as the remaining energy $(E_b)_K - h\nu_K$] through the Auger effect. (Notice that for intuitive convenience we are treating the binding energies as positive potentials, whereas they are actually negative.) Assuming that the atom opts entirely for the Auger effect, it may eject an electron from any shell outside of that in which the original vacancy occurred, in this case the K-shell. If an M-shell electron is ejected, it will have a kinetic energy T_M equal to

$$T_M = (E_b)_K - (E_b)_L - (E_b)_M \qquad (7.34a)$$

where $(E_b)_M$ is the binding energy in the M shell.

Now the atom has two electron vacancies, one in the L- and one in the M-shell. Let us assume that two N-shell electrons move in to fill those vacancies, and that the atom emits two more Auger electrons. If they both happened to be ejected from the N-shell, the atom would then have *four* N-shell vacancies. One of the those Auger electrons would have the kinetic energy

$$T_{N1} = (E_b)_L - 2(E_b)_N \qquad (7.34b)$$

and the other would have

$$T_{N2} = (E_b)_M - 2(E_b)_N \qquad (7.34c)$$

Thus the total kinetic energy of the three Auger electrons generated so far would be equal to

$$T_A = T_M + T_{N1} + T_{N2} = (E_b)_K - 4(E_b)_N \qquad (7.34d)$$

This process is repeated, increasing the number of electron vacancies by one for each Auger event that occurs, until all the vacancies are located in the outermost shell(s). The total amount of kinetic energy carried by all the Auger electrons together is equal to the original-shell binding energy $(E_b)_K$ minus the sum of the binding energies of all the final electron vacancies. As these are subsequently neutralized by electrons from the conduction band, those electrons as they approach will acquire kinetic energies equal to the outer-shell binding energies of the vacancies they fill. Thus *all* of $(E_b)_K$ in this example ends up as electron kinetic energy, contributing to the kerma. If an x-ray $h\nu_K$ had been emitted, then the remainder of $(E_b)_K$ would have become electron kinetic energy.

It should be mentioned that since an Auger chain reaction or "shower" suddenly produces a multiply charged ion, which may have a net positive charge even in excess of 10 elementary charges, the resulting local Coulomb-force field can be quite disruptive to its molecular or crystalline surroundings.

Returning now to consideration of fluorescence x-rays, it is shown in Chapter 9, Section II.A, that there are several levels in the L or higher shells from which the K-shell replacement electron may come, although some specific transitions are quantum-mechanically forbidden to occur. As a result $h\nu_K$ has several closely grouped values that may be represented for present purposes by a mean value $h\bar{\nu}_K$. Figure

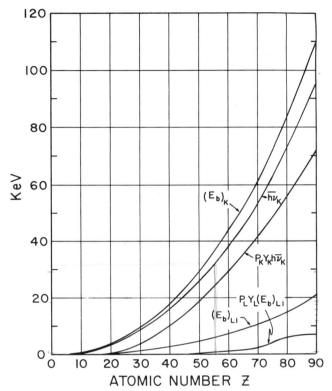

FIGURE 7.15. Electron binding energies $(E_b)_K$ in the K-shell and $(E_b)_{L1}$ in the $L1$-shell; weighted mean fluorescence x-ray energy $h\bar{\nu}_K$ in the K-shell; and the products $P_K Y_K \cdot h\bar{\nu}_K$ and $P_L Y_L (E_b)_{L1}$. The latter provides an upper-limit estimate of $P_L Y_L h\bar{\nu}_L$. Taken or derived from tables by Lederer and Shirley (1979).

7.15 contains a graph of $h\bar{\nu}_K$ vs. Z, which may be compared with the uppermost curve of K-shell binding energy $(E_b)_K$. Naturally $h\bar{\nu}_K < (E_b)_K$, because $(E_b)_K$ represents the difference in potential energy between an electron in the K-shell and one completely away from the atom, while fluorescence photons result from smaller transitions.

In addition to the fluorescence yields, Fig. 7.14 contains a second kind of function: P_K is the fraction (τ_K/τ) of all photoelectric interactions that occur in the K-shell, for photons for which $h\nu > (E_b)_K$. (This is the fraction obtainable from the height of the K-edge step, as mentioned earlier in relation to Fig. 7.13b). Likewise $P_L = \tau_L/\tau$ for photons where $(E_b)_{L1} < h\nu < (E_b)_K$. The product $P_K Y_K$ then is the fraction of all photoelectric events in which a K-fluorescence x-ray is emitted by the atom, and $P_L Y_L$ is the corresponding quantity for the L-shell, for the appropriate ranges of $h\nu$. The product $P_K Y_K \cdot h\bar{\nu}_K$ then represents the mean energy carried away from the atom by K-fluorescence x-rays, per photoelectric interaction in all shells combined, where

$h\nu > (E)_K$. An upper limit of a similar L-shell quantity $P_L Y_L \cdot h\bar{\nu}_L$ can be estimated as $P_L Y_L(E_b)_{L1}$. Both of these quantities are plotted in Fig. 7.15, and their use will be shown in subsequent discussion.

The probability of any other fluorescence x-ray except those from the K-shell being able to carry energy out of an atom is negligible for $h\nu > (E_b)_K$. For that case all the rest of the binding energy $(E_b)_K$, and all of the binding energy involved in photoelectric interactions in other shells, may be assumed to be given to Auger electrons. Thus we can write for the mean energy transferred to charged particles per photoelectric event

$$h\nu - P_K Y_K \cdot h\bar{\nu}_K \tag{7.35}$$

The photoelectric mass energy-transfer coefficient is thus given by

$$\frac{\tau_{tr}}{\rho} = \frac{\tau}{\rho}\left[\frac{h\nu - P_K Y_K h\bar{\nu}_K - (1 - P_K) P_L Y_L h\bar{\nu}_L}{h\nu}\right] \tag{7.36a}$$

for $h\nu > (E_b)_K$.

For photons having energies lying between the K and the highest L edge, [i.e., $(E_b)_{L1} < h\nu < (E_b)_K$], the corresponding equation for τ_{tr}/ρ can be written as

$$\frac{\tau_{tr}}{\rho} = \frac{\tau}{\rho}\left[\frac{h\nu - P_L Y_L \cdot h\bar{\nu}_L}{h\nu}\right] \tag{7.36b}$$

where $P_L Y_L \cdot h\bar{\nu}_L$ can be approximated by $P_L Y_L(E_b)_{L1}$, as plotted in Fig. 7.15; this quantity is insignificant except in high-Z materials.

It should be noted that even though fluorescence x-rays may carry some energy out of the atom of their origin, the distance that such an x-ray can penetrate through the medium before undergoing another photoelectric interaction will be severely limited. For example, the K-fluorescence from lead averages $\cong 76$ keV, for which the mass energy-absorption coefficient in lead is $\cong 0.23$ m^2/kg, and the broad-beam 10th-value layer is about 1 mm. For L fluorescence the photon penetration distance in lead is of the order of $\frac{1}{100}$ as great.

Figure 7.16 shows the mass energy-transfer coefficients for carbon and lead, corresponding to the attenuation coefficients shown in Fig. 7.13. Notice that the curve for $(\mu_{tr}/\rho)_{Pb}$ is practically equal to $(\tau_{tr}/\rho)_{Pb}$ for $h\nu \lesssim 0.1$ MeV, and that the size of the K-edge step is somewhat less here than in Fig. 7.13, due to the loss of K-fluorescence energy as indicated by Eq. (7.36a).

IV. PAIR PRODUCTION

Pair production is an absorption process in which a photon disappears and gives rise to an electron and a positron. It can only occur in a Coulomb force field, usually that near an atomic nucleus. However it can also take place, with lower probability, in the field of an atomic electron. This latter process is usually called "triplet production," because the host electron that provides the Coulomb field also acquires significant kinetic energy in conserving momentum. Thus two electrons and a positron are ejected from the site of the interaction. A minimum photon energy of $2m_0c^2$

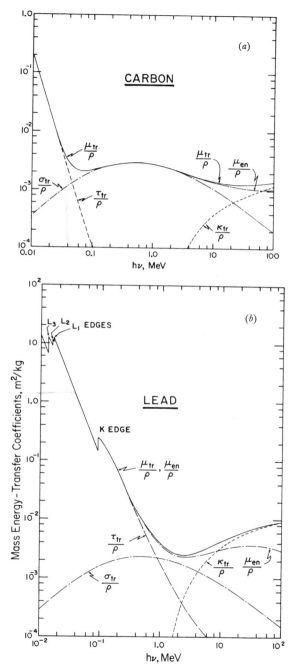

FIGURE 7.16. Mass energy-transfer coefficients for carbon (*a*) and lead (*b*). τ_{tr}/ρ indicates the contribution of the photoelectric effect, σ_{tr}/ρ that of the Compton effect, and κ_{tr}/ρ that of pair production. μ_{tr}/ρ represents their sum. The total mass energy-absorption coefficient (μ_{en}/ρ) is also shown. Note that these μ_{en}/ρ data for $h\nu > 10$ MeV do not take into account in-flight annihilation. Data after Hubbell (1969).

147

= 1.022 MeV is obviously required for pair production to occur in the nuclear field. $4m_0c^2$ is the threshold for triplet production, because of momentum-conservation considerations to be discussed later.

A. Pair Production in the Nuclear Coulomb Force Field

Figure 7.17 illustrates schematically a pair-production event in a nuclear field. The incident photon $h\nu$ gives up all of its quantum energy in the creation of the electron–positron pair with kinetic energies T^- and T^+. The energy-conservation equation, ignoring the vanishingly small kinetic energy given to the nucleus, is simply

$$h\nu = 2m_0c^2 + T^- + T^+$$

$$= 1.022 \text{ MeV} + T^- + T^+ \tag{7.37}$$

The electron and positron do not necessarily receive equal kinetic energies, but their average is given by

$$\overline{T} = \frac{h\nu - 1.022 \text{ MeV}}{2} \tag{7.38}$$

For $h\nu$ values well above the threshold energy $2m_0c^2$, the electrons and positrons are strongly forward directed. Their average angle of departure relative to the original photon direction is roughly

$$\overline{\theta} \cong \frac{m_0c^2}{\overline{T}} \quad \text{(radians)} \tag{7.39}$$

For example, for $h\nu = 5$ MeV, we have $\overline{T} = 1.989$ MeV and $\overline{\theta} \cong 0.26$ radians = 15°.

From a theory due to Bethe and Heitler, the atomic differential cross section $d(_a\kappa)$ for the creation of a positron of energy T^+ (and a corresponding electron of energy $h\nu - 2m_0c^2 - T^+$) is given by

$$d(_a\kappa) = \frac{\sigma_0 Z^2 P}{h\nu - 2m_0c^2} dT^+ \quad \text{(cm}^2\text{/atom)} \tag{7.40}$$

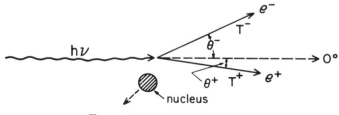

FIGURE 7.17. Pair production in the Coulomb force field of an atomic nucleus. An incident photon of quantum energy $h\nu$ vanishes, giving rise to a positron–electron pair. The atom participates in conservation of momentum, but receives negligible kinetic energy $T_a \cong 0$.

where

$$\sigma_0 = \frac{r_0^2}{137} = \frac{1}{137}\left(\frac{e^2}{m_0c^2}\right)^2 = 5.80 \times 10^{-28} \text{ cm}^2/\text{electron},$$

and parameter P is a function of $h\nu$ and Z. P is displayed graphically in Figure 7.18 as a function of the fraction of the total kinetic energy that resides with the positron. A slight expected asymmetry in energy distributions between the positron and electron was neglected in deriving these P-values, which thus appear symmetrical about $T^+/(h\nu - 2m_0c^2) = 0.5$. Nuclear attraction and repulsion tend to give the positron slightly more energy than the electron, the difference being less than $0.0075Z$ MeV (Evans, 1955).

The total nuclear pair-production cross section per atom may be gotten by integrating $d(_a\kappa)$ from Eq. (7.40) over all values of T^+:

$$_a\kappa = \int_{T^+} d(_a\kappa) = \sigma_0 Z^2 \int_0^{(h\nu - 2m_0c^2)} \frac{P\, dT^+}{h\nu - 2m_0c^2}$$

$$= \sigma_0 Z^2 \int_0^1 P\, d\left(\frac{T^+}{h\nu - 2m_0c^2}\right) = \sigma_0 Z^2 \overline{P} \qquad (7.41)$$

Evidently $_a\kappa$ is proportional to the atomic number squared. The dependence of $_a\kappa$ upon $h\nu$ is roughly logarithmic through the $\overline{P}$-term, tending to become a constant

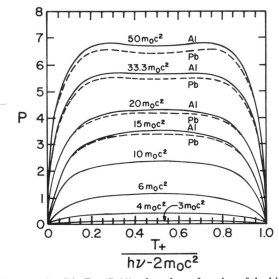

FIGURE 7.18.   The quantity P in Eq. (7.41), plotted as a function of the kinetic-energy fraction given to the positron. The small difference between lead and aluminum shows the small amount of Z-dependence. [After Davisson and Evans (1952). Reproduced with permission of R. D. Evans and the American Physical Society.]

independent of $h\nu$ for very large $h\nu$ because of electron screening of the nuclear field (see Fig. 7.13).

The mass attenuation coefficient for nuclear pair-production is obtained from Eq. (7.41) as

$$\frac{\kappa}{\rho} = {}_a\kappa \frac{N_A}{A} \qquad (cm^2/g) \tag{7.42}$$

Again, since Z/A is roughly constant ($= 0.45 \pm 0.05$) except for hydrogen, κ/ρ $\tilde{\propto} Z$.

B. Pair Production in the Electron Field

In the kinematics of pair production in the electron field (i.e., triplet production), the photon divides its energy between the positron–electron pair produced and the host electron. The energy conservation equation becomes

$$h\nu = 1.022 \text{ MeV} + T^+ + T_1^- + T_2^- \tag{7.43}$$

and the average kinetic energy of the three particles is

$$\overline{T} = \frac{h\nu - 1.022 \text{ MeV}}{3} \tag{7.44}$$

As mentioned earlier, the threshold for this process is $4m_0c^2 = 2.044$ MeV, even though the energy being converted into mass is still $2m_0c^2$, the same as for nuclear-field pair production. It can be shown, as follows, that the higher threshold is required by conservation of momentum, as first derived by Perrin (1933).

In Fig. 7.19a a photon of energy $h\nu$ is shown approaching an electron e_1^- assumed to be at rest in the laboratory frame of reference, R. For convenience the same two particles are considered in Fig. 7.19b with respect to a moving frame of reference R', in which the momentum of the photon–electron system is null. The velocity of R' relative to R is $+\beta c$, that is, R' moves to the right with constant velocity. This makes the electron appear to move to the left with the same speed, i.e., $v = -\beta c$.

The resulting momentum of the electron is $-m\beta c = -m_0\beta c/\sqrt{1 - \beta^2}$, where m is the electron's relativistic mass with respect to R'. The photon's momentum relative to R' is $h\nu'/c$. Thus for null momentum we can write

$$\frac{h\nu'}{c} - \frac{m_0\beta c}{\sqrt{1 - \beta^2}} = 0 \tag{7.45}$$

The Doppler effect causes the frequency ν' of the photon relative to the moving frame of reference to be less than ν, according to the relation

$$\nu' = \nu \sqrt{\frac{1 - \beta}{1 + \beta}} \tag{7.46}$$

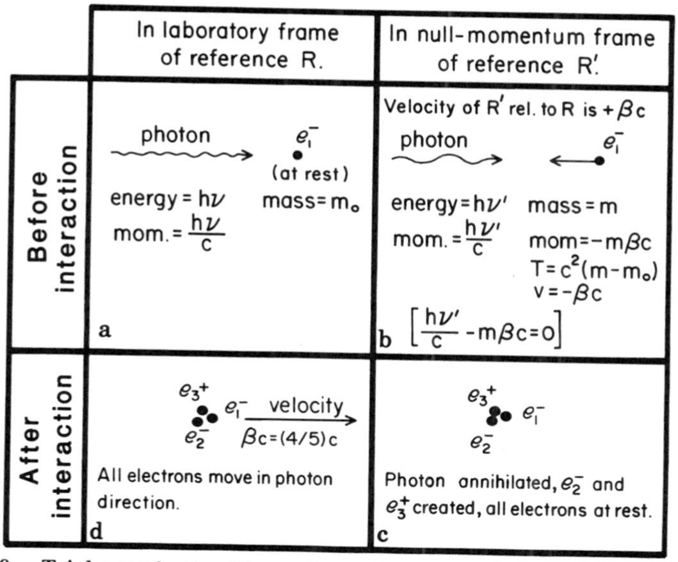

	In laboratory frame of reference R.	In null-momentum frame of reference R'.

Before interaction	photon $\longrightarrow$ e_1^- (at rest)
	
	energy = $h\nu$ mass = m_o
	
	mom. = $\dfrac{h\nu}{c}$
	
	a
		Velocity of R' rel. to R is $+\beta c$
		
		photon $\longrightarrow$ $\longleftarrow e_1^-$
		
		energy = $h\nu'$ mass = m
		
		mom. = $\dfrac{h\nu'}{c}$ mom. = $-m\beta c$
		  $T = c^2(m - m_o)$
		  $v = -\beta c$
		
		$\left[\dfrac{h\nu'}{c} - m\beta c = 0\right]$
		
		b

After interaction	e_3^+ e_1^- velocity $\longrightarrow$ e_2^- $\beta c = (4/5)c$ All electrons move in photon direction. d	e_3^+ e_1^- e_2^- Photon annihilated, e_2^- and e_3^+ created, all electrons at rest. c

FIGURE 7.19. Triplet-production kinematics at the minimum photon energy threshold, $h\nu = h\nu_{min}$. Diagrams at left apply to the laboratory frame of reference R, those at right to moving frame of reference R'. The momentum of the photon–electron system is zero in R'.

Substitution of Eq. (7.46) to eliminate ν' in Eq. (7.45) allows solution for β:

$$\beta = \frac{\alpha}{1 + \alpha} \tag{7.47}$$

in which

$$\alpha \equiv \frac{h\nu}{m_0 c^2} \tag{7.48}$$

The minimum photon energy, $h\nu_{min}$, necessary for triplet production can be derived by noting that the sum of the photon energy $h\nu'_{min}$ and the electron kinetic energy T relative to R' must just equal the total rest mass of the electron and positron created. That is,

$$h\nu'_{min} + m_0 c^2 \left(\frac{1}{\sqrt{1 - \beta^2_{min}}} - 1\right) = 2 m_0 c^2 \tag{7.49}$$

where

$$h\nu'_{min} = h\nu_{min}\sqrt{\frac{1 - \beta_{min}}{1 + \beta_{min}}}, \qquad \beta_{min} = \frac{\alpha_{min}}{1 + \alpha_{min}}, \qquad \alpha_{min} \equiv \frac{h\nu_{min}}{m_0 c^2}$$

This equation can be solved for β_{min}, which is found to have the value $\frac{4}{5}$. Thus $h\nu_{min}$ = $4m_0c^2$.

It is interesting to observe that, in the moving frame of reference R', the two electrons and the positron all must be at rest after a minimum-$h\nu$ event, as shown in Fig. 7.19c. This is so because all of the available quantum and kinetic energy has been spent in mass creation, leaving none for motion. As a consequence, in the laboratory frame of reference all three particles in the triplet move together in the original photon's direction with velocity $(\beta c)_{min} = \frac{4}{5}c$, as shown in Fig. 7.19d.

For higher incident photon energy than $4m_0c^2$ the three particles may share the excess energy and depart the point of the interaction in various directions, so long as the null momentum is preserved relative to R'. Perrin has shown that the kinetic energy of each of the particles, relative to the laboratory system, lies within the limits given by

$$T = \frac{\alpha^2 - 2\alpha - 2 \pm \alpha\sqrt{\alpha(\alpha - 4)}}{2\alpha + 1} \tag{7.50}$$

This reduces to $2m_0c^2/3$ for the threshold case in which $\alpha = 4$, meaning that the particles in Fig. 7.19d each have a kinetic energy equal to $\frac{1}{3}$ of the $2m_0c^2$ energy not needed for mass creation. For 10-MeV photons Eq. (7.50) predicts that the product particles each have energies between 3 keV and 8.7 MeV.

The atomic cross section for triplet production (i.e., for all the atomic electrons combined) is small compared to the nuclear pair-production cross section for the same atom. The ratio is given approximately by

$$\frac{_a\kappa(\text{electrons})}{_a\kappa(\text{nucleus})} \cong \frac{1}{CZ} \tag{7.51}$$

in which C is a parameter depending only on $h\nu$. C is unity for $h\nu \rightarrow \infty$, and rises slowly with decreasing energy to $\cong 2$ at 5 MeV (see discussion given by Evans, 1955). Thus in Pb the triplet cross section is only 1% or so of the pair-production cross section, rising to 5-10% for $Z = 10$.

For most purposes in radiological physics and dosimetry it will suffice to combine the separate cross sections for pair and triplet production into a single cross section for both, usually still called the pair-production cross section. Thus

$$\left(\frac{\kappa}{\rho}\right)_{\text{pair}} = \left(\frac{\kappa}{\rho}\right)_{\text{nuclear}} + \left(\frac{\kappa}{\rho}\right)_{\text{electron}} \tag{7.52}$$

C. Pair-Production Energy-Transfer Coefficient

The fraction of the incident photon's energy that is transferred to the kinetic energy of the charged particles, both for nuclear and electron pair production, is $(h\nu - 2m_0c^2)/h\nu$. Therefore the mass energy-transfer coefficient for pair production is given by

$$\frac{\kappa_{tr}}{\rho} = \frac{\kappa}{\rho}\left(\frac{h\nu - 2m_0c^2}{h\nu}\right) \tag{7.53}$$

V. RAYLEIGH (COHERENT) SCATTERING

Rayleigh scattering is called "coherent" because the photon is scattered by the combined action of the whole atom. The event is elastic in the sense that the photon loses essentially none of its energy; the atom moves just enough to conserve momentum. The photon is usually redirected through only a small angle. Therefore the effect on a photon beam can only be detected in narrow-beam geometry. Rayleigh scattering contributes nothing to kerma or dose, since no energy is given to any charged particle, nor is any ionization or excitation produced.

The photon scattering angle depends on both Z and $h\nu$: $\frac{2}{3}$ of the photons are scattered at angles smaller than these, according to Fano (1953a):

$h\nu$	$h\nu = 0.1$ MeV	1 MeV	10 MeV
Al	15°	2°	0.5°
Pb	30°	4°	1.0°

It is seen that Rayleigh scattering has more practical importance at low energies, partly because the scattering angle is greater.

The atomic cross section for Rayleigh scattering is given by

$$_a\sigma_R \propto \frac{Z^2}{(h\nu)^2} \quad (\text{cm}^2/\text{atom}) \tag{7.54}$$

or in mass units

$$\frac{\sigma_R}{\rho} \propto \frac{Z}{(h\nu)^2} \quad (\text{cm}^2/\text{g or m}^2/\text{kg}) \tag{7.55}$$

Typical ratios of Rayleigh to total attenuation coefficients (σ_R/μ) are shown in the following table, derived from the tables of Hubbell (1969):

Element	$h\nu = 0.01$ MeV	0.1 MeV	1.0 MeV
C	0.07	0.02	0
Cu	0.006	0.08	0.007
Pb	0.03	0.03	0.03

The relative importance of Rayleigh scattering is seen to be fairly small, as it contributes only a few percent or less of the narrow-beam attenuation coefficient. Pronounced trends vs. Z and $h\nu$ tend to be obscured by variations in the competing interactions—photoelectric effect and Compton effect. However, for low Z (e.g., carbon) a gain is evident with decreasing photon energy.

The mass attenuation coefficient for Rayleigh scattering is shown in relation to the other interaction coefficients in Fig. 7.13. Rough agreement with Eq. (7.55) can be seen.

VI. PHOTONUCLEAR INTERACTIONS

In a photonuclear interaction an energetic photon (exceeding a few MeV) enters and excites a nucleus, which then emits a proton or neutron. (γ, p) events contribute directly to the kerma, but the relative amount remains less than 5% of that due to pair production. Thus it has been commonly neglected in dosimetry considerations.

(γ, n) interactions have greater practical importance because the neutrons thus produced may lead to problems in radiation protection. This is the case for clinical x-ray generators (Linacs, microtrons, betatrons) in which electrons are accelerated to 10 MeV or more. The x-ray beam will be slightly contaminated with neutrons, to a degree depending on accelerator energy and design. A 25-MV x-ray beam will usually have an order-of-magnitude greater neutron contamination than a 10-MV beam, because of the correspondingly greater (γ, n) interaction cross section. The biological consequences of these neutrons in a radiotherapy patient are probably negligible in comparison with the effects of the predominating photon beam. Nevertheless, as a precaution, governmental regulatory agencies are placing limitations on allowable neutron levels in radiotherapy x-ray beams.

The presence of (γ, n) neutrons must be taken into account in shielding design, especially since neutrons can escape through mazes much more readily than photons can. Moreover, neutrons can activate accelerator hardware, especially in the target region. Such hardware may require a time delay before approaching for service, and should always be monitored first for γ- and β-activity. Some low level of radioactivation may also occur in the body tissues of radiotherapy patients, due either to incident neutrons or to photonuclear interactions occurring in the body itself.

All of these consequences of (γ, n) interactions can be regarded as unwanted side effects of the use of higher-energy radiotherapy x-ray beams, offset by the increasingly favorable spatial distributions of dose in the body that can be achieved by such beams. Swanson (1979) has provided useful estimates of (γ, n) neutron production in accelerators. Anderson (1984) presents additional discussion of the relevant physics of photonuclear interactions.

VII. TOTAL COEFFICIENTS FOR ATTENUATION, ENERGY TRANSFER, AND ENERGY ABSORPTION

A. Mass Attenuation Coefficient

The total mass attenuation coefficient for γ-ray interactions, neglecting photonuclear interactions, can be written, in units of cm^2/g or m^2/kg, as

$$\frac{\mu}{\rho} = \frac{\tau}{\rho} + \frac{\sigma}{\rho} + \frac{\kappa}{\rho} + \frac{\sigma_R}{\rho} \tag{7.56}$$

in which τ/ρ is the contribution of the photoelectric effect, σ/ρ that of the Compton effect, κ/ρ that of pair production, and σ_R/ρ that of Rayleigh scattering.

For the practical application of Eq. (7.56) as a definition of the mass "narrow-beam" attenuation coefficient (see Chapter 3), it should be noted that the term $\sigma_R/$

ρ is appropriately included only where beam geometry allows the escape (i.e. non-detection) of the Rayleigh-scattered rays. Since this type of scattering usually deflects photons through only small angles, very narrow beam geometry is required to observe the effects of Rayleigh scattering.

B. Mass Energy-Transfer Coefficient

The total mass energy-transfer coefficient for γ-ray interactions, neglecting any (γ, p) photonuclear contribution, is given in units of cm^2/g or m^2/kg by

$$\frac{\mu_{tr}}{\rho} = \frac{\tau_{tr}}{\rho} + \frac{\sigma_{tr}}{\rho} + \frac{\kappa_{tr}}{\rho}$$

$$= \frac{\tau}{\rho}\left[\frac{h\nu - p_K Y_k h\bar{\nu}_K}{h\nu}\right] + \frac{\sigma}{\rho}\left[\frac{\overline{T}}{h\nu}\right] + \frac{\kappa}{\rho}\left[\frac{h\nu - 2m_0c^2}{h\nu}\right] \tag{7.57}$$

for photons having $h\nu$ above the K-edge in the elemental absorbing medium, and neglecting L-fluorescence in comparison with K-fluorescence. For $h\nu$ lying between the K- and L-edges, Eq. (7.57) is replaced by

$$\frac{\mu_{tr}}{\rho} = \frac{\tau_{tr}}{\rho} + \frac{\sigma_{tr}}{\rho}$$

$$= \frac{\tau}{\rho}\left[\frac{h\nu - p_L Y_L h\bar{\nu}_L}{h\nu}\right] + \frac{\sigma}{\rho}\left[\frac{\overline{T}}{h\nu}\right] \tag{7.58}$$

since neither K-fluorescence nor pair production is relevant in that case. The terms in Eqs. (7.57) and (7.58) have been defined in Eqs. (7.35) and (7.36) for the photoelectric effect, Eqs. (7.20), (7.22), and (7.24) for the Compton effect, and Eq. (7.53) for pair production.

C. Mass Energy-Absorption Coefficient

The mass energy-absorption coefficient μ_{en}/ρ is related to the mass energy-transfer coefficient by

$$\frac{\mu_{en}}{\rho} = \frac{\mu_{tr}}{\rho}(1 - g) \tag{7.59}$$

in which g represents the average fraction of secondary-electron energy that is lost in radiative interactions, that is, bremsstrahlung production and (for positrons) in-flight annihilation. The evaluation of g will be discussed in Chapter 8, Section I.G. For low values of Z and $h\nu$, g approaches zero and $\mu_{en}/\rho \cong \mu_{tr}/\rho$. For increasing Z or $h\nu$, g increases gradually, so that, for example, in Pb with $h\nu = 10$ MeV, $\mu_{en}/\rho = 0.74\,\mu_{tr}/\rho$.

It should be pointed out that, while μ/ρ and μ_{tr}/ρ are based only on the $h\nu$ and Z actually present at the point of photon interaction, μ_{en}/ρ must also be based on an assumption about the medium through which the secondary electrons pass in slowing down. Conventionally the interaction point is assumed to be surrounded by the same homogenous medium, at least out to a distance equal to the maximum electron range. Thus g in Eq. (6.59) is evaluated for the same surrounding material as assumed for μ_{tr}/ρ. It is possible to conceive of situations (e.g. near an interface) where the radiation yield of the electrons would be altered and the conventional value of μ_{en}/ρ could no longer predict how much energy would be spent in ionization and excitation by the secondary electrons.

D. Coefficients for Compounds and Mixtures

For compounds or intimate mixtures of elements the Bragg rule conveniently applies to mass attenuation and energy-transfer coefficients:

$$\left(\frac{\mu}{\rho}\right)_{mix} = \left(\frac{\mu}{\rho}\right)_A f_A + \left(\frac{\mu}{\rho}\right)_B f_B + \cdots \qquad (7.60)$$

and

$$\left(\frac{\mu_{tr}}{\rho}\right)_{mix} = \left(\frac{\mu_{tr}}{\rho}\right)_A f_A + \left(\frac{\mu_{tr}}{\rho}\right)_B f_B + \cdots \qquad (7.61)$$

where $f_A, f_B, \ldots$, are the weight fractions of the separate elements ($A, B, \ldots$) present.

This same rule also applies approximately to the mass energy-absorption coefficient, so long as radiative losses are small. That is,

$$\left(\frac{\mu_{en}}{\rho}\right)_{mix} \cong \left(\frac{\mu_{en}}{\rho}\right)_A f_A + \left(\frac{\mu_{en}}{\rho}\right)_B f_B + \cdots$$

$$\cong \left(\frac{\mu_{tr}}{\rho}\right)_A (1 - g_A) f_A + \left(\frac{\mu_{tr}}{\rho}\right)_B (1 - g_B) f_B + \cdots \qquad (7.62)$$

where the second statement is based on Eq. (7.59), and where g_A is the radiation yield fraction for element A, and so on.

Equation (7.62) would be exact if the electrons originating in atoms of element A confined their paths to traversing only other atoms of the same element. However, the electrons actually pass through the different elements present in proportion to their weight fractions. Thus we may write an exact equation to replace Eq. (7.62) by expanding the radiation-yield terms accordingly to give

$$\left(\frac{\mu_{en}}{\rho}\right)_{mix} = \left(\frac{\mu_{tr}}{\rho}\right)_A (1 - f_A g_A - f_B g_B - \cdots) f_A$$

$$+ \left(\frac{\mu_{tr}}{\rho}\right)_B (1 - f_A g_A - f_B g_B - \cdots) f_B + \cdots$$

$$= \left(\frac{\mu_{tr}}{\rho}\right)_{mix} (1 - f_A g_A - f_B g_B - \cdot \cdot \cdot \cdot)$$

$$\equiv \left(\frac{\mu_{tr}}{\rho}\right)_{mix} (1 - g_{mix}) \tag{7.63}$$

Values of g_A, g_B, . . . can be obtained from tables of μ_{tr}/ρ and μ_{en}/ρ, together with Eq. (7.59).

E.   Tables of Photon Interaction Coefficients

Appendix D.1 contains tables of K–N interaction and energy-transfer cross sections in units of cm^2/e, for the energy range 1 keV to 100 MeV. These data apply to the Compton effect in all media, assuming free electrons.

Appendix D.2 provides photon interaction cross sections per atom for several representative elements, compounds, and mixtures over the same energy range. Besides giving data for the photoelectric effect, Compton effect, pair production, and Rayleigh (coherent) scattering, their combined effect is given with and without Rayleigh scattering. Appendix D.3 tabulates mass attenuation coefficients μ/ρ, mass energy-transfer coefficients μ_{tr}/ρ, and mass energy absorption coefficients μ_{en}/ρ. The last have been corrected for radiative losses due to positron in-flight annihilation as well as bremsstrahlung. μ_{en}/ρ values for a few additional materials also are given in Appendix D.4.

There are several other available tables of photon interaction data that deserve mention here:

1.   McMaster et al. (1969) give a compilation of individual interaction cross-section data for $Z = 1$ to 83, 86, 90, 92, and 94, with $h\nu$ covering the range 1 keV to 1 MeV. Total attenuation coefficients are also included.

2.   Storm and Israel (1970) have provided a very useful table of atomic cross sections for $Z = 1–100$ and $h\nu = 1$ keV to 100 MeV. In our terminology their table columns give the photon energy E, $_a\sigma$, $_a\sigma_{en}$, $_a\sigma_R$, $_a\kappa$(nuclear), $_a\kappa$(electron), $_a\kappa_{en}$(nuclear) + $_a\kappa_{en}$(electron), $_a\tau$, $_a\tau_{en}$, $_a\mu$, $_a\mu - _a\sigma_s - _a\sigma_R$, and $_a\mu_{en}$. The Compton-effect cross sections include binding corrections, but positron in-flight annihilation is not accounted for in $_a\kappa_{en}$ or $_a\mu_{en}$. This reference also contains some other useful tables, including (a) atomic energy levels, (b) K- and L-fluorescent x-ray energies, (c) weighted-average K and L x-ray energies, (d) relative intensities of K and L x-rays, (e) theoretical vs. experimental photoelectric cross sections, and (f) relative shell contributions to photoelectric cross sections.

3.   Hubbell et al. (1980) give tables of photon cross sections for all the individual interactions, for $h\nu = 1$ MeV to 100 GeV and $Z = 1–100$. Total attenuation coefficients are also given. The Compton effect includes electron binding corrections.

4.   Hubbell (1982) updates all his previous compilations in abbreviated form, i.e., listing only μ/ρ and μ_{en}/ρ for 40 elements and 45 mixtures and compounds.

Several ICRP (1975) body compositions (blood, bone, brain, lung, skin, and soft-tissue) are included. In-flight annihilation is taken into account in μ_{en}/ρ up to $h\nu$ = 10 MeV, and extrapolated to 20 MeV.

PROBLEMS*

1. Is the mass Compton coefficient (either for attenuation or energy transfer) larger in carbon or lead? (See Figs. 7.13a, b, 7.16a, b.) Why?

2. Why is Rayleigh scattering not plotted in Fig. 7.16a, b, although quite significant in Fig. 7.13a, b?

3. On the basis of the K–N theory, what is the ratio of the Compton interaction cross sections per atom for lead and carbon?

4. Calculate the energy of the Compton-scattered photon at φ = 0°, 45°, 90°, and 180° for $h\nu$ = 50 keV, 500 keV, and 5 MeV.

5. What are the corresponding energies and angles of the recoiling electrons for the cases in problem 4?

6. Calculate for 1-MeV photons the total K–N cross section from Eq. (7.15), and derive the Compton mass attenuation coefficient for copper, expressed in cm²/g and m²/kg.

7. What is the maximum energy, and what is the average energy, of the Compton recoil electrons generated by 20-keV and 20-MeV γ-rays?

8. Calculate the energy of a photoelectron ejected from the K-shell in tin by a 40-keV photon. Calculate τ_{tr}/ρ; you may estimate from Fig. 7.15.

9. What is the average energy of the charged particles resulting from pair production in (a) the nuclear field and (b) the electron field, for photons of $h\nu$ = 2 and 20 MeV?

10. A narrow beam containing 10^{20} photons at 6 MeV impinges perpendicularly on a layer of lead 12 mm thick, having a density of 11.3 g/cm³. How many interactions of each type (photoelectric, Compton, pair, Rayleigh) occur in the lead?

11. Assuming that each interaction in problem 10 results in one primary photon being removed from the beam, how much energy is removed by each type of interaction?

12. How much energy is transferred to charged particles by each type of interaction in problem 10?

SOLUTIONS TO PROBLEMS

1. Carbon, because of larger electron density ($N_A Z/A$).

2. Rayleigh scattering transfers no energy to charged particles.

*Refer to the Appendix tables for required coefficients.

3. 82/6, since all electrons are assumed to be unbound and to have the same interaction cross section.

4. At

$$\varphi = 0°: h\nu' = h\nu;$$
$$45°: h\nu' = 0.0486, 0.389, 1.293 \text{ MeV};$$
$$90°: h\nu' = 0.0455, 0.253, 0.464 \text{ MeV};$$
$$180°: h\nu' = 0.0418; 0.169, 0.243 \text{ MeV}.$$

Also compare with Fig. 7.3.

5. At $\theta = 90°$, $T = 0$ for all $h\nu$. For $h\nu = 0.05$ MeV, $T = 1.39 \times 10^{-3}$, 4.46×10^{-3}, and 8.18×10^{-3} MeV at $\theta = 65.5°$, $42.3°$, and $0°$, respectively. For $h\nu = 0.5$ MeV, $T = 0.111$, 0.247, and 0.331 MeV at $\theta = 50.7°$, $26.8°$ and $0°$, respectively. For $h\nu = 5$ MeV, $T = 3.71$, 4.54, and 4.76 MeV at $\theta = 12.6°$, $5.30°$, and $0°$, respectively.

6. $_e\sigma = 2.112 \times 10^{-25}$ cm²/electron; $(\sigma/\rho)_{Cu} = 0.0580$ cm²/g $= 0.00580$ m²/kg.

7. At

$$20 \text{ keV}: T_{max} = 1.45 \text{ keV}, \quad \overline{T} = 0.721 \text{ keV}$$
$$20 \text{ MeV}: T_{max} = 19.75 \text{ MeV}, \quad \overline{T} = 14.5 \text{ MeV}$$

8. $T = 10.8$ keV; $\tau_{tr}/\rho = 0.99$ m²/kg.

9. At

$$h\nu = 2 \text{ MeV}: \quad \overline{T} = 0.489, 0 \text{ MeV}.$$
$$h\nu = 20 \text{ MeV}: \overline{T} = 9.49, 6.33 \text{ MeV}.$$

10. Photoelectric: 1.00×10^{18}; Compton: 1.793×10^{19}; pair: 2.556×10^{19}, Rayleigh: $\cong 6 \times 10^{16}$.

11. Photoelectric: 9.6×10^5 J; Compton: 1.72×10^7 J; pair: 2.46×10^7 J; Rayleigh: 6×10^4 J.

12. Photoelectric: 9.5×10^5 J; Compton: 1.11×10^7 J; pair: 2.04×10^7 J; Rayleigh: 0.

CHAPTER **8**

Charged-Particle
Interactions in Matter

I. INTRODUCTION

Charged particles lose their energy in a manner that is distinctly different from that of uncharged radiations (x- or γ-rays and neutrons). An individual photon or neutron incident upon a slab of matter may pass through it with no interactions at all, and consequently no loss of energy. Or it may interact and thus lose its energy in one or a few "catastrophic" events.

By contrast, a charged particle, being surrounded by its Coulomb electric force field, interacts with one or more electrons or with the nucleus of practically every atom it passes. Most of these interactions individually transfer only minute fractions of the incident particle's kinetic energy, and it is convenient to think of the particle as losing its kinetic energy gradually in a frictionlike process, often referred to as the "continuous slowing-down approximation" (CSDA). The probability of a charged particle passing through a layer of matter without any interaction is nil. A 1-MeV charged particle would typically undergo $\sim 10^5$ interactions before losing all of its kinetic energy.

From the stochastic viewpoint, it is impossible to predict even crudely how far an *individual* photon or neutron will penetrate through matter, since only one or a few randomly occurring interactions are needed to dissipate all of its quantum or kinetic energy. Charged particles, however, can be roughly characterized by a common *pathlength*, traced out by most such particles of a given type and energy in a specific medium. Because of the multitude of interactions undergone by each charged particle in slowing down, its pathlength tends to approach the expectation value that

160

would be observed as a mean for a very large population of identical particles. That expectation value, called the *range*, will be discussed later in the chapter. Note that because of scattering, all identical charged particles do not follow the same path, nor are the paths straight, especially those of electrons because of their small mass.

II. TYPES OF CHARGED-PARTICLE COULOMB-FORCE INTERACTIONS

Charged-particle Coulomb-force interactions can be simply characterized in terms of the relative size of the classical *impact parameter b* vs. the atomic radius *a*, as shown in Fig. 8.1. The following three types of interactions become dominant for $b \gg a$, $b \sim a$, and $b \ll a$, respectively.

A. "Soft" Collisions ($b \gg a$)

When a charged particle passes an atom at a considerable distance, the influence of the particle's Coulomb force field affects the atom as a whole, thereby distorting it, exciting it to a higher energy level, and sometimes ionizing it by ejecting a valence-shell electron. The net effect is the transfer of a very small amount of energy (a few eV) to an atom of the absorbing medium.

Because large values of b are clearly more probable than are near hits on individual atoms, "soft" collisions are by far the most numerous type of charged-particle interaction, and they account for roughly half of the energy transferred to the absorbing medium.

In condensed media (liquids and solids) the atomic distortion mentioned above also gives rise to the polarization (or density) effect, which will be discussed in Section III.E.

Under certain conditions a very small part of the energy spent by a charged particle in soft collisions can be emitted by the absorbing medium as coherent bluish-white

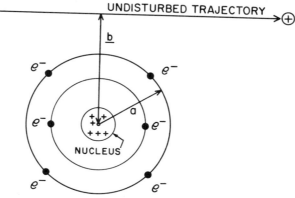

FIGURE 8.1. Important parameters in charged-particle collisions with atoms: *a* is the classical atomic radius; *b* is the classical impact parameter.

light called *Čerenkov radiation*. If the velocity v ($= \beta c$) of a charged particle traversing a transparent dielectric material of refractive index n exceeds c/n (the velocity of light in the medium), Čerenkov radiation is emitted at an angle ξ relative to the particle direction, where

$$\xi = \arccos \left(\frac{1}{\beta n}\right) \tag{8.1}$$

The Čerenkov photons thus form a conical wavefront of half angle $90° - \xi$ behind the particle, much like the shock wave trailing a supersonic object passing through air.

The energy emitted in the form of Čerenkov radiation comprises only a negligibly small fraction ($<0.1\%$) of that spent by the charged particle in atomic excitation and ionization through soft collisions, and it is usually unimportant in radiological physics. However, in high-energy nuclear physics, Čerenkov counters are useful instruments for detecting charged particles and measuring their velocities.

It has been sometimes pointed out that the Čerenkov effect is related to the polarization effect, since both depend in their theoretical treatments upon the dielectric constant of the absorbing medium. However, the polarization effect *decreases* the energy lost by a charged particle in traversing a given mass thickness of condensed (vs. gaseous) matter, while the production of Čerenkov radiation tends to *increase* the particle's energy loss. Thus the relating of these two effects may be confusing in the context of radiological physics. The Čerenkov effect is mentioned here only to put it in proper perspective.

B. Hard (or "Knock-On") Collisions ($b \sim a$)

When the impact parameter b is of the order of the atomic dimensions, it becomes more likely that the incident particle will interact primarily with a single atomic electron, which is then ejected from the atom with considerable kinetic energy and is called a delta (δ) ray. In the theoretical treatment of the knock-on process, atomic binding energies have been neglected and the atomic electrons treated as "free." δ-rays are of course energetic enough to undergo additional Coulomb-force interactions on their own. Thus a δ-ray dissipates its kinetic energy along a separate track (called a "spur") from that of the primary charged particle.

The probability for hard collisions depends upon quantum-mechanical spin and exchange effects, thus involving the nature of the incident particle. Hence, as will be seen, the form of stopping-power equations that include the effect of hard collisions depends on the particle type, being different especially for electrons *vs.* heavy particles.

Although hard collisions are few in number compared to soft collisions, the fractions of the primary particle's energy that are spent by these two processes are generally comparable.

It should be noted that whenever an inner-shell electron is ejected from an atom by a hard collision, characteristic x rays and/or Auger electrons will be emitted just as if the same electron had been removed by a photon interaction, as discussed in

Chapter 7. Thus some of the energy transferred to the medium may be transported some distance away from the primary particle track by these carriers as well as by the δ rays.

C. Coulomb-Force Interactions with the External Nuclear Field (**b ≪ a**)

When the impact parameter of a charged particle is much smaller than the atomic radius, the Coulomb-force interaction takes place mainly with the nucleus. This kind of interaction is most important for electrons (either + or −) in the present context, so the discussion here will be limited to that case. In all but 2–3% of such encounters, the electron is scattered *elastically* and does not emit an x-ray photon or excite the nucleus. It loses just the insignificant amount of kinetic energy necessary to satisfy conservation of momentum for the collision. Hence this is not a mechanism for the transfer of energy to the absorbing medium, but it is an important means of *deflecting* electrons. It is the principle reason why electrons follow very tortuous paths, especially in high-Z media, and why electron backscattering increases with Z. In doing Monte Carlo calculations of electron transport through matter, it is often assumed for simplicity that the energy-loss interactions may be treated separately from the scattering (i.e., change-of-direction) interactions. The differential elastic-scattering cross section per atom is proportional to Z^2 (see Evans, 1955, Chapter 19). This means that a thin foil of high-Z material may be used as a scatterer to spread out an electron beam while minimizing the energy lost by the transmitted electrons in traversing a given mass thickness of foil.

In the other 2–3% of the cases in which the electron passes near the nucleus, an *inelastic* radiative interaction occurs in which an x-ray photon is emitted. The electron is not only deflected in this process, but gives a significant fraction (up to 100%) of its kinetic energy to the photon, slowing down in the process. Such x-rays are referred to as *bremsstrahlung*, the German word for "braking radiation."

This interaction also has a differential atomic cross section proportional to Z^2, as was the case for nuclear elastic scattering. Moreover, it depends on the inverse square of the mass of the particle, for a given particle velocity. Thus bremsstrahlung generation by charged particles other than electrons is totally insignificant. As a practical consequence, the spectroscopy of x rays generated by proton beams colliding with matter reveals the presence of only the characteristic x-ray lines resulting from the knock-on collisions, with no detectable bremsstrahlung background. This of course is useful in x-ray analysis for trace elements.

Although bremsstrahlung production is an important means of energy dissipation by energetic electrons in high-Z media, it is relatively insignificant in low-Z (tissuelike) materials for electrons below 10 MeV. Not only is the production cross section low in that case, but the resulting photons are penetrating enough so that most of them can escape from objects several centimeters in size. Thus they usually carry away their quantum energy rather than expending it in the medium through a further interaction.

In addition to the foregoing three modes of kinetic energy dissipation (soft, hard, and bremsstrahlung interactions), a fourth channel is available only to antimatter (i.e., positrons): *in-flight annihilation*. In this process (see Berger, 1961) the positron is annihilated in encountering an electron before stopping. The remaining kinetic energy of the positron at that instant is given to one or both of the annihilation photons, so that their individual quantum energies may exceed the usual 0.511 MeV. The average fraction of a positron's kinetic energy that is spent in this type of radiative loss is said to be comparable to the fraction going into bremsstrahlung production (Berger, 1961). As noted in Chapter 6, the value of the energy absorption coefficient for pair production is decreased by in-flight annihilation of the positrons produced, and Hubble has taken this effect into account in his tables (see Appendixes D.2–D.4) by referring to Berger's 1961 calculations.

D. Nuclear Interactions by Heavy Charged Particles

A heavy charged particle having sufficiently high kinetic energy (~ 100 MeV) and an impact parameter less than the nuclear radius may interact inelastically with the nucleus. When one or more individual nucleons (protons or neutrons) are struck, they may be driven out of the nucleus in an *intranuclear cascade* process, collimated strongly in the forward direction. The highly excited nucleus decays from its excited state by emission of so-called *evaporation* particles (mostly nucleons of relatively low energy) and γ-rays. Thus the spatial distribution of the absorbed dose is changed when nuclear interactions are present, since some of the kinetic energy that would otherwise be deposited as local excitation and ionization is carried away by neutrons and γ-rays. Sondhaus and Evans (1969) and Cowan (1969) have discussed these processes. Raju et al. (1969) have provided tabular data indicating that, for example, 100-MeV protons incident on 5 g/cm^2 of graphite deposit an average absorbed dose only 2.5% less than that which would have resulted if no nuclear interactions occurred. This 2.5% is the maximum dose deficit in that example, assuming the escape of all the kinetic energy carried by a proton into a nuclear interaction, which is certainly an overestimate of the energy losses.

One special case where nuclear interactions by heavy charged particles attain first-order importance relative to Coulomb-force interactions is that of π^- *mesons (negative pions)*. These particles have a mass 273 times that of the electron, or 15% of the proton mass. They interact by Coulomb forces to produce excitation and ionization along their track in the same way as any other charged particle, but they also display some special characteristics:

1. Being only moderately heavy, π^--mesons scatter much less than do electrons, but more than protons. The rms scattering angle resulting from passage of a heavy charged particle through a thin slab of material is approximately inversely proportional to the particle's mass, and results from many small-angle nuclear scattering events. Thus the pion typically scatters at about a 7 times larger angle than a proton.

2. Negative pions are unstable, decaying to negative muons (μ^-) with a half-life of 2.54×10^{-8} s. Half of a beam of 50-MeV pions will decay over a 5-m flight path in vacuum. Muons decay to electrons ($\tau_{1/2} \simeq 2.2\ \mu s$).

3. When a negative pion reaches the end of its path in tissue, it is absorbed and annihilated by a nucleus (usually oxygen), which then releases about 100 MeV in the form of available kinetic energy of nuclear fragments. The rest mass of the pion is 140 MeV; the other 40 MeV is spent by the escaping fragments in overcoming the nuclear binding energy. Of the 100 MeV of kinetic energy available, 70 MeV is given to neutrons and 30 MeV to several charged particles (protons, α's, and heavier fragments), the tracks of which appear as a "star" in a photographic emulsion. This is called "star production". The neutrons carry away their energy, but the charged particles greatly enhance the dose near the end of the negative pion's track. These secondary particle tracks are very dense and biologically effective, and this mechanism for dose delivery to a tumor is of interest for cancer radiotherapy applications (Raju and Richman, 1972).

The effect of nuclear interactions is conventionally not included in defining the *stopping power* or *range* of charged particles, as in the following sections. Nuclear interactions by heavy charged particles are usually ignored in the context of radiological physics and dosimetry, but if necessary they can be corrected for by methods discussed by Bichsel (1968).

Internal nuclear interactions by electrons are negligible in comparison with the production of bremsstrahlung.

III. STOPPING POWER

The expectation value of the rate of energy loss per unit of path length x by a charged particle of type Y and kinetic energy T, in a medium of atomic number Z, is called its *stopping power*, $(dT/dx)_{Y,T,Z}$. The subscripts need not be explicitly stated where that information is clear from the context. Stopping power is typically given in units of MeV/cm or J/m (1 MeV/cm $\equiv 1.602 \times 10^{-11}$ J/m). Dividing the stopping power by the density ρ of the absorbing medium results in a quantity called the *mass stopping power* $(dT/\rho\ dx)$, typically in MeV cm^2/g or J m^2/kg (1 MeV cm^2/g = 1.602×10^{-14} J m^2/kg).

When one is interested in the fate of the energy lost by the charged particle, stopping power may be subdivided into "collision stopping power" and "radiative stopping power." The former is the rate of energy loss resulting from the sum of the soft and hard collisions, which are conventionally referred to as "collision interactions." Radiative stopping power is that owing to radiative interactions, as discussed in Section II.C. Unless otherwise specified, however, radiative stopping power may be assumed to be based on bremsstrahlung production alone. (The effect of in-flight annihilation, which is only relevant for positrons, is accounted for separately.) Energy spent in radiative collisions is carried away from the charged-particle track by the photons, while that spent in collision interactions produces ionization and excitation contributing to the dose near the track.

The *mass collision stopping power* can be written as

$$\left(\frac{dT}{\rho dx}\right)_c = \left(\frac{dT_s}{\rho dx}\right)_c + \left(\frac{dT_h}{\rho dx}\right)_c \tag{8.2}$$

where subscripts c indicate collision interactions, s being soft and h hard.

The terms on the right can be rewritten as

$$\left(\frac{dT}{\rho dx}\right)_c = \int_{T'_{min}}^{H} T' Q_c^s \, dT' + \int_{H}^{T'_{max}} T' Q_c^h \, dT' \tag{8.3}$$

in which:

1. T' is the energy transferred to the atom or electron in the interaction.
2. H is the somewhat arbitrary energy boundary between soft and hard collisions, in terms of T'.
3. T'_{max} is the maximum energy that can be transferred in a head-on collision with an atomic electron, assumed unbound. For a heavy particle with kinetic energy less than its rest-mass energy $M_0 c^2$,

$$T'_{max} \simeq 2m_0 c^2 \left(\frac{\beta^2}{1 - \beta^2}\right) = 1.022 \left(\frac{\beta^2}{1 - \beta^2}\right) \text{MeV} \tag{8.4}$$

which for protons equals 20 keV for $T = 10$ MeV, or 0.2 MeV for $T = 100$ MeV. For positrons incident, $T'_{max} = T$ if annihilation does not occur. However, in the case of electrons the primary and the struck electron are indistinguishable after the collision, according to the Dirac theory. Thus by convention the electron coming away with the greater energy is always referred to as the primary, and $T'_{max} \equiv T/2$.

4. T'_{max} is related to T'_{min} by

$$\frac{T'_{max}}{T'_{min}} \simeq \left(\frac{2m_0 c^2 \beta^2}{I}\right)^2 = \left(\frac{(1.022 \times 10^6 \text{ eV})\beta^2}{I}\right)^2 \tag{8.5}$$

in which I is the *mean excitation potential* of the struck atom, to be discussed later.

5. Q_c^s and Q_c^h are the respective differential mass collision coefficients for soft and hard collisions, typically in units of cm^2/g MeV or m^2/kg J.

A. The Soft-Collision Term

The soft-collision term in Eqs. (8.2) and (8.3) was derived by Bethe, for either electrons or heavy charged particles with z elementary charges, on the basis of the *Born approximation* which assumes that the particle velocity ($v = \beta c$) is much greater than the maximum Bohr-orbit velocity (u) of the atomic electrons. The fractional error in the assumption is of the order of $(u/v)^2$, and Bethe's formula is valid for $(u/v)^2 \sim (Z/137\beta)^2 \ll 1$. This appears to be a rather severe restriction, but the formula is found to be practically applicable even where this inequality is not well satisfied.

The Bethe soft-collision formula can be written as

$$\left(\frac{dT_s}{\rho dx}\right)_c = \frac{2Cm_0c^2z^2}{\beta^2}\left[\ln\left(\frac{2m_0c^2\beta^2H}{I^2(1-\beta^2)}\right) - \beta^2\right] \tag{8.6}$$

where $C \equiv \pi(N_AZ/A)\,r_0^2 = 0.150Z/A$ cm^2/g, in which N_AZ/A is the number of electrons per gram of the stopping medium, and $r_0 = e^2/m_0c^2 = 2.818 \times 10^{-13}$ cm is the classical electron radius. We can further simplify the factor outside the bracket by defining it as

$$k \equiv \frac{2Cm_0c^2z^2}{\beta^2} = 0.1535\,\frac{Zz^2}{A\beta^2}\,\frac{\text{MeV}}{\text{g/cm}^2} \tag{8.7}$$

where $m_0c^2 = 0.511$ MeV, the rest-mass energy of an electron.

The bracket factor in Eq. (8.6) and other following stopping power formulae is dimensionless, thus requiring the quantities m_0c^2, H, and I occurring within it to be expressed in the same energy units, usually eV. Only the factor k controls the dimensions in which the stopping power is to be expressed.

The mean excitation potential I is the geometric-mean value of all the ionization and excitation potentials of an atom of the absorbing medium. The influence of chemical binding on the I-value for atoms in a compound was studied by T. J. Thompson, whose results have been summarized by Berger and Seltzer (1983). The effect is significant in some cases for H, C, N, and O, and those authors employ a simple approximate means for taking this into account in computing I for compounds.

In general I for elements cannot be calculated from atomic theory with useful accuracy, but must instead be derived from stopping-power or range measurements. Bloch has estimated that $I \propto Z$, but actually I/Z shows variations vs. Z, and tends to increase at low Z. Appendixes B.1 and B.2 list some I-values according to Berger and Seltzer (1983). That reference contains an extensive review of I, electron and positron stopping-power and range information, and a comprehensive list of relevant references.

Since I only depends on the stopping medium, but not on the type of charged particle, experimental determinations have been done preferentially with cyclotron-accelerated protons, because of their availability with high β-values and the relatively small effect of scattering as they pass through layers of material. The paths of electrons are too crooked to allow their use in accurate stopping power determinations.

B. The Hard-Collision Term for Heavy Particles

The form of the hard-collision term in Eqs. (8.2) and (8.3) depends on whether the incident charged particle is an electron, positron, or heavy particle. We will treat the case of heavy particles first, having masses much greater than that of an electron, and will assume that $H \ll T'_{\text{max}}$. The hard-collision term may be written as

$$\left(\frac{dT_h}{\rho dx}\right)_c = k\left[\ln\left(\frac{T'_{\text{max}}}{H}\right) - \beta^2\right] \tag{8.8}$$

This can be combined with Eq. (8.6) to obtain the mass collision stopping power for combined soft and hard collisions by heavy particles:

$$\left(\frac{dT}{\rho dx}\right)_c = k\left[\ln\left(\frac{2m_0c^2\beta^2 T'_{max}}{I^2(1-\beta^2)}\right) - 2\beta^2\right] \tag{8.9}$$

which can be simplified further by substituting for T'_{max} from Eq. (8.4)

$$\left(\frac{dT}{\rho dx}\right)_c = 2k\left[\ln\left(\frac{2m_0c^2\beta^2}{(1-\beta^2)I}\right) - \beta^2\right]$$

$$= 0.3071 \frac{Zz^2}{A\beta^2}\left[13.8373 + \ln\left(\frac{\beta^2}{1-\beta^2}\right) - \beta^2 - \ln I\right] \tag{8.10}$$

Several important features of this formula should be pointed out.

1. DEPENDENCE ON THE STOPPING MEDIUM

There are two expressions influencing this dependence, and both decrease the mass collision stopping power as Z is increased. The first is the factor Z/A outside the bracket, which makes the formula proportional to the number of electrons per unit mass of the medium. This decreases by about 20% in going from C to Pb (see Appendix B.1).

The second is the term $-\ln I$ in the bracket, which further decreases the stopping power as Z is increased. The size of the decrease depends on the particle velocity, however, due to the influence of the β^2 terms in the bracket. For example, $-\ln I$ causes $(dT/\rho dx)_c$ to be 48% lower for Pb than for C at $\beta = 0.1$ (~ 5-MeV proton), and only 24% lower at $\beta = 0.85$ ($\cong 850$-MeV proton). Thus the term $-\ln I$ provides the stronger variation with Z, and the combined effect of the two Z-dependent expressions is to make $(dT/\rho dx)_c$ for Pb less than that for C by $\cong 40$–60% within the β-range 0.85–0.1, respectively.

2. DEPENDENCE ON PARTICLE VELOCITY

The strongest dependence on velocity comes from the inverse β^2 (outside of the bracket), which rapidly decreases the stopping power as β increases. That term loses its influence as β approaches a constant value at unity, while the sum of the β^2 terms in the bracket continues to increase. The stopping power gradually flattens to a broad minimum of 1–2 MeV cm²/g at $T/M_0c^2 \cong 3$, and then slowly rises again with further increasing T. Figure (8.2) illustrates this behavior for several stopping media, but does not show the high-energy rise, since the abscissa extends only to $T/M_0c^2 = 1$ (equivalent to a proton energy of 938 MeV).

The factor $1/\beta^2$ implies that the stopping power increases in proportion to $1/T$ without limit as particles slow down and approach zero velocity. Actually the validity of the stopping-power formula breaks down for small β, as will be discussed in Section III.C. However, the steep rise in stopping power that does occur (see Fig. 8.2) accounts for the "Bragg peak" observed in the energy-loss density near the end of a charged particle's path.

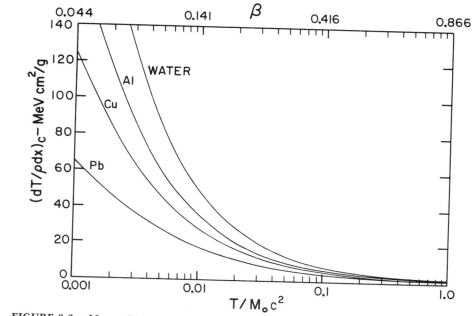

FIGURE 8.2. Mass collision stopping power $(dT/\rho dx)_c$ for singly charged heavy particles, as a function of β (upper scale) or of their kinetic energy T normalized by the rest mass M_0c^2. For protons $T/M_0c^2 = 1$ at $T = 938$ MeV. For particles with z charges, multiply ordinate by z^2. From data of Bichsel (1968).

3. DEPENDENCE ON PARTICLE CHARGE

The factor z^2 means that a doubly charged particle of a given velocity has 4 times the collision stopping power as a singly charged particle of the same velocity in the same medium. In Fig. 8.2, for example, an α-particle with $\beta = 0.141$ would have a mass collision stopping power of 200 MeV cm^2/g, compared with the 50 MeV cm^2/g shown for a singly charged heavy particle in water.

4. DEPENDENCE ON PARTICLE MASS

There is none. Particle mass does not appear in Eq. (8.10). All heavy charged particles of a given velocity and z will have the same collision stopping power.

5. RELATIVISTIC SCALING CONSIDERATIONS

For any particle, $\beta = v/c$ is related to the kinetic energy T by

$$T = M_0c^2\left[\frac{1}{\sqrt{1 - \beta^2}} - 1\right] \quad \text{and} \quad \beta = \left[1 - \left(\frac{1}{(T/M_0c^2) + 1}\right)^2\right]^{1/2} \quad (8.11)$$

The kinetic energy required by any particle to reach a given velocity is proportional to its rest energy, M_0c^2. This explains the abscissa in Fig. 8.2. The rest energies of some heavy particles are listed in Table 8.1.

TABLE 8.1.   Rest Energy and Charge of Heavy
Particles

Particle	M_0c^2 (MeV)	z
Muon	105.66	1
Pion	139.60	1
Proton	938.28	1
Neutron	939.57	0
Deuteron	1875.63	1
Triton	2808.95	1
α-particle	3727.41	2

It will be useful to digress here briefly into a discussion of charged particle acceleration. The kinetic energy T accumulated by a charged particle as it is accelerated through an electrical potential difference P (volts) is proportional to the number z of elementary charges it carries, but is independent of its mass. However, the heavier the particle, the slower it will be going at a given T, as indicated in Eq. (8.11). A simple one-step accelerator (e.g., a Van de Graaff) can in principle accelerate all singly charged particles to a kinetic energy (eV) that is numerically equal to the applied voltage, and an α particle to twice that energy. Thus a 10-MV potential can accelerate a proton to a kinetic energy of 10 MeV ($\beta = 0.1448$), a deuteron also to 10 MeV ($\beta = 0.1029$), or an α-particle to 20 MeV ($\beta = 0.1032$). It will be seen that β is nearly the same for the deuteron and α, since their z/M_0c^2 values are similar (see Table 8.1). A linear accelerator can, in principle, accelerate any charged particle to s times the kinetic energy it could be given by a single application of the potential difference, where s is the number of times that voltage is applied to the particle in the accelerator. A cyclotron, on the other hand, is limited by magnetic considerations to delivering particles having maximum kinetic energies proportional to z^2/M_0c^2. This is twice as great for a proton or an α-particle as for a deuteron.

6.   SAMPLE CALCULATION WITH EQ. (8.10)

Bichsel (1968) tabulated β, and a function $f(\beta)$ that equals the sum of all except the medium-dependent term $\ln I$ inside the brackets in Eq. (8.10).* He also provided values of I, $\ln I$, and Z/A for a number of elements.† For a 10-MeV proton, for example, $\beta = 0.14484$, $f(\beta) = 9.9733$, and if the absorber is copper having $I = 322$ eV, then $\ln I = 5.7746$ and $Z/A = 0.4564$, giving 28.05 MeV cm^2/g for Eq. (8.10) in that case. An α-particle of 39.726 MeV has the same velocity or β as a 10-MeV proton; hence Eq. (8.10) gives 112.21 MeV cm^2/g for an α-particle. This is four times the value obtained for the proton, since $z = 2$ for the α, and the terms in the bracket are unchanged.

---

*These tables include data for protons, electrons, muons, pions, and α-particles.
†The values of I provided by Berger and Seltzer (1983) differ slightly, and are to be preferred as the most up-to-date authoritative tabulation. See Appendixes B.1 and B.2 for some excerpted values.

A correction to Eq. (8.10) for atomic shell effects becomes significant for small β, as discussed in the next section.

C. Shell Correction

The Born approximation assumption, which underlies the stopping-power equation, is not well satisfied when the velocity of the passing particle ceases to be much greater than that of the atomic electrons in the stopping medium. Since K-shell electrons have the highest velocities, they are the first to be affected by insufficient particle velocity, the slower L-shell electrons are next, and so on. The so-called "shell correction" is intended to account for the resulting error in the stopping-power equation (8.10). As the particle velocity is decreased toward that of the K-shell electrons, those electrons gradually decrease their participation in the collision process, and the stopping power is thereby decreased below the value given by Eq. (8.10). When the particle velocity falls *below* that of the K-shell electrons, they cease participating in the collision stopping-power process. Equation (8.10) then underestimates the stopping power because that equation contains too large an I-value. (The proper I-value would ignore the K-shell contribution.)

Bichsel (1968) extended the earlier work of M. C. Walske to estimate the combined effect of all i shells into a single approximate correction C/Z, to be subtracted from the bracketed terms in Eq. (8.10). The corrected formula for the mass collision stopping power for heavy particles then becomes

$$\left(\frac{dT}{\rho dx}\right)_c = 2k \left[\ln \left(\frac{2m_0c^2\beta^2}{(1 - \beta^2)I} \right) - \beta^2 - \frac{C}{Z} \right]$$

$$= 0.3071 \frac{Zz^2}{A\beta^2} \left[13.8373 + \ln \left(\frac{\beta^2}{1 - \beta^2} \right) - \beta^2 - \ln I - \frac{C}{Z} \right] \quad (8.12)$$

The correction term C/Z is the same for all charged particles of the same velocity β, including electrons, and its size is a function of the medium as well as the particle velocity. C/Z is shown in Fig. 8.3 for protons in several elements.

A second correction term, δ, to account for the *polarization* or *density effect* in condensed media, is sometimes included also in Eq. (8.12). We have not done so because it is negligible for all heavy particles within the energy range of interest in radiological physics. For protons up to 800 MeV the effect on the stopping power is 0.1% or less. For electrons it is important, however, and it will be discussed in that connection.

D. Mass Collision Stopping Power for Electrons and Positrons

The formulae for the mass collision stopping power for electrons and positrons are gotten by combining Bethe's soft collision formula (8.6) with a hard-collision relation based on the Møller cross section for electrons or the Bhabha cross section for positrons, as discussed by Evans (1955) and Kase and Nelson (1978). The resulting formula, common to both particles, in terms of $\tau \equiv T/m_0c^2$, is

$$\left(\frac{dT}{\rho dx}\right)_c = k \left[\ln \left(\frac{\tau^2(\tau + 2)}{2(I/m_0c^2)^2} \right) + F^\pm(\tau) - \delta - \frac{2C}{Z} \right] \quad (8.13)$$

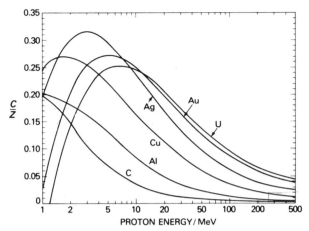

FIGURE 8.3. Semiempirical shell corrections of Bichsel for selected elements, as a function of the proton energy (ICRU, 1984a). Reproduced with permission from H. Bichsel and the International Commission on Radiological Units and Measurements.

in which, for electrons,

$$F^-(\tau) \equiv 1 - \beta^2 + \frac{\tau^2/8 - (2\tau + 1)\ln 2}{(\tau + 1)^2} \qquad (8.13a)$$

and for positrons,

$$F^+(\tau) \equiv 2\ln 2 - \frac{\beta^2}{12}\left\{23 + \frac{14}{\tau + 2} + \frac{10}{(\tau + 2)^2} + \frac{4}{(\tau + 2)^3}\right\} \qquad (8.13b)$$

Here C/Z is the previously discussed shell correction and δ is the correction term for the polarization or density effect, to be discussed in the next section.

E. Polarization or Density-Effect Correction

The polarization effect influences the soft collision process, which is an energy-transferring interaction between a passing charged particle and a relatively distant atom. In gases the atoms are spaced widely enough so that they undergo interactions independently of one another. However, in condensed media (liquids or solids) the density is increased by a factor of $\sim 10^3$–10^4 over that of a gas at atmospheric pressure, and the average atomic spacing is less than $\frac{1}{10}$ as great as in the gas. In this situation the dipole distortion of the atoms near the track of the passing particle weakens the Coulomb force field experienced by the more distant atoms, thus decreasing the energy lost to them. Because of this, the mass collision stopping power is decreased in condensed media.

Sternheimer has provided the most information about this phenomenon in a series of papers culminating in a generalized treatment (Sternheimer et al., 1982). This paper gives a formula and tables of data for calculating δ, the correction term to be subtracted in the bracket term as shown in Eq. (8.13) to correct for the polarization effect. δ is a function of the composition and density of the stopping medium, and of the parameter $\chi \equiv \log_{10}(p/m_0c) = \log_{10}(\beta/\sqrt{1-\beta^2})$ for the particle, in which p is its relativistic momentum mv, and m_0 its rest mass. δ may be taken as zero below a threshold value χ_0 in a given nonmetal. However, a small nonzero value of $\delta \cong 0.1$ exists in metals even for very low-energy particles, because of conduction electrons (the so-called "zero-energy" polarization effect).

Figure 8.4 shows that δ increases almost linearly as a function of χ above $\chi \cong 1$ for a variety of condensed media, being somewhat larger for low-Z than for high-Z media at a given χ-value. δ only begins to become important above the rest-mass energy of the particle. This accounts for the relative insignificance of the polarization effect, except for electrons, in normally encountered energy ranges. The size of the polarization effect for electrons, expressed as a percentage decrease in mass collision stopping power in solids or liquids compared with gases of the same Z, is shown in Table 8.2. It increases roughly as the logarithm of T above a few MeV of electron energy, and decreases gradually with increasing Z.

Useful tabulations of stopping power information for electrons have been provided by Berger and Seltzer (1983) and the ICRU (1984a) for numerous elements and compounds, for $T = 10$ keV to 1000 MeV. Appendix E contains tables of electron stopping powers, ranges, radiation yields (to be discussed in Section III.G), and density-effect corrections δ, excerpted from Berger and Seltzer's report (1983), for

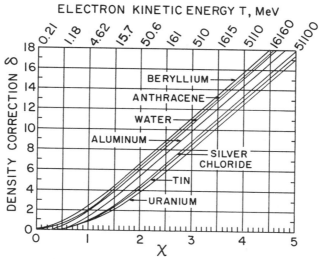

FIGURE 8.4.   Density-effect correction δ as a function of χ and electron kinetic energy T. After Sternheimer (1952). Reproduced with permission from R. M. Sternheimer and the American Physical Society.

TABLE 8.2.   Polarization Effect for Electrons

T (MeV)	Effect[a] (%)		
	C	Cu	Au
0.1	0	0	0
1.0	3	1.5	0.7
5	9	7	5
10	12	10	8
50	20	18	15

[a] Decrease in mass collision stopping power for condensed media vs. gases.

the stopping media H_2, He, C, N, O, Al, Si, Cu, Sn, Pb, air, water, A-150 plastic, muscle, fat, bone, polystyrene, Lucite, polyethylene, Teflon, LiF and CaF_2. Table 8.3, also derived from Berger and Seltzer (1983), relates mass collision stopping powers for positrons to those tabulated for electrons. The positron stopping power is evidently somewhat greater than that for electrons below 0.5 MeV, the reverse being true above that energy.

Figure 8.5 illustrates the influence of the polarization effect on electron (or positron) mass collision stopping powers vs. kinetic energy above 0.5 MeV. The same trends previously discussed for heavy particles in Section III.B.2 are also followed for electrons and positrons [Eq. (8.13)]. The steep rise for $\beta < m_0c^2$ is not shown, but the minimum at $\cong 3\,m_0c^2$ is evident, as is the continuing rise at still higher energy. The dashed curves are without correction for the polarization effect (i.e., they are for gaseous materials), while the solid curves show the corresponding corrected stopping powers for condensed media.

The polarization effect is particularly relevant to radiological physics measurements in which ionization chambers are used in electron or photon beams above ~ 2 MeV. Relating the absorbed dose in the gas to that in the solid surrounding medium

TABLE 8.3.   Ratio of Mass Collision Stopping Power for Positrons to that for Electrons[a]

T (MeV)	Ratio				
	C	Al	Cu	Ag	Pb
0.01	1.10	1.12	1.14	1.16	1.19
0.1	1.04	1.04	1.05	1.05	1.06
0.5	0.990	0.989	0.988	0.988	0.987
1.0	0.979	0.977	0.975	0.974	0.972
10	0.972	0.971	0.970	0.969	0.963
100	0.974	0.974	0.973	0.972	0.972
1000	0.976	0.976	0.975	0.975	0.974

[a] After Berger and Seltzer (1983).

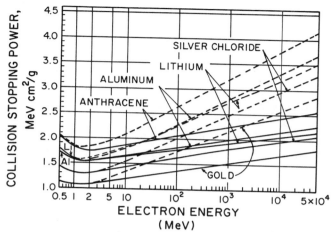

FIGURE 8.5. Mass collision stopping power for electrons in anthracene, Al, Li, AgCl, and Au, with (solid curves) and without (dashed curves) correction for polarization effect. After Sternheimer (1952). Reproduced with permission from R. M. Sternheimer and the American Physical Society.

through the application of cavity theory (Chapter 10) requires knowledge of the stopping powers, which are influenced by the polarization effect in the solid. This application will be discussed further in Chapter 13.

F. Mass Radiative Stopping Power

As mentioned in Section II.C, only electrons and positrons are light enough to generate significant bremsstrahlung, which depends on the inverse square of the particle mass for equal velocities. The rate of bremsstrahlung production by electrons or positrons is expressed by the *mass radiative stopping power* $(dT/\rho dx)_r$, in units of MeV cm^2/g, which can be written as

$$\left(\frac{dT}{\rho dx}\right)_r = \sigma_0 \ \frac{N_A Z^2}{A} \ (T + m_0 c^2)\overline{B}_r \tag{8.14}$$

where the constant $\sigma_0 = \frac{1}{137} (e^2/m_0 c^2)^2 = 5.80 \times 10^{-28}$ cm^2/atom [see also Eq. 7.40)], T is the particle kinetic energy in MeV, and $\overline{B}_r$ is a slowly varying function of Z and T having a value of $\frac{16}{3}$ for $T \ll 0.5$ MeV, and roughly 6 for $T = 1$ MeV, 12 for 10 MeV, and 15 for 100 MeV. $\overline{B}_r Z^2$ is dimensionless.

The derivation of Eq. (8.14) according to the theory of Bethe and Heitler is discussed by Evans (1955). Berger and Seltzer (1983) have provided extensive tables of $(dT/\rho dx)_r$, some of which are contained in Appendix E, Column 3.

It can be seen in comparing Eq. (8.14) with Eq. (8.6) that the mass radiative stopping power is proportional to $N_A Z^2/A$, while the mass collision stopping power is proportional to $N_A Z/A$, the electron density. Thus their ratio would be expected to be proportional to Z.

Equation (8.14) also shows proportionality to $T + m_0 c^2$, or to T for $T \gg m_0 c^2$. The corresponding energy dependence of the collision stopping power is not obvious from its formula, but can be seen in Fig. 8.6. Above $T = m_0 c^2$ it varies only slowly as a function of T. Thus the ratio of radiative to collision stopping power will be roughly proportional to T at high energies. For nonrelativistic electrons ($T \ll m_0 c^2$), Eq. (8.14) reduces to the Sommerfeld theory, in which the radiative stopping power is independent of T (see Evans, 1955) and $\bar{B}_r = \frac{16}{3}$.

The ratio of radiative to collision stopping power is often expressed in the form

$$\frac{(dT/\rho dx)_r}{(dT/\rho dx)_c} \cong \frac{TZ}{n} \tag{8.15}$$

in which T is the kinetic energy of the particle, Z is the atomic number of the medium, and n is a constant variously taken to be 700 or 800 MeV. Comparison with the tables in Appendix E shows that 700 ± 100 MeV best represents the value of n for T above 3 MeV, and $n \cong [700 + 200 \log_{10} (T/3)] \pm 100$ MeV for $0.01 < T < 3$ MeV. The radiative and collision stopping powers are roughly equal when $TZ \cong 700$ ($+100$ for Pb, or -100 for C) MeV.

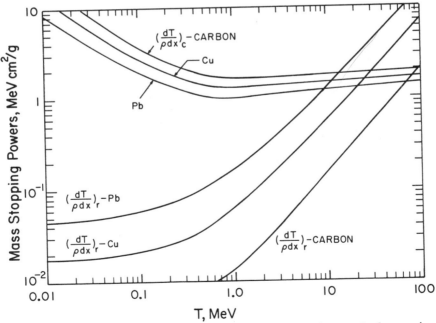

FIGURE 8.6. Mass radiative and collision stopping powers for electrons (and approximately for positrons) in C, Cu, and Pb. (From data of Bichsel, 1968.)

Figure 8.6 shows the stopping power trends vs. energy and Z. The collision stopping power is relatively independent of Z, so that any ratio of $(dT/\rho dx)_c$ for one medium to that for another is only weakly dependent on T. Also, above 1 MeV the variation of $(dT/\rho dx)_c$ itself vs. T is very gradual, and becomes even flatter in condensed media when the polarization effect is corrected for. The radiative stopping power clearly shows an approximate proportionality to Z and T above ~ 3 MeV, as indicated by Eq. (8.15) and the near-constancy of $(dT/\rho dx)_c$ in that energy range. The points of equality for radiative vs. collision stopping power in Fig. (8.6) are seen to fall near the values predicted by Eq. (8.15).

The total mass stopping power is the sum of the collision and radiative contributions:

$$\frac{dT}{\rho dx} = \left(\frac{dT}{\rho dx}\right)_c + \left(\frac{dT}{\rho dx}\right)_r \tag{8.16}$$

Along with its parts, $dT/\rho dx$ is tabulated as a function of T for a given stopping medium and type of charged particle; in Appendix E, for electrons. For heavier particles $(dT/\rho dx)_r \cong 0$, so $(dT/\rho dx) = (dT/\rho dx)_c$ almost exactly.

G. Radiation Yield

The *radiation yield* $Y(T_0)$ of a charged particle of initial kinetic energy T_0 is the total fraction of that energy that is emitted as electromagnetic radiation while the particle slows and comes to rest. For heavy particles $Y(T_0) \simeq 0$. For electrons the production of bremsstrahlung x-rays in radiative collisions is the only significant contributor to $Y(T_0)$. For positrons, in-flight annihilation would be a second significant component, but this has been customarily omitted in calculating $Y(T_0)$.

Berger and Seltzer have calculated $Y(T_0)$ for electrons, and their results are listed in the sixth column of the tables in Appendix E. The left-hand column of kinetic energies is to be interpreted as T_0 in relation to the range and radiation yield.

If we define $y(T)$ as

$$y(T) \equiv \frac{(dT/\rho dx)_r}{(dT/\rho dx)} \tag{8.17}$$

for an electron of instantaneous kinetic energy T, then the radiation yield $Y(T_0)$ for the electron of higher starting energy T_0 is an average value of $y(T)$ for T varying from 0 to T_0, as given by

$$Y(T_0) = \bar{y}(T_0) = \frac{\int_0^{T_0} y(T)\, dT}{\int_0^{T_0} dT} = \frac{1}{T_0} \int_0^{T_0} y(T)\, dT \tag{8.18}$$

The *amount* of energy radiated per electron is simply $Y(T_0) \cdot T_0$.

In Chapter 2, Section V.B, the concept of $\overline{W}$ was discussed and defined in terms of a quantity g_i [see Eq. (2.21)]. Its mean value g appears in the relation $\mu_{en}/\rho = (\mu_{tr}/\rho)(1 - g)$ in Chapter 7 [Eq. (7.59)]. g is also the average value of $Y(T_0)$ for all of the electrons and positrons of various starting energies T_0 present. Assuming that only Compton interactions occur, given a photon energy $E\gamma$,

$$g = \overline{Y}(T_0) = \int_0^{T_{max}} Y(T_0) \left(\frac{d\sigma}{dT_0}\right)_{E\gamma} dT_0 \Big/ \int_0^{T_{max}} \left(\frac{d\sigma}{dT_0}\right)_{E\gamma} dT_0 \tag{8.19}$$

in which σ is the Compton (Klein–Nishina) interaction cross section (e.g., in cm^2/e) and $(d\sigma/dT_0)_{E\gamma}$ is the differential cross section (cm^2/e MeV), as shown graphically in Chapter 7, Fig. 7.9, and T_{max} is the maximum electron energy.

H. Stopping Power in Compounds

The mass collision stopping power, the mass radiative stopping power, and their sum the mass stopping power can all be well approximated for intimate mixtures of elements, or for chemical compounds, through the assumption of *Bragg's Rule* (ICRU, 1984a). It states that atoms contribute nearly independently to the stopping power, and hence their effects are additive. This neglects the influence of chemical binding on I, as noted in Section III.A. In terms of the weight fractions f_{Z_1}, f_{Z_2}, of elements of atomic numbers Z_1, Z_2, etc. present in a compound or mixture, the mass stopping power $(dT/\rho dx)_{mix}$ can be written as

$$\left(\frac{dT}{\rho dx}\right)_{mix} = f_{Z_1}\left(\frac{dT}{\rho dx}\right)_{Z_1} + f_{Z_2}\left(\frac{dT}{\rho dx}\right)_{Z_2} + \cdots \tag{8.20}$$

where all stopping powers refer to a common kinetic energy and type of charged particle.

Appendix B.2 lists I-values for some compounds as reported by Berger and Seltzer (1983), which were selected from their Table 5.5. Data with an asterisk were derived by those authors from the formula (also based on Bragg's rule)

$$\frac{Z}{A} \ln I = \sum_i \left[f_{Z_i} (Z/A)_i \ln I_i \right] \tag{8.21a}$$

where $Z/A = \Sigma_i f_{Z_i}(Z/A)_i$ for the compound, and I is the compound's mean excitation potential. The elemental I_i-values employed were those in Berger and Seltzer's Table 5.1, which included approximate corrections for binding in compounds. Data in Appendix B.2 without asterisks are I values wholly or in part derived from experiments with the compounds.

A rough approximation to the polarization correction δ can also be gotten from the Bragg rule as

$$\delta = \frac{\sum_i f_{Z_i} (Z/A)_i \delta_i}{Z/A} \tag{8.21b}$$

I. Restricted Stopping Power

The mass collision stopping power $(dT/\rho dx)_c$ expresses the average rate of energy loss by a charged particle in all hard, as well as soft, collisions. The δ-rays resulting from hard collisions may be energetic enough to carry kinetic energy a significant distance away from the track of the primary particle. More importantly, if one is calculating the dose in a small object or thin foil transversed by charged particles (as will be discussed in Section V.A), the use of the mass collision stopping power will overestimate the dose, unless the escaping δ-rays are replaced (i.e., unless δ-ray CPE exists).

The *restricted stopping power* is that fraction of the collision stopping power that includes all the soft collisions plus those hard collisions resulting in δ rays with energies less than a cutoff value Δ. The mass restricted stopping power in MeV cm²/g, will be symbolized here as $(dT/\rho dx)_\Delta$. An alternative and very important form of restricted stopping power is known as the *linear energy transfer*, symbolized as L_Δ (ICRU, 1980). The usual units for L_Δ are keV/μm, so that

$$L_\Delta \text{ (keV/}\mu\text{m)} = \frac{\rho}{10}\left[\left(\frac{dT}{\rho dx}\right)_\Delta (MeV \; cm^2/g)\right] \tag{8.21c}$$

Linear energy transfer is of greatest relevance in radiobiology and microdosimetry.

If the cutoff energy Δ is increased to equal T'_{max} [$T/2$ for electrons, T for positrons, and Eq. (8.4) for heavy particles], then

$$\left(\frac{dT}{\rho dx}\right)_\Delta = \left(\frac{dT}{\rho dx}\right)_c \tag{8.21d}$$

and

$$L_\Delta \equiv L_\infty \tag{8.21e}$$

The *unrestricted linear energy transfer* L_∞ is an important reference parameter in radiation protection dosimetry, as shown in Chapter 2, Section V.

The calculation of $(dT/\rho dx)_\Delta$ for heavy particles makes use of Eq. (8.9), substituting Δ(eV) for T_{max}. Inserting the binding correction from Eq. (8.12) gives (in MeV cm²/g)

$$\left(\frac{dT}{\rho dx}\right)_\Delta = k\left[\ln\left(\frac{2m_0c^2\beta^2\Delta}{I^2(1-\beta^2)}\right) - 2\beta^2 - \frac{2C}{Z}\right] \tag{8.21f}$$

For electrons and positrons this quantity is given by the following equation (ICRU, 1984a) in which $\tau \equiv T/m_0c^2$ and $\eta \equiv \Delta/T$.

$$\left(\frac{dT}{\rho dx}\right)_\Delta = k\left\{\ln\left[\frac{\tau^2(\tau+2)}{2(I/m_0c^2)^2}\right] + G^\pm(\tau, \eta) - \delta - \frac{2C}{Z}\right\} \tag{8.21g}$$

For electrons

$$G^- (\tau, \eta) = -1 - \beta^2 + \ln[4(1 - \eta)\eta] + (1 - \eta)^{-1} \qquad (8.21h)$$
$$+ (1 - \beta^2)[\tau^2\eta^2/2 + (2\tau + 1)\ln(1 - \eta)]$$

and for positrons, substituting $\xi \equiv (\tau + 2)^{-1}$,

$$G^+ (\tau, \eta) = \ln4\eta - \beta^2[1 + (2 - \xi^2)\eta - (3 + \xi^2)(\xi\tau/2)\eta^2 \qquad (8.21i)$$
$$+ (1 + \xi\tau)(\xi^2\tau^2/3)\eta^3 - (\xi^3\tau^3/4)\eta^4]$$

$G^-(\tau, 1/2) = F^-(\tau)$ in Eq. (8.13a) and $G^+(\tau, 1) = F^+(\tau)$ in Eq. (8.13b). Thus for $\Delta = T/2$ in the case of electrons or $\Delta = T$ for positrons, Eq. (8.13) and (8.21g) become identical, verifying Eq. (8.21d). ICRU (1984a) provides a table of L_Δ/L_∞ values for T from 0.01 to 100 MeV; $\Delta = 1$, 10 and 100 keV; in C, Al, Cu, Ag, Pb, water and air; for electrons and positrons. Note that the symbol $S(T,\Delta)$ is substituted for $(dT/pdx)_\Delta$ in Chapter 10, and L/p is used in Chapter 13, corresponding to the usage of Spencer and Attix (1955) and AAPM (1983), respectively.

IV. RANGE

The concept of charged particle *range* was introduced in Section I. It may be defined as follows:

The range $\Re$ of a charged particle of a given type and energy in a given medium is the expectation value of the pathlength p that it follows until it comes to rest (discounting thermal motion).

A second, related quantity, the *projected range*, is defined thus:

The projected range $\langle t \rangle$ of a charged particle of a given type and initial energy in a given medium is the expectation value of the farthest depth of penetration t_f of the particle in its initial direction.

Both of these quantities are nonstochastic and are usually stated in units of mass/area (e.g., g/cm^2). They customarily exclude the effects of internal nuclear interactions. The concepts of p and t_f are elucidated in Fig. 8.7.

A. CSDA Range

Experimentally the range can be determined (in principle) for an optically transparent medium such as photographic emulsion by microscopically following each particle track in three dimensions, and obtaining the mean pathlength of many such identical particles of the same starting energy. A closely similar but not identical quantity is called the *CSDA range* (Berger and Seltzer, 1983), which represents the

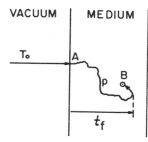

VACUUM | MEDIUM

T_0

A

B

P

t_f

FIGURE 8.7. Illustrating the concepts of *pathlength p* and *farthest depth of penetration*, t_f, for an individual electron. p is the total distance along the path from the point of entry A to the stopping point B. Note that t_f is not necessarily the depth of the terminal point B.

range in the continuous slowing down approximation. In terms of the mass stopping power, the CSDA range is defined as

$$\Re_{CSDA} \equiv \int_0^{T_0} \left(\frac{dT}{\rho dx}\right)^{-1} dT \tag{8.22}$$

where T_0 is the starting energy of the particle. If $dT/\rho dx$ is in MeV cm^2/g and dT in MeV, then $\Re_{CSDA}$ is thus given in g/cm^2.

$\Re_{CSDA}$ is the quantity tabulated, for example, in column 5 of the electron tables in Appendix E, as well as in the proton range tables of Bichsel (1968, Table IX), of Janni (1966) (who employed different nomenclature), and more recently of Anderson and Ziegler (1977). For all practical purposes $\Re_{CSDA}$ can be taken as identical to the range $\Re$ as defined above. Their small and subtle difference, due to the occurrence of discrete and discontinuous energy losses, has been discussed by Fano (NAS-NRC, 1964) and Bichsel (1968). The effect is expected to make the CSDA range slightly underestimate the actual range, by 0.2% or less for protons and by a somewhat greater (but undetermined) amount for electrons.

Figure 8.8 gives the CSDA range $\Re_{CSDA}$ for protons in C, Cu, and Pb. ($\Re_{CSDA}$) for carbon can be approximately represented ($\pm 5\%$) in g/cm^2 by

$$(\Re_{CSDA}) \simeq \frac{T_0^{1.77}}{415} + \frac{1}{670} \tag{8.23}$$

for proton kinetic energies 1 MeV $< T_0 <$ 300 MeV. Because of the decrease in the stopping power with increasing atomic number, the range (in mass/area) is greater for higher Z. Thus $\Re_{CSDA}$ in Pb is $\cong$ 3 times larger than for carbon at a proton energy of 1 MeV, decreasing to 2 times at 300 MeV. The proton range at a given energy is roughly proportional to Z^x, where $x \cong 0.4$ at 1 MeV, gradually falling to 0.3 at 30 MeV and 0.2 at 300 MeV.

The range of other heavy particles can be obtained from a proton table or estimated from Fig. 8.8 by recalling (from Section III.B.5) that:

a. All particles with the same velocity have kinetic energies in proportion to their rest masses [see Eq. (8.11)].

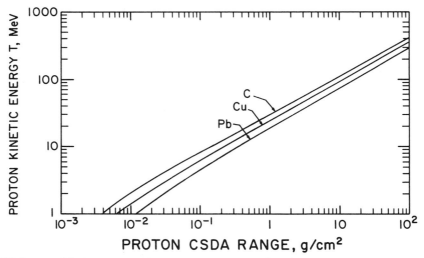

FIGURE 8.8. CSDA range (abscissa) vs. proton kinetic energy (ordinate) for C (graphite), Cu, and Pb.(From data of Bichsel, 1968).

b. All singly charged heavy particles with the same velocity have the same stopping power [see Eqs. (8.7) and (8.12)].

c. Consequently the range of singly charged heavy particles of the same velocity is proportional to their rest mass, since a proportional amount of energy must be disposed of.

For example, a deuteron with a kinetic energy of 20 MeV has the same velocity and stopping power as a 10-MeV proton. However, since the deuteron carries twice as much kinetic energy, it requires twice as much track length to dissipate that energy. An α-particle needs about 40 MeV to reach the same velocity as the 10-MeV proton. However, the z^2 dependence makes the stopping power for the α-particle 4 times that of the proton. The range needed to dissipate 40 MeV at 4 times the rate that the proton expends its energy is therefore about the same as the range of the 10-MeV proton.

In general the procedure for finding the CSDA range of a heavy particle of rest mass M_0 (see Table 8.1) and kinetic energy T_0 is to enter proton CSDA range tables (such as those of Anderson and Ziegler, 1977) at a proton energy $T_0^P = T_0 M_0^P / M_0$, where M_0^P is the proton's rest mass. If the tabulated proton CSDA range is $\mathfrak{R}_{\text{CSDA}}^P$, the other particle's range $\mathfrak{R}_{\text{CSDA}}$ is then obtained from

$$\mathfrak{R}_{\text{CSDA}} = \frac{\mathfrak{R}_{\text{CSDA}}^P M_0}{M_0^P z^2} \tag{8.24}$$

Equation (8.23) can be used in roughly approximating $\mathfrak{R}_{\text{CSDA}}^P$.

B. Projected Range

The projected range $\langle t \rangle$, defined at the beginning of Section IV, is most easily visualized in terms of flat layers of absorbing medium struck perpendicularly by a beam of charged particles. One counts the number of incident particles that penetrate the slab as its thickness is increased from zero to ∞ (or to a thickness great enough to stop all the incident particles).

$\langle t \rangle$ may be defined in that case as

$$\langle t \rangle \equiv \frac{\int_0^\infty t \cdot t_f(t)\, dt}{\int_0^\infty t_f(t)\, dt} = \frac{\int_0^\infty t \dfrac{dN(t)}{dt}\, dt}{\int_0^\infty \dfrac{dN(t)}{dt}\, dt} = -\frac{1}{N_0}\int_0^\infty t \cdot t_f(t)\, dt \qquad (8.25)$$

where N_0 is the number of incident particles minus those that undergo nuclear reactions, $N(t)$ is the number of particles penetrating a slab of thickness t, and $t_f(t) = dN(t)/dt$ is the differential distribution of farthest depths of penetration t_f. $dN(t)/dt$, which is the slope of the curve of penetrating particles vs. t, is always negative or zero.

Figure 8.9 shows typical graphs of the number of particles penetrating through slabs of varying thickness t. All particles are assumed to be monoenergetic and perpendicularly incident.

(a) HEAVY PARTICLES, NO NUCLEAR INTERACTIONS.

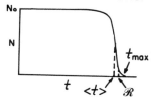

(b) HEAVY PARTICLES UNDERGOING NUCLEAR INTERACTIONS.

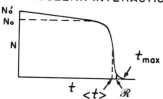

ELECTRONS

(c)

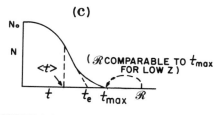

MONOENERGETIC PHOTONS (EXPONENTIAL)

(d)

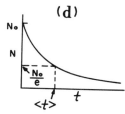

FIGURE 8.9. Numbers of monoenergetic charged particles or photons penetrating through a slab thickness t of absorbing medium. Scattered photons are assumed to be ignored in d. $\langle t \rangle$ is the projected range, t_e is the extrapolated penetration depth, t_{max} is the maximum penetration depth, and R is the range ($\cong R_{CSDA}$).

Figure 8.9a shows the penetration of heavy particles in the absence of nuclear interactions. Practically no reduction in numbers of particles is observed until the projected range $\langle t \rangle$ is approached, where a steep decrease to zero occurs. The value of t beyond which no particles are observed to penetrate is called t_{max}, the *maximum penetration depth*. For a proton or heavier particle this is only slightly less than the maximum pathlength, since t_{max} represents those particles which happen to suffer little scattering. The range $\Re$ (the mean value of the pathlength) is generally not more than 3% greater than $\langle t \rangle$ for protons (Bichsel, 1968).

Figure 8.9b illustrates the same situation for the case where nuclear interactions are present, causing the steady decline of N with increasing t from its initial value N_0' to N_0, which is equal to N_0' minus the number of particles undergoing nuclear reactions, and is approximately the number reaching the knee of the curve. Note that Eq. (8.25) calculates the projected range $\langle t \rangle$ on the basis of N_0, not N_0'. Likewise the CSDA range, which closely approximates the range $\Re$, is customarily calculated from Eq. (8.22) without including nuclear interactions, which are usually (but not always) negligible.

C. Straggling and Multiple Scattering

One can see from Fig. 8.9a and b that there is typically a distribution of farthest depths of penetration, t_f, by individual particles, giving rise to an S-shaped descending curve. This results from the combination of two effects: *multiple scattering* (which is predominant), and *range straggling*—a consequence of stochastic variations in rates of energy loss. Range straggling alone also affects pathlengths, giving rise to a less-pronounced distribution than is observed in t_f. A related effect, *energy straggling*, is the spread in energies observed in a population of initially identical charged particles after they have traversed equal path lengths. It will be somewhat exaggerated if the particles have passed through a layer of material, since multiple scattering then causes individual differences in path length as well. Multiple scattering in a foil also spreads an initially parallel beam of heavy charged particles into a conical angular distribution in accordance with Moliere's theory, as discussed by Bichsel (1968).

D. Electron Range

The electron CSDA range is calculated from Eq. 8.22, and the projected range from (8.25), the same as for heavy charged particles. However, it should be evident in Fig. 8.9c that these quantities are of marginal usefulness in characterizing the depth of penetration of electrons (or positrons). Scattering effects, both nuclear and electron–electron, cause the particles to follow such tortuous paths that $t_f(t)$ is smeared out from very small depths up to $t = t_{max} \cong 2\langle t \rangle$.

For low-Z media, t_{max} is comparable to $\Re$ (or $\Re_{CSDA}$), which is a convenience in the practical application of range tables. $\Re$ increases as a function of Z, as seen for protons in Fig. 8.8. A similar increase also occurs for electrons. However, a corresponding increase in the incidence of nuclear elastic scattering also takes place and *tends to make $\langle t \rangle$ and t_{max} roughly independent of Z for electrons and positrons* (Evans, 1955). Table 8.4 illustrates this effect, which can be seen in the static trend of t_{max} as Z is increased

TABLE 8.4. Comparison of Maximum Penetration Depth t_{max} with CSDA Range[a] for Electrons of Energy T_o

T_o (MeV)	Z	t_{max} (mg/cm^2)	$\mathfrak{R}_{CSDA}$ (mg/cm^2)	$t_{max}/\mathfrak{R}_{CSDA}$
.05	13 (Al)	5.05	5.71	.88
.10	13 (Al)	15.44	18.64	.83
.15	13 (Al)	31.0	36.4	.85
.05	29 (Cu)	5.42	6.90	.79
.10	29 (Cu)	17.1	22.1	.77
.15	29 (Cu)	34.0	42.8	.79
.05	47 (Ag)	5.04	7.99	.63
.10	47 (Ag)	15.6	25.2	.62
.15	47 (Ag)	30.2	48.4	.62
.05	79 (Au)	4.73	9.88	.48
.10	79 (Au)	14.3	30.3	.47
.15	79 (Au)	27.6	57.5	.48

[a] After Bichsel (1968), based on experimental results of Gubernator and Flammersfeld, and CSDA ranges of Berger and Seltzer (1964). Reproduced with permission from H. Bichsel and Academic Press, Inc.

from 13 to 79. $\mathfrak{R}_{CSDA}$ meanwhile increases by roughly $\frac{2}{3}$. Hence the curve shown in Fig. 8.9c remains roughly the same for media of different atomic numbers, with $\mathfrak{R}$ approximately coinciding with t_{max} for low Z, and $\mathfrak{R}$ gradually moving away to the right of t_{max} as Z increases.

The final column in Table 8.4 gives the ratio $t_{max}/\mathfrak{R}_{CSDA}$, which decreases from about 0.85 to 0.48 as Z goes from 13 to 79. This ratio shows very little energy dependence in the range $50 \leq T_0 \leq 150$ keV. This trend is continued at higher energies as well, judging from the calculations of Spencer (1959), which are excerpted in Table 8.5. That table contains values of $t_{max}/\mathfrak{R}_{CSDA}$ for electrons of 0.025 MeV $\leq T_0 \leq$

TABLE 8.5. $t_{max}/\mathfrak{R}_{CSDA}$ as Calculated by Spencer (1959) for a Plane Perpendicular Source of Electrons of Incident Energy T_o[a]

T_o (MeV)	$Z = 6$ (C)	13 (Al)	29 (Cu)	50 (Sn)	82 (Pb)
0.025	.95	.90	.80	—	—
0.05	.95	.87$_5$	.77$_5$	.72$_5$	—
0.1	.95	.87$_5$	.77$_5$	.70	.60
0.2	.95	.87$_5$	.75	.67$_5$	—
0.4	.95	.87$_5$	.75	.67$_5$	—
0.7	.95	.87$_5$	.75	.67$_5$	.55
1.0	.95	.87$_5$	.77$_5$	.67$_5$	.57$_5$
2	.95	.90	.77$_5$	.70	.60
4	.95	.90	.80	.75	—
10	.95	.92$_5$	.85	.80	—

[a] t_{max} was chosen as the tabulated penetration depth at which the dose first becomes zero. Data are not available where a dash is shown.

10 MeV in C, Al, Cu, Sn, and Pb. It is evident from a comparison of Tables 8.4 and 8.5 at $T_0 = 0.05$ and 0.1 MeV that the calculations agree reasonably well with experimental results for Al and Cu. Calculations for Sn and Pb (respectively) are significantly higher than measurements with Ag and Au, however, even after making allowances for the small Z-differences. The cause of this discrepancy is not known, but presumably resides in the calculation method for high-Z media. Spencer predicts $(t_{max}/\Re_{CSDA}) = 0.95$ for carbon at all energies. This is consistent with the statement earlier in this section that t_{max} is comparable to (i.e., probably $\cong 5\%$ less than) $\Re_{CSDA}$ for electrons in low-Z media.

Figure 8.10 is a graph of $\Re_{CSDA}$ vs. T_0 for electrons in carbon. Note the proportionality to T_0 above 2 MeV and to T_0^2 below 0.1 MeV.

The quantity t_0, also shown in Fig. 8.9c, is commonly called the *extrapolated range*, and is obtainable from experimental data by extrapolation of the straight portion of the descending curve to the axis. It has no physical significance except as a fairly well-defined experimental parameter for characterizing the penetrating power of charged particles for which multiple scattering is important, especially electrons.

E. Photon "Projected Range"

For comparison with the charged-particle penetration curves, Fig. 8.9d gives a corresponding curve for monoenergetic γ- or x-rays, where scattered photons are ignored. It is exponential vs. depth, with t_{max} at $t = \infty$. The concept of projected range $\langle t \rangle$ is even less useful here than it is for electrons as an indication of how far an individual ray will penetrate. Nevertheless if Eq. (8.25) is applied to the photon pen-

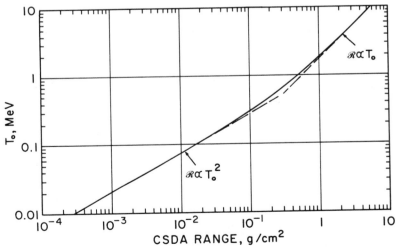

FIGURE 8.10.   CSDA range ($\cong 1.05 t_{max}$) of electrons in carbon. Note dependence upon T_0 above 2 MeV and upon T_0^2 below 0.1 MeV. t_{max} is comparable for higher Z-values as well. Data after Berger and Seltzer (1983); see Appendix E tables.

etration curve, employing $N(t) = N_0 e^{-\mu t}$, one obtains $\langle t \rangle = 1/\mu$, which is known as the *mean free path* or *relaxation length* of the photons in the medium. As noted in Chapter 7, it is the mean distance traveled by the individual photons in a large homogeneous population before each undergoes its first interaction. When $t = \langle t \rangle$, $N = N_0/e$.

V. CALCULATION OF ABSORBED DOSE

A. Dose in Thin Foils

1. SIMPLEST CASE

Consider a parallel beam of charged particles of kinetic energy T_0 perpendicularly incident on a foil of atomic number Z. We assume that the foil is thin enough so that:

a. the collision stopping power remains practically constant and characteristic of T_0, and

b. every particle passes straight through the foil, that is, scattering is negligible.

At the same time we will assume that:

c. the net kinetic energy carried out of the foil by δ rays is negligible, either because the foil is thick compared to the average δ-ray range, or because the foil is sandwiched between two foils of the same Z to provide CPE for the δ rays.

Backscattering may be ignored, as it is insignificant for heavy particles, and the average energy deposited by electrons in a thin foil is practically the same whether they are backscattered or transmitted (see Section V.D).

For heavy charged particles it is usually feasible to satisfy all of these requirements reasonably well if the foil thickness is only a few percent or less of the range. For electrons assumption **b** is the weakest, but may still give an adequate approximation in thin low-Z foils. Corrections for failure of each of these assumptions will be addressed later.

The energy lost in collision interactions by a fluence of Φ (charged particles/cm^2) of energy T_0 passing perpendicularly through a foil of mass thickness ρt (g/cm^2) is

$$E = \Phi \left(\frac{dT}{\rho dx}\right)_c \rho t \left(\frac{\text{MeV}}{\text{cm}^2}\right) \tag{8.26}$$

where $(dT/\rho dx)_c$ (MeV cm^2/g particle) is the mass collision stopping power of the foil medium, evaluated at T_0, and ρt is the particle pathlength through the foil.

Under assumption **c** the energy thus lost by the particles remains in the foil as energy imparted. Hence the absorbed dose in the foil can be gotten by dividing Eq. (8.26) by the mass per unit area of the foil:

$$D = \frac{\Phi(dt/\rho dx)_c\, \rho t}{\rho t} = \Phi \left(\frac{dT}{\rho dx}\right)_c \quad (\text{MeV/g})$$

$$= 1.602 \times 10^{-10}\, \Phi \left(\frac{dT}{\rho dx}\right)_c \text{Gy} \qquad (8.27)$$

in which the foil mass thickness ρt cancels, leaving the dose as simply the product of fluence and mass collision stopping power. This cancellation is very important, meaning that the dose in the foil is *independent of its thickness* as long as the particles travel straight through and do not lose enough energy to cause the stopping power to change significantly. Within these limitations, even tilting the foil away from the perpendicular does not alter the dose.

2. ESTIMATING δ-RAY ENERGY LOSSES

In the case where the foil is comparable in thickness to the range of the δ rays produced in it, assumption **c** may not be satisfied unless the target foil is sandwiched between "buffer" foils of the same material. Otherwise δ rays leaving will carry out energy, and other δ rays from adjacent but dissimilar materials may carry a different amount of energy in, producing a non-CPE situation for the δ rays in which the dose may differ from that given by Eq. (8.27).

If such a foil is isolated so that only the primary charged particles (no δ rays) are incident on it, one can estimate the dose in it by modifying Eq. (8.27). The mass collision stopping power is replaced by the corresponding restricted stopping power, $(dT/\rho dx)_\Delta$, as discussed in Section III.I. Here $(dT/\rho dx)_\Delta$ is that portion of the collision stopping power that includes only the interactions transferring less than the energy Δ. Thus if one chooses Δ to be the energy of those δ rays having, say, $\langle t \rangle = \rho t$, then one discards *all* the energy given to δ rays having projected ranges greater than the foil thickness. This will roughly account for the energy carried out of a thin isolated foil by δ rays, and provide an improved estimate of the average dose remaining in the foil.

In most cases it is difficult to fully isolate a foil with respect to incoming δ rays. Thus it is usually simpler and more accurate to use the sandwich method to provide δ-ray CPE in the foil than to estimate δ-ray energy losses.

3. ESTIMATING PATH LENGTHENING DUE TO SCATTERING IN THE FOIL

The average pathlength of heavy charged particles penetrating a foil in which only a few percent of the incident kinetic energy is lost is not significantly longer than a straight path through the foil in the direction of the entering particles. This is evident from the fact that the entire range of protons is usually not more than 3% greater than the projected range (see Section IV.B). Therefore a correction to Eq. (8.27) for path lengthening is not necessary for heavy particles.

For electrons, however, significant path lengthening results from multiple scattering, and a correction to Eq. (8.27) may be indicated. That is, the factor t in the numerator, which represents the mean electron pathlength traversed, becomes greater than the foil thickness t in the denominator, and should be given a modified symbol t'. Thus t'/t becomes greater than unity, and constitutes a correction factor for Eq. (8.27) to take account of path lengthening.

Birkhoff (1958) has discussed such a correction devised by Yang (1951), but suggested that on the basis of comparison with the Monte Carlo calculations of Hebbard and Wilson (1955) the Yang pathlength increase is probably too large by a factor of 2, and should be modified accordingly. Figure 8.11 gives values of $100(t' - t)/t$, the mean percentage path increase of electrons traversing a foil of mass thickness ρt (g/cm^2). In order to make the figure common to all foil media, the foil thickness is normalized by dividing it by the *radiation length* for the medium, which is the mass thickness in which electron kinetic energy would be diminished to $1/e$ of its original value due to radiative interactions only. That is, the normalized (dimensionless) foil thickness ξ is given by

$$\xi = \frac{\rho t}{X_0} \tag{8.28}$$

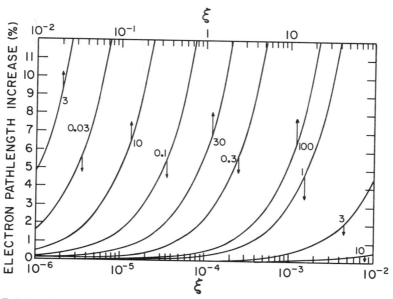

FIGURE 8.11.   Percentage increase in mean electron pathlength relative to normalized foil thickness ξ [= foil mass thickness ρt divided by radiation length of the medium; see Eq. (8.28)]. Data were calculated from the "modified Yang theory" according to Birkhoff (1958), given by $50t/w^2$ in Birkhoff's terminology. For a given energy and foil material the percentage increase in pathlength is proportional to foil thickness in the Yang approximation. Numbers on curves give electron energies in MeV.

where X_0 is the radiation length in the same units as ρt (g/cm^2). Seltzer and Berger (1985) have provided a table of X_0-values for 31 elements, of which a few are reproduced in Table 8.6.

As an example of the use of Fig. 8.11, consider a fluence of 10^{10}/cm^2 1-MeV electrons perpendicularly incident on a copper foil 0.01 g/cm^2 thick. X_0 for Cu is 13.04 g/cm^2 (from Table 8.6), giving $\xi = 7.7 \times 10^{-4}$. Figure 8.11 indicates that the mean electron pathlength will be 2.4% greater than 0.01 g/cm^2, increasing the absorbed dose in the foil by the same amount. The mass collision stopping power is 1.293 MeVcm^2/g, remaining constant within 0.1% while traversing the foil (see Appendix E). Ignoring δ-ray effects, the absorbed dose is thus increased from 2.07 Gy to 2.12 Gy by path lengthening due to electron scatter in the foil.

For applying Eq. (8.28) to compounds with elemental weight percentages f_{Z_i}, a mean value of X_0 is obtained from

$$\frac{1}{\overline{X}_0} = \frac{f_{Z_1}}{(X_0)_{Z_1}} + \frac{f_{Z_2}}{(X_0)_{Z_2}} + \cdots \tag{8.29}$$

B. Mean Dose in Thicker Foils

In foils that are thick enough to change the stopping power significantly (i.e. cause failure of assumption **a** in Section V.A.1, but not to stop the incident particles) one makes use of charged-particle CSDA range tables instead of stopping-power tables to calculate the average absorbed dose, which of course will no longer be uniform in depth through the foil. δ-ray effects may be neglected (that is, assumption **c** is satisfied), since the foil thickness is now large compared to most δ-ray ranges.

Assumption **b**, however, requiring straight tracks through the foil, will not be satisfied for this case, especially for electrons. As pointed out before, the resulting path-lengthening error is small ($\sim 1\%$) for heavy particles, and that correction will not be discussed here. The student is referred to Kase and Nelson (1978) or Evans (1955) for relevant information if such a correction is required. We will, however,

TABLE 8.6.   Radiation Lengths for Selected Elements[a]

Element	Z	X_o (g/cm^2)
H	1	63.04
He	2	94.39
C	6	43.35
Al	13	24.46
Cu	29	13.04
Sn	50	8.919
Pb	82	6.496
U	92	6.124

[a]After Seltzer and Berger (1985).

discuss next the calculation of the dose for the case of heavy charged particles passing straight through thicker foils.

1. DOSE FROM HEAVY PARTICLES

Using appropriate heavy-particle range tables such as those of Anderson and Ziegler (1977), one first enters the table to find the CSDA range (g/cm^2) of the incident beam of particles having kinetic energy T_0, in the appropriate foil material. The foil mass thickness *in the beam direction* is then subtracted, to find the residual CSDA range of the exiting particles. The range table is again entered to find the corresponding residual kinetic energy, T_{ex}, interpolating as necessary. Thus the energy spent in the foil by each particle is

$$\Delta T = T_0 - T_{ex} \quad (\text{MeV}) \tag{8.30}$$

and the energy imparted per unit cross-sectional area of particle beam is

$$E = \Phi \, \Delta T \quad (\text{MeV/cm}^2) \tag{8.31}$$

where Φ is the fluence.

The average absorbed dose is then obtained by dividing Eq. (8.31) by the mass thickness ρt if the beam passes through perpendicularly, or $\rho t / \cos \theta$ if the beam makes an angle θ with the perpendicular to the foil plane. Thus

$$D = 1.602 \times 10^{-10} \, \frac{\Phi \, \Delta T \cos \theta}{\rho t} \, \text{Gy} \tag{8.32}$$

2. DOSE FROM ELECTRONS

In this case we combine the technique of using range tables with that in which the path lengthening is corrected for. A further complication arises from the effect of bremsstrahlung production on the range. To avoid needless complication let us assume that the beam is perpendicularly incident; it will be obvious from the preceding section how to modify the calculation for a tilted foil.

The first step is to estimate the true mean pathlength for the electrons, which is done by the method discussed in Section V.A.3. If the foil is too thick to be covered by Fig. 8.11, this method is probably inadequate and computer radiation transport calculations should be employed. However, the percentage path lengthening in thicker foils may be roughly estimated by noticing that it is proportional to foil thickness in this approximation.

Using electron range tables such as those in Appendix E, one enters at the incident kinetic energy T_0 and obtains the corresponding CSDA range. From this the true mean pathlength of the electrons is subtracted to obtain the residual range of the exiting electron. The table is then reentered to obtain the residual kinetic energy T_{ex}. The energy lost by the particle is just $T_0 - T_{ex}$.

Some of this energy is carried away by bremsstrahlung x-rays, which can usually be assumed to make a negligible contribution to the energy imparted (or the dose) in the foil. To estimate the production of x-rays (which we will assume all escape), the ''radiation yield'' column in the Berger–Seltzer tables in Appendix E is employed. As explained before, the radiation yield $Y(T)$ of an electron of kinetic energy T is the fraction of T that is spent in radiative collisions as the electron slows down and stops. Consequently the energy fraction spent in collision interactions is $1 - Y(T)$. The energy spent in collision interactions in the foil is

$$\Delta T_c = (T_0 - T_{ex})_c = \{T_0[1 - Y(T_0)] - T_{ex}[1 - Y(T_{ex})]\}_c \qquad (8.33)$$

where $Y(T_0)$ and $Y(T_{ex})$ are obtained from column 6 in Appendix E. For a fluence Φ the average dose in the foil of mass thickness ρt is given in grays by

$$\overline{D} = 1.602 \times 10^{-10} \frac{\Phi \, \Delta T_c}{\rho t} \, \text{Gy} \qquad (8.34)$$

As an example of the calculation of the mean dose deposited by electrons in thicker foils, consider the case of a fluence of $10^{10}/\text{cm}^2$ 10-MeV electrons perpendicularly incident on a Pb layer 1 mm (1.13 g/cm^2) thick. From Table 8.6, the value of the radiation length for lead is $X_0 = 6.496$ g/cm^2, so the normalized foil thickness is 0.174. The pathlength increase is 8.5%, from Fig. 8.11; hence the mean pathlength is 1.23 g/cm^2.

Entering the electron range table for lead in Appendix E at $T_0 = 10$ MeV, we find $(R_{CSDA})_0 = 6.133$ g/cm². The residual range of the exiting electrons is $(R_{CSDA})_{ex} = 4.90$ g/cm², having a corresponding residual kinetic energy $T_{ex} = 7.29$ MeV.

The radiation yield of a 10-MeV electron is $Y(T_0) = 0.3162$, and that of a 7.29-MeV electron is $Y(T_{ex}) = 0.2607$ (see column 6 in Appendix E). Equation (8.33) gives

$$\Delta T_c = 10(1 - 0.3162) - 7.29(1 - 0.2607)$$

$$= 10(0.6838) - 7.29(0.7393) = 1.449 \, \text{MeV}$$

The average absorbed dose, from Eq. (8.34), is therefore

$$\overline{D} = 1.602 \times 10^{-10} \frac{1 \times 10^{10} \times 1.449}{1.13} = 2.05 \, \text{Gy}$$

If both path lengthening and the change in stopping power had been ignored, the corresponding approximate dose would have been about 6% less [from Eq. (8.27)]:

$$D = 1.602 \times 10^{-10} \times 1.201 \, \frac{\text{MeV cm}^2}{\text{g}} \times 10^{10} \, \text{cm}^{-2} = 1.92 \, \text{Gy}$$

C. Mean Dose in Foils Thicker than the Maximum Projected Range of the Particles

If the charged particles cannot penetrate through the foil of mass thickness ρt, then there will be a layer of unirradiated material beyond their stopping depth. If Φ particles/cm^2 of energy T_0 are perpendicularly incident and backscattering is negligible (as we have assumed throughout Section V), then the energy imparted in the foil per cm^2 equals the energy fluence (except for the correction for radiative losses):

$$E = \Phi T_0[1 - Y(T_0)] \quad (\text{MeV/cm}^2) \tag{8.35}$$

where the radiation yield $Y(T_0)$ is zero for heavy particles.

The average absorbed dose in the foil is given by

$$\overline{D} = 1.602 \times 10^{-10} \times \frac{\Phi T_0[1 - Y(T_0)]}{\rho t} \text{ Gy} \tag{8.36}$$

The dose of course changes radically with depth in the foil, as will be discussed in Section V.E.

If the radiative losses are considerable and the foil thickness is great enough, the dose throughout the foil may be significantly enhanced by the resulting x-ray field. A very crude estimate of the reabsorbed fraction of the energy invested in these x-rays can be gotten by calculating

$$\exp\left[-\frac{\mu_{en}}{\rho} \cdot \frac{\rho t}{2}\right] \tag{8.37}$$

where μ_{en}/ρ for the foil material is to be evaluated at some mean x-ray energy, say $0.4 T_0$ for thick-target bremsstrahlung. Multiplying the $Y(T_0)$ in Eq. (8.35) or (8.36) by the above exponential term roughly corrects for x-ray absorption, assuming the rays must pass through half the foil thickness to escape. An accurate treatment of this problem requires computer calculations, taking account of x-ray distributions vs. angle and energy.

D. Electron Backscattering

As noted before, the effect of particle backscattering on dose calculation has been neglected throughout Section V so far. For heavy particles this is justified by the fact that they are seldom scattered through large angles. For electrons, backscattering due to nuclear elastic interactions can be an important cause of dose reduction, especially for high Z, low T_0, and thick target layers. In this connection, an infinitely thick foil with respect to the backscattering of a perpendicularly incident beam of charged particles will be provided by a thickness of $t_{max}/2$ (i.e., half of the maximum penetration depth as defined in Section IV.B). Particles penetrating beyond that depth in a thicker layer obviously cannot return to the surface.

Electrons incident on a thin foil, in which a backscattering event is equally likely to occur in the first or the last infinitesimal layer of the foil, require no backscattering correction to the absorbed dose. On average, backscattering can be assumed to occur in the *midplane* of the foil. The energy spent in the foil by an electron reflected from the midplane is the same as if it passed straight through without backscattering. The energy distribution vs. depth in the foil is thus shifted toward the entry surface, but the average absorbed dose through the foil remains the same to a first approximation.

For thicker foils a backscattering correction requires a knowledge of what fraction of the incident energy fluence is redirected into the reverse hemisphere. For electrons perpendicularly incident on infinitely thick layers, this fraction may be called the *electron energy backscattering coefficient*, $\eta_e(T_0, Z, \infty)$. The measurement of η_e is best accomplished by calorimetry, comparing the known incident energy flux (i.e., the number of primary electrons multiplied by their individual energy) with the heating of the target. An example of such data has been provided by Wright and Trump (1962) for the energy range $T_0 = 1$ to 3.5 MeV, as shown in Fig. 8.12. The results of Schuler (1958) with 2-MeV electrons are in reasonable agreement. More extensive experiments of this type for other T_0, Z, and foil thicknesses less than as well as greater than $t_{max}/2$ are needed to allow accurate electron backscattering corrections to be applied more generally.

For lack of additional data on electron energy backscattering, one can make use of information on backscattered-electron *numbers* as an upper limit on the backscattered energy. For electrons with incident energies $T_0 \geq 1$ MeV, the backscattering coefficient $\eta(T_0, Z, \infty)$ (i.e., the fractional number of perpendicularly incident electrons that are backscattered from an infinitely thick layer of atomic number Z) has been given by Tabata (1967) as

$$\eta(T_0, Z, \infty) = 1.28 \exp\left[-11.9 Z^{-0.65}(1 + 0.103 Z^{0.37} T_0^{0.65})\right] \qquad (8.38)$$

which applies for T_0 at least up to 22 MeV, although it tends to underestimate small values of $\eta \leq 2\%$. This formula predicts that η increases with Z and decreases with

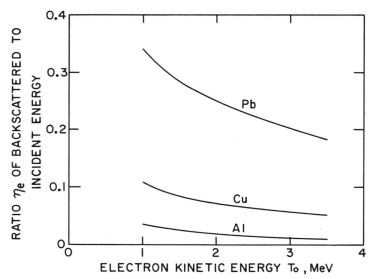

FIGURE 8.12. Fraction η_e of incident energy flux carried away by backscattered electrons. Primary electrons are perpendicularly incident, with individual kinetic energy T_0, on infinitely thick ($> t_{max}/2$) layers of the indicated scattering materials. After Wright and Trump (1962).

increasing electron energy. For example, at $T_0 = 1$ MeV, η is given as 0.45 for lead, 0.21 for copper, and 0.074 for aluminum, while at $T_0 = 3$ MeV these figures are reduced to 0.31, 0.13, and 0.040 respectively.

For electrons below $T_0 = 1$ MeV, Eq. (8.38) probably underestimates η. The experimental results of Bothe (1949), obtained with 0.37- and 0.68-MeV electrons, showed practically no energy dependence, yielding for copper the value $\eta \cong 0.43$. By comparison, for copper Eq. (8.38) gives 0.26 for $T_0 = 0.37$ MeV and 0.23 for $T_0 = 0.68$ MeV. Other backscattering data reviewed by Baily (1980) provide a variety of values, yielding no clear consensus on the true electron-backscattering picture for $T_0 < 1$ MeV. The role played by the numerous low-energy secondary electrons (δ-rays) that emerge from the scatterer along with the backscattered primaries may be an important source of variability in experimental results, especially for lower T_0. Tabata arbitrarily chose not to count any electrons that were backscattered with energies less than 50 eV, thus eliminating most secondaries.

As mentioned above, $\eta_e(T_0, Z, \infty)$ should be less than $\eta(T_0, Z, \infty)$, because each backscattered electron has less kinetic energy than it had when it was incident on the scattering material. Comparison of Eq. (8.38) with Fig. 8.12 tends to verify this. For example, 1-MeV electrons on Pb have a value of $\eta_e = 0.34$ from Fig. 8.12, while $\eta = 0.45$ from Eq. (8.38). Thus the average fractional energy per backscattered electron from Pb is about 0.75 of T_0 in that case, but decreases to 0.58 at $T_0 = 3$ MeV.

Tabata also measured $\eta(T_0, Z, t)$ as a function of the foil thickness t, but only for $T_0 = 6.08$ MeV and $Z = 29, 47$, and 79. The ratio $\eta(T_0, Z, t)/\eta(T_0, Z, \infty)$ was found to increase continuously with increasing t from 0 to $t_{max}/2$, and to have a value of about 0.6 to 0.8 for $t = t_{max}/4$. This shows that layers of material nearer the entry surface are more important in electron backscattering than are the deeper layers, as one might expect, but that the process is not confined to a thin surface layer.

E.   Dose vs. Depth for Charged-Particle Beams

Figure 8.9a, b, and c illustrated how the number of charged particles penetrating through a layer of some absorbing medium varies with the layer thickness. The variation of absorbed dose vs. depth in a medium shows quite different characteristics. The shape of this function depends on particle type and energy, the medium being penetrated, and the geometry of the beam.

1.   THE BRAGG CURVE

Heavy charged particles (protons and heavier) penetrating a material in which nuclear interactions are negligible show a dose-vs.-depth distribution in the shape of the classical *Bragg curve*, as illustrated in Fig. 8.13a. This is a consequence of the $\propto T_0^2$ dependence of the range at low energies (see, e.g., Figs. 8.8 and 8.10), which in turn results from the $\propto \beta^{-2}$ dependence of the stopping power. This means that if a particle spends the first half of its initial kinetic energy along a pathlength x, the remaining half of the energy will be spent in distance $\cong x/3$, thus crowding the spatial

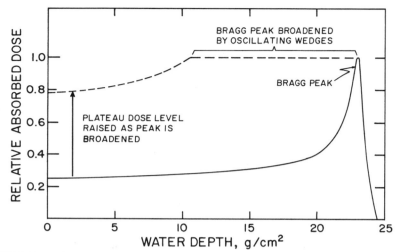

FIGURE 8.13a.   Dose vs. depth for 187-MeV protons in water, showing Bragg peak. The dashed curve demonstrates the effect of passing the beam through optimally designed, variable-thickness absorbers such as oscillating wedges. (After Karlsson, 1964. Reproduced with permission from Strahlentherapie.)

rate of energy expenditure toward the end of the track. The dose decreases from its maximum as the particles run out of energy and stop. This descending limb of the Bragg curve roughly coincides with the corresponding curve of particles vs. depth.

The highly localized dose maximum shown in Fig. 8.13a suggests the possible usefulness of such a beam for delivery of therapeutic doses of ionizing radiation to tumors at some depth in the body while minimizing dose to overlying normal tissues. This possibility was discussed by Raju et al. (1969). They pointed out that the Bragg peak of heavy particles is *too* localized, and needs to be "smeared out" in depth if tumors even 1 cm in diameter are to be uniformly dosed. Such devices as oscillating wedges can be used to produce a distribution of incident energies, resulting in a roughly square-topped Bragg peak as in Fig. 8.13a, but at the expense of increasing the "plateau" dose level relative to the Bragg peak dose.

As mentioned earlier, negative pions are captured by atoms of tissue when they stop, causing the atomic nuclei to emit neutrons, γ-rays, and heavy charged particles. The latter particles, being of relatively short range, enhance the dose in the vicinity of the Bragg peak. Figure 8.13b shows the resulting enhanced Bragg curve, in comparison with the corresponding curve for positive pions that are not captured.

2. DOSE VS. DEPTH FOR ELECTRON BEAMS

As noted before, the small mass of electrons makes them scatter easily. As a result, they do not give rise to a Bragg peak near the end of their projected range as heavy particles do. Instead, a diffuse maximum is reached at roughly half of the maximum

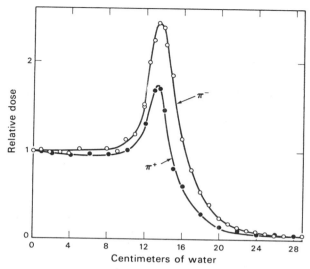

FIGURE 8.13b.   Dose vs. depth in water for 65-MeV positive and negative pion beams. The absorbed dose is enhanced for the negative beam, especially around the Bragg peak, by nuclear capture and annihilation with emission of energetic particles. (After Raju and Richman, 1972. Reproduced with permission from the North Holland Physics Publishing Co.)

penetration depth, as shown in Fig. 8.14a for "broad" beams of electrons of several incident energies. An electron beam is defined as broad if its radius upon entry is at least equal to its CSDA range. Figure 8.14b shows the effect of decreasing the radius below that value (indicated as ∞ in the figure), for a 10-MeV beam. The curve shape is evidently affected very strongly.

3. CALCULATION OF ABSORBED DOSE AT DEPTH

At any point P at depth x in a medium w where the charged-particle fluence spectrum is known, the absorbed dose can be calculated as

$$D_w = 1.602 \times 10^{-10} \int_0^{T_{max}} \Phi_x(T)\left(\frac{dT}{\rho dx}\right)_{c,w} dT \qquad (8.39)$$

where $\Phi_x(T)$ is the differential charged-particle fluence spectrum, excluding δ rays, in particles/cm^2 MeV; $(dT/\rho dx)_{c,w}$ is the mass collision stopping power for medium w, in units of MeV cm^2/g particle, given as a function of kinetic energy T; T is in MeV; and D_w is given in grays, since 1.602×10^{-10} Gy = 1 MeV/g.

The exclusion of δ rays from $\Phi_x(T)$ is based on the assumption that CPE exists at P for the δ rays. Thus any energy carried out of a small volume around P by δ rays will be replaced by other δ rays from elsewhere. The use of the mass collision stopping power, rather than a restricted stopping power, is consistent with this assumption. δ-ray CPE requires that the medium and the particle fluence be ho-

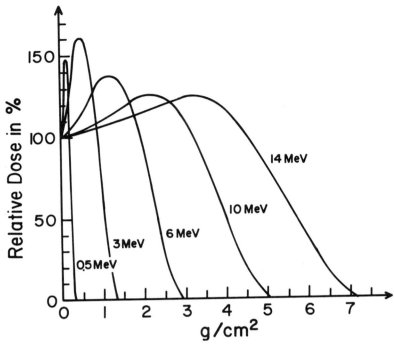

FIGURE 8.14a. Dose vs. depth in water for broad electron beams of the indicated incident energies. (After Holm, 1969. Reproduced with permission of N. W. Holm and Academic Press.)

mogeneous within the maximum δ-ray range from P. In practice this assumption is usually adequately satisfied because most δ rays tend to have short ranges ($\lesssim 1$ mm) in condensed media.

The problem of determining $\Phi_x(T)$ at the point of interest is, of course, nontrivial, generally requiring radiation-transport calculations for a good solution. However, an estimate can be obtained rather easily from range tables for a monoenergetic plane-parallel beam of heavy charged particles incident on a homogeneous medium, since scattering and energy straggling are small effects. One enters the range tables at initial energy T_0, determining the range $\mathfrak{R}$. From this the depth x is subtracted to obtain the remaining range $\mathfrak{R}_r$ of the particle when it reaches depth x. Then the table is reentered at range $\mathfrak{R}_r$ to determine the remaining kinetic energy T_r. The particle fluence Φ_x at depth x in this simple case is taken to be the same as the Φ_0 incident on the surface (neglecting nuclear interactions), and all the particles are assumed to have energy T_r (MeV). Thus the integral in Eq. (8.39) can be dispensed with, and the dose (Gy) is given by

$$D_x = 1.602 \times 10^{-10} \; \Phi_0 \left(\frac{dT}{\rho dx} \right)_{c,w} \tag{8.40}$$

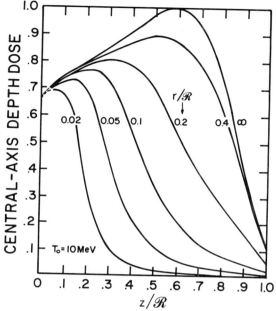

FIGURE 8.14b. Dose vs. depth in water for circular electron beams of radius r at incidence. $\mathfrak{R}$ = CSDA range, z = depth in phantom. T_0 = 10 MeV. (After Berger, 1981. Reproduced with permission from M. J. Berger and the American Institute of Physics.)

where Φ_0 is in particles/cm^2 and $(dT/\rho\,dx)_{c,w}$ is the mass collision stopping power for the medium w, evaluated at T_r. This method begins to fail when x approaches the particle range, making $\Phi_x < \Phi_0$ (see Fig. 8.9a).

For the case of a broad beam of monoenergetic electrons (see preceding section) of energy $T_0 > 1$ MeV (see Fig. 8.10) perpendicularly incident on a semi-infinite homogeneous low-Z medium, one can roughly estimate the most probable energy of the electrons at depth. Since the range is proportional to the kinetic energy for megavolt electrons, the modal energy decreases from T_0 to 0 approximately linearly with depth as x goes from 0 to the range $\mathfrak{R}$. However, the electron fluence at depth is *not* easily estimated, mainly because of multiple scattering. Thus dose calculations on the basis of electron fluence generally require radiation transport calculations (see Nelson, 1980).

The problem of measuring dose in a medium by inserting a small sensor or probe (e.g., a cavity ion chamber) at the point of interest involves cavity theory, which will be discussed in Chapter 10. Chapter 13 will deal with in-phantom dosimetry, including practical application of cavity theory. The usefulness of the above method for estimating the electron modal energy vs. depth will become apparent there, as it provides an effective energy at which stopping-power ratios (used in cavity theory) can be evaluated.

PROBLEMS

1. Compare the passage of charged and uncharged particles through matter. What are the approximate probabilities of a single charged particle achieving a pathlength equal to twice its range, or of a single photon having a pathlength twice as great as the mean free path $1/\mu$? (Assume the photon is totally absorbed in its first interaction.)

2. Describe the general types of interactions that contribute to the collision stopping power, $(dT/\rho dx)_c$.

3. A 200-keV electron passes through a thin sample of fused silica for which the index of refraction is $n = 1.46$. At what angle is the Čerenkov radiation (if any) emitted, relative to the electron direction? What is the half angle of the conical ''shock'' wavefront (relative to the backward direction)?

4. Consider a small mass of tissue irradiated by negative pions.

    (a) Calculate the absorbed dose in grays due to star production only, at a point in a region throughout which 7×10^7 pions stop per gram (assuming CPE for the star fragments).

    (b) Use Eqs. (2.1) and (2.2) to obtain the value of the kerma.

5. What is the maximum energy that can be transferred to an electron in a hard collision by a 25-MeV (a) electron (according to convention), (b) positron, (c) proton, (d) α-particle?

6. Redo problem 5 for the case where each of the particles has the same *velocity* as a 25-MeV proton.

7. What are the soft and hard components of the mass collision stopping power for an 800-MeV triton in copper? (Assume $H = 10^2$ eV.) Does the total agree with Eq. (8.10)?

8. (a) At what kinetic energy would an α-particle have the same velocity as the particle in problem 7?

    (b) What is the mass collision stopping power of such an α-particle in Cu?

9. A cyclotron is capable of accelerating protons to 100 MeV, maximum.

    (a) What are the approximate maximum kinetic energies to which deuterons and α-particles can be accelerated?

    (b) Compute the mass collision stopping power in water for such an α-particle. Ignore the shell correction.

10. Calculate the mass collision stopping power for a 20-MeV proton in lead, without the shell correction.

11. Calculate the mass collision stopping powers for an electron and for a positron with a kinetic energy of 50 MeV in aluminum. (Include the polarization-effect correction.)

12. Estimate the approximate mass radiative stopping power for the electrons in problem 11. Also, what would it be for lead in place of aluminum?

13. From Appendix E, how much energy (J) is emitted as x-radiation by 10^{15} electrons entering a layer of tin at $T_0 = 10$ MeV and exiting at $\overline{T} = 7$ MeV?

14. From Eq. (8.23) and following discussion, what is the approximate value of the range (g/cm^2) of a 30-MeV proton in iron?

15. (a) At what energy would a deuteron have the same velocity as the proton in problem 14?

    (b) What would be this deuteron's range in iron?

16. What is the dose (Gy) in a thin LiF dosimeter struck by a fluence of 3×10^{11} e/cm^2 with $T_0 = 20$ MeV? (Ignore δ-rays.)

17. What is the average dose (Gy) in an aluminum foil 0.3 g/cm^2 thick, from being irradiated perpendicularly by 10^9 e/cm^2 of energy $T_0 = 3$ MeV? (Let x-rays escape.)

SOLUTIONS TO PROBLEMS

1. The charged particle has $\cong 0$ probability of reaching twice its range, while the photon has a probability of $e^{-2} = 0.14$ of traveling a distance $2/\mu$ without an interaction.

3. $\xi = 9.9°$, $90° - 9.9° = 80.1°$.

4. (a) 0.336 Gy.

   (b) 0.336 Gy; note that

   $$\epsilon_{tr}^n = \epsilon_{tr} = (R_{in})_u - (R_{out})_u^{non-r} + \Sigma Q$$

   $$\frac{d\epsilon_{tr}}{dm} = 7 \times 10^7[0 - 70 \text{ MeV} + 100 \text{ MeV}] = 2.1 \times 10^9 \text{ MeV/g};$$

   40 MeV spent in overcoming nuclear binding energy is part of the remaining products' rest mass.

5. (a) 12.5 MeV.

   (b) 25 MeV.

   (c) 0.0552 MeV.

   (d) 0.0138 MeV.

6. (a) 6.8 keV.

   (b) 13.6 keV.

   (c) 0.0552 MeV.

   (d) 0.0552 MeV.

7. (a) 1.08 MeV cm²/g.

   (b) 1.49 MeV cm²/g.

   (c) 2.57 MeV cm²/g (agrees).

8. **(a)**   1062 MeV.

    (b)   10.3 MeV cm^2/g.

9. **(a)**   Deuteron: 50 MeV; α-particle: 101 MeV.

    (b)   86 MeV cm²/g.

10. 11.6 MeV cm²/g.

11. Electron: 1.79 MeV cm^2/g; positron: 1.74 MeV cm^2/g.

12. 1.6 MeV cm^2/g for Al (vs. 1.76 in Appendix E); 8 MeV cm^2/g for Pb, (vs. 6.87 in Appendix E).

13. 168 J.

14. 1.5 g/cm^2.

15. **(a)**   60 MeV.

     (b)   3.1 g/cm².

16. 79.5 Gy.

17. 0.256 Gy.

CHAPTER 9

X-Ray Production
and Quality

I. INTRODUCTION

The scope of this chapter is limited to the physics of x-ray generation and beam-quality description. The specifics of various types of x-ray machines and electron accelerators have been adequately dealt with in other texts such as that of Johns and Cunningham (1983).

The word "quality" as applied to an x-ray beam ordinarily may be taken as synonymous with "hardness", i.e., penetrating ability. In the earlier days of radiotherapy, before megavolt x- or γ-ray beams became generally available, the effectiveness of x-ray treatment of deep-seated tumors depended upon the ability of the orthovoltage (< 300-kV) x-rays to penetrate to the tumor while limiting the dose to overlying tissues. For that application, the more strongly penetrating the beam, the higher its quality. The same term is still applied to x-ray beam hardness even in cases where penetrating power should not necessarily be maximized (e.g., in diagnostic radiology).

"Quality" of radiation is also used in the more general sense of *energy spectral distribution*, or in the special meaning of *biological effectiveness*.

II. X-RAY PRODUCTION AND ENERGY SPECTRA

A. Fluorescence X-Rays

Fluorescence (also called "characteristic") x-ray production has been discussed to some extent in Chapters 5 (in connection with the electron capture and internal conversion) and 7 (in its association with the photoelectric effect). It was also mentioned in Chapter 8 that when hard collisions occur between charged particles and inner-shell electrons, the filling of the resulting shell vacancy generates fluorescence x-rays. Only a small fraction ($\lesssim 1\%$) of the charged-particle energy spent in collision interactions goes into fluorescence x-ray production, however.

1. FLUORESCENCE YIELD

The probability that a fluorescence x-ray will escape from the atom of its origin is called the *fluorescence yield*, symbolized by Y_K for a K-shell vacancy, and so on. Y_K and Y_L are plotted vs. Z in Fig. 7.14. Evidently, escaping fluorescence x-rays are practically nonexistent for elements with atomic numbers less than 10, and the K-shell yield increases rapidly with Z to about 0.95 for tungsten ($Z = 74$), the most common x-ray tube target.

For the L-shell the yield remains relatively low, and since the L-shell binding energy also is small (12.1 keV for the $L1$ shell in tungsten—see Table 9.1), L-shell fluorescence is of little practical importance as an x-ray production process. Only K-shell fluorescence need be considered here.

2. INITIATING EVENT

The initiating event in K-fluorescence x-ray production is the removal of a K-shell electron by one of the processes mentioned above. Thus the minimum energy that must be supplied is the K-shell binding energy, $(E_b)_K$. Appendix B.1 lists $(E_b)_K$ and $(E_b)_{L1}$ for all the elements. A photon of quantum energy $h\nu \geq 69.5$ keV, for example, can generate K-fluorescence in tungsten through the photoelectric effect.

An electron of kinetic energy $T > 69.5$ keV can do likewise by ejecting the K-shell electron in a hard collision. Notice that the electron is *not* required to have an incident energy exceeding *twice* the binding energy to accomplish this, even though an electron is conventionally supposed to be able to give no more than half its energy to another electron, as discussed in Chapter 8, Section III.D. That formalism, as applied in the electron stopping-power equation, merely acknowledges that the incident electron and the struck electron are indistinguishable after the collision, and the one departing with the most energy is therefore *designated, post facto*, as having been the incident electron. The fact that an incident electron with $T > (E_b)_K$ can remove a K-shell electron proves, however, that kinetic-energy transfers up to T must occur in electron–electron collisions, as one would expect from momentum-conservation considerations.

Although electron beams are the most common means of generating fluorescence x-rays, they appear in that case against a very strong background of bremsstrahlung continuous-spectrum x-rays. If it is desired to have a relatively pure fluorescence x-ray source with greatly reduced bremsstrahlung background, either heavy-particle excitation or x-ray excitation of fluorescence by the photoelectric effect may be employed. Both methods are used for trace-element fluorescence analysis (Gilfrich et al., 1973). Larson et al. (1955) designed an x-ray-excited fluorescence source that was said to be suitable for dosimeter calibrations. Compton-scattering limits the beam purity in that case, and the output dose rate is low.

When heavy particles such as protons or α-particles are used to excite x-ray fluorescence, one might suppose from momentum-conservation considerations that the minimum energy necessary to ionize the K-shell would be controlled by Eq. (8.4), or

$$T'_{max} = \frac{4 M_0 m_0 T}{(M_0 + m_0)^2} > (E_b)_K \qquad (9.1)$$

where T'_{max} is the maximum energy that can be transferred by a heavy particle of rest mass M_0 and kinetic energy T to a free electron of mass m_0 at rest. Thus, on this basis, a proton ($M_0 = 1836 m_0$) would have to have an energy 460 times the binding energy E_b to eject an electron from its shell. However, it is found that this threshold does not apply for ionization of strongly bound electrons by heavy particles. That is because the binding energy, in effect, increases the mass of the electron, thereby allowing larger energy transfers. A thorough discussion has been provided by Merzbacher and Lewis (1958). Figure 9.1 gives cross sections for fluorescence x-ray production by protons.

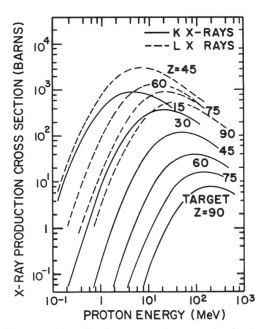

FIGURE 9.1. Atomic cross sections for fluorescence x-ray production by protons. (From Gordon and Kraner, 1971. Reproduced with permission from Brookhaven National Laboratory.)

TABLE 9.1   Electron Binding Energies E_b in Tungsten[a]

Shell $\downarrow$	$(E_b)_K$ (keV)	Shell $\downarrow$	$(E_b)_L$ (keV)	Shell $\downarrow$	$(E_b)_M$ (keV)	Shell $\downarrow$	$(E_b)_N$ (keV)
K	69.525	L_{I}	12.098	M_{I}	2.820	N_{I}	0.595
		L_{II}	11.541	M_{II}	2.575	N_{II}	0.492
		L_{III}	10.204	M_{III}	2.281	N_{III}	0.424
				M_{IV}	1.871	N_{IV}	0.256
				M_{V}	1.809	N_{V}	0.242
						N_{VI}	0.036
						N_{VII}	0.034

3. *K*-FLUORESCENCE PHOTON ENERGY

Following the creation of a *K*-shell vacancy, an electron from another higher shell will fill it, and may emit a fluorescence photon having a quantum energy equal to the difference in the two energy levels involved. Again citing the example of tungsten, Table 9.1 lists the binding energies for the *K*-, *L*-, *M*-, and *N*-shells, having 1, 3, 5, and 7 subshells, respectively. Quantum mechanical selection rules allow transitions to the *K*-shell mainly from the levels shown in boxes.

The resulting transitions to the *K*-shell, the designation of the resulting fluorescence lines, and their quantum energies and relative frequencies of occurrence are shown in Table 9.2. It will be seen that the fluorescence line known as α_1 occurs at 59.321 keV with relative strength 100, α_2 at 57.984 keV with relative strength 57.6,

TABLE 9.2   *K*-Shell X-Ray Fluorescence Energies in Tungsten[a]

Transition	Designation	Energy (keV)		Relative No. of Photons	
K-L_{III}	α_1	59.321		100	
K-L_{II}	α_2	57.984		57.6	
K-M_{II}	β_3	66.950 ⎫		10.8 ⎫	
K-M_{III}	β_1	67.244 ⎪ $\cong 67.2$		20.8 ⎪ 32.1	
K-M_{IV}	$\beta_{5/1}$	67.654 ⎪		0.233 ⎬	
K-M_{V}	$\beta_{5/2}$	67.716 ⎭		0.293 ⎭	
K-N_{II}	$\beta_{2/1}$	69.033 ⎫		2.45 ⎫	
K-N_{III}	$\beta_{2/2}$	69.101 ⎪		4.77 ⎪	
K-N_{IV}	$\beta_{4/1}$	69.269 ⎬ 69.276 $\cong 69.1$		0.127 ⎬ 8.4	
K-N_{V}	$\beta_{4/2}$	69.283 ⎭			
K-O_{II}	$\beta_{2/3}$	69.478 ⎫ 69.484		1.07 ⎭	
K-O_{III}	$\beta_{2/4}$	69.489 ⎭			

[a] After Storm and Israel (1970). Reproduced with permission from Academic Press.

$\beta_3 + \beta_1 + \beta_{5/1} + \beta_{5/2}$ at about 67.2 keV with combined relative strength 32.1, and all the other lines closely grouped around 69.1 keV with combined relative strength 8.4. With typical spectroscopic resolution the lines appear as two closely spaced doublets separated by about 10 keV, the α-doublet being about four times as strong as the β. This general pattern is typical of other x-ray targets as well.

If a narrower energy spectral distribution than the combined $\alpha + \beta$ line array is desired, a filter having its K-edge between the α- and β-lines will discriminate against the latter.

X-ray fluorescence lines are often used for energy calibration of photon spectrometers.

4. DIRECTIONAL DISTRIBUTIONS OF FLUORESCENCE VS. BREMSSTRAHLUNG

Since fluorescence is emitted in a secondary transition process following a primary ionization event, there is no angular correlation between the direction of the incident particle and that of the fluorescence photon. Fluorescence is emitted isotropically with respect to both energy and intensity, neglecting attenuation of rays in escaping the target. Bremsstrahlung x rays, on the other hand, are emitted anisotropically, tending to go more and more closely in the electron's direction with increasing energy. In thin targets in which electron scattering can be neglected, bremsstrahlung production shows strong angular dependence and a minimum value at 180°. Figure 9.2 compares the directional distributions for K-fluorescence and bremsstrahlung x rays generated in a thin silver foil by 50- and 500-keV electrons. It is evident that the ratio of K-fluorescence to bremsstrahlung is a maximum at 180°. This is generally true irrespective of Z, T, or target thickness, although the angular dependence of bremsstrahlung x rays becomes much less pronounced for thick targets. Motz et al. (1971) and Dick et al. (1973) have investigated high-intensity K-fluorescent x-ray sources based on this principle.

5. DEPENDENCE OF FLUORESCENCE OUTPUT ON ELECTRON BEAM ENERGY

The energy of the incident electron beam also influences the intensity of fluorescence x-ray production. If T is below the K binding energy, no K-lines appear. For $T > (E_b)_K$ all the K-lines are generated with fixed relative strengths, shown in Table 9.2 for tungsten, regardless of how much higher T may be. However, the efficiency for K-fluorescence production increases rapidly at first for $T > (E_b)_K$, reaches a maximum, and then decreases slowly as T continues to rise.

Figure 9.3 shows this trend for thick targets. For thin targets the maxima occur at lower energies, and of course the K-fluorescent x-ray outputs are also lower, as reported by Motz et al. (1971). Since the bremsstrahlung output from a thick target continues to increase with T without limit (as will be discussed in the next section), the ratio of K-fluorescence to bremsstrahlung x-ray output must also reach a maximum and then decrease for still higher T. Measuring at 180°, Motz et al. report

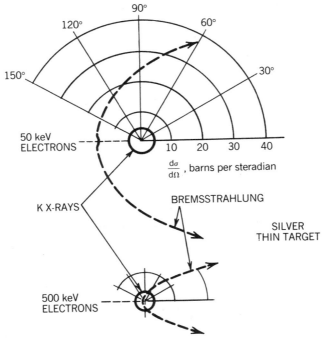

FIGURE 9.2. Comparison of the directional distributions of *K* x-rays (solid curves) and bremsstrahlung (dashed curves) for 50- and 500-keV electrons incident on a thin silver target. The relative magnitudes are shown in terms of differential cross sections for *K*-shell ionization and bremsstrahlung production, per unit solid angle in which the photons are emitted. (From Dick et al., 1973. Reproduced with permission of C. E. Dick and The American Institute of Physics.)

achieving maximum fluorescence x-ray "purities" (i.e., *K*-photons/total photons) of 56–86%, depending upon *Z*.

Table 9.3 roughly compares the *K*-fluorescence outputs and beam purities attainable by (a) the photoelectric effect (using x rays to excite the fluorescer), (b) using electrons with 180° geometry, and (c) using heavy ions. The last method is seen to reach the highest-purity beams, with outputs comparable to those gotten with electrons. The output with photoelectric excitation is evidently several orders of magnitude lower.

At the time of this writing none of these methods for fluorescence x-ray beam generation is in common use for dosimetry applications, probably because all require special apparatus. Instead, heavily filtered bremsstrahlung x-ray beams are usually employed, e.g., for dosimeter energy-dependence measurements. It will be shown, however, that the spectral widths of such beams are much greater than for *K*-fluorescence lines, with a resulting loss of energy resolution.

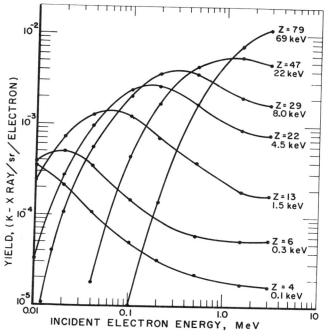

FIGURE 9.3. Dependence of K x-ray yield from thick targets of $Z = 4$ to 79 on incident electron energy. The approximate mean energy of the K fluorescence is also given for each curve. (From Sparrow and Dick, 1976. Reproduced with permission from C. E. Dick.)

TABLE 9.3. Comparison of Different Excitation Sources for K X-ray Production[a]

	Excitation Source	Maximum Output (K photons/sr s)	Beam Purity (%)
a.	*X-ray Photons*		
	300 kV, 10 mA	$\sim 10^{10}$	> 90
b.	*Electrons*		
	300 kV, 10 mA	$\sim 10^{14}$	50–95
	1000 A, pulsed	$\sim 10^{19}$	50–95
c.	*Heavy Ions*		
	2 MeV, 1 mA, DC	$\sim 10^{14}$	> 95
	10 A, pulsed	$\sim 10^{18}$	> 95

[a] After Motz et al. (1971). Reproduced with permission from J. W. Motz and The American Institute of Physics.

209

B. Bremsstrahlung X Rays

1.   PRODUCTION EFFICIENCY

The practical generation of bremsstrahlung x rays is done by accelerating an electron beam and allowing it to strike a metallic target. Equation (8.15) shows that the ratio of mass radiative stopping power to mass collision stopping power is proportional to TZ. This means that high-Z targets convert a larger fraction of the electron's energy into bremsstrahlung x rays than lower-Z targets. Tungsten ($Z = 74$) is a common choice, as it has not only a high atomic number, but a high melting point as well. The energy that is not radiated as bremsstrahlung is of course spent in producing ionization and excitation by collision interactions. This energy nearly all degrades to heat in the target, except for the very small fraction emitted as fluorescence x rays. Thus target cooling is required. In a thin target (i.e., in the present context, one in which the electron beam is not appreciably scattered and loses so little energy that the stopping power is unchanged) the approximate fraction of the total energy lost that goes into bremsstrahlung x-ray production is (from Eq. 8.15)

$$\frac{(dT/\rho dx)_r}{(dT/\rho dx)} = \frac{(dT/\rho dx)_r}{(dT/\rho dx)_c + (dT/\rho dx)_r} = \frac{TZ}{n + TZ} \tag{9.2}$$

where T is the electron energy in MeV, and the value of n for tungsten is 775 at 100 MeV, 786 at 10 MeV, 649 at 1 MeV, 371 at 0.1 MeV, and 336 at 0.01 MeV. Figure

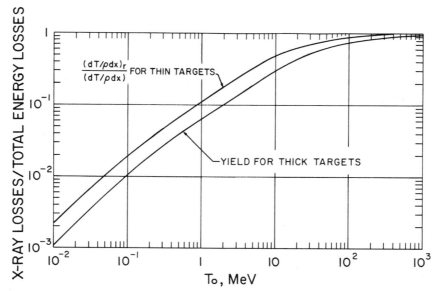

FIGURE 9.4.   Fraction of electron energy losses that are spent in bremsstrahlung x-ray production in thin (upper curve) or thick (lower curve) tungsten targets (data after Berger and Seltzer, 1983). Upper curve: Eq. (9.2); lower curve: radiation yield (fraction of the incident electron kinetic energy T_0 that goes into x-ray production as the particle slows to a stop in a thick target).

9.4 shows in the upper curve the value of Eq. (9.2), from the tables of Berger and Seltzer (1983). This ratio rises roughly linearly with increasing T (= the incident energy T_0), asymptotically approaching unity. At 1 GeV, 99% of the energy lost in a thin W foil goes into x-ray production.

However, the overall energy x-ray production efficiency remains small in thin targets at all electron energies, since most of T_0 is retained by the electron and carried out the back of the target foil. Only in thick targets, in which the electrons are stopped, or semithick ones, in which a large part of the electrons' energy is spent, can reasonable efficiencies be attained. The lower curve of Fig. 9.4 expresses this, indicating the *radiation yield*, or fraction of T_0 spent in generating bremsstrahlung x-rays as the electron is brought to a stop in a thick tungsten target. The ordinate of this curve at each T_0 represents the average value of the upper curve from $T = 0$ to T_0, since an incident electron descends in energy through all the intermediate T-values as it slows down in the target.

It can be seen from Fig. 9.4, for example, that a 100-keV electron beam spends only 1% of its energy on bremsstrahlung production in a thick tungsten target. The other 99% is spent in collision interactions, of which <1% generates fluorescence x-rays and the rest heats the target.

2. UNFILTERED BREMSSTRAHLUNG ENERGY SPECTRUM

a. For $T_0 \ll m_0 c^2$

The shape of the unfiltered bremsstrahlung radiant energy spectrum, generated in a thin target of any atomic number Z by an electron beam of incident energy $T_0 \ll m_0 c^2$, is shown in Fig. 9.5a. It will be seen that the maximum photon energy $h\nu_{max}$ is T_0, the kinetic energy of the incident electrons. This relationship is known as Duane and Hunt's law (1915).

This figure also shows that the radiant-energy spectrum is constant over the energy range from $0 \leq h\nu \leq h\nu_{max}$. Thus, for example, the number of photons emitted per unit energy interval at energy $h\nu$ is twice the number at $2h\nu$, assuming both energies to be less than $h\nu_{max}$.

It is not obvious why electrons impinging on a thin target should generate a spectrum of this simple shape, but it can be visualized intuitively by means of an argument based on the classical impact parameter (see Chapter 8, Section II). When the impact parameter b is equal to 0, the electron has a direct hit on the nucleus and gives all of its energy T_0 to create a photon $h\nu_{max}$. (We need not consider here the more probable nuclear elastic scattering process, which competes with x-ray production for all impact parameters.) As the impact parameter increases, the area in an annulus of radius b and width db increases proportionally, as shown in Fig. 9.6. The differential interaction cross section therefore also increases in proportion to b, as does the number of photons generated in a given annulus. However, the strength of the interaction, hence the quantum energy of the x-rays produced, certainly decreases as b increases. If we *assume* that $h\nu \propto 1/b$, then the number of photons and their quantum

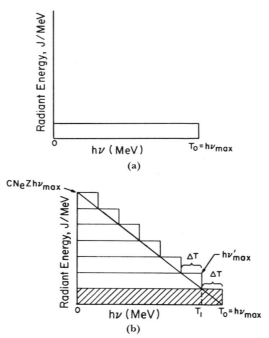

FIGURE 9.5.   Bremsstrahlung radiant-energy spectrum from (a) a thin target, (b) a thick target irradiated by electrons of incident energy $T_0 \ll m_0 c^2$.

energy will be reciprocal, and a flat radiant-energy spectrum such as that in Fig. 9.5a will result.

Thick targets can be simplistically regarded as a stack of imaginary thin target foils, adequate in aggregate depth to stop the electron beam. As the beam passes through successive foils, the electrons lose their kinetic energy gradually by many

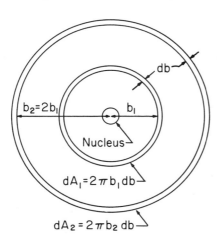

FIGURE 9.6.   Classical explanation of the thin-target x-ray spectrum generated by nonrelativistic electrons. Consider a beam of electrons of kinetic energy T_0 entering the page perpendicularly, and each passing the nucleus at some distance (impact parameter) b. The differential interaction cross section when $b = b_1$ is proportional to the area $dA_1 = 2 \pi b_1$ db. For $b = b_2 = 2b_1$, $dA_2 = 2 dA_1$. Thus twice as many photons (N_2) come from interactions in dA_2 as the N_1 from dA_1. If the magnitude of the interaction (i.e., the x-ray quantum energy hv produced) is assumed to be proportional to $1/b$, then $hv_1 = 2 hv_2$. Therefore $N_1 hv_1 = N_2 hv_2$, and the x-ray radiant-energy spectrum should be flat, as it is observed to be.

small collision interactions. Radiative losses are negligible as a mechanism for reducing the beam energy for $T_0 \ll m_0 c^2$.

The foils in the stack need not all be taken to be the same thickness, but instead are assumed to become progressively thinner with increasing depth, so that each one reduces the beam energy by the same amount. The collision stopping power increases approximately as $1/T$ ($\propto 1/\beta^2$) for decreasing energies (see Chapter 8, Section III.B.2); therefore the foil thicknesses must be successively decreased in proportion to T to maintain constant energy expenditure in each one through collision interactions. The amount of energy spent by the electron beam in x-ray production per foil must therefore decrease with depth in proportion to the foil thickness, since the Sommerfeld nonrelativistic radiative stopping power is independent of T.

These considerations explain the shape of Fig. 9.5b. The electron beam enters the first target foil at kinetic energy T_0, and generates an amount of x-ray energy proportional to the area of the shaded rectangular block. In passing through that foil it loses energy ΔT, nearly all through collision interactions, and then enters the second foil with energy $T_1 = T_0 - \Delta T$. The amount of x-ray energy it generates in the second foil is represented by the area of the second block, which is drawn to have the same height as the first, but with a maximum photon energy $h\nu'_{max} = T_1$. Thus the x-ray energy emitted from the second foil is T_1/T_0 times that from the first, and so on for subsequent foils.

It will be instructive to derive an approximate equation for the total bremsstrahlung production in a thick target. The Sommerfeld formula for the mass radiative stopping power for nonrelativistic electrons can be gotten from Eq. (8.14) by setting $T = 0$ and $\overline{B}_r = \frac{16}{3}$:

$$\left(\frac{dT}{\rho dx} \right)_r = 5.80 \times 10^{-28} \frac{N_A Z^2}{A} (0.511) \left(\tfrac{16}{3} \right)$$

$$= 9.52 \times 10^{-4} \frac{Z^2}{A} \text{ MeV cm}^2/\text{g} \qquad (9.3)$$

The radiant energy R_n of the bremsstrahlung emitted from the nth foil in the stack of N foils is equal to the product of Eq. (9.3), the number of incident electrons N_e, and the nth-foil thickness. Thus

$$R_n = 9.52 \times 10^{-4} \frac{Z^2}{A} N_e \left[\left(\frac{T_0 - (n-1) \Delta T}{T_0} \right) \rho t_1 \right] \text{ MeV} \qquad (9.4)$$

where ρt_1 = mass thickness of the 1st foil, in g/cm^2, and the bracketed factor is that of the nth foil,

$\quad T_o$ = electron energy incident on the 1st foil (MeV),

$\quad \Delta T$ = energy loss by collision interaction in any foil (MeV),

$\quad n$ = number of the foil, counting from the front (incident) side,

$\quad N_e$ = number of electrons incident, and

$\quad Z, A$ = atomic number and atomic weight, respectively.

The total radiant energy from all N foils is the summation of Eq. (9.4):

$$R = 9.52 \times 10^{-4} \frac{Z^2 N_e}{A} \left[\rho t_1 \sum_{n=1}^{N} \left(\frac{T_0 - (n-1)\, \Delta T}{T_0} \right) \right] \text{MeV} \qquad (9.5a)$$

where the bracketed factor is simply the total mass thickness of the stack of foils. This may be set equal to the range $\Re$ of the electrons, which we can assume have straight tracks for ease of visualization. Substitution in Eq. (9.5a) gives

$$R = 9.52 \times 10^{-4} \frac{Z^2 N_e}{A} \Re \text{ MeV} \qquad (9.5b)$$

For nonrelativistic electrons Fig. 8.10 indicates that $\Re \propto T_0^2$. Numerical examination of the range data listed in Appendix E for high-Z media at $T_0 \sim 0.1$ MeV indicates that

$$\frac{Z}{A} \Re \cong k T_0^2 \qquad (9.6)$$

where $\Re$ is given in g/cm^2, T_0 in MeV, and k is a constant of proportionality roughly equal to 1 g/cm^2 MeV^2

Substituting Eq. (9.6) into Eq. (9.5b) gives

$$R \cong 1 \times 10^{-3} \, N_e \, Z T_0^2 \text{ MeV} \qquad (9.7)$$

where the constant includes k and has the units MeV^{-1}. This approximate formula can be verified by comparison with the radiation yields tabulated in Appendix E, remembering that $Y(T_0) = R/T_0 N_e$. Thus, for example, for $Z = 82$ and $T_0 = 0.1$ MeV, Eq. (9.7) equals 8.2×10^{-4} MeV per electron, while $Y(T_0) T_0 = 1.162 \times 10^{-3}$. The crude agreement (30%) is adequate, considering the approximations involved in Eq. (9.7). The tabulated yield values are of course the more correct.

Nevertheless Eq. (9.7) provides a useful estimate of the bremsstrahlung radiant energy generated in a thick target, in terms of number and energy of electrons delivered to the target and its atomic number. It will be seen that the unfiltered x-ray output is proportional to the charge delivered to the target in the x-ray tube (i.e., current $\times$ time), as well as the atomic number of the target and the square of the electron kinetic energy (or x-ray tube voltage).

Returning now to the unfiltered thick-target spectrum shown in Fig. 9.5b, it will be seen that the array of rectangular areas (representing the x-ray outputs of all the imaginary individual foils comprising the thick target) can be fitted by a triangular envelope called the *Kramers spectrum* (Kramers, 1923), having the formula

$$R'(h\nu) = C \, N_e \, Z \, (h\nu_{\max} - h\nu), \qquad (9.8)$$

where $R'(h\nu)$ is the differential radiant-energy spectral distribution of bremsstrahlung generated in the thick target of atomic number Z, typically in J/MeV; $h\nu_{\max} = T_0$ is the maximum photon energy (MeV); C is a constant of proportionality; and $R'(h\nu) = C \, N_e \, Z(h\nu)_{\max}$ for $h\nu = 0$. The area under the triangle represents the total radiant energy of the unfiltered bremsstrahlung, and can be seen from Fig. (9.5b) to have the value

$$R = \frac{C}{2} N_e Z(h\nu)^2_{max} = \frac{C}{2} N_e Z T_0^2 \qquad (9.9)$$

Comparison with Eq. (9.7) shows that the constant $C/2$ has a value around 1×10^{-3} MeV^{-1} when R and T_0 are both expressed in MeV. R may of course be converted into joules while leaving T_0 in MeV by use of the relation 1 MeV = 1.602 $\times 10^{-13}$ J; hence

$$R \cong 1.6 \times 10^{-16} N_e Z T_0^2 \text{ J} \qquad (9.10)$$

The constant C in Eq. (9.8) evidently has a value around 3×10^{-16} J/MeV^2 if $R'(h\nu)$ is given in J/MeV, as shown in Fig. 9.5b.

It is helpful in interpreting Eqs. (9.8)–(9.10) to observe the graphical effect of changing the parameters. Figure 9.7a shows the effect of doubling N_e or Z. The curve slope is doubled; hence the ordinate is doubled at every energy. The area under the curve (i.e., the total radiant energy) is likewise multiplied by 2. In Fig. 9.7b the effect of doubling $T_0 = h\nu_{max}$ is indicated. The curve slope remains constant in this case, while the area under the curve quadruples, as shown by the construction in dashed lines. Combined changes in N_e and T_0, such as may occur in pulsed x-ray generators, may be handled graphically by changing both the slope and the intercept on the abscissa accordingly, in each of a set of time subdivisions during a pulse, then summing the resulting spectra for the whole pulse.

The simple triangular spectra shown in Figs. 9.5b and 9.7 are never observed experimentally, for two reasons. Firstly, the fluorescence x-ray lines are superimposed, assuming the electron energy exceeds the shell binding energy. Moreover, the lower-energy photons are preferentially removed by photoelectric-effect inter-

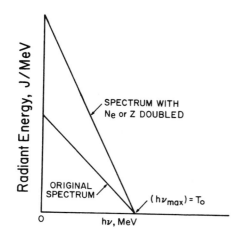

FIGURE 9.7a.   Effect of doubling N_e or Z on the unfiltered bremsstrahlung x-ray spectrum.

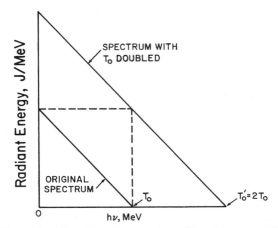

FIGURE 9.7b.   **Effect of doubling $T_0 = h\nu_{max}$ on the unfiltered bremsstrahlung x-ray spectrum.**

actions within the target material itself, the exit window of the x-ray tube, and such additional filters as may be added. The effects of such filtration on the spectrum will be discussed in Section III. However, it should be mentioned here that the exponent of T_0 in Eq. (9.10) is effectively increased from 2 to around 3 by filtration that cuts off the lower-energy portion of the Kramers spectrum.

b.   For $T_0 \gtrsim m_0c^2$

For relativistic electrons the generation of bremsstrahlung can no longer be adequately described by the Sommerfeld equation, and the more general Bethe–Heitler formula (8.14) applies. The differential cross section $d\sigma_r$ for the emission of a photon with quantum energy between $h\nu$ and $h\nu + d(h\nu)$, by an electron of kinetic energy T, is given in cm^2/atom by

$$d\sigma_r = 5.80 \times 10^{-28} \frac{B_r Z^2}{h\nu} \left(\frac{T + m_0c^2}{T} \right) d(h\nu) \tag{9.11}$$

Hence the photon output spectrum has the form

$$\frac{d\sigma_r}{d(h\nu)} \propto \frac{B_r}{h\nu} \tag{9.12}$$

and the radiant energy spectrum is proportional to B_r, which is a gradually decreasing dimensionless function having a value around 20 at $h\nu/T = 0$, and 0 at $h\nu/T = 1$. The curve shape between these limits depends on T, as shown by Evans (1955, p. 603), based on Heitler's calculations.

Figure 9.8 gives the energy-flux density spectrum (which has the same shape as the radiant-energy spectrum) from a moderately thick (1.5 mm) tungsten wire target struck by 11.3-MeV electrons (range = 3.5 mm) as measured by Motz et al. (1953) using a Compton spectrometer. Also shown are the Bethe–Heitler theoretical spectra

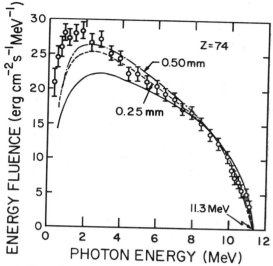

FIGURE 9.8. Bremsstrahlung intensity (energy-flux density) spectrum in the 0° direction for 11.3-MeV electrons on a 1.5-mm tungsten target, as measured with a Compton spectrometer (points). The Bethe–Heitler thin-target spectrum, modified by the photon absorption in window materials, is shown by the solid curve (lower). The dashed curves show corresponding theoretical spectra for 10-mil ($\frac{1}{4}$-mm) and 20-mil ($\frac{1}{2}$-mm) tungsten targets corrected for attenuation in the target material as well. (After Motz et al., 1953. Reproduced with permission from J. W. Motz and The American Physical Society.)

for a thin target and for 0.25- and 0.50-mm targets, each corrected for photon attenuation in the target and windows. This accounts for the low-energy decrease in all the curves, which would otherwise extrapolate to the $h\nu = 0$ axis along more or less straight lines with slopes established by the curve trends above 3 MeV.

It can be seen by comparing this figure with Fig. 9.5a,b that there is less difference between thick- and thin-target spectra at high generating energies such as 11.3 MeV than at low energies ($T_0 \lesssim m_0c^2$). Moreover, they both are bowed upward in Fig. 9.8, in contrast to the straight-line spectrum for the low T_0 and thick target in Fig. 9.5b. This upward bowing comes from the function B_r of Heitler [see Eq. (9.12) above].

3. BREMSSTRAHLUNG DIRECTIONAL DEPENDENCE

The bremsstrahlung spectral shape for thin targets is isotropic, i.e., is independent of direction relative to that of the electron beam. However, the bremsstrahlung intensity in that case depends strongly on direction, the x rays tending to be emitted with an appreciable sideways component for low-energy electron beams, and more strongly forward as T_0 is increased. This trend was shown in Fig. 9.2. For still higher energies the bremsstrahlung x rays are emitted close to the 0° direction, as indicated in Fig. 9.9.

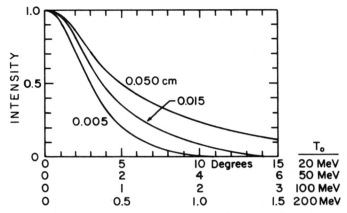

FIGURE 9.9. Ratio of bremsstrahlung intensity at angle θ to that at $\theta = 0$ for three thicknesses of tungsten target, as calculated by Schiff (1946). Note that the curves for different energies T_0 differ only by a scale factor that is inversely proportional to T_0. (Reproduced by permission of The American Physical Society.)

The narrowness of this forward bunching of rays is seen from Fig. 9.9 to be directly proportional to T_0. For example, the x rays from a 0.05-cm tungsten target reach half their central-axis intensity at $\theta = 5°$ for $T_0 = 20$ MeV, and 0.5° for 200 MeV. This means that the x-ray output in the 0° direction increases with T_0 more strongly than does the output in all directions. At $\theta = 0°$ the x-ray energy fluence tends to increase as T_0^4 for $T_0 \sim 1$ MeV, as $T_0^{2.3}$ at ~ 10 MeV, and as T_0^2 at ~ 100 MeV (NCRP, 1977).

It was mentioned earlier (Section II.B.2.a) that, due to the effect of beam filtration at low energies, the radiant energy emitted in all directions varied roughly as T_0^3. This is also observed with respect to the x-ray energy fluence at $\theta = 90°$, the sideways beam ordinarily employed for $T_0 < 300$ keV. For higher values of T_0 the exponent for 90° emission gradually decreases from 3 to about $\frac{1}{2}$ at 100 MeV (NCRP, 1977).

The forward peaking at high energies necessitates the use of a conical beam-flattening filter in linac x-ray beams for radiotherapy applications, even though the phenomenon becomes less pronounced for thicker targets (see Fig. 9.9). Such a filter attenuates the beam less strongly as a function of distance away from its central axis, thus producing a beam of more uniform intensity over a useful area. Exact alignment of such a filter is of course critical.

For thick targets and orthovoltage energies (≤ 300 kV) the x-ray intensity as a function of direction is controlled by photon attenuation in the target. The photoelectric attenuation coefficient in the high-Z, high-density metal becomes so large that only the photons originating near the surface can escape. Even 0.1 mm of tungsten attenuates 100-keV photons by half, and lower-energy rays are absorbed even more strongly. Thus the differing degree of target filtration in various directions creates spectral dependence upon direction that thin-target, unfiltered x rays do not exhibit.

These considerations, together with the small range of low-energy electrons in penetrating the target (~ 0.01 mm for 100-keV electrons on tungsten), and the need for providing a means of carrying away heat, dictate the use of front-surface targets slanted toward an exit window on the side of the x-ray tube for T_0 up to about 0.3 MeV. For higher electron energies the x-ray beam is usually taken out at 0°, after passing through a perpendicular target.

III. X-RAY FILTRATION AND BEAM QUALITY

An unfiltered x-ray beam contains fluorescence x rays, characteristic of the target atomic number, as well as bremsstrahlung. The upper curve in Fig. 9.10 illustrates this for a thick tungsten target bombarded by 100-keV electrons, assuming the emission of all photons created. The K-fluorescence lines are shown almost completely resolved (see Table 9.2) at the correct energies, and with the correct relative heights

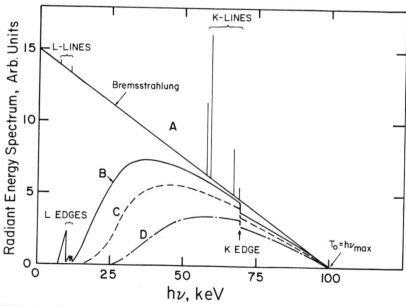

FIGURE 9.10. X-ray spectrum from 100-keV electrons on a thick tungsten target. Upper curve A: Unfiltered. B: Filtered through 0.01 mm W in escaping the target. C: Additionally filtered through 2 mm Al. D: Filtered through 0.15 mm Cu and 3.9 mm Al in addition to inherent target filtration. To avoid confusion, the K-fluorescence lines are not shown in curves B, C, and D, but are attenuated from their heights in curve A in the same proportion as the bremsstrahlung is attenuated at the same energies.

(which are arbitrary with respect to the bremsstrahlung spectrum). The *L*-lines are not shown, but their energy range is indicated.

A. X-Ray Filtration

1. FOR $T_0 \leq 300$ keV

Figure 9.10 also illustrates (in curve B) the filtering effect on the x rays of passing through 0.01 mm of tungsten, as might occur in escaping from the target. The *K*-fluorescence lines are still present, attenuated by a few percent, but have been deleted from curves B, C, and D to avoid confusion in the graph. Note the influence of the *K* binding energy at 69.5 keV: the photoelectric attenuation is greater just above than below it, causing a discontinuity in the spectrum.

Curve C in Fig. 9.10 shows the additional attenuating effect of 2 mm of aluminum, and curve D of 0.15 mm Cu + 3.9 mm Al.

In calculating curves B, C and D from curve A, the narrow-beam attenuation coefficients (μ/ρ) are used. For such added filtration, narrow-beam geometry is usually well approximated, and hence μ/ρ is appropriate (see Fig. 3.2). For internal target filtration (curve B) photon scattering is negligible, since the photoelectric effect dominates. The fluorescence photons resulting from those interactions are inconsequential in comparison with the strong fluorescence generated through direct *K*-shell ionization by the incident electrons. Thus that case also can be treated as though the geometry were narrow-beam.

The principal result of adding filters to an x-ray beam is evidently to remove photons preferentially at energies where the attenuation coefficient is largest. The photoelectric effect is the dominating interaction by photons below a few hundred keV (see Fig. 7.1), and since the photoelectric interaction coefficient varies approximately as $(1/h\nu)^3$ in this energy range [see Eq. (7.31)] except at the binding energies, the lower end of the spectrum therefore appears to be gradually "peeled off" by adding more and more filtration. The result is to narrow the spectral distribution progressively, crowding it closer and closer to the applied kilovoltage, T_0. In other words, it becomes more like a monoenergetic single-line spectrum at T_0, the more heavily it is filtered. The x-ray beam is said to be "hardened" by such filtration, as the "softer", more easily attenuated photons have been filtered out.

The most common x-ray filtering media are lead, tin, copper, and aluminum, which may be used singly or in combination. The advantage of combination filters (Thoraeus, 1932) is that they are generally capable of narrowing the spectrum to any desired degree while preserving more of the x-ray output than can be achieved with a single filtering material. The higher-*Z* filters provide strong filtering action but cause discontinuities at the shell binding energies. The lower-*Z* filters tend to smooth the resulting spectrum. This trend can be seen in Fig. 9.10.

It is important in using combination filters that they be positioned in the beam in descending order of *Z*, going in the direction of the rays. This allows each filter to remove the fluorescence x rays that originate in the higher-*Z* filter upstream from it. Aluminum ($h\nu_K = 1.5$ keV) is best for the final filter. Copper ($h\nu_K = 9$ keV) fluorescence also is low enough in energy not to be detectable in most cases. However, neither tin ($h\nu_K = 29$ keV) nor lead ($h\nu_K = 85$ KeV) should be used without sufficient following filtration to remove the fluorescence, unless those photons are desired as part of the output.

Filter thicknesses are conventionally specified in millimeters, although it is usually preferable physically to measure the area (e.g., 10×10 cm^2) and weight of a filter, and thus determine its average mass thickness (g/cm^2 or kg/m^2). The thickness can then be stated in millimeters for any reference density of the metal, which may be found to differ somewhat from that of the actual filter. The densities in Appendix B.1 may be used where standard values have not been specified. In any case the millimeter thickness of filters should be related to a density.

2. FOR $T_0 \gtrsim 300$ keV

At higher energies the photoelectric effect becomes less important than the Compton effect (see Fig. 7.1), and the total coefficient is less energy-dependent, as evident in Fig. 7.13a,b. Thus the filtering of an x-ray spectrum generated by megavolt electrons mainly removes the photons below a few hundred keV without greatly modifying the spectral shape at higher energies. However, the use of a thick high-Z filter such as lead on a multimegavolt x-ray beam tends to filter out the highest-energy photons (>4 MeV) through pair production, as well as the lowest through the photoelectric effect. Podgorsak et al. (1975) have shown that this can decrease the penetrating power of a radiotherapy x-ray beam in the body or a low-Z phantom. In such a medium pair production is unimportant as a mechanism for attenuation, and the highest-energy photons (up to $\cong 60$ MeV) are the most penetrating (see Fig. 7.13a).

B. X-Ray Beam-Quality Specification

The quality of an x-ray beam can be specified in terms of either its spectrum or its attenuation characteristics in a reference medium. Bear in mind however that a beam may not be uniform in quality over its cross-sectional area, because of differences in filtration (e.g., in escaping the target).

1. SPECTRA

Spectra can be either (a) estimated from theoretical considerations (including the effect of filtration), as already outlined, or (b) derived by Laplace transformation from a measured narrow-beam attenuation curve, as described by Greening (1950), or (c) measured directly by some type of spectrometer [GeLi, SiLi, scintillator, bent-crystal (Birks, 1970), or Compton (Motz et al., 1953), etc.]. Method (b) is relatively difficult and provides little improvement over spectra derivable by method (a). The GeLi detector is probably the method of choice for obtaining well-resolved spectra, including the fluorescence peaks, for T_0 below a few hundred keV. At still higher energies large scintillators are probably preferable, as GeLi detectors of obtainable size become too transparent to the upper end of the spectrum, requiring large corrections. These devices are discussed in Chapter 15. Birks's bent-crystal method is preferable for transient phenomena, as the entire spectrum is registered instantaneously on film.

An excellent example of the application of the GeLi method has been provided by Seelentag et al. (1979), who measured 135 x-ray spectra for various filtrations and T_0-values from 10 to 300 keV. Fig. 9.11a shows the spectrum measured for T_0 = 100 keV with added filtration, of 2 mm Al, Fig. 9.11b shows the corresponding spectrum for 0.15 mm Cu and 3.9 mm Al, and Fig. 9.11c shows the spectrum for a filtration of 2 mm Sn, 0.5 mm Cu, and 4 mm Al. In each figure two curves are given: The solid curve represent the numbers of photons per unit energy interval [e.g., Eq. (1.17)], while the dashed curve represents the exposure per unit energy interval [e.g., Eq. (2.27)]. These spectra can be related in shape as follows: The photon-number spectrum is multiplied by $h\nu$ at each energy to get the radiant-energy spectrum (not shown); that in turn is multiplied by $(\mu_{en}/\rho)_{air}$ at each energy to get the exposure spectrum [since $\overline{W}/e$ = constant in Eq. (2.27)]. All the curves in Figs. 9.11a–c have been arbitrarily normalized to unity at the maximum ordinate value.

Figure 9.11d compares the theoretically estimated bremsstrahlung spectrum with that measured by a GeLi spectrometer for T_0 = 100 keV and filtration with 2 mm Al. The solid curve reproduces curve C from Fig. 9.10; the dashed curve was derived from the solid curve in Fig. 9.11a by multiplying it by $h\nu$ and renormalizing to the theoretical curve at 60 keV. The shapes of these bremsstrahlung radiant-energy spectra are seen to be closely comparable, indicating that the theoretical estimate is quite reasonable in that case.

A quantitative estimate of the fluorescence output is also possible by means of the K-shell ionization cross section (see Kolbenstvedt, 1967, and Dick et al., 1973), but that is not treated here.

2. ATTENUATION CURVES AND HALF-VALUE LAYERS

a. $T_0 \gtrsim 300$ keV.

As noted above, it is possible (with some limitations) to derive an x-ray spectrum from the shape of an attenuation curve. This means that the latter curve shape must be a ''signature'' for the related spectrum. That is, each x-ray beam spectrum is uniquely related to an attenuation-curve shape in a given medium. Thus attenuation data can be used to characterize x-ray beams.

To standardize such data the following conventions are generally followed:

- Pure aluminum or copper is used as the attenuating medium, Al being preferred for $T_0 \lesssim 120$ keV and Cu for higher energies $\lesssim 0.5$ MeV.
- Narrow-beam geometry is required (i.e., scattered rays from the attenuator must not reach the detector).
- The detector (e.g., ion chamber) must be air-equivalent, that is, must give a constant response per unit of exposure, independent of photon energy.

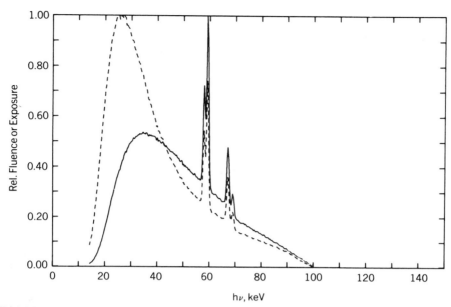

FIGURE 9.11a. Measured spectrum for 100-keV electrons on a thick tungsten target, with filtration in 2 mm Al added to a 3-mm Be window tube. Solid curve: photon numbers spectrum; dashed curve: exposure spectrum. (Seelentag et al., 1979. Reproduced with permission from the authors and the Gesellschaft für Strahlen-und Umweltforschung mbH, Munich.)

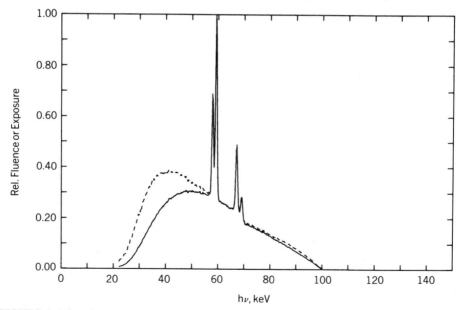

FIGURE 9.11b. Same as Fig. 9.11a, but for a filter of 0.15 mm Cu + 3.9 mm Al. (From Seelentag et al., 1979. Reproduced with permission from the authors and the Gesellschaft für Strahlen- und Umweltforschung mbH, Munich.)

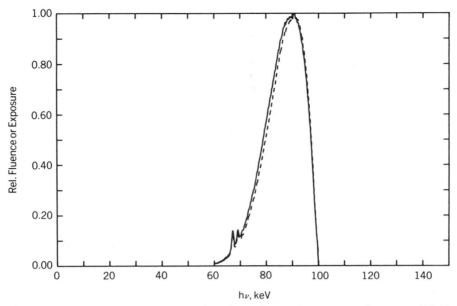

FIGURE 9.11c.   Same as Fig. 9.11a, but for a filter of 2 mm Sn + 0.5 mm Cu + 4 mm Al. Note that the intensity of this beam is too low to be seen if it were plotted on Fig. 9.10 with the same vertical scale as the other curves. (From Seelentag et al., 1979. Reprinted with permission from the authors and the Gesellschaft für Strahlen- und Umweltforschung mbH, Munich.)

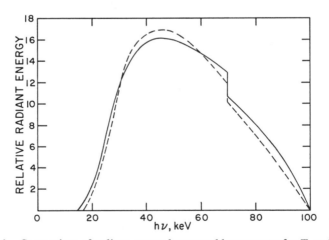

FIGURE 9.11d.   Comparison of radiant-energy bremsstrahlung spectra for $T_0 = 100$ keV, thick tungsten target, filter 2 mm Al. Solid curve: derived from measured spectrum in Fig. 9.11a; dashed curve: theoretical, same as curve C in Fig. 9.10. The two curves are arbitrarily normalized at 60 keV.

224

The third requirement means that the detector response is proportional to the area remaining under the exposure spectrum, as a function of attenuator thickness. The choice of an air-equivalent detector is arbitrary, but is based on the widespread availability of such ion chambers. Energy-independent photon counters or energy-fluence meters are not as common or convenient to use. The shape of an attenuation curve, for a given x-ray beam and medium, depends on the quantum-energy dependence of the detector response.

Figure 9.12 shows the approximate attenuation curves that would result if the x-ray beams in Figs. 9.11a–c were attenuated in aluminum, using an air-equivalent detector to measure the x-rays transmitted. Also shown (curve D) is the attenuation curve resulting from monoenergetic 100-keV x rays. The steeper the curve, the softer is the x-ray beam; and the greater the curvature, the broader the spectrum. The progressive hardening and narrowing of the spectrum with increasing filtration is evident here. The heaviest filter produces a curve that is practically exponential (see curve C) with a slope approaching that of a monoenergetic 100-keV beam. Still greater filtration would bring the slope still closer, but with still further reduction in an already low beam intensity.

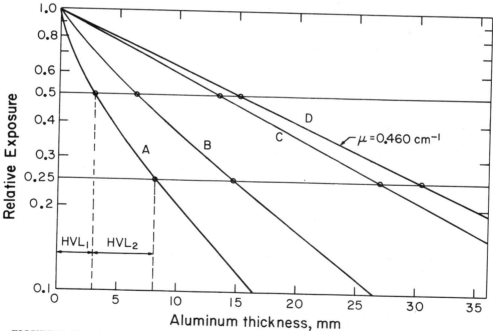

FIGURE 9.12. Approximate exposure-attenuation curves in aluminum for $T_0 = 100$-keV x-rays from a thick tungsten target, filtered by (A) 2 mm Al; (B) 0.15 mm Cu + 3.9 mm Al; and (C) 2 mm Sn + 0.5 mm Cu + 4 mm Al. (From data of Seelentag et al., 1979.) Also shown for comparison is the attenuation of 100-keV photons in aluminum (curve D). The first and second half-value layers are shown for curve A.

The attenuation curves in Fig. 9.12, and their related x-ray spectra, can be reasonably well specified for radiological applications in terms of their *first and second half-value layers*, HVL_1 and HVL_2. HVL_1 *is defined as the thickness required to reduce the exposure by half, in narrow-beam geometry*; HVL_2 *is the thickness necessary to reduce it by half again under the same conditions.* In Fig. 9.12 the circled points indicate where the curves cross the values 0.5 and 0.25 of relative exposure. The first and second half-value layers are indicated for curve A. Table 9.4 lists the HVL_1 and HVL_2 values for all the curves.

The last column gives the *homogeneity coefficient, defined as the ratio* HVL_1/HVL_2. This approaches unity as the spectrum is narrowed by filtration to approach monochromaticity, in which case attenuation is exponential, giving a straight curve on such a semilogarithmic plot.

The necessity for specifying HVL_2 as well as HVL_1 in characterizing an x-ray beam is illustrated in Fig. 9.13. Three attenuation curves are shown: for a 100-kV x-ray beam lightly filtered by 3 mm Al, a 50-kV beam heavily filtered by 0.1 mm Pb + 4 mm Al, and a monoenergetic beam at 37 keV. All have the same first half-value layer in aluminum: 3.8 mm. However, their second half-value layers are, respectively, 5.82, 4.13, and 3.8 mm. Their homogeneity coefficients are therefore 0.66, 0.92, and 1.00. HVL_1 alone evidently cannot provide the required information about the breadths of the spectra, which in this case differ greatly. HVL_2 (or the homogeneity coefficient) provides this information in a compact and convenient form, although with less detail than the entire spectrum would convey. Those spectra were measured by Seelentag et al. (1979). The 100-keV spectrum is very broad, extending down to 15 keV. The 50-keV spectrum is much narrower, extending only to 20 keV.

Another quantity that is sometimes used in beam-quality specification is the *equivalent photon energy,* $h\nu_{eq}$. This is defined as *the quantum energy of a monoenergetic beam having the same* HVL_1 *as the beam being specified.* In the case shown in Fig. 9.13, $h\nu_{eq} = 37$ keV for both of the other beams A and B. The equivalent photon energy clearly gives no more information than HVL_1, but gives it in a form that is especially useful in describing heavily filtered beams approaching monochromaticity. Stating the applied voltage T_0 in addition to $h\nu_{eq}$ also conveys some sense of the spectral width, which is roughly $2(T_0 - h\nu_{eq})$ for heavily filtered beams.

TABLE 9.4.   Half-Value Layers and Homogeneity Coefficients for the Aluminum Attenuation Curves in Fig. 9.12

Curve	Energy (keV)	Filter (mm)	HVL_1 (mm Al)	HVL_2 (mm Al)	HC (Al)
A	100	2 Al	3.02	5.12	0.59
B	100	0.15 Cu + 3.9 Al	6.56	8.05	0.81
C	100	2 Sn + 0.5 Cu + 4 Al	13.4	13.5	0.99
D	100[a]	none	15.1	15.1	1.00

[a] Monoenergetic.

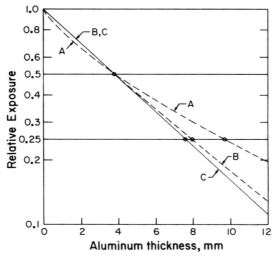

FIGURE 9.13. An example of the attenuation of three dissimilar x-ray beams having practically the same value of HVL_1 (3.8 mm) in aluminum. Curve A: 100 kV, 3 mm Al filter, $HVL_2 = 5.82$ mm. Curve B: 50 kV, 0.1 mm Pb + 4 mm Al filter, $HVL_2 = 4.13$ mm. Curve C: monoenergetic 37-keV beam, $HVL_2 = 3.8$ mm. Note that 37 keV is the equivalent photon energy for both beams A and B. (HVL data after Seelentag et al., 1979.)

Note that the values of $h\nu_{eq}$ derived from different attenuating media are not necessarily identical for broad spectra, but they converge to a common value as the beam is hardened by heavy filtration.

Figure 9.14 gives values of $h\nu_{eq}$ as a function of HVL_1 for aluminum and copper attenuators. The value of $h\nu_{eq}$ can be alternatively obtained by the following procedure:

$$\frac{X}{X_0} = 0.5 = e^{-(\mu/\rho)_{eq} \cdot HVL_1 \cdot \rho}$$

$$\left(\frac{\mu}{\rho}\right)_{eq} = \frac{0.6931}{\rho \cdot HVL_1} \ cm^2/g$$

(9.13)

where HVL_1 is to be expressed in centimeters. The value of $h\nu_{eq}$ corresponding to $(\mu/\rho)_{eq}$ can then be obtained by interpolation in the tables of Appendix D.3, where the μ/ρ data include Rayleigh (coherent) scattering.

b. $T_0 \gtrsim 300$ keV

In the higher-energy x-ray region where the photoelectric effect is unimportant, the preceding discussion of attenuation and half-value layer is not relevant. Specification of a spectrum is still the most rigorous means of beam characterization, bearing in mind that the spectrum may not be uniform over the beam area, especially if a high-Z beam-flattening filter is used.

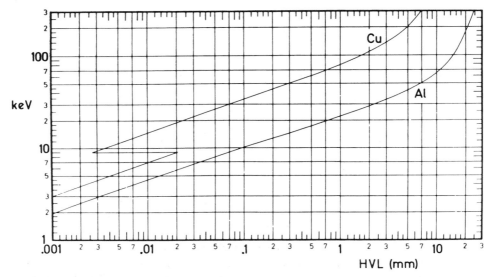

FIGURE 9.14. Equivalent photon energy vs. HVL$_1$ in copper or aluminum. (From Seelentag, et al., 1979. Reprinted with permission from the authors and the Gesellschaft für Strahlen- und Umweltforschung mbH, Munich.)

Routine specification of the hardness of radiotherapy x-ray beams is usually given in the form of a curve of absorbed dose in a water phantom vs. depth, for a 10 × 10-cm^2 beam as specified at the depth of maximum dose (D_{max}), and for a source-to-surface distance (SSD) of 1 m. The depth (from the phantom surface) at which the dose is reduced to $D_{max}/2$ is sometimes substituted for the whole curve as an abbreviated means of quality specification.

Figure 9.15 shows a family of such curves for a variety of beams. Values of $D_{max}/2$ are seen to range from 22 cm for curve A (22 MV, SSD 70 cm) down to 2.7 cm for Curve F (120 kV, 2 mm Al, SSD 15 cm). The depth of D_{max} of course increases with energy as the range of the secondary electrons increases.

Characterization of megavolt photon beams may be complicated by the presence of secondary electrons, which can originate in source hardware, beam collimator, filters, shaping blocks and their supporting tray, and the air through which the beam passes. Such electron contamination tends to reduce or eliminate the so-called "skin-sparing" advantage of megavolt photon beams for radiotherapy. Improvements in beam purity and skin sparing can be achieved through (a) reduction in beam size to allow electrons to scatter out, (b) magnetic removal of electrons, (c) use of a medium-to-high-Z filter that backscatters electrons without generating appreciable additional photoelectrons or pairs, and/or (d) replacing the air through which the beam passes by helium in a thin plastic bag. These measures have been discussed at length elsewhere (Biggs and Russell, 1983; Attix et al. 1983). The magnet is the most effective for the multimegavolt region.

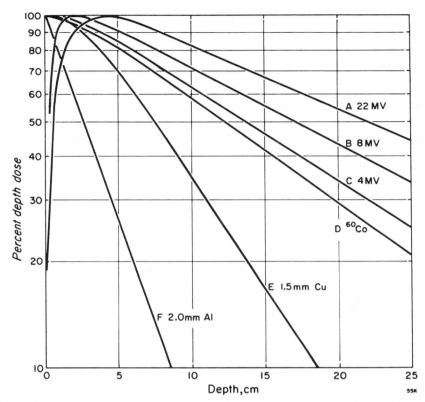

FIGURE 9.15. Variation of absorbed dose vs. depth in a water phantom for the following 10 × 10-cm^2 photon beams: A, 22 MV, 70-cm SSD; B, 8 MV, 100-cm SSD; C, 4 MV, 100-cm SSD; D, ^{60}Co γ-rays, 100-cm SSD; E, 200 keV, HVL$_1$ = 1.5 mm Cu, 50-cm SSD; F, 120 kV, HVL$_1$ = 2.0 mm Al, 15-cm SSD. (From Johns and Cunningham, 1983. Reproduced with permission from J. R. Cunningham, and Charles C Thomas, Publisher.)

PROBLEMS

1. A 100-MeV proton beam of 10^{14} p/s is perpendicularly incident on a rhodium foil 25 μm in thickness. Estimate the production rate of K and L x-rays (use Fig. 9.1).

2. Compare the K x-ray yield per electron in thick targets of gold, silver, and copper for $T_0 = 0.1$ and 1.0 MeV. Sum over all directions, neglecting attenuation.

3. At what electron energy does the collision stopping power equal the radiative stopping power in tungsten?

4. Using the curves in Fig. 9.4, estimate the amount of bremsstrahlung x-ray energy (J) generated when 10^{16} electrons having $T_0 = 1$ MeV are perpendicularly incident on (a) a tungsten foil 0.025 mm thick, or (b) a thick tungsten target. Assume that the mass stopping power is 1.13 MeV cm^2/g.

5. An imaginary pulsed x-ray machine spends 50% of the pulse length at $T_0 = 90$ keV with a beam current of $i = 15$ mA, 25% at 60 keV with $i = 20$ mA, and 25% at 40 keV with $i = 10$ mA.

   (a) Graphically construct the time-averaged unfiltered bremsstrahlung spectrum in arbitrary units.

   (b) Calculate the attenuation in passing through 1 mm Cu + 2 mm Al, and draw the resulting filtered spectrum.

   (c) Redraw (b) as a photon fluence spectrum and as an exposure spectrum, normalizing to the same maximum ordinate value.

6. A linear accelerator generates an x-ray beam with 20-MeV electrons perpendicularly incident on a tungsten target 0.05 cm thick. Design a copper beam-flattening filter that would produce the maximum uniform intensity throughout a 20×20-cm^2 beam at a distance of 1 m. The filter is to be located 10 cm from the target. (Use Fig. 9.9, and assume that the effective x-ray energy is $\cong 0.4$ T_0.)

7. Calculate a spectrum to compare with the measured photon fluence spectrum in Fig. 9.11c.

8. Calculate the equivalent photon energies for the beams described by curves A, B, and C in Fig. 9.12. Compare with Fig. 9.14.

SOLUTIONS TO PROBLEMS

1. L: 1.3×10^{13}/s; K: 1.6×10^{12}/s.

2.

T_0	$Z = 29$	47	79
0.1	2.5×10^{-2}	5.7×10^{-3}	1.3×10^{-4}
1.0	3.0×10^{-2}	7.0×10^{-2}	6.3×10^{-2}

3. 10.6 MeV.

4. (a) 8.9 J, (b) 97 J.

6. 4.3 cm at center; 0 thickness at edge, at a radius of 1.414 cm. Thicknesses at intermediate radii according to Fig. 9.9.

8. A: 34 keV; B: 48 keV; C: 85 keV.

CHAPTER **10**

Cavity Theory

I. BRAGG–GRAY THEORY

The basis for cavity theory is contained in Eq. (8.27) of Chapter 8. If a fluence Φ of identical charged particles of kinetic energy T passes through an interface between two different media, g and w, as shown in Fig. 10.1a, then one can write for the absorbed dose on the g side of the boundary

$$D_g = \Phi \left[\left(\frac{dT}{\rho dx} \right)_{c,g} \right]_T \tag{10.1}$$

and on the w side,

$$D_w = \Phi \left[\left(\frac{dT}{\rho dx} \right)_{c,w} \right]_T \tag{10.2}$$

where $[(dT/\rho dx)_{c,g}]_T$ and $[(dT/\rho dx)_{c,w}]_T$ are the mass collision stopping powers of the two media, evaluated at energy T. Usually we may omit the brackets and subscript T, evaluation at an appropriate energy T being implied.

Assuming that the value of Φ is continuous across the interface (i.e., ignoring backscattering) one can write for the ratio of absorbed doses in the two media adjacent to their boundary

$$\frac{D_w}{D_g} = \frac{(dT/\rho dx)_{c,w}}{(dT/\rho dx)_{c,g}} \tag{10.3}$$

231

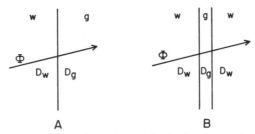

FIGURE 10.1. (*A*) A fluence Φ of charged particles is shown crossing an interface between media w and g. Assuming Φ to be continuous across the boundary, the dose ratio D_w/D_g equals the corresponding ratio of mass collision stopping powers. (*B*) A fluence Φ of charged particles passes through a thin layer of medium g sandwiched between regions containing medium w. Assuming Φ to be continuous across layer g and both interfaces, the dose ratio D_w/D_g is again equal to the corresponding ratio of mass collision stopping powers.

W. H. Bragg (1910) and L. H. Gray (1929, 1936) applied this equation to the problem of relating the absorbed dose in a probe inserted in a medium to that in the medium itself. Gray in particular identified the probe as a gas-filled cavity, whence the name "cavity theory". The simplest such theory is called the Bragg–Gray (B–G) theory, and its mathematical statement, referred to as the *Bragg-Gray relation*, will be developed next.

Suppose that a region of otherwise homogeneous medium w, undergoing irradiation, contains a thin layer or "cavity" filled with another medium g, as in Fig. 10.1*b*. *The thickness of the g-layer is assumed to be so small in comparison with the range of the charged particles striking it that its presence does not perturb the charged-particle field.* This assumption is often referred to as a "Bragg–Gray condition". It depends on the scattering properties of w and g being sufficiently similar that the mean path length (g/cm^2) followed by particles in traversing the thin g-layer is practically identical to its value if g were replaced by a layer of w having the same mass thickness. Similarity of backscattering at w–g, g–w, and w–w interfaces is also implied.

For heavy charged particles (either primary, or secondary to a neutron field), which undergo little scattering, this B–G condition is not seriously challenged so long as the cavity is very small in comparison with the range of the particles. However, for electrons even such a small cavity may be significantly perturbing unless the medium g is sufficiently close to w in atomic number.

Bragg–Gray cavity theory can be applied whether the field of charged particles enters from outside the vicinity of the cavity, as in the case of a beam of high-energy charged particles, or is generated in medium w through interactions by indirectly ionizing radiation. In the latter case it is also assumed that no such interactions occur in g. All charged particles in the B–G theory must originate elsewhere than in the cavity. Moreover charged particles entering the cavity are assumed not to stop in it.

A second B–G condition, incorporating these ideas, can be written as follows: *The absorbed dose in the cavity is assumed to be deposited entirely by the charged particles crossing it.*

This condition tends to be more difficult to satisfy for neutron fields than for photons, especially if the cavity gas is hydrogenous, thus having a large neutron-interaction cross section. The heavy secondary charged particles (protons, α-particles, and re-coiling nuclei) also generally have shorter ranges than the secondary electrons that result from interactions by photons of quantum energies comparable to the neutron kinetic energies. Thus we see that the first B–G condition is the more difficult of the two to satisfy for photons and electrons, while the second B–G condition is the more difficult to satisfy for neutrons.

Under the terms of the two B–G conditions, the ratio of absorbed doses in the adjacent medium w to that in the cavity g is given by Eq. (10.3) for each mono-energetic component of the spectrum of charged particles crossing g. For a differential energy distribution Φ_T (particles per cm^2 MeV) the appropriate average mass col-lision stopping power in the cavity medium g is

$$
{}_m\overline{S}_g \equiv \frac{\displaystyle\int_0^{T_{max}} \Phi_T \left(\frac{dT}{\rho dx}\right)_{c,g} dT}{\displaystyle\int_0^{T_{max}} \Phi_T \, dT}
$$

$$
= \frac{1}{\Phi} \int_0^{T_{max}} \Phi_T \left(\frac{dT}{\rho dx}\right)_{c,g} dT = \frac{D_g}{\Phi} \tag{10.4}
$$

and likewise, for a thin layer of wall material w that may be inserted in place of g,

$$
{}_m\overline{S}_w \equiv \frac{\displaystyle\int_0^{T_{max}} \Phi_T \left(\frac{dT}{\rho dx}\right)_{c,w} dT}{\displaystyle\int_0^{T_{max}} \Phi_T \, dT}
$$

$$
= \frac{1}{\Phi} \int_0^{T_{max}} \Phi_T \left(\frac{dT}{\rho dx}\right)_{c,w} dT = \frac{D_w}{\Phi} \tag{10.5}
$$

Combining Eqs. (10.4) and (10.5) gives for the ratio of absorbed dose in w to that in g, which is the B–G relation in terms of absorbed dose in the cavity:

$$
\boxed{\frac{D_w}{D_g} = \frac{{}_m\overline{S}_w}{{}_m\overline{S}_g} \equiv {}_m\overline{S}_g^w} \tag{10.6}
$$

If the medium g occupying the cavity is a gas in which a charge Q (of either sign) is produced by the radiation, D_g can be expressed (in grays) in terms of that charge as

$$
D_g = \frac{Q}{m} \left(\frac{\overline{W}}{e}\right)_g \tag{10.7}
$$

where Q is expressed in coulombs, m is the mass (kg) of gas in which Q is produced, and $(\overline{W}/e)_g$ is the mean energy spent per unit charge produced (J/C; see Chapter 2, Section V.B, and Chapter 12, Section VI). By substituting Eq. (10.7) into Eq. (10.6), we obtain the B–G relation expressed in terms of cavity ionization:

$$D_w = \frac{Q}{m}\left(\frac{\overline{W}}{e}\right)_g \cdot {}_m\overline{S}{}_g^w \qquad (10.8)$$

This equation allows one to calculate the absorbed dose in the medium immediately surrounding a B–G cavity, on the basis of the charge produced in the cavity gas, provided that the appropriate values of m, $(\overline{W}/e)_g$, and ${}_m\overline{S}{}_g^w$ are known.

Note that Q is generally greater than the charge Q' *collected* from the ion chamber, because of ionic recombination (as discussed in Chapter 12, Section V), requiring a correction.

m may be less than the total mass of gas contained in an ion chamber, if some of the volume is not active in providing measurable charge—for example, if some of the electrical lines of force terminate on a grounded guard ring. In most cases the value of m must be inferred from a chamber calibration in a known radiation field, a subject that is addressed in Chapter 13.

B–G theory also may be applied to solid- or liquid-filled "cavities" g, using Eq. (10.6) to calculate D_w from a value of D_g measured in some way. For example, medium g might be a thin plastic film that gradually darkens as a known function of absorbed dose. Thus D_g could be determined after an exposure by means of a densitometer measurement. However, it is relatively difficult to satisfy the B–G conditions with condensed cavity media, since the cavity thickness must be only ~0.001 times as great as for a gas-filled cavity at 1 atm to obtain a comparable mass thickness of g. Thus a 1-mm gas-filled cavity is comparable to a 1-μm layer of a condensed medium.

So long as ${}_m\overline{S}{}_g^w$ is evaluated for the charged-particle spectrum Φ_T that crosses the cavity, as in Eqs. (10.4)–(10.6), the B–G relation requires neither charged-particle equilibrium (CPE) nor a homogeneous field of radiation. However, the charged-particle fluence Φ_T must be the same in the cavity and in the medium w at the place where D_w is to be determined.

If CPE does exist in the neighborhood of a point of interest in the medium w, then the insertion of a B–G cavity at the point may be assumed not to perturb the "equilibrium spectrum" of charged particles existing there, since by definition a B–G cavity satisfies the B–G requirements. Thus a B–G cavity approximates an evacuated cavity in this respect. The presence of an equilibrium spectrum of charged particles allows some simplification in estimating Φ_T and hence ${}_m\overline{S}{}_g^w$, as will be seen later in Spencer's derivation of the B–G relation.

The medium w surrounding the cavity of an ionization chamber is ordinarily just the solid chamber wall itself, and one often refers to the B–G theory as providing a relation between the doses in the gas and in the wall.

II. COROLLARIES OF THE BRAGG–GRAY RELATION

Two useful corollaries of the B–G relation can be readily derived from it. The first relates the charge produced in different gases contained in the same chamber, while the second relates the charge in the same gas contained by different chamber walls.

A. First Bragg-Gray Corollary

A B–G cavity chamber of volume V with wall medium w is first filled with gas g_1 at density ρ_1, then with gas g_2 at density ρ_2. Identical irradiations are applied, producing charges Q_1 and Q_2, respectively. The absorbed dose in gas g_1 can be written as

$$D_1 = D_w \cdot {}_m\bar{S}_w^{g_1} = \frac{Q_1}{\rho_1 V}\left(\frac{\overline{W}}{e}\right)_1, \tag{10.9}$$

and the dose in gas g_2 as

$$D_2 = D_w \cdot {}_m\bar{S}_w^{g_2} = \frac{Q_2}{\rho_2 V} \cdot \left(\frac{\overline{W}}{e}\right)_2 \tag{10.10}$$

The ratio of charges therefore becomes

$$\frac{Q_2}{Q_1} = \frac{\rho_2 V}{\rho_1 V} \cdot \frac{(\overline{W}/e)_1}{(\overline{W}/e)_2} \cdot \frac{{}_m\bar{S}_w^{g_2}}{{}_m\bar{S}_w^{g_1}} \tag{10.11}$$

which reduces to the first B–G corollary:

$$\frac{Q_2}{Q_1} = \frac{\rho_2}{\rho_1} \cdot \frac{(\overline{W}/e)_1}{(\overline{W}/e)_2} \cdot {}_m\bar{S}_{g_1}^{g_2} \tag{10.12}$$

Note that Eq. (10.12) does not depend explicitly upon the wall material w, implying that the same value of Q_2/Q_1 would be observed if the experiment were repeated with different chamber walls. This is true as long as the spectrum Φ_T of charged particles crossing the cavity is not significantly dependent on the kind of wall material. For example, the starting spectrum of secondary electrons produced in different wall media by γ-rays is the same if the γ-energy is such that only Compton interactions can occur. Although different wall media modify the starting electron spectrum somewhat differently as the electrons slow down (to be discussed in Section III), the resulting *equilibrium spectrum* that crosses the cavity in different thick-walled ion chambers is sufficiently similar that Q_2/Q_1 is observed to be nearly independent of the wall material in this case.

B. Second Bragg-Gray Corollary

A single gas g of density ρ is contained in two B–G cavity chambers that have thick walls (exceeding the maximum charged-particle range), and that receive identical irradiations of penetrating x- or γ-rays, producing CPE at the cavity. The first chamber has a volume V_1 and wall material w_1, the second has a volume V_2 and wall w_2. The absorbed dose in the wall of the first chamber, adjacent to its cavity, can be written as

$$D_{w_1} \overset{\text{CPE}}{=} (K_c)_{w_1} = \Psi \left(\frac{\overline{\mu_{en}}}{\rho} \right)_{w_1}$$

$$= D_1 \cdot {}_m\overline{S}_g^{w_1} = \frac{Q_1}{\rho V_1} \left(\frac{\overline{W}}{e} \right)_g \cdot {}_m\overline{S}_g^{w_1} \qquad (10.13)$$

where Ψ = photon energy fluence,
$(\mu_{en}/\rho)_{w_1}$ = mean mass energy-absorption coefficient of wall w_1 for those photons,
$\quad D_1$ = absorbed dose in gas g in the first chamber,
$\quad Q_1$ = charge produced in the first chamber.
The corresponding equation for the second chamber is

$$D_{w_2} \overset{\text{CPE}}{=} (K_c)_{w_2} = \Psi \left(\frac{\overline{\mu_{en}}}{\rho} \right)_{w_2}$$

$$= D_2 \cdot {}_m\overline{S}_g^{w_2} = \frac{Q_2}{\rho V_2} \left(\frac{\overline{W}}{e} \right)_g \cdot {}_m\overline{S}_g^{w_2} \qquad (10.14)$$

The ratio of the ionizations in the two chambers is obtained from Eqs. (10.13) and (10.14) as

$$\frac{Q_2}{Q_1} = \frac{V_2}{V_1} \cdot \frac{(\mu_{en}/\rho)_{w_2}}{(\mu_{en}/\rho)_{w_1}} \cdot \frac{{}_m\overline{S}_g^{w_1}}{{}_m\overline{S}_g^{w_2}} \qquad (10.15)$$

where the constancy of $(\overline{W}/e)_g$ for electron energies above a few keV allows its cancellation.

A further simplification of the final factor to ${}_m\overline{S}_{w_2}^{w_1}$ can be made only if the charged-particle spectrum Φ_T crossing the cavity is the same in the two chambers [see Eqs. (10.4)–(10.6)]. The Compton-interaction case cited in the preceding section allows such a simplification, for example. If such a cancellation of stopping powers thus eliminates g from Eq. (10.15), the same value of Q_2/Q_1 should result irrespective of the choice of gas.

An equation similar to (10.15) can be obtained for neutron irradiations in place of photons by substituting kerma factors F_n for the mass energy-absorption coefficients [see Eq. (2.9a)]:

$$\frac{Q_2}{Q_1} = \frac{V_2}{V_1} \cdot \frac{(\overline{F}_n)_{w_2}}{(\overline{F}_n)_{w_1}} \cdot \frac{{}_m\overline{S}_g^{w_1}}{{}_m\overline{S}_g^{w_2}} \cdot \frac{(\overline{W}/e)_1}{(\overline{W}/e)_2} \qquad (10.16)$$

The ratio $\overline{W}/e$ may have to be retained here if w_1 and w_2 differ sufficiently to produce heavy charged-particle spectra that have somewhat different $\overline{W}/e$ values even in the same gas. Otherwise it can be canceled as in Eq. (10.15).

III. SPENCER'S DERIVATION OF THE BRAGG–GRAY THEORY

In laying the groundwork for developing an improved cavity theory, L. V. Spencer re-derived the B–G theory by a different (though more restricted) approach that is valuable in providing additional insight into the nature of the spectrum when charged-particle equilibrium exists (Spencer and Attix, 1955).

Consider a small cavity filled with medium g, surrounded by homogeneous medium w that contains a homogeneous source emitting N identical charged particles per gram, each with kinetic energy T_0 (MeV). The cavity is assumed to be far enough from the outer limits of w that CPE exists. Both B–G conditions are assumed to be satisfied by the cavity, and bremsstrahlung generation is assumed to be absent.

The absorbed dose at any point in the undisturbed medium w where CPE exists can be stated as

$$\overset{\text{CPE}}{D_w \; = \; K_w \; = \; NT_0} \qquad \text{(MeV/g)} \qquad (10.17)$$

where 1 MeV/g = 1.602×10^{-10} Gy

An equilibrium charged-particle fluence spectrum Φ_T^e (cm^{-2} MeV^{-1}) exists at each such point, and the absorbed dose can be written in terms of this spectrum as

$$D_w \; = \; \int_0^{T_0} \Phi_T^e \left(\frac{dT}{\rho dx}\right)_w dT \qquad (10.18)$$

where $(dT/\rho dx)_w$ has the same value as the mass collision stopping power for w, in the absence of bremsstrahlung generation.

It will be seen that the value of Φ_T^e that satisfies the integral equation formed by setting Eqs. (10.17) and (10.18) equal is

$$\Phi_T^e \; = \; \frac{N}{(dT/\rho dx)_w} \qquad (10.19)$$

Evidently the equilibrium spectrum for an initially monoenergetic source of charged particles is directly proportional to the number released per unit mass, and is inversely proportional, at each energy $T \leq T_0$, to the mass stopping power in the medium in which the particles are allowed to slow down and stop. Figure 10.2 is a graph of the equilibrium spectrum of primary electrons that results from Eq. (10.19) when it is applied (twice) to the example of two superimposed sources of N electrons per gram each, one emitting at $T_0 = 2$ MeV and the other at $T_0 = 0.2$ MeV, in a water medium. This is not a realistic spectrum, however, as δ-ray production (which would cause the lower limb of the spectrum to turn up instead of down; see Fig. 10.4 in Section V below) has been ignored. δ-ray effects will be discussed in the next section. The present approximation to the equilibrium spectrum, as stated by Eq. (10.19), is based on the *continuous slowing-down approximation* (CSDA) referred to in Sections I and IV.A of Chapter 8.

We will now digress briefly from Spencer's derivation to provide additional insight

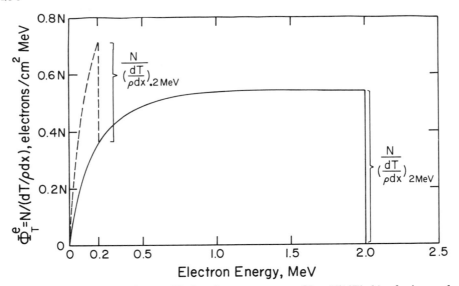

FIGURE 10.2. Example of an equilibrium fluence spectrum, $\Phi_T^e = N/(dT/\rho dx)$, of primary electrons under CPE conditions in water, assuming the continuous-slowing-down approximation. Solid curve: The distributed source emits N electrons of $T_0 = 2$ MeV per gram of water. Dashed curve: A second source of N e/g at $T_0 = 0.2$ MeV is added. Note that this doubles the differential fluence below 0.2 MeV. δ-ray production has been ignored in deriving this spectrum.

into the nature of the equilibrium fluence, Φ^e, which can be obtained from the following integration of Φ_T^e:

$$\Phi^e = \int_0^{T_0} \Phi_T^e \, dT = \int_0^{T_0} \frac{N \, dT}{(dT/\rho dx)_w} = N\Re_{\text{CSDA}}$$

$$= \rho N \frac{\Re_{\text{CSDA}}}{\rho} \qquad (10.20)$$

where $\Re_{\text{CSDA}}$ is the CSDA range in medium w of the charged particles of starting energy T_0 [see Eq. (8.22)]. Whether N is given in particles per gram and $\Re_{\text{CSDA}}$ in g/cm^2, or ρN is in particles per cm^3 and $\Re_{\text{CSDA}}/\rho$ in centimeters, the equilibrium fluence is given in particles per cm^2 by their product. The basis for the *Fano theorem*, to be discussed in Section VII, is contained in Eq. (10.20), namely, that Φ^e is independent of the density of the medium. Bragg (1910) stated his original cavity theory in terms of charged-particle ranges instead of stopping powers, in accordance with their reciprocal relationship as shown in Eq. (10.20).

Returning now to Spencer's derivation of the B–G theory, one can say that since the same equilibrium fluence spectrum of charged particles, Φ_T^e, crosses the cavity as exists within medium w, the absorbed dose in the cavity medium g can be written in the same form as Eq. (10.18):

$$D_g = \int_0^{T_0} \Phi_T^e \left(\frac{dT}{\rho dx}\right)_g dT = N \int_0^{T_0} \frac{(dT/\rho dx)_g}{(dT/\rho dx)_w} dT \tag{10.21}$$

Hence the ratio of the dose in the cavity to that in the solid w is obtained from Eqs. (10.17) and (10.21):

$$\frac{D_g}{D_w} = \frac{1}{T_0} \int_0^{T_0} \frac{(dT/\rho dx)_g}{(dT/\rho dx)_w} dT = {}_m\overline{S}_w^g \tag{10.22}$$

which is the same as the B–G relation shown in Eq. (10.6), considering Spencer's added assumptions of monoenergetic starting energy T_0, charged-particle equilibrium, and zero bremsstrahlung. The equivalence of ${}_m\overline{S}_w^g$, as employed in Eq. (10.22), to the reciprocal of ${}_m\overline{S}_g^w$ as defined in Eq. (10.6) may not be immediately obvious, and will be explained in Section IV.

The foregoing Spencer treatment of B–G theory can be generalized somewhat to accommodate bremsstrahlung generation by electrons and its subsequent escape. Equation (10.17) is rewritten as

$$\overset{\text{CPE}}{D_w} = (K_c)_w = NT_0 [1 - Y_w(T_0)] \tag{10.23}$$

where $(K_c)_w$ is the collision kerma and $Y_w(T_0)$ is the radiation yield (which is defined in Section III.G of Chapter 8) for medium w.

Equations (10.18) and (10.21), respectively, are changed to

$$D_w = \int_0^{T_0} \Phi_T^e \left(\frac{dT}{\rho dx}\right)_{c,w} dT \tag{10.24}$$

and

$$D_g = \int_0^{T_0} \Phi_T^e \left(\frac{dT}{\rho dx}\right)_{c,g} dT \tag{10.25}$$

where $(dT/\rho dx)_{c,w}$ and $(dT/\rho dx)_{c,g}$ are the mass collision stopping powers in media w and g, respectively. The equilibrium fluence, as given by Eq. (10.19), remains unchanged; hence one can rewrite Spencer's statement of B–G theory in Eq. (10.22) in the following form to take account of bremsstrahlung:

$$\frac{D_g}{D_w} = \frac{1}{T_0[1 - Y_w(T_0)]} \int_0^{T_0} \frac{(dT/\rho dx)_{c,g}}{(dT/\rho dx)_w} dT = {}_m\overline{S}_w^g \tag{10.26}$$

The quantities necessary for the numerical evaluation of this equation are tabulated in Appendix E for electrons in several media.

IV. AVERAGING OF STOPPING POWERS

For the special case treated by Spencer in the foregoing derivation, the spectrum of primary charged particles crossing the cavity is known, being given by Eq. (10.19).

However, the evaluation of $_m\overline{S}_w^g$ in Eq. (10.22) is seen to be a simple average of the ratio of stopping powers throughout the energy range 0 to T_0, apparently unweighted by Φ_T^e. In fact the fluence weighting is implicit, as can be seen by applying Spencer's assumptions to Eqs. (10.4) and (10.5): Setting $T_{max} = T_0$ for the upper limit of integration, assuming CPE and the absence of bremsstrahlung generation, Eq. (10.4) becomes

$$_m\overline{S}_g \equiv \frac{\int_0^{T_0} \Phi_T^e \left(\frac{dT}{\rho dx}\right)_g dT}{\int_0^{T_0} \Phi_T^e \, dT} = \frac{1}{\Phi^e} \int_0^{T_0} \Phi_T^e \left(\frac{dT}{\rho dx}\right)_g dT$$

$$= \frac{N}{\Phi^e} \int_0^{T_0} \frac{(dT/\rho dx)_g}{(dT/\rho dx)_w} dT = \frac{D_g}{\Phi^e} \tag{10.27}$$

where Eq. (10.19) has been substituted for Φ_T^e inside the integral. A similar equation can be written for $_m\overline{S}_w$ from Eqs. (10.5) and (10.19). The mean mass-stopping-power ratio $_m\overline{S}_w^g$ can then be obtained as shown in Eq. (10.22) through the application of Eq. (10.17), which clearly depends on the existence of an equilibrium spectrum.

   Since the Spencer B–G treatment was limited to only a single starting energy (T_0) of the charged particles, it will be useful to extend it to distributions of starting energies, such as are generated by photons in a statistically large number of Compton events. Consider a homogeneous source of charged particles throughout medium w, emitting a continuous distribution of starting energies: Let N_{T_0} charged particles of energy T_0 to $T_0 + dT_0$ be emitted per gram of w and per MeV interval, where $0 \le T_0 \le T_{max}$. Assume that CPE exists, and that bremsstrahlung may be produced and it escapes. The absorbed dose in w is given by

$$D_w \overset{CPE}{=} (K_c)_w = \int_{T_0=0}^{T_{max}} N_{T_0} T_0 [1 - Y_w(T_0)] \, dT_0 \tag{10.28}$$

while the dose in the cavity medium g is

$$D_g = \int_{T_0=0}^{T_{max}} dT_0 \int_{T=0}^{T_0} \Phi_T^e \left(\frac{dT}{\rho dx}\right)_{c,g} dT$$

$$= \int_{T_0=0}^{T_{max}} N_{T_0} \, dT_0 \int_{T=0}^{T_0} \frac{(dT/\rho dx)_{c,g}}{(dT/\rho dx)_w} dT \tag{10.29}$$

Thus for a continuous distribution of charged-particle starting energies the ratio of absorbed doses in cavity and wall is given by

$$\frac{D_g}{D_w} = \frac{\int_0^{T_{max}} N_{T_0} \, dT_0 \int_0^{T_0} \frac{(dT/\rho dx)_{c,g}}{(dT/\rho dx)_w} \, dT}{\int_0^{T_{max}} N_{T_0} \, T_0 \, [1 - Y(Y_0)] \, dT_0} \equiv {}_m\overline{\overline{S}}{}_w^g \qquad (10.30)$$

where the double bar on ${}_m\overline{\overline{S}}{}_w^g$ signifies integration over the T_0 distribution, as well as over T for each T_0-value.

Where CPE does not exist in the vicinity of the cavity, mean stopping powers can be calculated as an average weighted by the differential charged-particle fluence distribution Φ_T crossing the cavity, as in Eqs. (10.4) and (10.5). Thus in general the mean stopping-power ratio for a B–G cavity can be expressed as

$$\frac{\frac{1}{\Phi} \int_0^{T_{max}} \Phi_T \left(\frac{dT}{\rho dx}\right)_{c,g} dT}{\frac{1}{\Phi} \int_0^{T_{max}} \Phi_T \left(\frac{dT}{\rho dx}\right)_{c,w} dT} = \frac{{}_m\overline{S}_g}{{}_m\overline{S}_w} = {}_m\overline{S}{}_w^g = \frac{D_g}{D_w} \qquad (10.31)$$

Since collision stopping powers for different media show similar trends as a function of particle energy, their ratio for two media is a very slowly varying function. This allows Eq. (10.31) to be reasonably well approximated through simple estimation. For example, one may first determine the average energy $\overline{T}$ of the charged particles crossing the cavity:

$$\overline{T} = \frac{\int_0^{T_{max}} \Phi_T \, T \, dT}{\int_0^{T_{max}} \Phi_T \, dT} = \frac{1}{\Phi} \int_0^{T_{max}} \Phi_T \, T \, dT \qquad (10.32)$$

and then look up the tabulated mass collision stopping powers for the media in question at that energy. The same procedure may be followed also if $\overline{T}$ can be estimated in some other way, or if the crossing electrons have a known, roughly monoenergetic energy, such as occurs at depth in a medium upon which monoenergetic charged particles are incident (e.g., see the footnote in Table 13.9, Chapter 13).

For an equilibrium spectrum resulting from charged particles of mean starting energy $\overline{T}_0$, the stopping powers may be looked up at the energy $\overline{T}_0/2$ for a crude (but often adequate) estimate of the mean stopping-power ratio required for the B–G relation. The average starting energy $\overline{T}_0$ of Compton-effect electrons can be calculated from Eq. (7.23).

V. SPENCER CAVITY THEORY

By the 1950s experiments had shown that the B–G cavity theory did not accurately predict the ionization in air-filled cavities, especially with walls of high atomic number. At the National Bureau of Standards, the preliminary results of Attix, De La Vergne, and Ritz (1958) suggested to Spencer that δ-ray production had to be taken into account (Spencer and Attix, 1955).

For example, the solid curves in Fig. 10.3 show the relative ionization measured per unit volume of air in flat, guard-ringed ion chambers with equilibrium-thickness walls of graphite, Al, Cu, Sn, and Pb, exposed to the 412-keV γ rays from ^{198}Au. It can be seen that the ionization decreases as the air-gap thickness is increased, the trend becoming more pronounced as Z increases. This is partly due to a gradual failure of lateral CPE, as electrons scattering out of the chamber edges are not fully replaced by electrons generated by γ-ray interactions in the 2.5-cm-wide guard-ring area, made of the same wall material.

The marks labeled Pb, Sn, Cu, Al, and C on the vertical axis of Fig. 10.3 are B–G-theory predictions calculated from the second B–G corollary (Eq. 10.15), for Pb/C, Sn/C, Cu/C, and Al/C chambers, normalized to the graphite-wall experimental value for small air-gap widths. Although the conditions for validity of the B–G theory should be most closely satisfied for cavities of negligible size, the ionization-density curves evidently do not approach the B–G values but instead tend toward higher values as the cavity size is reduced. The Spencer theory (dashed curves) comes significantly closer to the experimental results, and predicts a rising curve even for small gaps (<2 mm) where the electron losses from the chamber edge were shown to be negligible.

In examining the inadequacy of the B–G theory it should be remembered that the stopping-power ratio in Eq. (10.15) is evaluated under the assumption of the CSDA, upon which collision stopping powers are based. Actually δ rays (energetic electrons) are produced in knock-on electron–electron collisions, and these δ rays join the flux of electrons crossing the cavity. Their presence enhances the equilibrium spectrum at the lower electron energies, since the kinetic energy of an electron undergoing a knock-on collision is immediately shared with the electron it hits. Thus an electron of energy T striking another may, for example, transfer $\frac{1}{4}$ of its energy to the resulting δ-ray. The electron flux will consequently be deficient by one electron in the energy region from $3T/4$ to T, and will be enriched by one electron in the region from 0 to $T/4$. The resulting equilibrium electron spectrum is further progressively enhanced as the energy is decreased because the Møller (1931) differential cross section for δ-ray production is inversely proportional to the square of the δ-ray energy.

Considering now Eq. (10.15), and approximating the last term by $_m\overline{S}\,{}^{w_1}_{w_2}$ to simplify the argument, we see that

$$\frac{(Q/V)_2}{(Q/V)_1} \overset{\propto}{\approx} {}_m\overline{S}\,{}^{w_1}_{w_2} \tag{10.33}$$

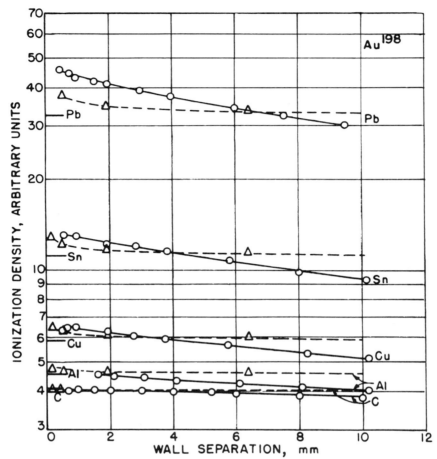

FIGURE 10.3. Comparison of measured ionization densities (solid curves) in flat air-filled ion chambers having various wall materials and adjustable gap widths, with Bragg–Gray theory (tick marks at left) and Spencer theory (dashed curves), for ^{198}Au γ rays. (After Attix, De La Vergne, and Ritz, 1958.)

or, letting chamber wall 1 be graphite and 2 be Pb, for example,

$$\frac{(Q/V)_{Pb}}{(Q/V)_{C}} \approx {_m}\bar{S}^{C}_{Pb} \tag{10.34}$$

That is, the ratio of ionization densities in the Pb/graphite chambers is approximately proportional to ${_m}\bar{S}^{C}_{Pb}$. That stopping-power ratio gradually increases with decreasing electron energy. Thus the presence of more low-energy electrons in the equilibrium spectrum as a result of δ-ray production gives $_m\bar{S}^C_{Pb}$ a larger value than it would have if evaluated by the CSDA assumption.

Spencer's goal in modifying the B–G cavity theory was not only to incorporate the δ-ray effect, but to do it in such a way that the observed variation of ionization density with cavity size could be accounted for, at least for cavities small enough to satisfy the B–G conditions.

To reach this goal while avoiding unnecessary complications that would make the calculations infeasible required a fairly simple model. By contrast, a more sophisticated theory was developed by Burch (1955) about the same time, but it proved to be too complicated for practical application. NCRP (1961) discusses and compares these theories.

Spencer's theory (Spencer and Attix, 1955; Spencer, 1965, 1971) starts with the same assumptions that he employed in rederiving the B–G theory: the two B–G conditions, the existence of CPE, and the absence of bremsstrahlung generation. The derivation specifically addresses the case of a distributed homogeneous source of monoenergetic electrons of initial energy T_0 (MeV), emitting N particles per gram throughout a homogeneous medium w.

The cavity, containing medium g (typically air), is characterized with respect to size by a parameter Δ, which was somewhat arbitrarily taken to be the mean energy of electrons having projected ranges just large enough to cross the cavity. [It might be argued in retrospect that Δ could have been identified instead as the mean energy necessary for the δ ray that is generated in the cavity *to escape from it*. This would decrease the Δ assigned to a given cavity by roughly a factor of $1/\sqrt{2} \cong 0.7$, because the range is proportional to T_0^2 (see Fig. 8.10). However, the theory is not very sensitive to the Δ-value.]

The equilibrium spectrum, $\Phi_T^{e,\delta}$, of electrons (including δ-rays) generated in the surrounding medium is arbitrarily divided into two components in Spencer's schematization:

a.   The "fast" group: electrons that have energies $T \geq \Delta$, and that can therefore transport energy. In particular they have enough energy to cross the cavity if they strike it.

b.   The "slow" group: electrons with $T < \Delta$. These are assumed to have *zero range*, i.e., to drop their energy "on the spot" where their kinetic energy falls below Δ. Hence they are assumed not to be able to enter the cavity, nor to transport energy.

The absorbed dose at any point in medium w where CPE exists is given by

$$D_w \overset{\text{CPE}}{=} NT_0 = \int_\Delta^{T_0} \Phi_T^{e,\delta} \cdot {}_mS_w(T, \Delta) \, dT \qquad (10.35)$$

where $_mS_w(T, \Delta)$ is the restricted stopping power for electrons of energy T in medium

w, which includes only energy losses to δ-rays not exceeding Δ [see Eq. (8.21g)]. Only these low-energy δ-rays contribute to the dose at the place where they are produced; the higher-energy δ-rays carry their energy elsewhere. The integral starts at Δ because electrons of lesser energy have been assumed to have no range.

The equilibrium spectrum, including δ rays, can be expressed in a form similar to that of Eq. (10.19):

$$\Phi_T^{e,\delta} = \frac{NR(T_0, T)}{(dT/\rho dx)_w} \tag{10.36}$$

where $R(T_0, T)$ is the ratio of the differential electron fluence including δ rays to that of primary electrons alone. Table 10.1 gives approximate values of $R(T_0, T)$ that were derived from tables provided by Spencer and Attix (1955). It can be seen that the equilibrium spectrum is enhanced manyfold at electron energies that are small fractions of T_0 (e.g., $\cong$ 20-fold at $T = 0.004 T_0$).

Figure 10.4 (McConnell et al, 1964) shows the effect of the δ rays on the shape of an equilibrium β-ray spectrum. In this case the medium is copper and the distributed source is ^{64}Cu, which emits both β^- and β^+ particles. The solid curve shows the equilibrium spectrum that results from Eq. (10.36). The points were measured with a spectrometer, corrected to include the β^+ particles (not detected by the spectrometer). Evidently the calculated spectrum accurately predicts the differential flux density down to 1 keV. At still lower energies the theoretical spectrum is only about one-half of that measured, possibly due to overestimation of the stopping power below the copper L-shell binding energy. The strong influence of δ rays on the equilibrium spectrum is well illustrated in these results, however.

TABLE 10.1. Approximate[a] Values of $R(T_0, T) = \Phi_T^{e,\delta}/\Phi_T^e$, the Ratio of the Differential Electron Fluences with and without δ-rays[b]

			$R(T_0, T)$		
T/T_0	C	Al	Cu	Sn	Pb
1.00	1.00	1.00	1.00	1.00	1.00
0.50	1.00	1.00	1.00	1.00	1.00
0.25	1.05	1.05	1.06	1.06	1.07
0.125	1.21	1.23	1.25	1.27	1.29
0.062	1.60	1.66	1.73	1.79	1.85
0.031	2.4	2.6	2.8	2.9	3.1
0.016	4.4	4.7	5.2	5.5	6.0
0.008	8.5	9.4	10.5	11.3	12.3
0.004	17	19	22	24	—

[a] Average of data for $T_0 = 1.31$, 0.65, and 0.33 MeV.
[b] Derived from Spencer and Attix (1955).

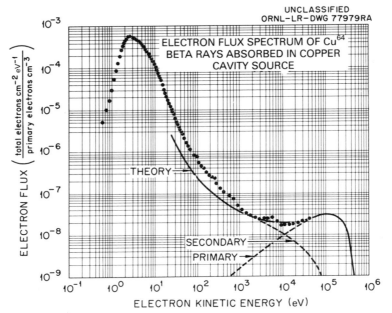

FIGURE 10.4. Equilibrium spectrum of ^{64}Cu β rays in copper. The "primary" curve is the equilibrium spectrum of primary β^-- and β^+-particles emitted by the distributed source. The "secondary" curve, extending into the solid curve labeled "theory", is the δ-ray contribution calculated by means of the factor $R(T_0, T)$. The solid curve combines the primaries and calculated secondaries. The points were measured with an electrostatic spectrometer. (After McConnell et al., 1964. Reproduced with permission from H. H. Hubbell, Jr. and the Oak Ridge National Laboratory.)

Substituting Eq. (10.36) into Eq. (10.35), we obtain the equation

$$D_w \overset{\text{CPE}}{=} NT_0 = N \int_\Delta^{T_0} \frac{R(T_0, T)}{(dT/\rho dx)_w} \cdot {}_mS_w(T, \Delta)\, dT \tag{10.37}$$

Note that if this integral had the lower limit 0 instead of Δ, then the relation

$$R(T_0, T) = \frac{(dT/\rho dx)_w}{{}_mS_w(T, \Delta)} \tag{10.38}$$

would satisfy the integral equation. To satisfy Eq. (10.37) as written requires that $R(T_0, T)$ must be somewhat greater than in Eq. (10.38), to properly account for the addition of the δ rays to the fast electron group.

A corresponding equation can be written for the dose D_g in the cavity:

$$D_g = N \int_\Delta^{T_0} \frac{R(T_0, T)}{(dT/\rho dx)_w} \cdot {}_mS_g(T, \Delta)\, dT \tag{10.39}$$

and the ratio of doses in cavity and wall is a statement of the Spencer cavity theory:

$$\frac{D_g}{D_w} = \frac{\int_\Delta^{T_0} \dfrac{R(T_0,T)}{(dT/\rho dx)_w} \cdot {}_mS_g(T,\Delta)\, dT}{\int_\Delta^{T_0} \dfrac{R(T_0,T)}{(dT/\rho dx)_w} \cdot {}_mS_w(T,\Delta)\, dT} \qquad (10.40)$$

where the denominator is shown in Eq. (10.37) to equal T_0. It is preferable in carrying out such calculations, however, to use the symmetrical form shown in Eq. (10.40) without relying on the denominator equaling T_0, since any errors that might be present in $R(T_0,T)$ or $(dT/\rho dx)_w$ will then tend to cancel.

Table 10.2 gives values of D_g/D_w calculated by Spencer for air cavities having Δ-values from 2.5 to 82 keV, in media of $Z = 6$ to 82 containing distributed monoenergetic electron sources of $T_0 = 1308, 654$, and 327 keV. For comparison the final column (also calculated by Spencer) provides the corresponding B–G-theory values,

TABLE 10.2 Values of D_g/D_w Calculated for Air Cavities by Spencer[a] from Spencer Cavity Theory, vs. Bragg–Gray Theory

			D_g/D_w						
			Spencer						
Wall Medium	T_0 (keV)	Δ (keV) = Range[b] (mm) =	2.5 0.015	5.1 0.051	10.2 0.19	20.4 0.64	40.9 2.2	81.8 7.2	Bragg–Gray
C	1308		1.001	1.002	1.003	1.004	1.004	1.005	1.005
	654		0.990	0.991	0.992	0.992	0.993	0.994	0.994
	327		0.985	0.986	0.987	0.988	0.988	0.989	0.989
Al	1308		1.162	1.151	1.141	1.134	1.128	1.123	1.117
	654		1.169	1.155	1.145	1.137	1.131	1.126	1.125
	327		1.175	1.161	1.151	1.143	1.136	1.130	1.134
Cu	1308		1.456	1.412	1.381	1.359	1.340	1.327	1.312
	654		1.468	1.421	1.388	1.363	1.345	1.329	1.327
	327		1.485	1.436	1.400	1.375	1.354	1.337	1.353
Sn	1308		1.786	1.694	1.634	1.592	1.559	1.535	1.508
	654		1.822	1.723	1.659	1.613	1.580	1.551	1.547
	327		1.861	1.756	1.687	1.640	1.602	1.571	1.595
Pb	1308		—	2.054	1.940	1.865	1.811	1.770	1.730
	654		—	2.104	1.985	1.904	1.848	1.801	1.796
	327		—	2.161	2.030	1.946	1.881	1.832	1.876

[a] Personal communication. These data replace those given in Table II of Spencer and Attix (1955), which did not take account of the polarization effect (see Chapter 8, Section III.E).
[b] In air.

which can be seen to agree most closely with the Spencer theory for the larger cavity sizes. The difference from unity generally increases with decreasing cavity size, because of the influence of more and more δ-rays (see Fig. 10.4) in the integrals of Eq. (10.40).

The Spencer cavity theory evidently gives somewhat better agreement with experimental observations for small cavities than does simple B–G theory, by taking account of δ-ray production and relating the dose integral to the cavity size. However, it still relies on the B–G conditions cited in Section I, and therefore fails to the extent that they are violated. In particular, in the case of cavities that are large (i.e., comparable to the range of the secondary charged particles generated by indirectly ionizing radiation), neither B–G condition is satisfied. This problem is discussed in the next section.

Equation (10.40) can be restated without the requirements for CPE or for the absence of bremsstrahlung by simply replacing $R(T_0, T)/(dT/\rho\, dx)_{w,g}$ with the actual crossing spectrum of charged particles, Φ_T^δ, which of course must include the δ-rays. This will only be useful if Φ_T^δ is known, however.

VI. BURLIN CAVITY THEORY

Burlin (1966, 1968) recognized the need for a γ-ray cavity theory that would bridge the gap between small cavities for which the B–G or Spencer theory could be applied, and very large cavities for which the wall influence is negligible.

Figure 10.5 illustrates this cavity-size transition. A region of homogeneous medium w is shown uniformly irradiated by γ-rays. Three cavities containing medium g are considered: small (satisfying the B–G conditions), intermediate, and large compared to the ranges of the secondary electrons present. Using the terminology of Caswell (1966), the absorbed dose in the small cavity (Fig. 10.5a) is delivered almost entirely by "crossers", i.e., secondary electrons completely traversing the cavity, such as e_1. The average absorbed dose in the intermediate-sized cavity in Fig. 10.5b is delivered partly by crossers, but also by "starters" like e_2 that originate in the cavity and stop in the wall, "stoppers" (e_3) starting in the wall and terminating in the cavity, and "insiders" (e_4) that start and stop within the cavity. Note that the dose in this

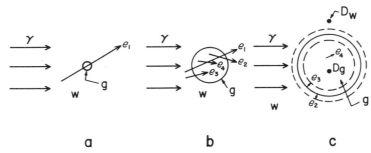

$$a \qquad\qquad b \qquad\qquad c$$

FIGURE 10.5. The cavity-size transition in Burlin theory (see text).

case will in general not be uniform throughout the cavity, but may depend on the distance inward from the wall.

If a cavity is made large enough so that the maximum-range stoppers from the wall can affect the dose in only a negligibly thin layer of cavity medium (the thickness of which is exaggerated in Fig. 10.5c), then the average dose in the cavity is practically all delivered by the insiders, e_4, which are generated by γ-ray interactions in the cavity medium g itself.

To arrive at a usefully simple theory Burlin made the following assumptions, either explicitly or implicitly:

1. The media w and g are homogeneous.

2. A homogeneous γ-ray field exists everywhere throughout w and g. (This means that no γ-ray attenuation correction is made in this theory for the presence of the cavity.)

3. Charged-particle equilibrium exists at all points in w and g that are farther than the maximum electron range from the cavity boundary.

4. The equilibrium spectra of secondary electrons generated in w and g are the same.

5. The fluence of electrons entering from the wall is attenuated exponentially as it passes through the medium g, without changing its spectral distribution.

6. The fluence of electrons that originate in the cavity builds up to its equilibrium value exponentially as a function of distance into the cavity, according to the same attenuation coefficient β that applies to the incoming electrons, as shown in Fig. 10.6 for the simple homogeneous case where $g = w$.

The Burlin cavity relation can be written in its simplest form as follows:

$$\frac{\overline{D}_g}{D_w} = d \cdot {}_m\overline{S}_w^g + (1 - d)\left(\frac{\overline{\mu_{en}}}{\rho}\right)_w^g \qquad (10.41)$$

where d is a parameter related to the cavity size that approaches unity for small cavities and zero for large ones, thus providing the proper values of Eq. (10.41) for the limiting cases; $\overline{D}_g$ is the average absorbed dose in the cavity medium g; $D_w = (K_c)_w$ is the absorbed dose in medium w under CPE conditions (i.e., not within electron range of the cavity); ${}_m\overline{S}_w^g$ is the mean ratio of mass collision stopping powers for g and w, obtained either on the basis of the B–G or Spencer theory; and $(\overline{\mu_{en}/\rho})_w^g$ is the mean ratio of the mass energy-absorption coefficients for g and w.

Burlin expressed d as the average value of Φ_w/Φ_w^e in the cavity (see Fig. 10.6):

$$d \equiv \frac{\overline{\Phi}_w}{\Phi_w^e} = \frac{\displaystyle\int_0^L \Phi_w^e\, e^{-\beta l}\, dl}{\displaystyle\int_0^L \Phi_w^e\, dl} = \frac{1 - e^{-\beta L}}{\beta L} \qquad (10.42)$$

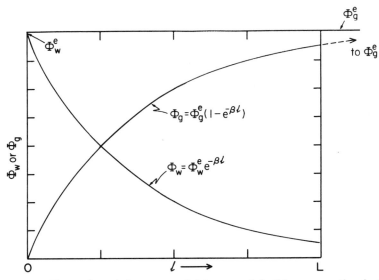

FIGURE 10.6. Illustration of the exponential-decay and -buildup assumption in the Burlin cavity theory. The equilibrium wall fluence of electrons, Φ_w^e, is shown decaying exponentially as they progress into a homogeneous cavity for which the wall w and cavity g media are assumed to be identical. The electrons under consideration are only those flowing from left to right. The buildup of the cavity-generated electron fluence Φ_g^e follows a complementary exponential, asymptotically approaching its equilibrium value $\Phi_g^e = \Phi_w^e$.

where l is the distance (cm) of any point in the cavity from the wall, along a mean chord of length L, which is taken as being equal to *four times the cavity volume V divided by its surface area S*, for convex cavities and diffuse (i.e., isotropic) electron fields. The corresponding relation for $1 - d$, representing the average value of Φ_g/Φ_g^e throughout the cavity, is

$$1 - d \equiv \frac{\overline{\Phi_g}}{\Phi_g^e} = \frac{\int_0^L \Phi_g^e (1 - e^{-\beta l})\, dl}{\int_0^L \Phi_g^e\, dl} = \frac{\beta L + e^{-\beta L} - 1}{\beta L} \tag{10.43}$$

Figure 10.6 deserves some additional explanation: A uniform γ-ray field is shown generating secondary electrons throughout the wall medium w and cavity medium g, which are assumed to be identical as well as homogeneous in this simple case. Considering only the electron fluence component flowing from left to right, the fluence Φ_w from the wall decays as $e^{-\beta l}$ from its initial equilibrium value of Φ_w^e, while the fluence Φ_g of electrons generated in the cavity builds up as $(1 - e^{-\beta l})$, approaching asymptotically its equilibrium value, $\Phi_g^e = \Phi_w^e$. These two functions, while they may not in fact be strictly exponential, must have a unit sum at all depths l in this homogeneous case, according to the Fano theorem, (to be discussed in Section VII). Likewise Eqs. (10.42) and (10.43) must sum to unity.

For the nonhomogeneous case where $g \neq w$, $(\Phi_w^e \neq \Phi_g^e)$. Moreover, if the β-value of the cavity medium for the wall electrons [Eq. (10.42)] is not the same as for the cavity-generated electrons [Eq. (10.43)], due to a difference in spectral distributions, then in general Eq. (10.43) will give a value

$$\frac{\overline{\Phi}_g}{\Phi_g^e} \equiv d' \neq (1 - d) \tag{10.44}$$

and hence

$$d' + d \neq 1 \tag{10.45}$$

The Burlin theory ignores this possible source of error in adopting assumptions 5 and 6.

In applications involving air-filled cavities Burlin (1966) evaluated β (cm^{-1}) from an empirical formula due to Loevinger:

$$\beta = \frac{16\rho}{(T_{\max} - 0.036)^{1.4}} \tag{10.46}$$

where ρ is the air density (g/cm^3) and $T_{\max}$ is the maximum value of the starting energies T_0 of the β-rays in MeV. More generally, Burlin et al. (1969) later suggested using a β-value satisfying

$$e^{-\beta t_{\max}} = 0.01 \tag{10.47}$$

That is, the maximum depth of electron penetration, $t_{\max}$, is to be arbitrarily taken as the depth to which only 1% of the electrons can travel. Janssens et al. (1974) have found that a constant of 0.04 in place of 0.01 in Eq. (10.47) improves the agreement with experimental results. $t_{\max}$ can be determined from Table 8.5 and the electron CSDA range tables in Appendix E, referring to the average starting energy $\overline{T}_0$ of the electrons.

The Burlin theory has been found to estimate the average dose in cavities fairly well over a wide range of sizes. It is particularly useful in relation to condensed-state dosimeters, which typically have dimensions that are comparable to the ranges of the electrons present. Ogunleye et al. (1980) measured the dose in stacks of LiF thermoluminescence dosimeters (TLDs), each 0.1 g/cm^2 thick, sandwiched between equilibrium-thickness walls of various media and irradiated perpendicularly by ^{60}Co γ-rays, as shown in Fig. 10.7. The data were normalized to the homogeneous case where the wall medium also consisted of solid LiF.

Figure 10.8 gives the relative average absorbed doses measured in each layer of four dosimeters in the stacks of 1, 2, 3, 5, and 7 layers. Evidently the dose varies with depth in the stack, decreasing a few percent from top to bottom in the case of the polystyrene wall medium, and rising more and more steeply with increasing depth for wall media of Al, Cu, and Pb. This pattern is primarily brought about by

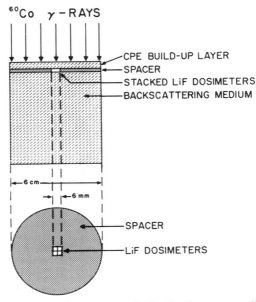

FIGURE 10.7. ⁶⁰Co γ-ray experiment to test the Burlin theory as applied to LiF TLD chips, each $0.38 \times 3.18 \times 3.18 \ mm^3$, $\rho = 2.64 \ g/cm^3$, stacked four per layer in 1, 2, 3, 5, and 7 layers. The CPE buildup layer and backscattering medium were both made of the same wall material, either LiF, polystyrene, Al, Cu, or Pb. The spacer was adjusted to equal the TLD stack thickness, and for the results presented here was made of LiF to produce a semi-infinite one-dimensional cavity. (After Ogunleye, et al., 1980. Reproduced with permission of The Institute of Physics, U.K.)

the Z-dependence of electron nuclear scattering. That is, in low-Z media electrons projected forward by γ-ray interactions tend to keep going in that direction, while in high-Z media they are more often backscattered.

The Burlin theory ignores all electron-scattering effects (as do the B–G and Spencer theories). Thus it would be to some extent fortuitous if such a simple theory were found to predict the average cavity dose accurately. Nevertheless it can be seen in Fig. 10.9 that fairly good agreement is obtained with the experimental results of Ogunleye et al., especially for the polystyrene and aluminum wall media. For multiple layers of dosimeters in Cu walls the theoretical prediction is about 1 % too high, while for Pb it is 3–4 % low.

In evaluating Eq. (10.42) to obtain the value of d for each dosimeter stack thickness, β/ρ has been taken here as 13.4 cm^2/g for LiF, obtained from the β-ray measurements of Paliwal and Almond (1976). The mean chord length L has been evaluated as 4V/S, which for a flat plate of infinite extent is equal to twice its thickness, or $L = 2t$. Ogunleye et al. (1980) had originally assumed that $L = 1.2t$, based on the average angle of Compton electron emission and straight electron tracks, obtaining relatively poor agreement. Horowitz et al. (1983) later showed that this value

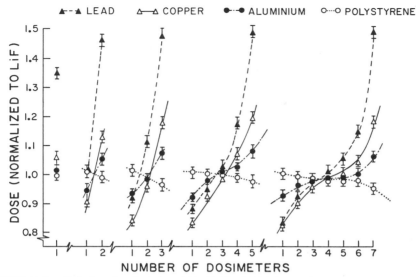

FIGURE 10.8. Relative absorbed dose in individual TLD layers in the experiment described in Fig. 10.7. ^{60}Co γ-rays pass from left to right in relation to this graph. (After Ogunleye et al., 1980. Reproduced with permission of The Institute of Physics, U.K.)

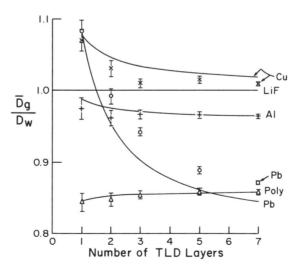

FIGURE 10.9. Comparison of the Burlin theory (solid curves) with the experiment referred to in Figs. 10.7 and 10.8. The application of the theory in this case, as described in the text, differs from that of Ogunleye et al. (1980).

was incorrect anyway, and that $L = 1.539t$ was the proper value based on those assumptions. However, it is more realistic to assume that at a depth in the wall medium that is sufficient to give rise to charged-particle equilibrium, a diffuse electron field will exist, calling for the application of 4V/S to obtain the mean chord length in the cavity. Note that this value will apply to a convex cavity that is front–back symmetrical, even if the electron field arrives isotropically only from the front hemisphere and is absent from the back. For the geometry of the experiment shown in Fig. 10.7 the monodirectional ^{60}Co γ-ray beam will tend to produce such a condition, especially in the low-Z media.

Several authors have attempted to refit the Burlin theory to this experiment.

Ogunleye (1982) applied the 4V/S rule to evaluate the mean chord length when the spacer in Fig. 10.7 was made of the wall material instead of LiF. He obtained fair agreement with the corresponding experimental results, which had not been explicitly presented in the paper by Ogunleye et al. (1980).

Horowitz and Dubi (1982) proposed a modification of the Burlin theory that depended on the idea that the average path length for escape of the electrons originating in the cavity was less than the average path length of electrons crossing the cavity. Horowitz et al. (1983) compared this modified theory with the results of Ogunleye et al. (1980), reporting improved agreement. However, Kearsley (1984a) pointed out that the improvement was brought about by the adoption of $L = 1.539t$ in place of $1.2t$, not by the effect of Horowitz and Dubi's modification to the theory. It was also shown by Janssens (1983, 1984) and Shiragai (1984) that the fundamental basis for the modification was erroneous.

Shiragai also tried various combinations of values of β and L in applying the Burlin theory to the experiment of Ogunleye et al. (1980), concluding that $L = 4V/S$ and $\beta/\rho = 18.5$ cm^2/g gave the best overall fit. Unfortunately, this large β/ρ value relates to tissue, not LiF, and hence may be regarded as physically inadmissible in the present case.

Burlin et al. (1969) extended the use of the Burlin cavity theory to fields of primary electrons by simply deleting the irrelevant last term in Eq. (10.41), leaving

$$\frac{\overline{D}_g}{D_w} = d \cdot {_m}\overline{S}_w^g \tag{10.48}$$

in which D_w is presumably the dose in the wall through which the electrons enter the cavity, since CPE does not exist anywhere. Because $d = 1$ for small cavities, this equation reduces to the B–G relation, while for very large cavities both d and $\overline{D}_g$ approach zero. The electrons can then deposit energy only in a superficial layer of the cavity, thus having a negligible effect on the average dose.

For the case of diffuse β-ray fields Burlin et al. used Eq. (10.42) to define d, where Φ_w^e is to be interpreted as the *entry fluence*, since there is no equilibrium fluence.

This theory can only be applied to diffuse electron fields, which are attenuated more or less exponentially. Broad electron beams in the megavolt range, for example, are not attenuated exponentially, as can be seen in Fig. 8.14. Thus agreement with measurements in that case should be expected only for d-values near unity, that is, where Eq. (10.48) reduces to the B–G theory.

The calculation of the absorbed dose deposited in layers of material by charged-particle beams is discussed in Chapter 8, Section V. Note that in comparing the dose deposited in a dosimeter layer by an electron beam with that in a layer of another medium, one should apply to each the appropriate Yang correction for path lengthening due to scattering (see Fig. 8.11).

A number of unusual approaches to cavity theories for electron beams have been reported in the literature; they need not be examined here. The reader is referred to a paper by O'Brien (1977) for a rational assessment of some of them, as well as a description of a Monte Carlo calculation applied to the problem. Note that δ-rays are not generated in the CASCADE code used by O'Brien, however.

The Burlin theory can also be simplistically applied to neutron fields by substituting a kerma-factor ratio in place of the energy-absorption-coefficient ratio in Eq. (10.41). However, the variation of d with cavity size will not necessarily be governed by exponential attenuation of the heavy secondary charged particles (p, α, and recoiling atomic ions), and the spectra and mixture of such particles generated in the cavity will generally differ from those in the wall medium.

VII. THE FANO THEOREM

In 1954 Fano pointed out that in many practical cases the B–G requirement for a small, nonperturbing cavity is ignored, and the use of walls and cavity that are *matched* in atomic composition is substituted, thus easing the size restriction. He noted that this substitution had never been rigorously justified, and attempted to provide such a justification. Unfortunately, his proof disregarded the influence of the polarization effect, which seriously undermines the validity of the Fano theorem for megavolt photons irradiating a gas-filled cavity in a matching solid wall. For that case a more general cavity theory that accounts for the difference in stopping power between condensed and gaseous media must be used, such as the B–G or Spencer theory.

Nevertheless the Fano theorem is an important statement in that it applies generally to neutrons, as well as to photons below about 1 MeV:

Fano's theorem: In an infinite medium of given atomic composition exposed to a uniform field of indirectly ionizing radiation, the field of secondary radiation is also uniform and *independent of the density* of the medium, as well as of density variations from point to point.

It follows from this that the charged-particle fluence at any point where CPE exists has a value that is independent of density variations within the volume of origin of the particles, (assuming negligible polarization effect).

Equation (10.20) provides a mathematical statement of the Fano theorem that is intuitively obvious, and that has its roots in an earlier enunciation of this theorem by Bragg (1912):

> Consider a unit of volume in the material through which the γ rays are passing, and suppose the γ rays to be of equal intensity at all places in the material: If this condition is not quite realized in experiment, we can easily allow for the defect. The sum total of the portions of the paths of β particles which are completed within the unit of volume in each second is proportional to two things, (a) the number of β rays originated in each unit of mass of the substance (this is nearly independent of the nature of the substance where γ rays are very penetrating), (b) the range, d. This would be true even if d were not actually the same for every ray but were only an average. This statement will perhaps be more obvious when it is considered that halving the density would halve the number of β rays springing up in each unit of volume, but double the range of each so that the number crossing each unit of volume in a second would be the same as before. In other words, the whole length of the tracks completed in a unit of volume depends only on the nature of the substance and not on its density or uniformity.

Fano's proof, which follows, employs the radiation transport equation, which has been generally discussed by Roesch (1968).

Fano first considered an infinite medium of uniform density, homogeneously irradiated by γ rays. Let $S(E, \mathbf{u})$ be the number of electrons of variable energy E and variable direction $\mathbf{u}$ that are generated per unit mass of the medium. $S(E, \mathbf{u})$ is evidently uniform throughout the medium. Denote by $k(E', E, \mathbf{u}' \cdot \mathbf{u}) \, dE' \, d\mathbf{u}'$ the probability that electrons of energy E will be scattered inelastically, so as to have energy E' and direction $\mathbf{u}'$, per unit mass thickness of material traversed (g/cm^2). Let $N(E, \mathbf{u})$ be the uniform fluence of electrons of each energy and direction.

The fluence balance at each location in the medium requires that all local increases and decreases of $N(E, \mathbf{u})$ cancel, as in the following equation:

$$S(E, \mathbf{u}) - N(E, \mathbf{u}) \int_0^E dE' \int_{4\pi} d\mathbf{u}' \, k(E', E, \mathbf{u}' \cdot \mathbf{u})$$

$$+ \int_E^\infty dE' \int_{4\pi} d\mathbf{u}' \, k(E, E', \mathbf{u} \cdot \mathbf{u}') N(E', \mathbf{u}') = 0 \qquad (10.49)$$

The first term is the source contribution to $N(E, \mathbf{u})$; the second is its depletion due to all mechanisms of energy loss, scattering, absorption, or other transformations; and the third represents the increase in $N(E, \mathbf{u})$ by processes that affect electrons of higher energy and/or different direction.

For comparison Fano next considered a medium of the same composition as before, but with density $\rho(\mathbf{r})$ varying from one point $\mathbf{r} = (x, y, z)$ to another. The fluence of electrons at $\mathbf{r}$ will now be indicated by $\Phi(\mathbf{r}, E, \mathbf{u})$. Another, more general, transport equation can be written in the same form as Eq. (10.49), but without assuming that CPE exists, i.e., that the sum of the terms equals zero. The rate of variation (if any) of $\Phi(\mathbf{r}, E, \mathbf{u})$ from point to point is instead assumed to be given by its gradient, $\mathbf{u} \cdot \mathrm{grad}$

$\Phi(\mathbf{r}, E, \mathbf{u})$. The new transport equation will be expressed in electrons per cm^3 instead of electrons per gram by multiplying it through by the local density, $\rho(\mathbf{r})$:

$$\mathbf{u} \cdot \text{grad } \Phi(\mathbf{r}, E, \mathbf{u}) = \rho(\mathbf{r})S(E, \mathbf{u})$$

$$- \Phi(\mathbf{r}, E, \mathbf{u})\rho(\mathbf{r}) \int_0^E dE' \int_{4\pi} d\mathbf{u} \, k(E', E, \mathbf{u}' \cdot \mathbf{u})$$

$$+ \rho(\mathbf{r}) \int_E^\infty dE' \int_{4\pi} d\mathbf{u}' \, k(E, E', \mathbf{u} \cdot \mathbf{u}')\Phi(\mathbf{r}, E', \mathbf{u}') \qquad (10.50)$$

If the solution $\Phi(\mathbf{r}, E, \mathbf{u})$ to Eq. (10.50) can be shown to be the same as the solution $N(E, \mathbf{u})$ to Eq. (10.49), the theorem will be proved, since that common solution will then apply regardless of density variations. If $N(E, \mathbf{u})$ is substituted for $\Phi(\mathbf{r}, E, \mathbf{u})$ in Eq. (10.50), the left side vanishes, since N has no gradient. The right side reduces to $\rho(\mathbf{r})$ times Eq. (10.49), which also equals zero. Thus, the electron fluence $\Phi(\mathbf{r}, E, \mathbf{u})$ is everywhere the same as the equilibrium fluence $N(E, \mathbf{u})$, and the theorem is proved.

VIII. OTHER CAVITY THEORIES

Spencer (1971) discussed in a general way two fundamentally different approaches to cavity theory:

a. The "surface" approach, in which one evaluates the total energy contribution in the cavity by each group of electrons that enter it. He indicated that this was the viewpoint adopted by Gray in developing his cavity theory.

b. The "volume" approach, in which one considers the energy deposition in each cavity volume element by electrons arriving from everywhere. Spencer found Bragg's development of cavity theory compatible with this idea. Fano's proof of the Fano theorem is also clearly an application of the volume approach in terms of electron fluence.

Janssens et al. (1974) modified the Burlin theory by recalculating the weighting factor d with more detailed consideration of the penetration of wall electrons into the cavity. Instead of assuming a constant spectrum and exponential attenuation of the electron fluence, they used range–energy relations applied to each electron energy, in the CSDA. Electron-backscattering effects were discussed but not included.

Janssens (1981) provided a modification of the Spencer theory in which the rate of energy loss in the cavity by low-energy electrons was related to cavity size, rather than simply assuming that electrons drop their energy on the spot as soon as T falls below the value of Δ. The mean rate of energy deposition per unit chord length was taken to be equal to the restricted stopping power $S(T, \Delta)$ when $T > 2\Delta$, or equal to the unrestricted collision stopping power $S(T)$ for $\Delta < T < 2\Delta$ (since the energy limit Δ is no longer effective), or equal to $(T/\Delta)S(T)$ for $T < \Delta$. In the latter case

T/Δ operates as a weighting factor for the stopping power that gradually de-emphasizes the influence of the short-range electrons.

Kearsley (1984b) focused attention on the effect of electron backscattering at the cavity–wall interface, for electrons both entering and leaving the cavity. He modified the Burlin theory accordingly, obtaining an expression of the same form as Eq. (10.41), but with weighting factors d_1 and d_2 in place of d and $d - 1$. The factors d_1 and d_2 include the influence of multiple backscattering, and assume exponential attenuation of electron fluence as in Burlin's theory. In the limit as the backscatter factors for the wall and cavity approach zero, $d_1 \rightarrow (1 - e^{-\beta L})/\beta L$ and $d_2 \rightarrow 1 - d_1$. The comparison of Kearsley's results with the experiment of Ogunleye et al. (1980) was handicapped by his use of $L = 1.2t$, which is unrealistically thin for that case as previously mentioned.

An outstanding feature of the Kearsley theory is its capability of predicting dose as a function of depth in the cavity, so that comparisons can be made with the individual layers of LiF dosimeters. Figure 10.10 shows remarkably good agreement with the results of Ogunleye et al. in this respect.

Luo Zheng-Ming (1980) has developed a cavity theory based on application of the electron transport equation in the cavity and in the surrounding medium. It is a very detailed theory that considers electron production in the cavity as well as the wall medium, and is applicable to all cavity sizes. The author compared this theory with the ion-chamber results of Attix et al. (1958) for 38-keV x-rays, obtaining good agreement.

It is arguable that the development of new and more complicated cavity theories may be reaching a period of diminishing return in competition with Monte Carlo computer methods, which are becoming more accessible and satisfactory and less expensive to run. Simple cavity theories will continue to be useful for approximate

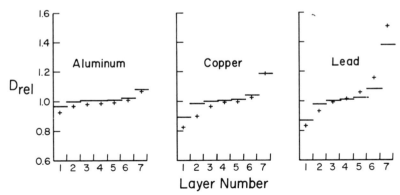

FIGURE 10.10. The average dose to a given layer of a seven-layer stack of LiF dosimeters divided by the equilibrium LiF dose, as calculated using the Kearsley model (bars) and as measured by Ogunleye et al. (+) for Al, Cu, and Pb walls. (After Kearsley, 1984b. Reproduced with permission from E. E. Kearsley and The Institute of Physics, U.K.)

solutions and estimates, but exact computations, especially for complex geometries and radiation fields, will likely be done by extensive use of computers with programs such as EGS (Ford and Nelson, 1978; Nelson, 1980) and its later improvements.

IX. DOSE NEAR INTERFACES BETWEEN DISSIMILAR MEDIA UNDER γ-IRRADIATION

Figure 10.8 clearly shows that the spatial distribution of absorbed dose in a medium near an interface with a different medium is a function of their relative atomic numbers and of the direction of the γ rays. Because of the substantial thickness of the LiF dosimeter layers relative to the range of the secondary electrons in this case, however, some detail was lost.

Dutreix and Bernard (1966) studied the ionization produced by ^{60}Co γ rays in a thin air-filled cavity as it was gradually moved from an equilibrium depth in carbon, through the carbon–copper interface, and to an equilibrium depth in the copper. The γ rays were perpendicularly incident either from the carbon or the copper side of the interface. The solid curves in Fig. 10.11 give their results, which may be interpreted as the variation vs. depth either of the electron fluence or of the absorbed dose in a low-Z (i.e., air) nonperturbing dosimeter. The ordinate is normalized to 100 at an equilibrium depth in the carbon.

Dutreix and Bernard have provided the following interpretation of these observations.

In case A, in which the γ rays pass from copper to carbon, the backscatter component of electrons in copper is seen to decrease gradually from its equilibrium value of B_{Cu} as the interface is approached. Its value is approximately zero at the interface if we assume negligible backscattering from carbon, so the electron flux there equals just the forward component, F_{Cu}. In the carbon beyond the interface, this component gradually decays to zero, while a new population of forward-moving electrons is generated in the carbon by γ-ray interactions, reaching its carbon equilibrium value at the maximum distance to which they can penetrate from the interface. It should be noted that the decay of F_{Cu} with depth is steeper than the carbon buildup curve, because the electrons emerge from the copper nearly isotropically due to scattering, while the electrons are generated in the carbon with a Compton angular distribution, as shown in Fig. 7.8. Consequently a minimum is created in the upper solid curve of total electron fluence, on the low-Z side of the boundary. The overall electron fluence transition, then, is from the equilibrium value in copper, dipping to a minimum on the low-Z side of the interface, then gradually rising to the equilibrium value in carbon.

The case of the reverse photon direction, shown in graph B, reveals a maximum instead of a minimum, again on the far side (now in the high-Z medium) of the interface. We see the forward-moving equilibrium electron fluence in the carbon remaining constant until the interface is reached, then decaying in the copper. The fluence of electrons that originate in the copper starts to build up at some distance

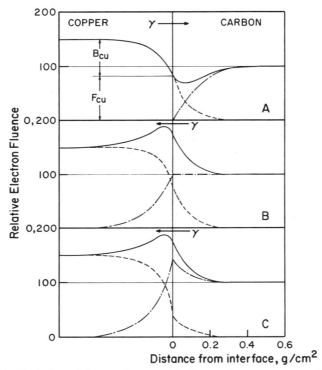

FIGURE 10.11 Variation of electron fluence with distance from a copper–carbon interface irradiated perpendicularly by ^{60}Co γ rays (Dutreix and Bernard, 1966). Solid curves: Ionization measured in a thin, flat air layer as it is gradually traversed through the interface by addition and removal of copper and carbon foils at the air-gap walls. Dashed curves: Electrons arising in copper. Dash–dotted curves: Electrons arising in carbon.

The arrows indicate the photon direction in each case: left to right in A, right to left in B and C. F_{Cu} is the fraction of the equilibrium fluence of electrons that flow with a component in the γ-ray direction in the copper; B_{Cu} is the backscattered component. In the carbon the backscattered component is small, and is assumed to be negligible here. (Reproduced with permission from J. Dutreix and The British Journal of Radiology.)

inside the carbon, due to backscattering in the copper. It is shown attaining the value B_{Cu} at the interface, then rising to its Cu-equilibrium value as the forward-moving fluence builds up.

The foregoing explanation of the processes that occur in case B does not take into account the electrons that originate in the carbon and backscatter from the copper. Chapter 8, Section V.D, gives a backscattering coefficient of 0.43 for electrons below 1 MeV striking copper. Thus, as can be seen in graph C, the forward fluence from the carbon is enhanced by 43% at the boundary, rather than remaining constant as shown in B. The curve indicating the fluence of electrons that originate in copper is diminished accordingly in graph C, so that the sum of the Cu and C electrons still agrees with the (solid) experimental curve.

It can be seen in Fig. 10.11 that the equilibrium fluence of electrons is about 50% higher in copper than in carbon. Equation (10.20) implies that it should be only about 20% higher. The number of electrons produced per gram by ^{60}Co γ-rays is proportional to $(\mu/\rho)_{Cu} = 0.0530$ cm^2/g and $(\mu/\rho)_C = 0.0578$ cm^2/g, and their mean energy is $1.25 \, (\sigma_{tr}/\sigma) = 0.580$ MeV. The CSDA ranges for electrons of this energy are obtainable from Appendix E as $\mathfrak{R}_{Cu} = 0.320$ g/cm^2 and $\mathfrak{R}_C = 0.245$ g/cm^2. Thus the ratio of equilibrium fluences should be

$$\frac{\Phi_{Cu}^e}{\Phi_C^e} = \frac{0.0530 \times 0.320}{0.0578 \times 0.245} = 1.20 \tag{10.51}$$

The excess observed by Dutreix and Bernard was probably caused by the presence of lower-energy scattered photons in the ^{60}Co γ-ray beam. Photons with an energy of, say, 0.2 MeV would produce more electrons and with longer ranges in copper than in carbon, due to the photoelectric effect. The presence of only about 5% of such photons in the beam could account for the results in Fig. 10.11.

Similar ^{60}Co γ-ray measurements by Wall and Burke (personal communication) are shown in Fig. 10.12, indicating the relative dose or electron fluence occurring in aluminum near an interface with gold or beryllium. The same general pattern is observed as in the copper–carbon results shown in Fig. 10.11: a *minimum* is observed just beyond the interface when the photons go from a higher-Z to a lower-Z medium;

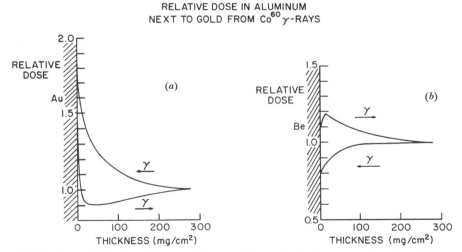

RELATIVE DOSE IN ALUMINUM
NEXT TO GOLD FROM Co^{60} γ-RAYS

FIGURE 10.12. Variation of dose and electron fluence in aluminum as a function of distance from an interface with (*a*) gold, (*b*) beryllium. Arrows indicate the direction of ^{60}Co γ rays. (After Wall and Burke, personal communication, 1970.)

a *maximum* is seen beyond the interface if the photons go from a lower-Z to a higher-Z medium. A bone–tissue interface will of course behave in a similar way.

Comparable results should be expected at higher photon energies, but with an expanded scale of distances from the interface as the secondary-electron ranges increase.

At lower energies the transient effects will conversely be crowded closer to the interface. At 100 keV, the transient effects in unit-density materials will be confined to the region within about 0.15 mm of the interface; at 30 keV that distance is reduced to 20 μm. At larger distances from the interface the fluence and dose will approximate their equilibrium values as CPE is closely achieved.

PROBLEMS

1. A boundary region between carbon and aluminum media is traversed by a fluence of 4.10×10^{11} e/cm^2 at an energy of 12.5 MeV. Ignoring δ-rays and scattering, what is the absorbed dose D_C in the carbon adjacent to the boundary, and what is the dose ratio D_{Al}/D_C?

2. A small air-filled cavity ion chamber has copper walls with thickness equal to the maximum electron range. The cavity volume is 0.100 cm^3, the air density is 0.001293 g/cm^3, and a given γ-ray exposure generates a charge (either sign) of 7.00×10^{-10} C.

   (a) What is the average absorbed dose in the cavity air?

   (b) Apply B–G theory to estimate the absorbed dose in the adjacent copper wall, assuming a mean energy $\overline{T} = 0.43$ MeV for the cavity-crossing electrons.

   (c) Suppose $\overline{T}$ is 34% in error and should have the value 0.65 MeV. Redo part (b). What was the resulting percentage error in D_{Cu}?

3. A "Bragg–Gray cavity" is generally characterized by two important assumptions. What are they?

4. Two air-filled cavity ionization chambers are identical except that one is aluminum and the other graphite. The walls are thicker than the maximum secondary-electron range for 1-MeV photons, which are negligibly attenuated. Calculate the approximate ratio of charge generated in the two chambers, assumed to be B–G cavities.

5. Consider a B–G cavity chamber with equilibrium thickness copper walls. It is first filled with a mass m of air, then by the same mass of hydrogen. Assuming identical γ-ray irradiations in the two cases, what is the charge ratio Q_{air}/Q_H? Assume ionic recombination has been corrected for, that $(\overline{W}/e)_H = 36.5$ J/C, and that the mean electron energy $\overline{T} = 0.80$ MeV.

6. (a) Compare the β/ρ value obtained from Eq. (10.47) with the value 13.4 cm^2/g gotten from Paliwal and Almond (1976) for the case of LiF irradiated by ^{60}Co γ-rays.

(b) What constant is needed on the right side of Eq. (10.47) in place of 0.01 to give exact agreement?

7. A layer of water 1 mm thick between two equilibrium-thickness layers of Teflon is irradiated by 2-MeV photons.

   (a) From Burlin theory calculate the approximate average dose in the water ($\overline{D}_{water}$) if the collision kerma in the adjacent Teflon is 10 Gy. Take $\mu_{en}/\rho = 0.0225$ cm^2/g for Teflon, use Eq. (10.47) as amended by Janssens et al. (1974) to obtain β, assume a diffuse electron field, and neglect γ-ray attenuation.

   (b) What are the small-cavity (B–G) and large-cavity limiting values for $\overline{D}_{water}$?

SOLUTIONS TO PROBLEMS

1. 116.2 Gy, 0.937.
2. **(a)** 0.1839 Gy.
   (b) 0.1397 Gy.
   (c) 0.1399 Gy, 0.2%.
3. (a) The cavity is small enough not to perturb the charged-particle field, and (b) the cavity dose is deposited entirely by crossing charged particles.
4. $Q_{Al}/Q_C = 1.10$.
5. $Q_{air}/Q_H = 0.466$.
6. 17.8 cm^2/g, 0.031.
7. **(a)** 11.8 Gy.
   (b) Small limit: 12.0 Gy, large limit: 11.6 Gy.

CHAPTER 11

Dosimetry Fundamentals

I. INTRODUCTION

Having covered in the preceding chapters all the necessary radiological physics upon which radiation dosimetry depends (except for some neutron physics that will be deferred until Chapter 16), we are now in a position to discuss radiation dosimetry itself.

A. What is Radiation Dosimetry?

Strictly, radiation dosimetry (or simply "dosimetry") deals with the measurement of the absorbed dose or dose rate resulting from the interaction of ionizing radiation with matter. More broadly it refers to the *determination* (i.e., by measurement or calculation) of these quantities, as well as any of the other radiologically relevant quantities such as exposure, kerma, fluence, dose equivalent, energy imparted, and so on. One often measures one quantity (usually the absorbed dose) and derives another from it through calculations based on the previously defined relationships. Energy spectrometry of ionizing radiations is a separate undertaking, but is often carried out in connection with a dosimetry problem, and may then be considered an integral part of it.

B. What is a Dosimeter?

A *dosimeter* can be defined generally as any device that is capable of providing a reading r that is a measure of the absorbed dose D_g deposited in its *sensitive volume V* by ionizing radiation. If the dose is not homogeneous throughout the sensitive volume, then r

is a measure of some kind of mean value $\overline{D}_g$. Ideally r is proportional to D_g, and each volume element of V has equal influence on the value of r, in which case $\overline{D}_g$ is simply the average dose throughout V. This idealization is often, but not always, well approximated in practical dosimeters. Most dosimeters do exhibit some degree of nonlinearity of r vs. D over at least some part of their dose range, or there may be poor coupling of the dose-measuring signal to the readout apparatus. For example, an ion chamber may contain regions from which the ions are incompletely collected, or all segments of a large scintillator may not deliver light to the photomultiplier with equal efficiency.

This discussion of course applies equally well to dose-rate measuring devices by substituting $d\overline{D}_g/dt$ for $\overline{D}_g$.

Ordinarily one is not interested in measuring the absorbed dose in a dosimeter's sensitive volume as an end in itself, but rather as a means of determining the dose (or a related quantity) for another medium in which direct measurements are not feasible. Interpretation of a dosimeter reading in terms of the desired quantity is the central problem in dosimetry, usually exceeding in difficulty the actual measurement. In some cases the dosimeter can be calibrated directly in terms of the desired quantity (e.g., exposure, or tissue dose), but such a calibration is generally energy-dependent unless the dosimeter closely simulates the reference material, as will be discussed in Section II.

C. Simple Dosimeter Model in Terms of Cavity Theory

A dosimeter can generally be considered as consisting of a sensitive volume V filled with medium g, surrounded by a wall (or envelope, package, container, capsule, buffer layer, etc.) of another medium w having a thickness $t \geq 0$, as shown in Fig. 11.1. Its resemblance to a cavity and its surroundings, such as those described in Chapter 10, is more than coincidental. A simple dosimeter can be treated in terms of cavity theory, the sensitive volume being identified as the "cavity", which may

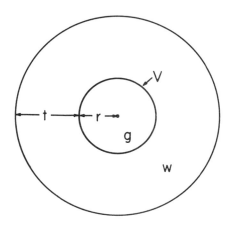

FIGURE 11.1. Schematic representation of a dosimeter as a sensitive volume V containing medium g, surrounded by a wall of medium w and thickness t.

contain a gaseous, liquid, or solid medium g, depending on the type of dosimeter. Cavity theory provides one of the most useful means of interpretation of dosimeter readings, as will be seen in the following sections.

The dosimeter wall can serve a number of functions simultaneously, including:

- being a source of secondary charged particles that contribute to the dose in V, and provide charged-particle equilibrium (CPE) or transient charged-particle equilibrium (TCPE) in some cases,
- shielding V from charged particles that originate outside the wall,
- protecting V from "hostile" influences such as mechanical damage, dirt, humidity, light, electrostatic or RF fields, etc., that may alter the reading,
- serving as a container for a medium g that is a gas, liquid, or powder, and
- containing radiation filters to modify the energy dependence of the dosimeter.

II. GENERAL GUIDELINES ON THE INTERPRETATION OF DOSIMETER MEASUREMENTS

A. For Photons and Neutrons

1. IMPORTANCE OF CPE OR TCPE

It may be recalled from Eqs. (2.13), (4.6), and (4.11) that under CPE and TCPE conditions, respectively,

$$D \overset{\text{CPE}}{=} K_c = \Psi \left(\frac{\mu_{en}}{\rho} \right) \tag{11.1}$$

and

$$D \overset{\text{TCPE}}{=} K_c(1 + \mu'\overline{x}) \equiv K_c\beta = \Psi \left(\frac{\mu_{en}}{\rho} \right) \beta \tag{11.2}$$

for photons. For neutrons, referring also to Eq. (2.8), one has the corresponding relationships:

$$D \overset{\text{CPE}}{=} K = \Phi F_n \tag{11.3}$$

and

$$D \overset{\text{TCPE}}{=} K(1 + \mu'\overline{x}) \equiv K\beta = \Phi F_n\beta \tag{11.4}$$

Consider now a dosimeter with a wall of medium w, thick enough to exclude all charged particles generated elsewhere, and at least as thick as the maximum range of secondary charged particles generated in it by the photon or neutron field. The dosimeter reading r provides us with a measure of the dose D_g in the dosimeter's sensitive volume. If the latter volume is small enough to satisfy the B–G condition of nonperturbation of the charged-particle field, and assuming that the wall is uniformly irradiated, CPE exists in the wall near the cavity. B–G or Spencer cavity theory can be used to determine the dose D_w there from that (D_g) in the sensitive volume. Then Eq. (11.1) or (11.3) permits the calculation of Ψ or Φ for the primary field from the value of D_w. More importantly, the dose D_x in any other medium x replacing the dosimeter and given an identical irradiation under CPE conditions can be gotten from

$$D_x \overset{\text{CPE}}{=} D_w \frac{\overline{(\mu_{en}/\rho)_x}}{\overline{(\mu_{en}/\rho)_w}} \qquad \text{for photons} \tag{11.5}$$

or

$$D_x \overset{\text{CPE}}{=} D_w \frac{\overline{(F_n)_x}}{\overline{(F_n)_w}} \qquad \text{for neutrons} \tag{11.6}$$

The exposure X (C/kg) for photons can in turn be derived from the absorbed dose D_{air} (for x = air) through this relation (from Eq. 4.8):

$$X \overset{\text{CPE}}{=} D_{air} \left(\overline{\frac{e}{W}}\right)_{air} = \frac{D_{air}}{33.97} \tag{11.7}$$

For higher-energy radiation ($h\nu \gtrsim 1$ MeV or $T_n \gtrsim 10$ MeV), where CPE fails but TCPE takes its place in dosimeters with walls of sufficient thickness, Eqs. (11.2) and (11.4) replace Eqs. (11.1) and (11.3), respectively. Relating D_w to Ψ or Φ then requires evaluation of the ratio $\beta = D/K_c$ for each case. However, the value of β is generally not much greater than unity (see Fig. 13.4) for radiation energies up to a few tens of MeV, and it is not strongly dependent on atomic number. Thus for media w and x not differing very greatly in Z, Eqs. (11.5) and (11.6) are still approximately valid. Equation (11.7) may be extended to higher energies, where TCPE exists, by dividing D_{air} by β.

If the dosimeter in question has too large a sensitive volume for the application of B–G theory, Burlin theory [Eq. (10.41)] can be substituted to calculate the equilibrium dose D_w in the wall medium at the point of interest, from the value of $\overline{D}_g$ given by the dosimeter reading. Then all of the preceding equations (11.1)–(11.7) are still operational. Note however that the sensitive-volume-size parameter d is required to be known in this case, and it may not follow exactly the simple forms suggested by Burlin and others, leading to uncertainty in dosimetry interpretation.

2. ADVANTAGES OF MEDIA MATCHING

There are clear advantages in matching a dosimeter to the medium of interest x, and also matching the media composing the wall (w) and sensitive volume (g) of the dosimeter to each other. The most obvious matching parameter is atomic composition, but the density state (gaseous vs. condensed) also influences the collision-stopping-power ratio of w to g for electrons by the polarization effect. More adaptable guidelines for media matching will be discussed in following subsections.

a. $w \cong g$

If the wall and sensitive-volume media of the dosimeter are identical with respect to composition and density, then $D_w = \overline{D}_g$ for all homogeneous irradiations.

To the extent that w and g are at least made similar to each other with respect to composition and density state (i.e., gaseous vs. condensed), the influence of cavity theory is kept minimal. Consequently the requirement for information about the radiation energy spectrum to allow accurate evaluation of the terms in, for example, the Burlin cavity relation (10.41) is lessened, allowing the use of convenient approximations without significant loss of accuracy in determining D_w from $\overline{D}_g$.

b. $w = g \cong x$

If a variety of homogeneous dosimeters ($w = g$) were available, it would be advantageous to choose one made of a material that matched the medium of interest, x, as closely as possible. If they were identical, then the dosimeter would be truly representative of that medium with respect to radiation interactions, and $D_x = D_w$ ($= \overline{D}_g$) in Eqs. (11.5) and (11.6). To the degree that the dosimeter simulates the medium x, the calculation of D_x through the application of one of those equations is again simplified by reducing the need for spectral information.

Unfortunately, dosimeters are only available in a finite variety, and there are other selection constraints besides composition that limit even further the choice of a dosimeter for a particular application. Cavity theories can be thought of as means of obtaining needed flexibility in matching dosimeters to media of interest, since they allow w to differ from g. For example, it may be easier to match only the wall w to the medium x, relying on cavity theory to calculate D_w from $\overline{D}_g$. Trying to match g to x is generally made more difficult by the additional dosimetric requirements imposed on the medium in the sensitive volume. Section III lists a number of these characteristics that impose added constraints on g.

The next three subsections will provide some practical approaches to media matching.

3. MEDIA MATCHING OF w AND g IN PHOTON DOSIMETERS

Since it is often infeasible in trying to devise a homogeneous dosimeter to make w and g actually similar in atomic composition, it will be helpful to point out the important parameters involved. The Burlin cavity relation (10.41) is useful in this connection:

$$\frac{\overline{D_g}}{D_w} = d \cdot {}_m\overline{S}_w^g + (1 - d)\left(\overline{\frac{\mu_{en}}{\rho}}\right)_w^g$$

It can be seen that the average dose $\overline{D}_g$ in the dosimeter's sensitive volume will be equal to the equilibrium dose D_w in the wall medium if

$${}_m\overline{S}_w^g = \left(\overline{\frac{\mu_{en}}{\rho}}\right)_w^g = 1 \tag{11.8}$$

independent of the value of d, which varies with the size of the dosimeter's sensitive volume. In other words, the matching criteria between the media w and g call for the respective matching of their mass collision stopping powers and their mass energy-absorption coefficients. When those parameters are each the same for the wall as for the medium in the sensitive volume V, the need to evaluate d in the Burlin equation (10.41) is eliminated, providing a substantial simplification.

Moreover, since $\overline{D}_g$ then remains equal to D_w, which is the CPE dose value in the wall medium at the point of interest, Eq. (11.5) may be used to calculate the dose in medium x from the observed value of D_w measured by the dosimeter.

The requirements given in Eq. (11.8) are still quite stringent and difficult to achieve, especially for a material w that is not identical to g in atomic composition. A more flexible and practicable matching relationship between media w and g is the following:

$${}_m\overline{S}_w^g = \left(\overline{\frac{\mu_{en}}{\rho}}\right)_w^g = n \tag{11.9}$$

where n is some constant, no longer required to be unity. In other words, the ratio of mass collision stopping powers for g/w is only required to be equal to the corresponding ratio of mass energy absorption coefficients. Under these conditions the Burlin equation simplifies to

$$\frac{\overline{D_g}}{D_w} = dn + (1 - d)n = n \tag{11.10}$$

irrespective of the value of d, as was the case for Eq. (11.8). However, now we see that $\overline{D}_g$ is n times as large as D_w.

To understand how the value of D_g depends on n, we write the following Burlin equations for two dosimeters containing the same sensitive volume medium g, and given the same photon irradiation. One is enclosed in wall w_1 and obeys Eq. (11.8), while the other is enclosed in w_2 and obeys Eq. (11.9):

$$\frac{\overline{D}_{g1}}{D_{w_1}} = d \cdot {}_m\overline{S}{}^g_{w_1} + (1 - d) \left(\frac{\mu_{en}}{\rho}\right)^g_{w_1} = 1 \tag{11.11}$$

$$\frac{\overline{D}_{g2}}{D_{w_2}} = d \cdot {}_m\overline{S}{}^g_{w_2} + (1 - d) \left(\frac{\mu_{en}}{\rho}\right)^g_{w_2} = n \tag{11.12}$$

But D_{w_1} and D_{w_2} are equilibrium absorbed doses in media w_1 and w_2, and are related by

$$\frac{D_{w_1}}{D_{w_2}} \overset{CPE}{=} \left(\frac{\mu_{en}}{\rho}\right)^{w_1}_{w_2} = n \tag{11.13}$$

the last equality having been derived from Eqs. (11.8) and (11.9). Comparison with Eq. (11.12) shows that

$$\overline{D}_{g2} = D_{w_1}$$

and Eq. (11.11) then provides the equality

$$\overline{D}_{g_1} = \overline{D}_{g2} \tag{11.14}$$

This proves that the dose in the dosimeter's sensitive volume is independent of the value of n so long as Eq. (11.9) is satisfied. This is because, under these conditions, the equilibrium dose in the wall is inversely proportional to n, thus maintaining $\overline{D}_g$ constant. Thus the reading of the dosimeter gives a value of $\overline{D}_g$ that is the same as if the wall were perfectly matched to g.

The practical case to which this approach is relevant occurs where photons interact only by the Compton effect in g and w. Then μ_{en}/ρ is nearly proportional to the number of electrons per gram, $N_A Z/A$. To a first approximation so is the mass collision stopping power of the secondary electrons. Consequently Eq. (11.9) is approximately satisfied, with $n \cong (Z/A)_g/(Z/A)_w$.

Example 11.1. A dilute aqueous chemical dosimeter (assume $=$ water) is enclosed in an equilibrium-thickness capsule of polystyrene and exposed to ^{60}Co γ-rays. Calculate the approximate ratio of $\overline{D}_g$ in this dosimeter to the dose (D_{water}) under CPE conditions in water, assuming $d = 1$ and $d = 0$.

Solution: $(\mu_{en}/\rho)_{water} = 0.0296 \text{ cm}^2/\text{g}$; $(\mu_{en}/\rho)_{poly} = 0.0288 \text{ cm}^2/\text{g}$. The average starting electron energy from the Compton effect is

$$\overline{T}_0 = \frac{\sigma_{tr}}{\sigma} \cdot 1.25 \text{ MeV} = 0.588 \text{ MeV}$$

The average equilibrium-spectrum electron energy is approximately

$$\overline{T} \cong \frac{\overline{T_0}}{2} = 0.3 \text{ MeV}$$

Thus

$$\left(\frac{dT}{\rho dx}\right)_{\text{water}, 0.3 \text{ MeV}} = 2.355 \text{ MeV cm}^2/\text{g}$$

$$\left(\frac{dT}{\rho dx}\right)_{\text{poly}, 0.3 \text{ MeV}} = 2.305 \text{ MeV cm}^2/\text{g}$$

$$\frac{\overline{D_g}}{D_{\text{poly}}} = d\frac{2.355}{2.305} + (1 - d)\frac{0.0296}{0.0288}$$

$$= 1.022\, d + 1.028\,(1 - d)$$

$$\frac{\overline{D_g}}{D_{\text{water}}} = \frac{\overline{D_g}}{D_{\text{poly}}} \cdot \frac{D_{\text{poly}}}{D_{\text{water}}} = \frac{\overline{D_g}}{D_{\text{poly}}}\left(\frac{\mu_{\text{en}}}{\rho}\right)_{\text{water}}^{\text{poly}}$$

$$= \left[d\frac{2.355}{2.305} + (1 - d)\frac{0.0296}{0.0288}\right]\frac{0.0288}{0.0296}$$

$$= d\frac{2.355}{2.305} \cdot \frac{0.0288}{0.0296} + (1 - d)$$

$$= 0.994d + (1 - d) = 1 - 0.006d$$

Thus we see that in this case $\overline{D_g}/D_{\text{water}}$ is equal to 0.994 when $d = 1$, rising to 1.000 for $d = 0$.

In this example polystyrene walls are seen to provide a close ($\leq 0.6\%$) match to the water in the dosimeter's sensitive volume.

4. MEDIA MATCHING FOR NEUTRON DOSIMETERS

Neutron interaction coefficients in general show no simple dependence upon atomic number, although elastic scattering in particular does depend simply on atomic mass, as will be discussed in Chapter 16. However, the approach that is always followed in matching media for neutron dosimetry is to try to use the same atomic composition, as far as possible, with special emphasis on matching the hydrogen content, since hydrogen has the largest elastic scattering cross section of any element.

For example, gaseous, liquid, and solid mixtures have been devised in attempts to simulate the mixture of important elements present in human muscle tissue. Practical tissue-equivalent (TE) plastics and gases substitute some carbon for oxygen, however, taking advantage of their comparable elastic-scattering characteristics. Thus the equation for neutrons that corresponds to Eq. (11.8), namely

$$_m\overline{S}^g_w = (\overline{F}_n)^g_w = 1 \tag{11.15}$$

may be roughly approximated for, say, a TE plastic chamber containing TE gas. Hence $\overline{D}_g \cong D_w$, and Eq. (11.6) can be used to deduce the dose in medium x (in this case tissue). Refinements and details of this method are discussed in Chapter 16.

5. MATCHING THE DOSIMETER TO THE MEDIUM OF INTEREST WHEN $w \neq g$

If the wall medium w differs from that in the sensitive volume, g, which of them is it more important to match to medium x? The answer again lies in the Burlin theory.

If $d = 1$ (small sensitive volume), then the indirectly ionizing radiation interacts only with the wall, which should therefore be matched as closely as possible to medium x, to minimize the need for spectral information in evaluating Eq. (11.5) or (11.6). In that case, for photons, D_x can be gotten from combining Eqs. (10.41) and (11.5) to obtain

$$\frac{\overline{D}_g}{D_x} = \frac{\overline{D}_g}{D_w} \cdot \frac{D_w}{D_x} = {}_m\overline{S}^g_w \left(\frac{\overline{\mu}_{en}}{\rho}\right)^w_x \tag{11.16}$$

and for the corresponding neutron case

$$\frac{\overline{D}_g}{D_x} = \frac{\overline{D}_g}{D_w} \cdot \frac{D_w}{D_x} = {}_m\overline{S}^g_w (\overline{F}_n)^w_x \tag{11.17}$$

If $d \cong 0$ in the Burlin equation (for a large sensitive volume), the wall influence on the dose in medium g is entirely lost. D_x can be gotten for photon irradiation by again combining Eqs. (10.41) and (11.5) to give

$$\frac{\overline{D}_g}{D_x} = \frac{\overline{D}_g}{D_w} \cdot \frac{D_w}{D_x} = \left(\frac{\overline{\mu}_{en}}{\rho}\right)^g_w \left(\frac{\overline{\mu}_{en}}{\rho}\right)^w_x = \left(\frac{\overline{\mu}_{en}}{\rho}\right)^g_x \tag{11.18}$$

and correspondingly for neutrons

$$\frac{\overline{D}_g}{D_x} = (\overline{F}_n)^g_x \tag{11.19}$$

Thus matching g to x will minimize the need for spectral information in evaluating D_x from these equations.

In the general case of intermediate-sized dosimeters ($0 < d < 1$) the full Burlin equation (10.41) may be used to obtain D_w from $\overline{D}_g$, and then Eq. (11.5) or (11.6) applied to calculate D_x.

6. CORRECTING FOR ATTENUATION OF RADIATION

Some attention should be paid to the difference in the attenuation of uncharged radiation in penetrating into the dosimeter and into the medium of interest, depending on the geometry. For example, if the dosimeter shown in Fig. 11.1 were immersed in a water medium (x) and irradiated with a γ-ray beam, the broad-beam attenuation could be calculated by application of μ_{en}/ρ in the straight ahead approximation, to the wall thickness t plus the radius r of the sensitive volume (see Chapter 3, Section V). That is, the photon energy fluence Ψ_{dos} reaching the center of the dosimeter, given Ψ_0 incident on its outer periphery, would be gotten from

$$\Psi_{dos} \cong \Psi_0 \exp\left[-\left(\frac{\mu_{en}}{\rho}\right)_w \rho_w t - \left(\frac{\mu_{en}}{\rho}\right)_g \rho_g r\right]$$

$$\cong \Psi_0 \left[1 - \left(\frac{\mu_{en}}{\rho}\right)_w \rho_w t - \left(\frac{\mu_{en}}{\rho}\right)_g \rho_g r\right] \quad (11.20)$$

where ρ_w and ρ_g are the densities of media w and g, respectively. On the other hand, the corresponding Ψ_{wat} reaching the center of the sphere of water that would replace the dosimeter if it were removed, and assuming the same Ψ_0 value, would be:

$$\Psi_{wat} \cong \Psi_0 \exp\left[-\left(\frac{\mu_{en}}{\rho}\right)_{wat} \rho_{wat}(t + r)\right] \cong \Psi_0 \left[1 - \left(\frac{\mu_{en}}{\rho}\right)_{wat} \rho_{wat}(t + r)\right]$$

$$(11.21)$$

Obviously if the dosimeter wall and sensitive volume were exactly water-equivalent with respect to μ_{en}/ρ and ρ, Eqs. (11.20) and (11.21) would be identical, indicating cancellation of attenuation effects. Otherwise the dosimeter reading should be multiplied by Ψ_{wat}/Ψ_{dos} to correct for the difference of attenuation in determining the dose to water at the dosimeter midpoint.

Where TCPE is present in place of CPE, the attenuation correction factor becomes $(\beta\Psi)_{wat}/(\beta\Psi)_{dos}$, which simplifies to Ψ_{wat}/Ψ_{dos} if β can be assumed to have approximately the same value in both media.

For neutrons, Eqs. (2.6) and (2.7) may be used to obtain a value of $(\mu_{tr}/\rho) = (\mu_{en}/\rho)$ that can serve as an effective broad-beam attenuation coefficient in the "straight-ahead" approximation. Equations (11.20) and (11.21) can then be used to calculate Φ_{dos} and Φ_{wat} from the same Φ_0 incident on each.

A Monte Carlo calculation, or just a more elegant volume-integral-type solution, would in principle give a more accurate result for this correction, for either photons or neutrons. However, for typical small-sized dosimeters where the correction is a few percent or less, the above approximation is usually sufficient.

An experimental check on the wall attenuation is sometimes feasible, and provides a very powerful means of verifying such calculations. Once the wall is made thicker than the charged-particle range, the observed variation of dosimeter reading is only a slow function of added wall thickness, due only to attenuation of the incident un-charged radiation. Furthermore, the reading decreases linearly with increasing thickness for small reading changes ($\lesssim 5\%$). Simply doubling the wall thickness by adding an appropriately shaped shell is often adequate to determine the attenuation correction. For example, if doubling the equilibrium wall thickness t to $2t$ were found to decrease the reading by 2%, one could conclude that the equilibrium wall thickness t alone also attenuated the photons or neutrons by about the same amount ($\cong 2\%$). This could be further established by adding still another shell thickness to verify the proportionality of the decrease in reading to thickness.

Also, for such small variations the correction for attenuation in the dosimeter radius r (in Fig. 11.1) can be estimated from the observed wall effect on the basis of proportionality to mass thickness. For example, if ρt were x (g/cm^2) and produced a 2% attenuation, then a ρr value of $x/2$ would result in another 1%, approximately.

Such simple procedures can often provide very useful information with minimal difficulty.

7. IMPORTANCE OF DOSIMETER WALL THICKNESS

It is helpful to decide in advance of making a measurement what its goal will be: To measure a quantity that depends on (a) the characteristics of the local photon or neutron field, or (b) the characteristics of the local secondary charged-particle field. If (a) is the objective, then the dosimeter should have a wall at least as thick as the maximum range of the charged particles present, to provide CPE or TCPE. If (b) is, then the dosimeter wall and sensitive volume should both be thin enough not to interfere with the passage of incident charged particles.

Both of these situations lend themselves to relatively straightforward dosimetric interpretation. For the thick-wall case, the dose in other media can be gotten through ratios of mass energy-absorption coefficients or neutron kerma factors, as shown in Eqs. (11.5) and (11.6). For a thin wall and thin detector, the dose in other media can be derived through B–G or Spencer cavity theory, i.e., stopping-power ratios.

If the wall is *neither* thick nor thin in relation to the range of the secondary electrons, an unfortunate situation arises where the dose in the sensitive volume either is due to a mixture of locally and distantly originating charged particles, or is deposited by a supply of secondary charged particles inadequate for equilibrium. Such mea-surements generally are not interpretable except through exotic computations, and are usually a waste of effort. They represent neither the uncharged- nor the charged-particle field at the undisturbed point of measurement. Such intermediate-walled dosimeters are to be avoided in practical dosimetry.

B. For Charged Particles

Charged-particle dosimetry calculations have been discussed in Chapter 8, Section V. However, the following summary statement is worth repeating: The absorbed dose at a point in a medium is gotten as the product of the charged-particle fluence (*not* the energy fluence) and the mass collision stopping power, assuming that CPE exists for the δ-rays. This product is to be summed over all energies in the primary (i.e., non-δ-ray) charged-particle spectrum.

The practical application of this statement is usually limited by a lack of information about the fluence and its spectrum, although transport calculations (especially Monte Carlo) are helping to remedy that deficiency. Nevertheless, dosimeter measurements are necessary at least to verify the calculations, and measurements are often easier and less expensive to carry out to a given level of accuracy.

Following are some important considerations in charged-particle dosimetry:

1. DOSIMETER SIZE

To measure the dose at a point in a medium, a dosimeter needs a sensitive volume small (or thin) enough to satisfy the B–G conditions, i.e., nonperturbation of the charged-particle field, and all dose to be deposited only by crossers. Moreover, the dosimeter wall should be thin enough so the dosimeter as a whole does not significantly perturb the field, but thick enough to serve any essential functions (e.g., containment) required by the dosimeter. Thin flat pillbox- or coin-shaped dosimeters, oriented perpendicular to the particle-beam direction, are often used to satisfy these requirements as closely as possible.

One may take as a rule of thumb that neither the wall thickness nor that of the sensitive volume should exceed ~ 1% of the range of the incident charged particles.

Where a significant spatial gradient of the charged-particle field exists, extrapolation of the dose in the sensitive volume to zero thickness (e.g., by means of an adjustable-gap ion chamber; see Chapter 12, Section III.B) may be necessary. Some typical electron and proton ranges in water are shown in Table 11.1. Ranges in other low-Z media are comparable, if given in mass units.

2. δ-RAY EQUILIBRIUM

One of the functions of the dosimeter wall is to generate δ rays to take the place of those that are generated in, and escape from, the sensitive volume. In other words

TABLE 11.1.   **Approximate CSDA Ranges of Electrons and Protons in Water**

	R (g/cm^2)	
T(MeV)	Electrons	Protons
0.01	0.00025	—
0.03	0.0018	—
0.1	0.014	—
0.3	0.084	—
1.0	0.44	0.0039
3	1.5	0.016
10	5.0	0.12
30	13.2	0.87
60	22.8	3.0

the wall should provide δ-ray CPE for the sensitive volume. This will occur if the wall matches the sensitive volume approximately with respect to atomic number and density state, is at least as thick as the maximum δ-ray range, and is uniformly irradiated throughout by the primary charged particles.

The importance of the wall as a δ-ray generator is greatest when the dose in free space is to be measured. In that case the escaping δ rays are not replaced at all unless the wall or other ambient media (including the air) provide them. The thinner the sensitive volume is, the more its dose is decreased by δ-ray losses, and the more dependent it becomes on the wall to supply δ-ray equilibrium. For heavy charged-particle beams the maximum δ-ray energy T'_{max} is roughly equal [from Eq. (8.4)] to $\beta^2/(1 - \beta^2)$, in MeV. Thus 10-MeV protons for example, generate δ rays of maximum energy $T'_{max} = 20$ keV, with a range in water of 9×10^{-4} g/cm^2, or 8 mm of air. The proton's range in this case is over 100 times greater. Thus δ-ray CPE is easily achieved for heavy-particle beams.

For electron beams of energy T the maximum δ-ray energy is $T/2$. Thus in principle it is not possible to provide full δ-ray CPE in a dosimeter in free space while keeping the wall thin enough not to perturb the primary beam. However, since the δ-ray spectrum is heavily weighted toward the lower energies, a much thinner wall ($\sim 1\%$ of the range of the primary electrons) may be adequate. Varying the wall thickness will show whether the chosen thickness is great enough so that the variation of reading vs t is either negligible or is extrapolatable to $t = 0$.

If the measurement is being made with the dosimeter immersed in a medium, little or no δ-ray effect may be seen when the wall is thickened or removed altogether, provided that the medium, the wall, and the sensitive volume are all similar in composition. If they do differ significantly, electron scattering effects are likely to dominate and obscure any thickness-dependent δ-ray influence.

3. CAVITY THEORY FOR ELECTRON BEAMS

At the time of this writing, there is no general and physically realistic cavity theory for relating the dose in a dosimeter to that in the medium at the point of measurement in an electron beam. The crux of the problem appears to be electron scattering, and a successful theory must account for it as a first-order effect.

For example, Harder (see below, Chapter 13, Section VI.B.1) has indicated that the dose in a homogeneous solid-walled, gas-filled cavity traversed by an electron beam may be either enhanced or diminished to some extent by electron scattering (ignoring the polarization effect), depending on the shape and orientation of the cavity. In the corresponding photon case described by the Fano theorem, the dose in the cavity is maintained constant irrespective of cavity geometry. Fano's theorem is not applicable to electron beams, since there is no distributed charged-particle source term [N in Eq. (10.20)] in that case.

Presumably condensed-state dosimeters should not exhibit the Harder effect to a significant degree, but they do show some tendency to ''trap'' electrons in a low-Z dosimeter surrounded by a higher-Z medium, due to multiple backscattering.

Kearsley has accounted for that effect in his photon cavity theory, but the electron-beam case has not been similarly treated yet at the time of this writing.

III. GENERAL CHARACTERISTICS OF DOSIMETERS

A. Absoluteness

An *absolute dosimeter* is one that can be assembled and used to measure the absorbed dose deposited in its own sensitive volume without requiring calibration in a known field of radiation. (It may, however, need some kind of calibration not involving radiation, such as electrical-heating calibration of a calorimetric dosimeter.)

Three types of dosimeters are now generally regarded as being capable of absoluteness:

- Calorimetric dosimeters.
- Ionization chambers.
- Fricke ferrous sulfate dosimeters.

These are not always employed as absolute dosimeters, however, because calibration offers certain advantages: A calibration can be stated in terms of some quantity of interest other than the absorbed dose in the sensitive volume, e.g., tissue dose or exposure. It can also provide traceability to an authoritative standardization laboratory such as the National Bureau of Standards. When an absolute dosimeter is used independently, it relies on its own accuracy instead of referring to a standard dosimeter in common with other radiation users. Thus an error may go undetected in an absolute dosimeter unless comparisons with others are carried out, or a calibration is obtained at a standardization laboratory. As in other fields of measurement, dosimetry standardization brings advantages not achieved by a multiplicity of individual absolute instruments.

The calorimetric dosimeter has the fundamental advantage of directly measuring the heat to which the absorbed dose degrades, without dependence on any coefficient of conversion, such as to ionization ($\overline{W}$) or to chemical yield (G). Thus if there is a hierarchy of dosimeter absoluteness, the calorimeter ranks at the top.

Other dosimeters may be considered absolute if designed as such; for example, proportional counters may be constructed with a built-in α-particle source that provides an inherent pulse-height calibration, rendering the dosimeter absolute in the sense that it does not need calibration in a known radiation field, other than the α beam it contains as an integral part.

Note that the absoluteness of a dosimeter is independent of its precision or its accuracy, characteristics to be discussed next. However, to be useful, an absolute dosimeter must be reasonably accurate and precise as well.

B. Precision and Accuracy

The concept of the *precision* or reproducibility of dosimeter measurements was discussed in Chapter 1, Section III.A; it has to do with random errors due to fluctuations in instrumental characteristics, ambient conditions, and so on, and the stochastic nature of radiation fields. Precision can be estimated from the data obtained in repeated measurements, and is usually stated in terms of the standard deviation. High precision is associated with a small standard deviation.

One should specify whether the standard deviation quoted for a set of measurements refers to the precision of individual readings [Eq. (1.4a)] or of their average value [Eq. (1.4b)]. The precision of a single measurement indicates how closely it is likely to agree with the expectation value of the quantity being measured. Likewise the precision of the average value of a cluster of repeated measurements expresses the likelihood of its agreement with the expectation value. For a sufficiently large number of readings, their average value coincides with the expectation value.

The *accuracy* of dosimeter measurements expresses the proximity of their expectation value to the true value of the quantity being measured. Thus it is impossible to evaluate the accuracy of data from the data themselves, as is done to assess their precision. Accuracy is a measure of the collective effect of the errors in all the parameters that influence the measurements. Estimation of the accuracy of an experimental determination is a tedious process, based mainly on "educated guessing." It is better done by the experimenter than by some later reviewer who lacks knowledge of the details. Note that in experiments that are limited to relative measurements, only the precision, not the accuracy, is important.

Although parametric errors are not random, but represent biases *either* up or down from their true values, their estimated magnitudes are usually combined as random errors if their direction is unknown and is believed to have equal probability of being too high or too low. The usual rules for the propagation of errors apply (see, e.g., Beers, 1953).

Clearly precision and accuracy are separate characteristics. Measurements may be highly precise but inaccurate, or vice versa, or may be strong in both or neither of these virtues. If one speaks of a dosimeter as being a high-precision instrument, one means that it is *capable* of excellent measurement reproducibility if properly employed. Poor technique, a hostile environment (e.g., high atmospheric humidity) or faulty peripheral equipment (e.g., ion-chamber cables or electrometer) may nevertheless cause poor reproducibility. A statement about the accuracy of a dosimeter refers to the freedom from error of its calibration, or of the parameters (such as the ion-chamber volume) that are relevant to its operation as an absolute instrument. Accuracy depends on the type of radiation being measured, and dosimeter calibrations are more or less specific in that respect. A dosimeter that is accurately calibrated to measure the exposure at one x-ray quality may be significantly in error at another.

The quantity that a dosimeter is inherently the most capable of measuring accurately, and that is the least influenced by changing the type or quality of the radiation, is the absorbed dose deposited in the dosimeter's own sensitive volume. This is discussed further in Section III. F.1.c below, and the N_{gas} approach to ion-chamber calibration is based on this idea, as discussed in Chapter 13, Section III.B.

C. Dose Range

1. DOSE SENSITIVITY

To be useful, a dosimeter must have adequate *dose sensitivity* $(dr/d\overline{D}_g)$ throughout the dose range to be measured. A constant dose sensitivity throughout the range provides a linear response (i.e., reading vs. dose, r vs. $\overline{D}_g$), that is desirable for ease of calibration and interpretation. However, single-valuedness of the function $r(\overline{D}_g)$, even if nonlinear, may be acceptable, though it requires that the calibration be carried out at a multiplicity of doses to provide a calibration curve.

2. BACKGROUND READINGS AND LOWER RANGE LIMIT

The lower limit of the useful dose range may be imposed by the *instrumental background* or zero-dose reading. This is the value of $r = r_0$ observed when $\overline{D}_g = 0$; sometimes it is referred to as "spurious response", since it is not caused by radiation. Examples of r_0 include charge readings due to ion-chamber insulator leakage, and thermoluminescence dosimeter readings resulting from response of the reader to infrared light emission by the dosimeter heater.

Clearly the instrumental background should be subtracted from any dosimeter reading. The usual procedure for determining this correction is to make measurements with the same dosimeter treated in the same way (including duration of the time) except for the absence of the applied radiation field. In this way the quantity one measures is r_0 plus the *radiation background* reading r_b. That is to say, if the radiation field to be measured is turned off during the background measurement, the ambient radiation field contributed by cosmic rays and by natural and man-made terrestrial sources will still affect the dosimeter, so the observed reading will be $r_0 + r_b$. In some applications, such as personnel dosimetry in radiation protection, this is the correct amount to be subtracted from a dose reading, since background radiation is not supposed to be included in personnel dose limits.

However, if for another purpose the total dose is to be measured, including radiation background, then r_0 should be determined either after a minimal time delay or after an appropriate storage period in a low-background (or known-background) environment such as a whole-body counter facility. The unshielded natural radiation-background tissue dose rate of about 0.3 mrad per day at sea level may already be low enough to be insignificant in comparison with the value of r_0 that is observed with short exposure times. A photographic film badge, for example, typically displays an instrumental background optical density approximating that of a 100-mrad reading, and even a 30-day exposure to natural background adds less than 10% to that reading.

If a background reading is very reproducible from run to run, subtracting it from a dosimeter reading may have little effect on the precision of the measurement. In many cases, however, the background reading exhibits significant nonreproducibility. As a rule of thumb, the lower limit of the practical dose range of a dosimeter is usually estimated to be the dose necessary to double the instrumental background reading. Evaluation of the precision of the measurements from repeated readings of both the radiation and the background will of course provide more quantitative information: If σ' is the standard deviation of the average of a group of radiation readings $\bar{r}$, and σ'_0 is the S.D. of the average of the background readings $\bar{r}_0$, then the S.D. of the net radiation reading $r - r_0$ is given by

$$\sigma'_{net} = \sqrt{(\sigma')^2 + (\sigma'_0)^2} \qquad (11.22)$$

(Note that these are not *percentage* standard deviations.)

If the background reading is negligibly small, then the lower dose limit is imposed by the capability of the dosimeter readout instrument to provide a readable value of r for the dose to be measured, $\overline{D}_g$. If r is less than 10% of full scale on analogue instruments, or contains fewer than three significant figures on digital readouts, the precision and accuracy may both become unsatisfactory. A more sensitive scale should then be used. Some dosimeter readout devices, notably electrometers, are designed to switch to the optimum-sensitivity range automatically.

If neither the background reading nor constraints on instrumental sensitivity provide a lower limit to the usable dose range, the stochastic nature of the radiation field itself will finally limit the precision of a small dose measurement as discussed in Chapter 1, Section III.A.

3. UPPER LIMIT OF THE DOSE RANGE

The upper limit of the useful dose range of a dosimeter may be imposed simply by external instrumental limitations, such as reading off scale on the least sensitive range of an electrometer. Alternatively some kind of inherent limit may be imposed by the dosimeter itself. Causes of this type include:

    a.   Exhaustion of the supply of atoms, molecules, or solid-state entities ("traps") being acted upon by the radiation to produce the reading.

    b.   Competing reactions by radiation products, for example in chemical dosimeters.

    c.   Radiation damage to the dosimeter (e.g., discoloration of light-emitting dosimeters, or damage to electrical insulators).

Usually the upper limit of the dose range is manifested by a decrease in the dose sensitivity $(dr/d\overline{D}_g)$ to an unacceptable value. It may be reduced to zero, or to a negative value, as in Fig. 11.2, which causes the dose-response function to become double-valued. In such a case other information is needed to decide which dose is represented by a large r-value, as shown in the figure. It is of course possible in principle to make use of the negative-slope part of a dose-response curve such as that in Fig. 11.2 for dosimetry purposes if it is sufficiently reproducible.

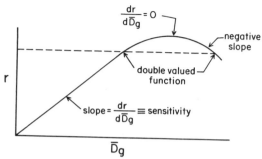

FIGURE 11.2 Illustrating a double-valued dose-response function resulting from a decrease in the dosimeter sensitivity at high doses.

D. Dose-Rate Range

1. FOR INTEGRATING DOSIMETERS

If a dosimeter is to be used for measuring the time-integrated dose (not the dose rate), then it is necessary that its reading not depend on the rate at which the dose is delivered, at least within the range of dose rates to be encountered.

Usually there will not be any low-dose-rate limitation except that imposed by the lower dose limits already discussed. For example a significant level of insulator leakage current in an ion chamber would give a background charge reading that would increase with time. Thus the measurement of a given dose would require subtraction of a larger background if it took a long time to accumulate (at a low dose rate) than if it were quickly delivered.

One case of a genuine low-dose-rate limitation is *reciprocity-law failure* in photographic film dosimeters. It occurs only with low-LET radiation (e.g., x rays or electrons) and is due to the necessity for several ionizing events to occur in a single grain of silver bromide to make it developable. Low-LET radiation can only create one ion pair at a time in a small volume like a AgBr grain in photographic emulsion, and after a time the ions can recombine. Thus the grain repairs itself at low enough dose rates, and never produces a *latent image*, that is, reaches a condition of developability. Consequently it never contributes to the opacity of the film, which is the parameter used to measure the dose. Biological damage by low-LET radiation exhibits similar time-repair characteristics.

The upper limit of dose-rate independence usually occurs when charged-particle tracks are created close enough together in space and time to allow the ions, electron–hole pairs, or active chemical products such as free radicals to interact between tracks. In an ion chamber this is called general or volume ionic recombination, as discussed in Chapter 12, Section V. Similar back reactions also occur in solid or liquid dosimeters, resulting in a loss of contribution to the reading r. However, track proximity may instead enhance the reading, for example by making more luminescence centers available for light production by the recombination of the charge carriers trapped along a given track in a thermoluminescence dosimeter.

2. FOR DOSE-RATE METERS

It is desirable in dose-rate-measuring dosimeters that the reading r be proportional to the dose rate $d\overline{D}_g/dt$, or at least be a single-valued function of it. "Jamming" or paralysis of an instrument, causing it to read zero or a small response at high dose rates, as can occur in Geiger–Müller counters when the dead time overlaps and becomes continuous, is intolerable, especially in personnel monitoring meters. The upper limit on the usable dose-rate range more usually takes the form of some kind of saturation of the reading vs. dose rate, due to ionic recombination or other results of track proximity, as discussed in the preceding section. The counting of two or more events as one when they occur temporally too close together in pulse-counting dosimeters also may cause saturation. Overloading of the resistor string that provides voltages to a photomultiplier tube can reduce the amplification of the light signal from a scintillation-type dosimeter at high dose rates. Other modes of saturation may also occur in various kinds of dosimeters.

In dose-rate measurements the *response time constant*, while not a limitation on the dose-rate range, is also an important consideration. It is defined as the time it takes for the reading in a constant field to rise to within $1/e$ of its steady-state value, or to decay to $1/e$ of that value upon removal from the field. A long time constant will cause a dose-rate meter to seek a mean reading value in a repetitively pulsed radiation field. Thus it will not indicate the actual dose rate existing either when the field is present (i.e., during the pulses) or when it is absent. For measuring single short radiation pulses, fast scintillators with photodiodes or electron channel multipliers in place of the slower photomultiplier tubes can provide nanosecond response time constants, making it possible to measure the pulse shape.

E. Stability

1. BEFORE IRRADIATION

The characteristics of a dosimeter should be stable with time until it is used. That includes "shelf life" and time spent *in situ* until irradiated (e.g., worn by personnel if a health-physics monitoring dosimeter.) Effects of temperature, atmospheric oxygen or humidity, light, and so on can cause a gradual change in the dose sensitivity or the instrumental background. Photographic, chemical, or solid-state dosimeters are generally more susceptible to these influences than ion chambers or counters. Protection from deleterious influences can often be designed into a dosimeter's envelope if the environmental cause of the problem is recognized. Film badges for example require sealing in a plastic bag to exclude humidity for use as personnel dosimeters in tropical climates. Some thermoluminescent dosimeters (TLDs, notably LiF) show a gradual sensitivity change during storage at room temperature due to a migration and rearrangement of the trapping centers in the crystalline phosphor, that can be controlled by special annealing.

2. AFTER IRRADIATION

The latent reading in some types of integrating dosimeters (e.g., photographic, chemical, solid-state) may be unstable to some extent, suffering "fading" losses during the time interval between irradiation and readout. Again, harsh ambient conditions of elevated temperature or humidity, direct sunlight or bright fluorescent lighting, and so on, may aggravate this effect.

If such time-dependent fading losses are unavoidable, it is advantageous to make them as reproducible as possible through standardization of laboratory technique so that a fading correction can be applied to the readings. Figure 11.3 outlines a protocol for measuring both the pre- and postirradiation instabilities of a group of identical dosimeters. An alternative scheme that is preferable especially for TLDs reverses this procedure, preparing (i.e., annealing) the dosimeters at various times t_p and reading out all groups in one session at the end of the experiment. This is preferable for TLDs and because it is especially difficult to obtain long-term constancy of TLD reading instruments, while it is straightforward to "prepare" TLDs that are made from a common batch of phosphor by annealing them identically at different times t_p.

F. Energy Dependence

1. Specification

Generally speaking, the *energy dependence* of a dosimeter is the dependence of its reading r, per unit of the quantity it is supposed to measure, upon the quantum or kinetic energy of the radiation, as illustrated in Fig. 11.4. Figure 11.4A gives the reading r obtained from an imaginary dosimeter vs. some dosimetric quantity J (such as exposure, absorbed dose in water under CPE conditions, etc.). Let us suppose that the calibration curves shown have been obtained at the three different radiation energies (or qualities) E_1, E_2, and E_3, as shown. In this example the dosimeter response is assumed to be linear at energy E_1, but becomes progressively more nonlinear at E_2 and E_3. The corresponding plots of r/J vs. J are shown in Fig. 11.4B. The *energy-dependence curves* for the two J-values J_1 and J_2 are given in Fig. 11.4C, and are seen

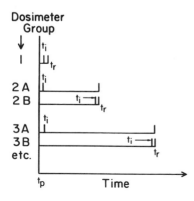

FIGURE 11.3.   Protocol for measuring pre- and postirradiation instability effects in integrating dosimeters, where a common dosimeter "preparation" time t_p is used. Group-1 dosimeters are promptly irradiated at time t_i, then promptly read out at time t_r. Groups 2A, 3A, . . . are irradiated promptly but stored various times before being read out at time t_r. Groups 2B, 3B, . . . are stored various times before being irradiated, then promptly read out. The A groups measure the postirradiation instability, and the B groups the preirradiation instability.

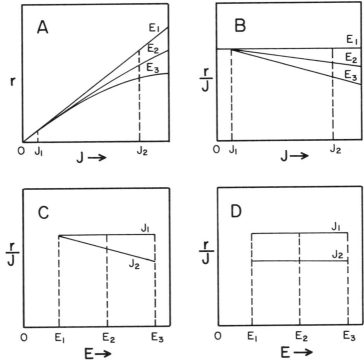

FIGURE 11.4. Illustration of the general concept of energy dependence of a dosimeter that provides a reading r as a result of an irradiation that is quantified in terms of the quantity J (representing exposure, absorbed dose in tissue, etc.). See discussion in the text.

to differ in this case for $E > E_1$. In measuring the quantities of size J_1 this imaginary dosimeter is evidently energy-independent, while at J_2 it is energy-dependent for radiation with energy above E_1.

If only a *single* curve of r vs. J, for instance the E_3 curve in Fig. 11.4A, were obtained at all energies, then the dosimeter would be energy-independent at all J-levels. For each value of J a horizontal line would result as in Fig. 11.4D, producing a family of such energy-independent r/J curves for different J-values. If the single energy-independent calibration curve were linear, such as the E_1 curve in Fig. 11.4A, then a common horizontal line would result in Fig. 11.4D, providing a single r/J value that would be applicable to all J-values and all radiation energies in this simplest case.

There are two common usages of the term "energy dependence" that are often encountered in the literature, usually without definition or clarification, and a third usage that is less common but more fundamental. These will be discussed in the following subsections.

a. Energy Dependence ≡ Dependence of the Dosimeter Reading, per Unit of X- or γ-ray Exposure, on the Mean Quantum Energy or Quality of the Beam, r/X vs. $\bar{E}$

This usage is commonly found in health-physics personnel monitoring or any application in which exposure is commonly referred to. ^{60}Co γ-rays are frequently used as the reference energy for normalization, producing energy-dependence curves looking typically like Fig. 11.5 for dosimeters made of materials higher than, equal to, and lower than *air* in atomic number (the medium to which exposure refers). The ordinate of such a curve is often found to be labeled "relative sensitivity," "relative response," or some other such nondescript term, while what is actually meant is shown in Fig. 11.5.

The rise in the top curve below about 0.1 MeV is caused by the onset of photoelectric effect in the sensitive volume of the dosimeter. The flat maximum usually occurs at about 30–50 keV, below which the curve may slowly descend due to attenuation in the dosimeter, onset of photoelectric effect in the reference material (air), and LET dependence of the dosimeter (see Section III.F.1.c below).

The shape of the curves in Fig. 11.5 can be estimated by:

$$\frac{\left(\dfrac{r}{X}\right)_{\bar{E}}}{\left(\dfrac{r}{X}\right)_{1.25}} \cong \frac{\left[\dfrac{(\mu_{en}/\rho)_g}{(\mu_{en}/\rho)_{air}}\right]_{\bar{E}}}{\left[\dfrac{(\mu_{en}/\rho)_g}{(\mu_{en}/\rho)_{air}}\right]_{1.25}} \qquad (11.23)$$

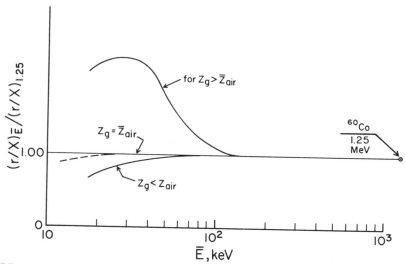

FIGURE 11.5.   Typical energy-dependence curves in terms of the response per unit exposure of x- or γ rays.

where the subscript g refers to the material in the dosimeter's sensitive volume. This equation is based on the assumptions that:

1. The dosimeter's sensitive volume is in charged-particle equilibrium, and the wall medium $w = g$.

2. Attenuation is negligible in the dosimeter, both for incident photons and for fluorescence photons generated in the dosimeter.

3. A given absorbed dose to the sensitive volume produces the same reading, irrespective of photon energy (i.e., the dosimeter is LET-independent).

These assumptions are all questionable and may require suitable corrections for their failure in specific cases. Matching the wall medium to the material in the dosimeter's sensitive volume, as discussed in Section II, can satisfy assumption 1. Substituting $(\tau/\rho)_g$ for $(\tau_{tr}/\rho)_g$ in $(\mu_{en}/\rho)_g$ [see Eqs. (7.57) and (7.59)] has the effect of assuming the local reabsorption of all fluorescence photons generated in the sensitive volume, thus providing an upper limit for the influence of that effect. Attenuation of photons entering the dosimeter can be simply estimated by the "straight-ahead approximation", as discussed in Chapter 3, Section V. Failure of assumption 3 is referred to as "LET dependence" of a dosimeter; more will be said about it presently. The total effect of assumptions 2 and 3 may cause a perfectly air-equivalent dosimeter to decrease its reading at low photon energies, as indicated by the dashed curve.

b. Energy Dependence ≡ Dependence of the Dosimeter Reading per Unit of Absorbed Dose in Water on the Photon or Electron-Beam Energy

This usage is commonly found in radiotheraphy literature, where "absorbed dose" always refers to water (or muscle tissue) unless otherwise specified. Inasmuch as water and tissue are not identical (see Fig. 2.2a), one should say which is meant, but since the differences are small ($\sim 1\%$) in the megavolt region, this choice frequently remains unspecified.

For x rays the equation that corresponds to Eq. (11.23), by which a homogeneous dosimeter's energy dependence can be estimated, is

$$\frac{(r/D_{\text{water}})_{\overline{E}}}{(r/D_{\text{water}})_{1.25}} \cong \frac{[(\mu_{en}/\rho)_g/(\mu_{en}/\rho)_{\text{water}}]_{\overline{E}}}{[(\mu_{en}/\rho)_g/(\mu_{en}/\rho)_{\text{water}}]_{1.25}} \qquad (11.24)$$

which depends on water as a reference material and ^{60}Co γ rays for normalization. Figure 11.6a illustrates this equation over the energy range from 1.25 to 50 MeV for LiF and bone-equivalent dosimeters. Because of the large secondary-electron ranges at these energies, this equation is only satisfied to the extent that TCPE is present, $g =$ wall w, and β is the same in water as in the dosimeter. Also, considerable x-ray attenuation occurs in the thick walls, and the size of the resulting dosimeter may be impractical anyway. In radiotherapy dosimetry these problems are usually avoided by doing the measurements in a phantom, letting it comprise most of the dosimeter's wall thickness, as discussed in Chapter 13.

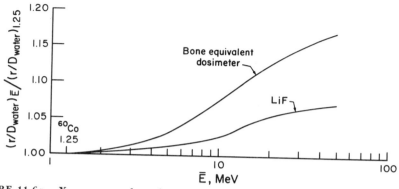

FIGURE 11.6a. X-ray energy dependence estimated from Eq. (11.24) for a LiF and a bone-equivalent dosimeter, in terms of response per unit absorbed dose in water, normalized to ^{60}Co γ rays.

The rising value of the curves in Fig. 11.6a with increasing photon energy of course results from the effect of pair production.

For electron beams of kinetic energy T (MeV), the corresponding equation for estimating energy dependence in terms of the dose to water, normalized to $T = 1$ MeV, is

$$\frac{\left(\dfrac{r}{D_{\text{water}}}\right)_T}{\left(\dfrac{r}{D_{\text{water}}}\right)_{1\,\text{MeV}}} \cong \frac{\left[\dfrac{(dT/\rho dx)_{c,g}}{(dT/\rho dx)_{c,\text{water}}}\right]_T}{\left[\dfrac{(dT/\rho dx)_{c,g}}{(dT/\rho dx)_{c,\text{water}}}\right]_{1\,\text{MeV}}} \qquad (11.25)$$

where $(dT/\rho dx)_{c,g}$ is the mass collision stopping power of the material g in the dosimeter's sensitive volume, and $(dT/\rho dx)_{c,\text{water}}$ that in water. This approximation assumes that:

1. CPE exists for δ-rays entering and leaving the sensitive volume.
2. The incident electrons lose only a very small fraction of their energy in traversing the dosimeter.
3. Electron scattering is the same in g as in water.
4. The reading per unit dose to the dosimeter's sensitive volume remains energy-independent ("LET-independent").

Items 1 and 3 are suspect, while 2 and 4 are easily satisfied in the energy region above 1 MeV. Figure 11.6b illustrates Eq. (11.25) for an air-cavity chamber, LiF, and bone-equivalent dosimeters. Clearly the lack of polarization effect in the gaseous air relative to water causes a large energy dependence in that case. Neither LiF nor a bone-equivalent dosimeter shows much dependence. This illustrates the fact that collision

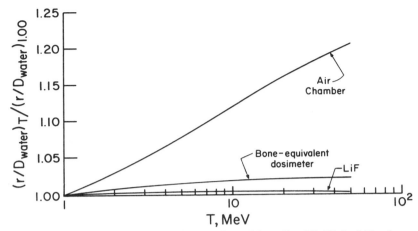

FIGURE 11.6b.   Electron-energy dependence estimated from Eq. (11.25) for LiF, a bone-equiv-alent dosimeter, and an air-filled ion chamber, in terms of response per unit absorbed dose in water, normalized to T = 1 MeV.

stopping-power ratios are insensitive to electron energy unless the polarization effect is involved.

c.   Energy Dependence ≡ Dependence of the Dosimeter Reading per Unit of Absorbed Dose to the Material in the Sensitive Volume Itself, on the Radiation Energy or Beam Quality

This kind of energy dependence is the most fundamental, inasmuch as it reflects the dosimeter's energy efficiency, i.e., the ability of the dosimeter to give the same read-ing for the same amount of absorbed energy in its own sensitive volume, regardless of radiation type or quality. It is often called "LET dependence" because it usually manifests itself as a change in reading per unit dose as a function of charged-particle track density, due to ionic recombination or other second-order effects that depend on the proximity of radiation products in the dosimeter. For example, ion chambers show such LET dependence only at radiation energies low enough ($\lesssim 10$ keV) so the value of $\overline{W}$ for the gas is no longer constant but begins to rise. This constancy for low-LET radiation provides the basis for ion-chamber calibrations in terms of the quantity N_{gas}, as will be discussed in Chapter 13, Section III.B.

Equations (11.23)–(11.25) can be modified to express the LET independence of a dosimeter by changing all the "air" or "water" subscript to "g", making all those equations reduce to unity identically for all energies.

2.   MODIFICATION

The energy dependence of a dosimeter can be changed to some extent, especially when the photoelectric effect is causing an overresponse. In that case a medium-Z

(e.g., tin), high-Z (e.g., lead), or composite filter can be incorporated into the design of the dosimeter capsule. The thickness t can be chosen to correct the overresponse at about 100 keV, using $e^{-\mu t}$ as a guide. Note that although the geometrical situation seems to call for broad-beam attenuation (e.g., by using μ_{en} in the straight-ahead approximation), the fluorescence photons tend to be re-absorbed in the filter before they can reach the sensitive volume. Thus the use of the narrow-beam coefficient gives a better estimate of the required thickness t.

Having determined the thickness needed to correct the response at 100 keV, it will be found to have been overcorrected at lower energies, the reading being essentially zero at 50 keV. This can be rectified by *perforating* the filter using the unfiltered height of the maximum overresponse as a guide. For example, if the dosimeter overresponded tenfold at its maximum at, say, 40 keV, and read zero at that energy with the solid filter in place, then 10% perforation area would be appropriate to restore the reading to its proper level at 40 keV. This would in turn cause a small overresponse again at 100 keV, necessitating some increase in t. Experimental testing is of course required to verify and finally adjust the design.

This approach to the modification of energy dependence adds weight and size, and introduces directional dependence to the dosimeter reading, influenced by the geometrical design. A sophisticated example of a design that minimizes the directional dependence is shown in Fig. 11.7, a photograph of the spherical dosimeter of Maushart and Piesch (1967).

Another, more powerful method of modifying the response function of pulse-detecting dosimeters, such as proportional counters or scintillators, was conceived by Hurst and Ritchie (1962). The pulse heights provide a measure of the energy of the particle that made the pulse, and the number of pulses of each height indicates the relative strength of that part of the radiation energy spectrum. Hurst and Ritchie proposed applying various weighting factors to different parts of the pulse-height spectrum by electronic amplification to obtain any desired adjustment in energy dependence. Their proposal preceded the microcomputer, necessitating a crude histogram approach, which can be easily improved upon today.

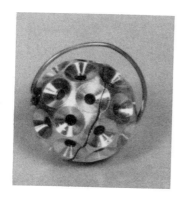

FIGURE 11.7.   A perforated filter to reduce the photoelectric overresponse of a dosimeter while retaining response to photons below $\cong 80$ keV. The spherical design minimizes directional dependence. (Maushart and Piesch, 1967. Courtesy of R. Maushart.)

G. Miscellany

A few other dosimeter characteristics deserve brief mention:

The *configuration* of a dosimeter sometimes is crucial to its use. It may be necessary to simulate as closely as possible the geometry of the test object. For example, a thin plastic-film dosimeter might best measure the dose in a layer of biological cells, while the Fricke chemical dosimeter would be appropriate for determining the average dose in a large volume such as a kidney-shaped container in an irradiated phantom. Finally, small size of a dosimeter is of primary importance in its application *in vivo* in patient or test animals.

A dosimeter needs a *relevant calibration* that is appropriate to the radiation type and quality, as well as to the quantity to be measured. A calibration in terms of the dose to the dosimeter's own sensitive volume is more generally applicable than other types of calibrations.

If different types of radiations coexist in the field to be measured, attention must be paid to the relative sensitivity of the dosimeter to the different components. It may be possible in specific cases to discriminate against one type of radiation (e.g., by attenuation) so that another may be measured without competition. The special problems encountered in measuring neutron and γ-ray doses simultaneously are especially difficult. These will be dealt with in Chapter 16.

There are many dosimeters in the literature that may be useful but have never become commercially available. Given a choice, a commercial system is usually easier to apply, so long as it satisfies other requirements. In particular, chemical dosimetry must still be done on the basis of local preparation, primarily because of shelf-life instability. Calorimetric dosimetry has also eluded commercial manufacture, so far.

The *reusability* of a dosimeter has several important implications. Reusable dosimeters such as thermoluminescent dosimeters can be individually calibrated; single-use dosimeters such as film badges cannot. The latter can only be batch-calibrated by irradiating and measuring representative samples. In that case the precision of measurements refers to the reproducibility of readings obtained from different members of the dosimeter batch after they have been given identical irradiations.

The advantage of reusability of a dosimeter depends on how difficult or convenient it is to restore it to its original condition. If it cannot be fully purged of the effects of an earlier dose, some of the advantage is lost. A shift in sensitivity, for example, means that dosimeters must be segregated on the basis of prior history and recalibrated before reusing. Economies that may be realized through reuse of dosimeters may thus be limited.

PROBLEMS

1. Name five purposes that the wall of a dosimeter may serve.
2. Estimate the energy dependence of the reading per unit exposure for LiF and CaF_2 TLDs, and draw these data as curves like those in Fig. 11.5.

3. A LiF TL dosimeter is enclosed in equilibrium-thickness capsules of Teflon and Lucite, for γ-ray energies of 0.2 and 1.25 MeV. Calculate the ratio of the average dose in the LiF in the dosimeter to the LiF dose under CPE conditions, for each capsule and energy, assuming $d = 1$ and 0 in Burlin theory (see Example 11.1). Which capsule gives the closer match to the LiF in the dosimeter?

4. A CaF_2 dosimeter is enclosed in equilibrium-thickness walls of Al to measure the dose to Si under TCPE conditions in a field of 6-MeV γ-rays. Neglecting x-ray attenuation, if the average dose in the CaF_2 is 30 Gy, what is the Si dose? Assume that the CaF_2 is (a) small (Burlin's $d = 1$) or (b) large ($d = 0$).

5. Suppose the CaF_2 in the dosimeter in Problem 4 were 2 mm thick and the aluminum wall were just equal to the electron range.

   (a) Estimate the x-ray attenuation to reach the dosimeter's center, using the straight-ahead approximation.

   (b) If it were immersed in water, what would be the corresponding attenuation in the water it displaced?

6. A LiF TLD chip gives a reading r after receiving an absorbed dose of 4.5 Gy to the LiF from ^{60}Co γ rays. Later the same reading is obtained after the chip is struck perpendicularly by a beam of 500-keV electrons on its 3.2×3.2-mm^2 face. The chip thickness is 0.9 mm. What is the electron fluence, neglecting backscattering?

SOLUTIONS TO PROBLEMS

1. Provides CPE; stops charged particles from outside; protects; contains; and adjusts energy dependence.

3. For $d = 1$:

Material	Energy (MeV)	$\bar{D}_g/D_{LiF}$
Teflon	0.2	1.008
	1.25	1.004
Lucite	0.2	0.948
	1.25	0.970

In all cases $\bar{D}_g/D_{LiF} = 1.000$ for $d = 0$. Teflon gives the better match.

4. (a) 31.6 Gy, (b) 30.5 Gy.

5. (a) 6.4%, (b) 2.5%.

6. 1.33×10^{10} e/cm^2.

CHAPTER **12**

Ionization Chambers

I. INTRODUCTION

The ionization chamber is the most widely used type of dosimeter for precise measurements, such as those required in radiotherapy. Such chambers are commercially available in a variety of designs for different applications, and may be constructed in a machine shop when special designs are required. If the ion-collecting gas volume can be determined by means other than calibration in a known field of ionizing radiation, the chamber becomes an absolute dosimeter, as pointed out in Chapter 11. This is, however, not usually practicable outside of national standards laboratories, and in any case it is preferable to work with dosimeters having calibrations traceable to such a laboratory.

In this chapter we will begin by discussing free-air ionization chambers. Chambers of this type, although seldom seen except in standards laboratories, experimentally demonstrate the concepts of exposure, CPE, and ion-chamber absoluteness.

II. FREE-AIR ION CHAMBERS

A. Conventional Designs

The definition of exposure, as given in Chapter 2, Section V, requires the measurement of all the ionization produced by collision interactions in air by the electrons resulting from x-ray interactions in a known mass of air. However, the experimental difficulty of doing this generally requires one to rely on charged-particle equilibrium,

292

as discussed in Chapter 4, Section IV. Only in one special design (discussed in Section II.B.1) is dependence upon this requirement to replace lost electrons avoided.

A number of different designs of free-air chambers have evolved in standardization laboratories in different countries, some cylindrical and some plane-parallel in geometry. We will first consider the plane-parallel type, such as that used at the National Bureau of Standards (NBS) in calibrating cavity ion chambers for constant x-ray-tube potentials from 50 to 300 kV.

Figure 12.1 is a schematic plan view of such a chamber (Wyckoff and Attix, 1957), which is enclosed in a Pb shielding box to exclude x rays scattering in from elsewhere. At the front the box is a tungsten-alloy diaphragm that is aligned with the x-ray beam central axis, and passes a beam of cross-sectional area A_0 in the plane of axial point P. This is the point where cavity chambers to be compared with the free-air chamber are centered, after the beam has been calibrated and the free-air chamber is removed. A monitoring ion chamber through which the beam passes allows normalization of individual irradiation runs to correct for fluctuations in beam intensity and for timing errors in the shutter (not shown).

The plate system inside the box consists of three coplanar plates on one side of the beam and a parallel high-voltage plate opposite. The plates are all parallel to the x-ray beam axis, and equidistant from it. The distance of the plates from the beam is designed to put them beyond the range of substantially all the secondary electrons originating in the beam (e.g., electron e_1 in Fig. 12.1).

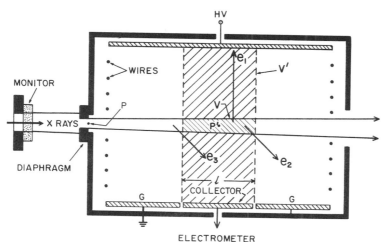

FIGURE 12.1.   Schematic plan view of a typical standard free-air ionization chamber. The x-ray beam passes midway between the high-voltage plate and the co-planar guard (G) and collector plates, operated at ground potential. The x-ray beam enters the chamber through a tungsten-alloy diaphragm with an aperture area A_0. The ionization desired for an exposure measurement is that produced by the electrons originating in volume V. The measured ionization is that collected from volume V'. CPE for volume V' makes the two ionizations equal.

To provide a uniform electric field between the plates, a set of wires* encircles the space between them at both ends and at the top and bottom. The chamber height from wire to wire equals the width from plate to plate. These wires are electrically biased in uniform steps to establish parallel equipotential planes between the plates. The guard electrodes also assist in producing field uniformity.

Under these conditions the electric lines of force (paths followed by + and − ions) go straight across the chamber, perpendicular to the plates. Ions of one sign produced within the larger shaded volume (V'), and not lost in ion recombination, are thus transported to the collector plate, electrically connected to the electrometer input. The dimension l is the collector length plus half the gap width between collector and guard plate at each end.

1.   CHARGED-PARTICLE EQUILIBRIUM

The collecting volume V' is penetrated by the x-ray beam passing through the aperture. The volume V is common to both V' and the volume occupied by the beam itself; V is shown crosshatched in the diagram. V is the actual volume of origin of the secondary electrons whose ionization we wish to measure.

The lateral dimensions of the chamber are great enough to accommodate electrons like e_1, which remain within V' and thus produce all their ionization where it will be collected and measured.

The electrons like e_2, which originate within the defined volume of origin V, may have paths that carry some of their kinetic energy out of V', where the remaining ionization they produce will not reach the collector, but will go to the grounded guard plate instead. This ionization must be replaced by other electrons such as e_3 that originate in the beam outside of volume V.

For x-ray tube potentials up to 0.5 MeV the electrons have nearly equal tendencies to move forward and backward in the chamber, due to their initial angular distribution being predominantly sideways to the beam direction, and the effect of scattering in the air. Thus the attenuation of the x-rays in the distance l, separating the place of origin of corresponding electrons e_2 and e_3, tends to cancel, and the charge compensation is nearly exact. Moreover, the effective center of origin of electrons is the geometric center P' of V and V'.

Consequently the volume V' as a whole is in charged-particle equilibrium. That is, the ionization produced by all of the electrons originating in the beam within V is equal to all of the ionization produced within V', and the correct amount of charge is thus measured (neglecting the small effects of scattered photons, bremsstrahlung, and ionic recombination, yet to be discussed).

Notice that the distance from the boundaries of V to each end of the lead box must be greater than the maximum electron range also, to avoid perturbing the CPE con-

---

*NBS uses parallel metal strips in place of wires, as they provide a somewhat stronger field-flattening effect.

dition. In summary, one can say that *the distance from the volume of origin V to an obstruction in any direction must exceed the electron range, to preserve CPE in the volume V'*.

Note also that elementary volumes within V' are not in CPE; only the volume V' as a whole satisfies CPE.

2. ACCURATE DEFINITION OF THE MASS OF AIR, *m*, IN THE DEFINITION OF EXPOSURE

Defining the mass of air, m, by which the measured charge is to be divided to obtain the exposure can be simplified by noticing that each photon passing through the defining aperture passes through the volume V, except for those attenuated or scattered away in the air. If the fluence is Φ_0 (photons/m^2) at the aperture of area A_0 (m^2), then $\Phi_0 A_0$ photons will enter. Ignoring air effects, the fluence Φ decreases in proportion to the inverse square of the distance from the source, as the beam proceeds through the chamber. Simultaneously the beam area A increases in proportion to the square of the distance from the source. Thus ΦA remains constant and equal to $\Phi_0 A_0$ through the chamber.

Evidently then the number of electrons produced by ΦA photons in traversing the volume V, of length l (m), will be constant, irrespective of the actual cross-sectional area A of the beam in V, so long as the path length of each x ray in passing through V is not significantly increased by the angle θ the x-ray makes with the central axis. In all practical cases the source is sufficiently distant so that $l/\cos\theta \simeq l$, and this error is negligible. Consequently one can replace the actual volume of origin V by a cylindrical volume $V_c = A_0 l$ (m^3), which is multiplied by the air density ρ (kg/m^3) to obtain the defined mass m (kg) of air.

The exposure at the aperture (point P) is thus determined by the measurement, which must be corrected upward by the air attenuation occurring in the distance between P and the midpoint P' in V. If Q (C) is the charge produced in V', the exposure at point P is given (in C/kg) by

$$X = \frac{Q}{m} e^{\mu x'} = \frac{Q}{l A_0 \rho} e^{\mu x'} \tag{12.1}$$

where x' is the distance from P to P', and μ is the air attenuation coefficient. The effect of scattered photons will be discussed in Section II.A.4.

3. PROOF THAT THE EXPOSURE IS DEFINED AT THE PLANE OF THE APERTURE

Although the foregoing argument is reasonable, a more rigorous proof of exactly what it is that is measured by a free-air chamber would be desirable.

Let A_0 be the aperture area, at distance y from the source S in Fig. 12.2. Ψ_0 is the energy fluence at point P in the plane of the defining aperture. A disc-shaped mass element of air $dm_0 = \rho A_0 \, ds$ is located at P.

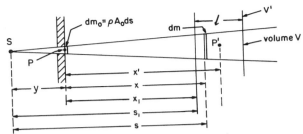

FIGURE 12.2.   The free-air-chamber geometry discussed in the proof.

The electrons resulting from x-ray interactions in dm_0, if allowed to dissipate all their energy in air, would produce a charge of either sign equal to

$$dQ_0 = dm_0 \; \Psi \left(\frac{\mu_{en}}{\rho}\right)_{air} \left(\frac{e}{\overline{W}}\right)_{air} = \rho A_0 \Psi_0 \left(\frac{\mu_{en}}{\rho}\right)_{air} \left(\frac{e}{\overline{W}}\right)_{air} ds \qquad (12.2)$$

Consider now a second elemental mass of air dm, at a distance s from the source, and a part of the volume V occupied by the beam and the collecting volume V':

$$dm = \rho A_0 \left(\frac{s}{y}\right)^2 ds \qquad (12.3)$$

dm is irradiated by an energy fluence $\Psi(s)$:

$$\Psi(s) = \Psi_0 \left(\frac{y}{s}\right)^2 e^{-\mu(s-y)} \cong \Psi_0 \left(\frac{y}{s}\right)^2 [1 - \mu(s-y)] \qquad (12.4)$$

where the approximation is very close for the small ($\sim 1\%$) attenuations that actually occur in typical free-air-chamber dimensions (< 30 cm). Thus the ionization produced by the electrons that originate in dm will be given by

$$dQ = dm \; \Psi(s) \left(\frac{\mu_{en}}{\rho}\right)_{air} \left(\frac{e}{\overline{W}}\right)_{air}$$

$$= \rho A_0 \left(\frac{s}{y}\right)^2 \Psi_0 \left(\frac{y}{s}\right)^2 [1 - \mu(s-y)] \left(\frac{\mu_{en}}{\rho}\right)_{air} \left(\frac{e}{\overline{W}}\right)_{air} ds$$

$$= dQ_0 [1 - \mu(s-y)] \qquad (12.5)$$

We assume that this charge is all collected and measured (i.e., that CPE exists for volume V', and that no ionic recombination occurs). The charge due to electrons from elemental mass dm is less than that from dm_0 by the amount of beam attenuation in the intervening air column.

The *total* charge Q generated by electrons originating in all of V is

$$Q = \rho A_0 \Psi_0 \left(\frac{\mu_{en}}{\rho}\right)_{air} \left(\frac{e}{\overline{W}}\right)_{air} \int_{s_1}^{s_1+l} [1 - \mu(s - y)] \, ds \qquad (12.6)$$

where s_1 is the distance from the x-ray source to the front plane of V. Letting $x = s - y$ and $x_1 = s_1 - y$, the above integral can be recast in the form

$$Q = k \int_{x_1}^{x_1+l} (1 - \mu x) \, dx = k \left[\frac{(1 - \mu x)^2}{-2\mu}\right]_{x_1}^{x_1+l}$$

$$= kl \left[1 - \mu\left(x_1 + \frac{l}{2}\right)\right]$$

$$= \rho A_0 l \Psi_0 \left(\frac{\mu_{en}}{\rho}\right)_{air} \left(\frac{e}{\overline{W}}\right)_{air} \left[1 - \mu\left(x_1 + \frac{l}{2}\right)\right] \qquad (12.7)$$

Since $x_1 + (l/2)$ is the distance from the aperture P to the midpoint P' of volume V, we see that Q is the charge due to the electrons originating in the cylindrical mass $\rho A_0 l$, exposed to the energy fluence Ψ_0 that exists at the aperture P, and corrected for attenuation in air through the distance from P to P'.

The exposure at point P (aperture) is

$$\frac{dQ_0}{dm_0} = \frac{\rho A_0 \Psi_0 \, (\mu_{en}/\rho)_{air} (e/\overline{W})_{air} \, ds}{\rho A_0 \, ds}$$

$$= \Psi_0 \left(\frac{\mu_{en}}{\rho}\right)_{air} \left(\frac{e}{\overline{W}}\right)_{air} \qquad (12.8)$$

The measured charge (assuming no recombination occurs) per unit mass in cylindrical volume $A_0 l$ is

$$\frac{Q}{m} = \frac{\rho A_0 l \, \Psi_0 \left(\frac{\mu_{en}}{\rho}\right)_{air} \left(\frac{e}{\overline{W}}\right)_{air} \left[1 - \mu\left(x_1 + \frac{l}{2}\right)\right]}{\rho A_0 l}$$

$$= \Psi_0 \left(\frac{\mu_{en}}{\rho}\right)_{air} \left(\frac{e}{\overline{W}}\right)_{air} \left[1 - \mu\left(x_1 + \frac{l}{2}\right)\right]$$

$$= \frac{dQ_0}{dm_0} \left[1 - \mu\left(x_1 + \frac{l}{2}\right)\right] \qquad (12.9)$$

Hence the exposure at point P is related to the value of Q/m by

$$X = \frac{dQ_0}{dm_0} = \frac{Q}{m} \left[1 - \mu\left(x_1 + \frac{l}{2}\right)\right]^{-1}$$

$$\cong \frac{Q}{m} \left[1 + \mu\left(x_1 + \frac{l}{2}\right)\right] \qquad (12.10)$$

where m is the mass of air in the cylindrical volume $A_0 l$. Typically $\mu \cong 2\text{-}3\%$ per meter of air, and $\mu(x_1 + l/2) < 0.01$.

4. SCATTERED X-RAYS IN THE CHAMBER

In the preceding treatment μ was taken to be the narrow-beam attenuation coefficient for the x-rays passing through air. This supposes that scattered photons do not result in measurable ionization in the chamber. That is not strictly the case, as can be seen from Fig. 12.3. Initially ignoring the plastic tube, we see that photons $h\nu_1$ and $h\nu_2$ are x-rays scattered out of the beam, which interact with other air atoms to launch electrons e_1 and e_2, respectively, thus producing excess ionization in the volume V'. Likewise photon $h\nu_3$, a bremsstrahlung x-ray emitted by electron e_3, may give rise to another electron e_4, which produces unwanted ionization, since the exposure is supposed to exclude ionization due to bremsstrahlung produced by the electrons that originate in the defined mass of air.

A method for determining the ionization contribution due to scattered and bremsstrahlung x-ray was described by Attix and De La Vergne (1954) as follows: A tube of nearly air-equivalent material such as Lucite, extending the full length of the ion-chamber enclosure, is positioned inside the chamber so that the x-ray beam passes through it from end to end without striking it. The tube must have walls thick enough to stop the electrons originating inside it, but thin with respect to attenuation of the scattered x rays, so that they may escape unimpeded. The plastic is completely coated with conducting graphite, and biased at half of the potential of the HV plate to minimize field distortion. The ratio of the ionization measured with the tube in place to that with the tube removed will approximate the fraction f_s of the total ionization that is contributed by scattered and bremsstrahlung x rays. In a chamber $\cong 50$ cm $\times$ 20 cm $\times$ 20 cm, $f_s \cong 0.003$ to 0.004 for 50–250-kV x-rays.

Wyckoff and Attix (1957) pointed out that the fraction f_e of the ionization Q in Eq. (12.1) that is lost due to a slight inadequacy in chamber plate separation (thus stopping some electrons short of their full range) tends to compensate for the f_s error. This balance can be exact at only one energy, however, as the sizes of the two errors vary in opposite directions as a function of x-ray energy. Nevertheless, for an optimum chamber size the net correction required for these combined errors can be minimized within a range of x-ray generating potentials. Equation (12.1) may be

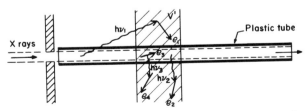

FIGURE 12.3. Measurement of the ionization due to scattered x-rays in a free-air chamber by the plastic-tube method.

corrected for the two effects through multiplication by $1 - f_s + f_e$, using data from the cited references.

5. OTHER CAUSES OF ELECTRIC-FIELD DISTORTION IN PARALLEL-PLATE CHAMBERS

As discussed in the introductory part of Section II.A, parallel-plate free-air chambers such as the NBS design must have a uniform electric field between the high-voltage plate and the collector-guard plates, to assure that the dimensions of the ion-collection volume V' and the length of the volume V are accurately known. The electrical lines of force must go straight across, perpendicular to the plates. To accomplish this, in addition to the graded-potential guard wires already mentioned, it is also important that:

a. all the plates be parallel to each other and to the beam axis, which must be perpendicular to the front and back boundaries of the volume V',

b. the collector and guard plates be coplanar, and

c. the collector be kept at the same electrical potential as the guards (usually at ground).

Even the contact potentials of the surfaces of these plates must be the same (e.g., electroplated with nonoxidizing metal) if local electric-field distortion near the gaps between them is to be avoided. Null-type electrometer circuits, which maintain the input potential at its initial value throughout the period of charge collection, are essential for this application. Figure 12.4 illustrates the distorting effects of noncoplanarity of the guard and collector plates, and Fig. 12.5 of having the collector surface at a different potential than that of the guard. Note that $\pm$HV averaging removes the error in Fig. 12.5, but not in Fig. 12.4.

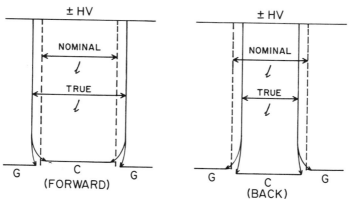

FIGURE 12.4. Effect of collector (C) misalignment with guards (G). At left, C moved forward of guards increases the effective length of the collecting volume over its nominal value l, independent of HV polarity. At right, the reverse case, with the collector recessed, results in the true collecting length being shorter than the nominal l.

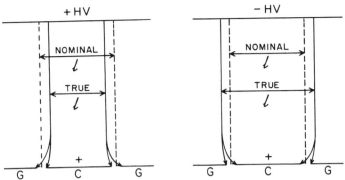

FIGURE 12.5 Effect of collector plate surface potential being higher ($\sim +1$ V) than guard plates. With $+$ HV the length of V' is less than nominal l; for $-$HV the length is greater than l. $\pm$HV averaging cancels the error. Where the potential of C is negative relative to the guards, the direction of the errors is reversed, but $\pm$HV averaging still cancels them.

B. Novel Free-Air-Chamber Designs

1. VARIABLE-LENGTH FREE-AIR CHAMBER (ATTIX, 1961; ATTIX AND GORBICS, 1968)

This chamber (see Fig. 12.6) consists of two telescoping cylinders with the x-ray beam passing along their axis through holes at the centers of the two flat end. The holes are covered by windows W of conducting plastic to keep out stray electrons and provide electrostatic shielding for the collecting electrode inside. The x-ray beam is defined by passing it through an aperture of known area in a fixed diaphragm, aligned with the chamber axis.

The ions formed throughout the chamber are collected on an off-center telescoping metal rod, correcting for ion recombination as necessary. The chamber shell is operated at high potential (e.g., ± 5000 V) and is enclosed in a Pb-lined box to keep out scattered x rays. The diameter of the collecting rod is made small enough, and its position far enough from the x-ray beam, that only a very small ($< 0.01\%$) loss of ionization results from electrons striking it.

The chamber dimensions are such that, in its collapsed condition (upper diagram), electrons originating in the x-ray beam where it crosses the fixed central plane cannot reach the walls in any direction. Likewise no electrons from the windows W are capable of reaching the central plane.

After an ionization measurement Q_1 is made in the collapsed condition, the chamber volume is expanded by a length ΔL (as much as twofold), while keeping the chamber midplane and the defining aperture fixed relative to the x-ray source. A second ionization measurement Q_2 is then made.

Referring to the diagram, the ionization component measured from the volume A' is the same as that from A except for a slight ($< 1\%$) increase due to decreased beam attenuation. The same can be said for the volumes B' and B, except that the

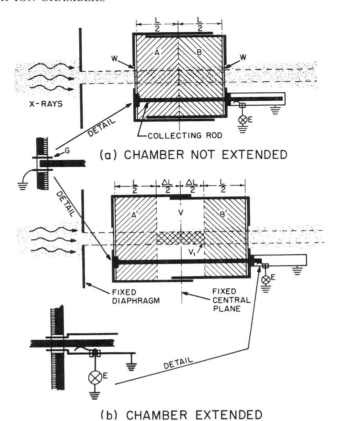

(a) CHAMBER NOT EXTENDED

(b) CHAMBER EXTENDED

FIGURE 12.6. The variable-length type of free-air chamber. The defining aperture and the midplane of the chamber both remain fixed with respect to the x-ray beam as the chamber is extended (Attix, 1961).

attenuation effect is in the reverse direction, canceling that for A' to A (assuming linear attenuation, which is accurate within 0.01% for attenuations <1%). Therefore the observed increase in ionization $(Q_2 - Q_1)$ must be due only to the electrons that originate in crosshatched volume V_1 in the center of the chamber. Those electrons will all run their full range in air and produce their full complement of ionization that will be measured directly in accordance with the definition of exposure. They need not remain in volume V to do this, since ions are collected from A' and B' as well.

If A_0 is the aperture area (m^2), ΔL is the length of chamber expansion (m), and ρ is the air density (kg/m^3), then the exposure at the aperture is given by

$$X = \frac{Q_2 - Q_1}{\rho A_0 \, \Delta L} \, e^{\mu x'} (1 - f_s + f_e) \qquad \text{(C/kg)} \qquad (12.11)$$

where x' is the distance from the aperture to the fixed central plane, μ is the narrow-beam attenuation coefficient for the x-rays in air, f_s is the fraction of $Q_2 - Q_1$ that is produced by scattered and bremsstrahlung x rays, and f_e is the fraction lost due to any electrons being stopped by the collecting rod and inadequate chamber radius.

The advantages of this design of free-air chamber over conventional designs are several:

1. There is no dependence of the measurement upon CPE. Since the electrons originating in V_1 cannot escape from the ion-collecting volume, there is no need for replacement of lost electrons.

2. There is no need for electric-field uniformity, plate alignment, or maintenance of the collector at ground potential.

3. The air mass can be defined more accurately, as the uncertainty in the length of the collecting volume in a conventional chamber is eliminated. ΔL can be determined by a precision screw, or even gauge blocks if desired.

It is necessary to cover the collecting-rod insulators at both ends of the chamber with conducting cups to avoid instability caused by charge collection on the insulator surfaces (Attix and Gorbics, 1968). In general it is a good idea to minimize the bare surface area of insulators facing into the collecting volume of *any* ion chamber, to avoid this kind of instability. This holds true for cavity chambers as well as free-air chambers. Laitano and Toni (1984) describe the use of this type of free-air chamber as a national x-ray standard.

2. HIGH-ENERGY FREE-AIR ION CHAMBERS

Free-air chambers are practical mainly with x-rays generated at energies between 10 and 300 keV. At higher energies the range of the secondary electrons in air becomes so great that the size of the chamber becomes prohibitively large. Wyckoff and Kirn (1957) described a large chamber (~ 1 m^3 between plates) capable of measuring 500-keV x-rays, and Wyckoff (1960) measured ^{60}Co γ rays with such a chamber in a pressure tank at 12 atm of air. In the latter case the results were compared to measurements made with a graphite-walled cavity ionization chamber, thus verifying the capability of the latter to determine exposure at this energy.

Joyet (1963) suggested employing a longitudinal magnetic field in a conventional free-air chamber to bend electron paths into spirals and thus prevent their striking the walls even for x-ray energies up to 50 MeV (see Fig. 12.7). Joyet pointed out that, as photons are increased in energy, the secondary electrons produced in Compton and pair-production events become more energetic but more forward directed. Thus the maximum side-directed (90°) component of the secondary-electron energy resulting from 50-MeV photons is only about 3 MeV, as shown by the dashed curve on the right ordinate of Fig. 12.8. The solid curve shows the magnetic field strength necessary to bend such electrons into spiral paths of radius 6 cm, which would prevent electrons from striking the wall in the chamber shown in Fig. 12.7.

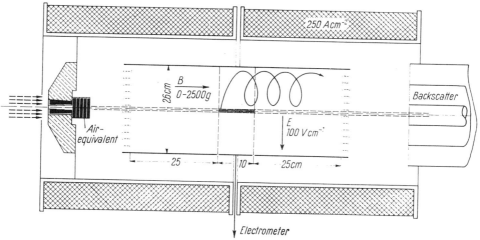

FIGURE 12.7. Schematic plan view of a parallel-plate free-air chamber with magnetic field and solid air-equivalent filters. (Joyet, 1963. Reproduced with permission from the *Journal of Applied Mathematics and Physics, Basel.*)

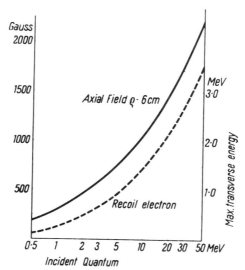

FIGURE 12.8. Maximum transverse energy $E_e \sin \varphi$ of the recoil electrons for incident quanta up to 50 MeV, and intensity of the magnetic field for the containment of the recoil electrons between the parallel plates. (Joyet, 1963. Reproduced with permission from the *Journal of Applied Mathematics and Physics, Basel.*)

The fatal flaw in this design is that it is not really a free-air chamber. To produce CPE in the collecting volume a sufficiently thick layer of solid "air-equivalent" material must be provided upstream to build up an equilibrium population of electrons passing through the ion-collecting region. (Up to 300 keV this is provided by the air space between the aperture and the collecting volume.) One may as well make a thick-walled cavity chamber out of the air-equivalent material instead, since the ionization measured by the Joyet chamber at high photon energies is primarily determined by the electrons generated by x-ray interactions in the air-equivalent filters shown in Fig. 12.7.

III. CAVITY IONIZATION CHAMBERS

Cavity ionization chambers come in many varieties, but basically consist of a solid envelope surrounding a gas- (usually air-) filled cavity in which an electric field is established to collect the ions formed by radiation. Cavity chambers offer several advantages over free-air ion chambers:

1.   They can be made very compact, even for high-energy use, since the range of the secondary electrons in the solid wall material is only $\sim 10^{-3}$ as great as in atmospheric air.

2.   They can measure multidirectional radiation fields, while free-air chambers require nearly monodirectional beams aligned to pass perpendicularly through the aperture.

3.   Through the application of cavity theory (Chapter 10), the absorbed dose can be determined in any material of which the cavity wall is made.

4.   Cavity chambers are capable of great variety in design, to permit dose measurements of charged particles and neutrons as well as photons. Free-air chambers are designed exclusively for x rays, mainly below 300 keV, and do not lend themselves to modification for other kinds of radiation.

5.   Gas cavities can be designed to be thin and flat to measure the dose at the surface of a phantom and its variation as a function of depth, or can be made very small to function as a probe to sample the dose at various points in a medium under irradiation.

6.   Collected charge can be measured in real time by connecting the chamber to an electrometer, or the chamber can be operated without cables if it is a condenser-type cavity chamber.

A. Thimble-Type Chambers

Spherical or cylindrical chambers (as shown schematically in Fig. 12.9) having gas volumes of 0.1–3 cm^3 are the most common forms of cavity ion chambers. Such chambers, especially the spherical designs, are reasonably isotropic in their sensitivity to radiation except for attenuation in the connecting "stem". Conventionally

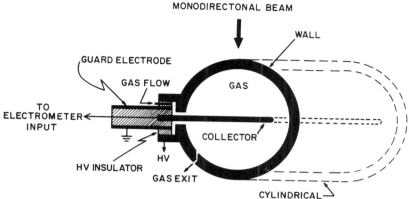

FIGURE 12.9. Fully guarded spherical thimble-type cavity ionization chamber. Cylindrical types may be regarded as elongated spherical chambers.

such "thimble" chambers, as they are sometimes called, are irradiated at right angles to the stem axis when monodirectional beams are measured. This not only avoids stem attenuation but also minimizes the length of the stem and cable that are irradiated, thus reducing the possible influence of radiation-induced electrical leakage in the cable insulation. Such effects will be discussed in Section IV.

1. FULLY GUARDED CHAMBERS

The high voltage (HV), usually ± 200–500 V, is shown in Fig. 12.9 applied to the chamber wall, with the collector connected to the electrometer input at or near ground potential. Alternative hookups are covered in Section IV. The insulator arrangement shown exemplifies a *fully guarded* ion chamber, by which is meant that electric current leaking through (or across the surface of) the HV insulator is intercepted by a grounded guard electrode ("guard ring") that extends completely through the insulator assembly in the stem. Thus this current cannot reach the collector and affect the measured charge. The inner insulator separating the collector from the guard electrode has practically no potential difference across it; thus little leakage occurs.

The insulator-and-guard assembly is shown in this design to be covered by an overhanging lip of the chamber wall. This is done to avoid instabilities caused by charge collection on the insulator surfaces. Without this covering lip the ions from a substantial fraction of the chamber volume would be delivered to the guard electrode instead of the collector, and that fraction would strongly depend on the pattern of ionic charge stuck on the surface of the insulators. The covering lip limits the affected gas volume only to the thin underlying crevice, thus practically eliminating this source of instability. A number of other designs can be used to accomplish this as well. Note that this same problem arose in the extendable free-air chamber and was solved in a similar way (Attix and Gorbics, 1968).

2. GAS FLOW

A gas connector is also shown in Fig. 12.9, allowing the chamber to be filled (and continuously replenished by flowing) with a gas other than air, or with pure dry air in place of ambient atmosphere. This feature is not present in most designs, but is important for neutron dosimetry, where tissue-equivalent and other special gases are employed, as discussed in Chapter 16. In using the gas-flow technique it is necessary to flush the chamber thoroughly at a relatively high gas-flow rate initially, then adjust the flow rate high enough to maintain gas purity without significantly increasing the pressure in the cavity above the ambient pressure. For proper operation, one should (a) vary the flow rate to find a ''plateau'' within which the measured charge is independent of flow rate; (b) beware of porous chamber walls (e.g., graphite), through which air will leak *inward* and contaminate the flow gas (Pearson et al., 1980); (c) avoid long runs of plastic tubing, which may contaminate the gas with plasticizer vapor; (d) check to see that the background ionization current is not a function of gas flow rate, since ions may be created by gas friction effects; and (e) if possible, use a separate gas-handling system (regulator, tubing, and flowmeter) for each gas, to avoid gas intermixing and unnecessarily long flushing delays when switching the ion chamber from one gas to another.

3. CHAMBER WALL THICKNESS

For dose measurements in fields of photons or neutrons under CPE or TCPE conditions, thus allowing relatability to K_c, thimble chamber walls should be made thick enough to (a) keep out of the cavity any charged particles that originate outside of the wall, and simultaneously (b) provide at the cavity an equilibrium charged-particle fluence and spectrum that is fully characteristic of the photon or neutron interactions taking place in the wall material. For photon fields the required wall thickness can be taken (conservatively) as being equal to the range (see Appendix E) of the maximum-energy secondary electrons set in motion by the photons in the wall itself or in other nearby media. In this connection it should be remembered that photoelectrons from nearby high-Z beam collimators may be more energetic than the maximum-energy Compton-recoil electrons generated in low-Z walls, in which case requirement (a) above is more stringent than (b).

The ionization charge Q produced in the mass m of gas is related to the absorbed dose in the cavity gas D_g by

$$D_g = \frac{Q}{m} \left(\frac{\overline{W}}{e} \right)_g \qquad (12.12)$$

where $(\overline{W}/e)_g$ for the gas has values to be discussed in Section IV.D for air and Section VI in general. D_g can in turn be related to the absorbed dose D_w in the inner layer of the wall through the application of appropriate cavity theory (Chapter 10), that is, a properly evaluated stopping-power ratio of wall to gas.

D_w is equal to $(K_c)_w$ under CPE conditions, and is proportional to it under TCPE conditions (see Chapter 11, Sect. II.A). Thus the measurement can be related to the photon energy fluence through Eqs. (11.1) and (11.2) or to the neutron fluence through Eqs. (11.3) and (11.4), for thick-walled ion chambers.

If the chamber is designed to measure the absorbed dose at a point of interest in a charged-particle field, the volume must be small, and the chamber wall must be thin, relative to the range of the incident particles. This applies whether the charged particles constitute the primary beam or are generated in the surrounding media by photon or neutron interactions. If the wall and cavity gas are approximately matched in atomic number, there will be a balance between δ rays escaping into the wall from the cavity gas and vice versa, assuming the wall is thick enough to provide such a δ-ray equilibrium. For practical purposes a wall thickness of $\cong 15$ mg/cm^2 (the range of a 100-keV electron) should suffice, as most δ rays resulting from electron–electron collisions have energies less than that. For heavy charged-particle beams the δ rays are still lower in energy, not exceeding the values given by Eq. (8.4). Thus it will be seen that the optimal wall thickness for charged-particle beam measurements is too thin for practical construction as a thimble chamber, and flat pillbox designs with thin plastic film windows suggest themselves.

Assuming δ-ray equilibrium, and assuming here that the small chamber accurately samples the charged-particle field without perturbing it (but see the necessary corrections in Chapter 13, Section VI.B), the dose in the cavity gas can be related to that in the irradiated medium at the point of measurement through application of B–G cavity theory, employing an average ratio of collision stopping powers evaluated for the spectrum of incident charged particles (excluding δ rays, since they are taken to be in equilibrium).

4. CHAMBER WALL MATERIAL

Air is of course a medium of special interest for photon dosimetry because of its role as the reference medium for the definition of exposure and its convenience as an ion-chamber gas. So-called "air-equivalent" chamber wall materials are often used. Air equivalence of the wall requires not only the matching of its mean mass energy-absorption coefficient to that of air for the photon spectrum present, but also the corresponding matching of the mean mass collision stopping powers for the secondary-electron spectrum present. These requirements cannot in general both be satisfied simultaneously, except that they are reasonably compatible where Compton effect is the dominant mode of photon interaction. If the photoelectric effect is important, its Z-dependence is so much stronger than that of the stopping power that the latter matching requirement is disregarded.

A less rigorous but more common statement of chamber-wall air equivalence with respect to photons is provided by the *effective atomic number* $\overline{Z}$, which must be further specified for the type of photon interaction being considered. For photoelectric effect the formula for $\overline{Z}$ has the form

$$\overline{Z} = \sqrt[m]{a_1 Z_1^m + a_2 Z_2^m + \cdots} \qquad (12.13)$$

where $a_1 = (f_1 Z_1/A_1)/\Sigma_i(f_i Z_i/A_i)$ is the fraction of the electrons present in the mixture that belong to atoms of atomic number Z_1, and so on; f_1 is the weight fraction of that element present; and m has a value of about 3.5 (Johns and Cunningham, 1983). On this basis $\overline{Z}_{air}$ is found to have a value of 7.8.

For dosimetry in charged-particle beams, the mean mass collision stopping power, derived by use of elemental weight fractions as weighting factors, is the most relevant quantity to be matched between the gas, wall, and reference media. The average charged-particle energy obtained from Eq. (10.32) is adequate to represent the charged-particle spectrum for this purpose.

Inasmuch as the wall must serve as an electrode, it must be electrically conducting, at least on the inside surface. Various plastics that are often employed as ion-chamber wall materials are generally electrical insulators; hence they need application of a conducting layer. Colloidal graphite in a water or alcohol base (the latter wets the plastic surface better) can be painted on in a dilute solution, dried, then polished with a cotton swab to maximize the electrical conductivity of the coating. Thin coats tend to adhere best, and have the least perturbing effect on the electron spectrum crossing the cavity.

Some special materials, such as A-150 tissue-equivalent plastic, are made volumetrically conducting as a result of incorporation of graphite during manufacture (Smathers et al., 1977).

The ion-collecting rod in a thimble chamber should be made of the same material as the wall if possible, as cavity theories do not deal with inhomogeneous wall media. However, the surface area of the rod is usually so much less than that of the wall that it will not have much influence unless the interaction cross sections in the rod are much larger than in the wall. For example, an aluminum rod is sometimes used in an air-equivalent-walled chamber to boost the photon response below ~ 100 keV by the photoelectric effect, thus compensating for the increasing attenuation of the x rays in the wall (also due to the photoelectric effect). Pure graphite pencil leads make convenient low-Z ion-collecting rods.

5. INSULATORS

Polystyrene, polyethylene, and Teflon are all excellent electrical insulators for ion-chamber use. Most other common plastics, such as PMMA (Lucite, Plexiglas), Nylon, and Mylar, are also acceptable in most cases. Teflon in particular is more readily damaged by radiation than the others, and should be avoided where total doses exceeding $\sim 10^4$ Gy are expected. However, its smooth "waxy" surface is the most tolerant of humidity in the air without allowing leakage currents to pass across.

Except for radiation-induced volumetric electrical leakage, most observed leakage is a surface phenomenon that is minimal for clean, polished surfaces and worsens where dirt and/or humidity are present. A fiber or hair bridging an insulator often is the cause of leakage, and a rubber syringe should be kept on hand for blowing away such debris. (The breath is too humid for this purpose.) One should avoid touching an insulator, especially with the fingers, as skin oil causes persistent leakage and is difficult to remove. Pure ethyl or methyl alcohol is sometimes helpful in cleaning insulators by wiping the surface with a cotton swab, then drying with a syringe. After such attempts one should not expect instant improvement; several hours may be needed for the insulator to return to normal. Remachining the surface of an insulator with a sharp, clean cutting tool, or replacing it entirely, may be necessary if leakage persists.

Note that mechanical stress of an insulator (e.g., bending a cable) can cause apparent leakage currents due to polarization effects, and rubbing the surface of an insulator can produce surface charges by the triboelectric effect that may take a long time to dissipate, during which leakage currents will be observed.

The effects of radiation on insulators are complicated and numerous. As in all irradiated media, atoms are ionized, but an electron may take some time to recombine if it is displaced an appreciable distance from the "hole" (ionized atom) and trapped there. The presence of an electric field during irradiation tends to align these electron–hole dipoles in a common direction, forming an *electret*. Gradual relaxation of the dipoles induces charges in the electrodes bounding the insulator, constituting a leakage current through the external circuit. This effect is sometimes called "soakage" of an insulator, as it gives the appearance of electric charge having been absorbed into the insulator, and gradually oozing out again (Liversage, 1952).

The forward projection of electrons in high-energy photon interactions can transport charge through an insulator and thus cause a high potential difference to develop between electrodes of a capacitor. Gross (1978) has studied this effect and applied it to the design of what he calls "Compton-current dosimeters."

Charged-particle beams incident on a thick insulator will build up charge wherever the particles stop at the end of their paths. It has been pointed out by Gross and Nablo (1967) and Galbraith et al. (1984) that when large blocks of insulating plastics such as acrylic or polystyrene are used as phantoms and irradiated to high doses by electron beams, the charge buildup due to stopped electrons may cause electric fields strong enough to influence the paths of primary or secondary electrons in the medium. This condition can persist for hours or even days, distorting the dose distribution in subsequent photon or electron irradiations.

At sufficiently high doses (~ 10–100 Gy) the resistivity of insulators decreases significantly, recovering gradually with a time constant of the order of hours, as discussed by Boag (1966). Thus an ion chamber should not be exposed to large doses before small ones are to be measured. Several investigators have studied the conductivity of insulators under irradiation, and the possible applicability of this effect as a dose-rate measuring parameter (Fowler, 1966).

Radiation can also damage organic insulators by chemical-bond breakage, causing the material to discolor and eventually to lose its mechanical integrity at very high doses—especially Teflon, as mentioned before.

6. CONDENSER-TYPE CHAMBERS

It is sometimes advantageous to design a thimble chamber to operate without external connections while being irradiated. One option for accomplishing this is to connect the chamber electrodes in parallel with a capacitor, built into the stem of

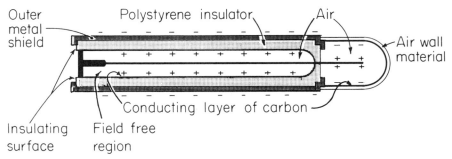

FIGURE 12.10. Schematic diagram of a Victoreen-type condenser ion chamber. Ions are produced in both of the air compartments, but there is no electric field to collect ions from the stem compartment at left, which behaves as a Faraday cage. The stem is designed to have the desired capacitance between inner and outer electrodes. (Johns and Cunningham, 1983. Reproduced with permission from J. R. Cunningham, and Charles C Thomas, Publishers.)

the chamber, as shown in Fig. 12.10. The capacitor (and chamber) are then charged up by temporarily connecting them across a potential P_1 (typically 300 V), which establishes an electric field in the chamber. When the chamber is irradiated, the positive ions are drawn to the wall and the negative ions to the collector (for the polarity shown in Fig. 12.10). Thus the charge stored in the capacitor–chamber combination is diminished, and the potential is decreased to a new value P_2. If the combined capacitance is C, the charge collected from the chamber during irradiation is

$$\Delta Q = Q_1 - Q_2 = C(P_1 - P_2) \tag{12.14}$$

ΔQ is most accurately determined as the difference between the charge Q_1 measured by connecting the unirradiated device across the input of a high-gain charge-integrating electrometer (see Section IV) and the charge Q_2 similarly measured after irradiation.

The radiation sensitivity of such a chamber is directly proportional to the chamber volume, and inversely proportional to C.

If the final voltage P_2 is allowed to fall too low, recombination of charge in the chamber can cause the collected charge ΔQ to be significantly less than the charge *produced* by ionization of the gas in the chamber, a matter to be discussed in Section V. This can be detected by observing a lack of proportionality between ΔQ and the irradiation time at a constant dose rate.

Some capacitor thimble chambers (e.g., the Victoreen *r*-meter) are designed to be used in conjunction with a companion string-type electrometer (including an internal voltage supply), which also has an internal capacitance comparable in value to that of the chamber and stem. Thus there is charge sharing to reach a common potential when the chamber and electrometer are connected. The reading of such an electrometer is viewed through an eyepiece, with the shadow of the fiber appearing against a scale labeled in roentgens, reading zero when fully charged. Such a chamber is to be calibrated in conjunction with its own electrometer, and must therefore be used exclusively with that electrometer when referring to that calibration. To correct consistently for the charge-sharing effect, the chamber is calibrated and used by always charging the electrometer initially to zero scale reading with the chamber connected, and again to zero before reconnecting the chamber following its irradiation.

B. Flat Cavity Chambers; Extrapolation Chambers

Flat cavity chambers have several special advantages:

1.   They can be constructed with thin foils or plastic membranes for one or both of the flat walls, causing only minimal attenuation or scattering of incident electrons or soft x-rays.

2.   The gas layer can be made as thin as $\cong 0.5$ mm, allowing sampling of the dose with good depth resolution, especially advantageous in regions where the dose changes rapidly with distance.

3.   In some designs the thickness of the gas layer is made variable, for example by an adjustable screw, thus allowing extrapolation of the ionization per unit gas-layer thickness to zero thickness. This in effect removes the influence of perturbation due to the presence of a finite cavity in a phantom, for example, and further increases resolution of dose vs. depth.

4.   The dose at the surface of a phantom can be measured by extrapolation (Velkley et al., 1975), and the buildup vs. depth can be observed by adding thin sheets of phantom medium over the entrance foil.

On the other hand, flat-geometry chambers are generally more complicated in design than thimble chambers, and more difficult to construct. Boag (1966) devised the chamber shown in Fig. 12.11 for electron-beam dosimetry. As shown, it contains three graphite-coated mica foils, but thinly aluminized Mylar would do as well. Capability for extrapolation of the air-layer thickness was not provided, but could be by using spacer rings or machining a screw around the rim. Such a chamber can

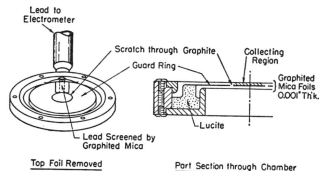

FIGURE 12.11.   Ionization chamber for dosimetry of fast-electron beams (Boag, 1966. Reproduced with permission of J. W. Boag and Academic Press.)

be used to study surface dose enhancement due to electron backscattering from a phantom, for example, since it contains no thick electrodes. The collecting electrode in this chamber is insulated from the surrounding guard electrode by a clean scratch through the colloidal graphite coating on one side of the middle foil. Notice that in this and most other flat chamber designs, the guard electrode serves primarily to provide a uniform electric field, thus allowing the radius of the collecting volume to be defined by the collecting-electrode radius plus the half-width of the insulating scratch or groove around it. In some flat-chamber designs the guard ring also stops leakage currents from the HV electrode, as in fully guarded thimble chambers.

Guarded flat chambers can be viewed as plane capacitors having a capacitance proportional to the area of the collecting volume, and inversely proportional to the plate separation. Thus a simple measurement of the chamber's capacitance, which can be done with a charge-calibrated electrometer and a calibrated variable voltage supply, can provide a check on the mechanical determination of the collecting volume:

$$C = \frac{\Delta Q}{\Delta P} = 8.85 \times 10^{-14} \frac{a}{s} \qquad (12.15)$$

where ΔQ is the charge measured (in coulombs) as a result of a voltage change of ΔP (in volts), a is the collecting area in cm^2, s is the plate separation in centimeters, C is given in farads, and the numerical constant has units of F/cm.

Commercially available flat chambers used to measure surface dose and dose buildup have been commonly designed with a thin foil entrance wall, but a thick conducting back wall comprising the collecting electrode and the surrounding guard electrode, as schematically shown in Fig. 12.12. When such a chamber is placed in a γ-ray beam, electrons are knocked out of the back electrode by the Compton effect,

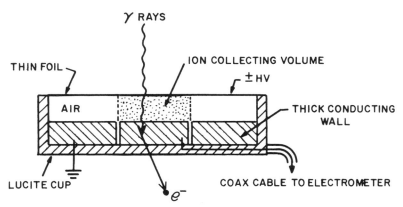

FIGURE 12.12. Schematic diagram of a flat chamber with thick back wall of conducting material, illustrating the cause of polarity differences observed in the measured output current resulting from γ radiation.

constituting a positive current entering the electrometer. If positive voltage is applied to the front foil, positive ions will arrive at the collecting electrode, adding to the Compton current. For negative applied voltage the negative ions are collected, and the net negative current sent to the electrometer is the difference between the ion current and the Compton current. Thus the true ion current may be obtained as the average of the currents measured with the two HV polarities. This effect, first explained by Richardson (1954), is most pronounced for a small plate separation and a thin front wall. As the front-wall thickness is increased, an equilibrium is gradually established for the electrons entering and leaving the collecting electrode, and the inequality between polarities disappears.

With charged-particle beams a comparable, but more complicated, effect is observed when the particles stop in the collecting electrode, or knock out δ rays.

These problems can be avoided by using chamber designs such as those shown in Fig. 12.11 and 12.13. The latter, recommended by the Nordic Association of Clinical Physics (1981), has a thin foil collector supported by (but insulated from) a thicker wall. Few charged particles can start or be stopped within such a thin collector.

Another kind of problem that may arise from faulty design of any type of ion chamber, but is more likely to affect flat chambers, is *extracameral ionization*, i.e., ionization that is collected from air spaces outside of the designated collecting volume. Such unwanted contributions of ionization can drastically affect the outcome of an experiment if unnoticed, especially in extrapolation chambers that are supposed to approach zero volume. Figure 12.14 illustrates two kinds of extracameral effect in a flat chamber, and how they may be avoided.

In Fig. 12.14a a flat chamber is shown, including an insulating plate painted on both sides with colloidal graphite, and a circular scratch made to separate the collector C from the guard ring G. A bare wire is shown attached to the collector and leading out to a coaxial-cable connection at the side, and thence to the electrometer input. It can be seen that since the radiation beam also irradiates the guard-ring area, air ions as shown (assuming +HV) may be collected by electric lines of force terminating on the wire, thus contributing measured charge from a region outside of the (speckled) collecting volume. In Boag's design (Fig. 12.11) this extracameral ion

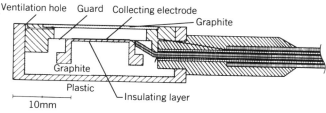

FIGURE 12.13. Flat chamber designed not to exhibit polarity-difference effects. The collecting electrode is very thin (<0.1 mm) and is mounted on a thin insulating layer (≅0.2 mm). (Mattsson, et al., 1981. Reproduced with permission from L. O. Mattsson and *Acta Radiologica Oncologie*.)

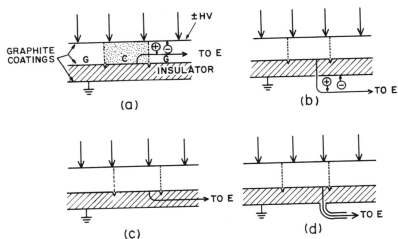

FIGURE 12.14. The extracameral ionization effect in flat pillbox chambers. The collector C and guard ring G are graphite coatings on an insulating plate, the back of which is also graphite-coated and grounded. (*a*) Bare wire connects collector to a coax cable, thence to the electrometer; (*b*) bare wire out the back; (*c*) wire buried in insulating plate; (*d*) coaxial cable all the way to the electrometer. (See text.)

collection was eliminated by covering the connecting lead with graphite-coated mica foil, as shown at left. Notice that the type of extracameral effect shown in Fig. 12.14*a* is particularly insidious because it cannot be detected by reversing the HV polarity; the polarity of the extracameral ionization follows that of the intended collecting volume.

In Fig. 12.14*b* a similar design is shown, except that now the wire passes from the collector *through* the insulating plate and out through a bare spot in the grounded graphite back surface, then to a coaxial connection at the side, leading to the electrometer. One might think that such an arrangement would not collect charge on the wire, since the HV lines of force do not reach it. However, all conductors have surface contact potentials, some as great as ~ 1 V. The difference in their magnitudes creates a weak electric field in any gas space between dissimilar surfaces, such as the wire and the graphite. Thus some of the ions created behind the chamber by the radiation field may be collected on the wire, although most will recombine for lack of sufficient electric field strength to separate them. Even so, the resulting extracameral charge collected may be considerable. In this case, however, the effect can be easily detected by HV polarity reversal, since the extracameral ion collection is unaffected. Thus it adds to the current in one polarity and subtracts in the other, and the ±average gives the correct current without the extracameral component.

In Fig. 12.14*c* the wire is shown sealed inside the insulating plate itself until it reaches the coaxial connector, and Fig. 12.14*d* shows the coaxial cable connecting directly to the back of the insulating plate. In either of these cases little or no extracameral effect will be observed.

C. Transmission Monitor Chambers

When radiation generators are not constant with time, due to power-line fluctuations for example, some kind of monitoring ionization chamber may be employed to allow normalization of results by dividing all radiation measurements by the corresponding monitor readings.

A thimble chamber can be used for this purpose, by simply positioning it at a convenient fixed location in the beam. However, a thin flat chamber through which the beam passes on its way to the point of measurement has the advantages that it can be permanently installed and that it can monitor specifically the segment of the beam that is of greatest interest, or can monitor the whole beam if preferred. If only a segment of the transmitted beam is to be monitored, a scribed collector can be used, as in Boag's design in Fig. 12.11. If the whole beam is to be monitored, the collimator should be placed upstream of the monitor chamber, and the chamber should have a collecting area that is larger than the beam.

A transmission chamber suitable for x-ray beam applications, rugged, and simple to contruct is shown in Fig. 12.15. This chamber should of course be well vented to the atmosphere to avoid plate distortion due to changes in barometric pressure. Relatively thick Lucite plates are shown, as they simplify construction by being self-supporting, but stretched foils could be substituted for electron beams or soft x-rays. Electrical contacts are made by bronze leaf springs that press against the inner colloidal graphite coatings when the plates are fixed in place. The graphite coatings on the outside surfaces are both grounded by contact with the aluminum rim. Electrical insulation for both the HV and collecting electrodes is provided by a border of bare Lucite around the edge, separating the graphited areas from the supporting rim. If beam uniformity or alignment is an issue, such a chamber can have its collector scribed into four quadrants, with as many bronze contacts leading out to coaxial connectors on the rim.

IV. CHARGE AND CURRENT MEASUREMENTS

A. General Considerations

The typical order of magnitude of charge or current to be measured from ionization chambers can be estimated from the fact that an exposure of 1 R generates a charge

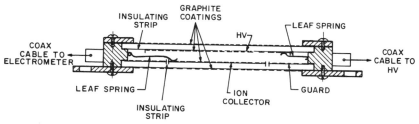

FIGURE 12.15. Simple design for a transmission ionization chamber. The size is optional, but the HV electrode should be larger in diameter than the ion collector, which in turn should cover the beam area to be monitored. (See text.)

of $\cong 3 \times 10^{-10}$ C in 1 cm^3 of room-temperature air at a pressure of 1 atm. In most practical cases, ion currents lie in the range 10^{-6} to 10^{-14} A. The measurement of such small currents, or the corresponding charges integrated over usual irradiation time intervals of seconds or minutes, requires careful technique and appropriate instrumentation, to be discussed next. A good general reference has been provided by Keithley et al. (1984).

1. ELECTROMETERS

Electrometers can be thought of simply as ultrahigh-impedance voltmeters. The gold-leaf electroscope, when equipped with a quantitative scale, qualifies as an early electrometer. Quartz-fiber electrometers are still in use with the Victoreen *r*-meter (Section III.A.6) and in self-reading pocket ion chambers. Greater sensitivity, and the convenience of electric meter readout, was provided by the vacuum-tube electrometer, many of which are still in use. The ultimate in electrometer sensitivity for measurement of the smallest currents and charges is achieved with a vibrating-reed electrometer, such as the Carey Model 31, which converts the DC input into an AC signal by means of an oscillating capacitance, and synchronously amplifies that single-frequency signal.

Most modern electrometers, however, are of the solid-state operational-amplifier type, which is entirely satisfactory for practically all ion-chamber applications. Some, such as the Keithley Model 602, have an analogue meter display which can be simultaneously read out with a separate digital voltmeter if desired. Others, such as the Keithley Model 616, have a direct digital readout. Such electrometers provide a variety of ranges of charge measurement by means of several built-in input capacitors, and several current ranges with built-in resistors.

For maximum flexibility of application it will be advantageous if the electrometer is designed with an inner chassis (and low-impedance terminal) that can be either grounded or biased at high voltage relative to the grounded case, as shown schematically in Fig. 12.16*a* and *b*. The front panel should also be equipped with both a coaxial and a triaxial terminal, or a triaxial terminal and a coaxial adaptor as in Fig. 12.16*c*. A separate adjustable dual-polarity HV source can then be used to bias either the ion-chamber collector or the chamber wall at any selected voltage and polarity relative to the other, as indicated in the figure. Applying a given negative voltage to the chamber wall with the collector at ground potential is of course equivalent to applying an equal positive voltage to the collector with the wall at ground. The guard ring remains at or near the same potential as the collector in either case, which is desirable to minimize leakage.

Some electrometers have a built-in battery power supply to bias the internal chassis with respect to the case, but this convenience is outweighed by the loss of such options as being able to check for ionic recombination (see Section V). Such internal batteries also tend to be forgotten as they gradually lose their voltage and allow more and more recombination to occur, and may eventually damage the electrometer by corrosion.

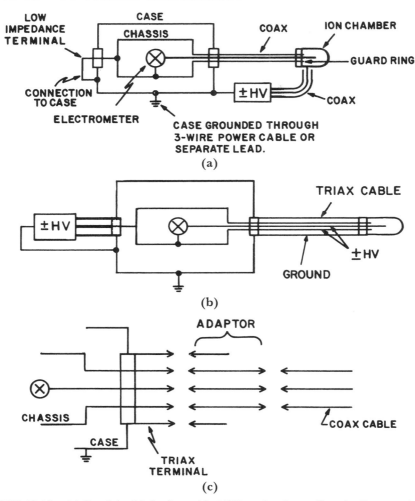

FIGURE 12.16. (*a*) Coaxial-cable hookup with ±HV on chamber wall, and collector and guard ring at ground potential. (*b*) Triaxial-cable hookup with ±HV on chamber collector and guard ring, and chamber wall grounded. (*c*) Adapter from triax terminal to coaxial cable. Note that the outer conductor of the triaxial terminal is not used.

Other special features may also be present in an electrometer; the manufacturer's instructions should be studied to be certain that the instrument is used correctly.

2. HIGH-VOLTAGE SUPPLIES

The HV power supply for biasing the ion chamber should be capable of providing, with front-panel controls, potentials from 0 to ±500 V for cavity chambers, or 0 to ±5000 V for free-air chambers. Good regulation against line-voltage fluctuations is essential, since HV fluctuations induce current to flow in the electrometer input circuit.

A free-air chamber having a voltage divider to bias the field-guarding wires requires sufficient output current for that purpose. Otherwise the HV supply should be equipped with a series resistor ($\sim 10^7$ Ω) inside the cabinet to limit the output current for safety. Note that measuring the output voltage then would require a voltmeter having an input impedance of at least 10^9 Ω. Moreover, instantaneous ionization currents greater than $\sim 10^{-6}$ A would cause substantial voltage depletion (> 10 V) on the ion chamber, requiring reduction or removal of the limiting resistor.

If a continuously adjustable HV supply is not available, a factor-of-two voltage change should be provided for assessing the degree of ionic recombination in the chamber, as discussed in Section V. A battery pack may be used for economy, but should be fully enclosed, output-limited for safety, and monitored regularly to verify its output voltage.

3. GENERAL OPERATING PRECAUTIONS

1.   The electrometer input-shorting switch should be routinely kept closed except when a measurement is underway, to ensure that it will not be unintentionally left open during any action that might create electrical transients, such as turning on the electrometer, connecting the HV, or changing the input cable connections. Leaving the switch open also risks running the electrometer off scale due to excess charge-collection. Instability or even damage may result in such cases.

2.   All parts of the electrical circuit connected to the electrometer input must be well insulated and electrostatically shielded, for example by use of coaxial or triaxial cables. Inadequate insulation results in electrical-charge leakage into or out of the system, observable as positive or negative background current when radiation is absent. Inadequate electrostatic shielding is apparent through sensitivity of the system to motion of nearby objects, such as a hand waved around the chamber or cable. If such trouble is observed, the input cable should be disconnected at the electrometer and a grounded metal cap placed over the terminal, to verify that the electrometer itself is stable with its input shorting switch open. Input-circuit components can then be connected one at a time to localize the cause of the problem. The HV source can also be removed and replaced with a grounding connection to ascertain whether it is causing the problem.

3.   All input-circuit cables should be of the nonmicrophonic type,* and should not be kinked, twisted, stepped on or flexed. Rough handling can cause large and variable background currents that may persist for hours. Small-diameter (e.g., Microdot X2) coaxial cables are relatively forgiving in this respect. Cable-connector insulators should not be touched, blown into with the breath, or allowed to get wet or dirty (see Section III.A.5).

*Ordinary coaxial cable can be made less microphonic by stripping off the outer cover and dousing the braided conductor with colloidal graphite.

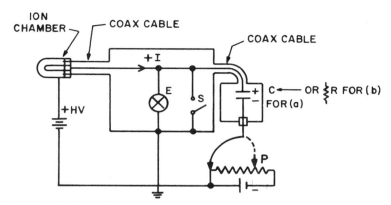

FIGURE 12.17. (*a*) Classical null method for measurement of charge with an electrometer (E). Potential *P* is supplied by a standard potentiometer, *S* is the input shorting switch, and *C* the known capacitance upon which charge *Q* is collected by the potential *P*, where $Q = CP$ when *E* is at null. (All polarities shown may be reversed.) (*b*) Classical null method for measurement of current with an electrometer. Known high-megohm resistor *R* replaces capacitor *C* in the circuit. The ionization current *I* passes through *R*, thus generating a potential drop *IR* that is equal in magnitude to the potential *P* when *E* is at null.

4. A single common electrical ground should be connected to all equipment cases and cable shields.

B. Charge Measurement

The classical electrometer circuit for measuring charge by a "null" method (i.e., using the electrometer only as a null-detecting voltmeter) is shown in Fig. 12.17*a*. An analogue readout is needed for this manual-adjustment method. Before discussing the operating procedure the capacitor *C* and the standard potentiometer will be described.

1. CAPACITORS

The capacitor *C* upon which the ionization charge is to be collected in Fig. 12.17*a* should be a high quality three-terminal polystyrene-dielectric type, that is, with a groundable metal case not connected to either lead. To cover the usual charge ranges it will be convenient to obtain at least four such capacitors (10^{-11}, 10^{-9}, 10^{-7}, and 10^{-5} F) and preferably the three intermediate decades also. These should be mounted inside (and grounded to) a metal box with the leads exiting through separate BNC connectors. The absolute values of such capacitors can be calibrated within 0.1% by means of a 1000-Hz precision AC capacitance bridge, such as the General Radio* Model 1615, the calibration of which should in turn be traceable to a standards laboratory. It is assumed in this procedure that the capacitors have "nonlossy" di-

*General Radio Co. West Concord, MA 01781, U.S.A.

electric, thus having the same capacitance value for DC electrometer use as that measured by the AC bridge. This is a good assumption for high-quality polystyrene capacitors such as Model SB or ST from Southern Electronics.* These capacitors do have a slight negative temperature coefficient, however, and should be used at approximately the same temperature as that at which they were calibrated. Otherwise their values are constant over long periods.

It is interesting (and sometimes disappointing) to find that expensive high-quality standard capacitors are generally designed for AC use, and may be very leaky and unusable for DC applications.

2.   STANDARD POTENTIOMETERS

To measure charge by the null method shown in Fig. 12.17a, not only must the value of capacitance C be known, but the potential P applied to it as well. A standard potentiometer such as the Rubicon Model 2704† can deliver known potentials in the ranges 0 to 0.2 V and 0 to 2.0 V, internally calibrated against a standard cell. The accuracy of the dial and slidewire settings should be verified at a standards laboratory, but are generally found to be closer than 0.1% to the true potentials.

Any highly stable and accurate, continuously adjustable voltage supply (e.g., Zener-diode stabilized) may be substituted, noting that higher voltages may be used with reciprocally lower capacitors C to measure a given range of charge values, since $Q = CP$.

3.   OPERATING PROCEDURE

The sequence of steps involved in a charge measurement by the circuit illustrated in Fig. 12.17a is as follows:

   1.   Select the value of C and the potentiometer range to accommodate the charge to be measured. For example, if the estimated ion current is 3×10^{-10} A and a 1-min irradiation time is desired, $Q \cong 2 \times 10^{-8}$ C. This can be collected on a capacitance of 10^{-7} F by P = 0.2 V, or on 10^{-9} F by 20 V.

   2.   Make a trial irradiation to select the most appropriate electrometer voltage-sensitivity scale, that is, where the needle takes at least several seconds to reach full scale, and the potentiometer can easily be manually adjusted to keep the needle near the null position (for conventional free-air chamber measurements) or at least continuously on scale. This kind of visual–manual operation is not feasible with a digital electrometer display.

   3.   With switch S closed, adjust the electrometer zeroing control to set the needle at an arbitrary "null" reading, which need not be zero; midscale may be more convenient. The input circuit is now at ground potential, and will be again whenever the electrometer indicates a null reading. Set P at zero.

   4.   With the radiation shutter closed, open switch S, isolating the input circuit

*Southern Electronics Co., Inc. 726 So. Flower St., Burbank, CA 91502, U.S.A.
†Rubicon Instruments, Penn Airborne Products Co., Industrial Blvd., Southampton, PA 18966, U.S.A.

at high impedance from ground. A slight offset from the electrometer null may be observed due to charge separation by contact potentials in the switch contacts. If so, readjust the electrometer zero to again read exactly null with S open. The input is now at ground potential, although insulated from ground.

5. Open the shutter to begin a timed irradiation of the ion chamber. Adjust P continuously to keep the needle on scale.

6. Immediately after the shutter closes, fine-adjust P to give an exact null reading on the electrometer. If the collected charge is positive, this will require a negative potential P to be applied to the lower side of C, as shown in Fig. 12.17a. Since the upper side of C must be at ground potential, the voltage across C is therefore equal to P, and the positive charge stored in C is $Q = CP$ (coulombs). Notice that since the input circuit is at the same potential (ground) at the end of the exposure as at the start, there can be no charge stored on the distributed capacitance of the input circuit. Consequently Q must be the entire charge (of either sign) collected in the chamber.

7. The background charge should be measured in the same manner for approximately the same elapsed time with the radiation source turned off.

4. "RACETRACK" TIMING

The following variation of the preceding method allows measurement of charge collected in a measured time interval without use of a shutter. Steps 1 and 2 in the foregoing section are unchanged.

3. With S closed, adjust the electrometer zeroing control to set the needle somewhat below the midscale point. Midscale will be taken as the null point. Set P at zero.

4. With the radiation beam already turned on, open S. As the needle crosses the midscale, start the stopwatch or timer. Adjust P to keep the needle on scale.

5. When the irradiation is long enough for desired timing accuracy, over-adjust P to move the electrometer needle below the midpoint. Then stop the timer as the needle again passes the midpoint. As in the preceding method, $Q = CP$. Although the input circuit is slightly offset from ground potential when the needle is at the midpoint null position, the offset is the same at the start and finish, so Q is still the total charge collected during the timed interval, none being trapped on the distributed capacitance.

5. AUTOMATIC FEEDBACK OPERATION

Clearly it would be more convenient, and probably more accurate, to arrange for the potentiometer in Fig. 12.17a to be automatically adjusted to make the electrometer reading remain constantly at its null setting. With modern high-gain electrometers this can be done very simply by means of a negative-feedback loop that also eliminates the need for the external potentiometer in the circuit, as illustrated in Fig. 12.18a. The open-loop gain G of the operational amplifier may be taken typ-

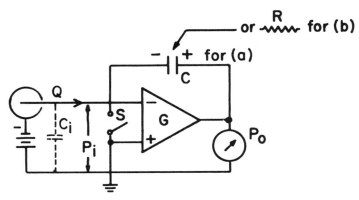

FIGURE 12.18. (*a*) Operational-amplifier electrometer circuit for charge measurement. (*b*) Operational-amplifier electrometer circuit for current measurement, for which the high-megohm resistor *R* replaces *C*.

ically as 10^5, meaning that if a small negative potential P_i is applied to the negative ("inverting") input terminal (the positive input terminal being grounded as shown), a positive potential of $P_0 = 10^5 P_i$ will simultaneously appear at the output terminal. Thus the potential across the capacitor C (with shorting switch S open) is $P_i + P_0$, with the indicated polarity.

Consider what happens when negative charge Q flows from the ion chamber: The input circuit is driven to a negative potential P_i, but as it does so the output potential rises to a 10^5 times greater positive potential, P_0, which is applied to capacitor C. The total potential across C is then $P_0 + P_i$, and it holds a charge $C(P_0 + P_i) = Q - C_i P_i$, where C_i is the distributed capacitance of the input circuit to ground. The input impedance of the operational amplifier may be assumed to be too high to allow the passage of any significant charge.

As a numerical example, let us assume that $G = 10^5$, $C = 10^{-9}$ F, $C_i = 10^{-10}$ F, and the negative charge from the ion chamber is $Q = 4 \times 10^{-9}$ C. Then $10^{-9} (P_0 + P_i) = 10^{-9} (10^5 + 1) P_i = 4 \times 10^{-9} - 10^{-10} P_i$, which may be solved to obtain $P_i = 3.999956 \times 10^{-5}$ V $\cong 4 \times 10^{-5}$ V; hence $P_0 \cong 4$ V. Thus the value of charge collected from the ion chamber is very accurately equal to the product of C and the output potential P_o, provided that the open-loop gain G is very large.

Because C is now a built-in capacitor in the electrometer, it should be calibrated *in situ*. In fact there are usually several capacitors of different values that can be switched into the circuit to change ranges in modern electrometers, and each needs calibration. Moreover, the output voltmeter in Fig. 12.18*a* is usually readable directly on a scale that is calibrated in coulombs in place of volts when charge is being measured. Thus the method of calibration basically is to inject a known charge into the electrometer's input terminal, and compare it with the resulting charge reading of the electrometer. This can be done accurately and easily for several points on each charge scale by the method shown in Fig. 12.19*a*, in which C_s is a high-quality ca-

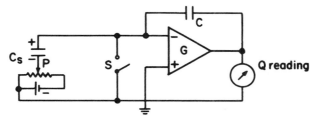

FIGURE 12.19a.   Calibration method for a charge-measuring feedback-controlled electrometer.

pacitor of known value. The calibrated polystyrene capacitors described in Section IV.B.1 may serve as C_s, and a potentiometer such as those discussed in Section IV.B.2 can be used for supplying P. The following steps should be followed:

1. With S shorted and P set at zero, adjust the electrometer scale or digital display to zero on the charge range to be calibrated. The electrometer's wiring diagram will show the nominal value of C employed for that range; C_s should be selected to be preferably of the same order of magnitude.

2. Open S; rezero as necessary. Adjust P from zero in stepwise fashion, for example, to 0.1 V, 0.2 V, . . . which will insert charges of $0.1C_s$, $0.2C_s$, . . . into the input circuit. The electrometer charge readings, if correct, should be identical to these values. One can thus quickly calibrate as many points as desired to verify linearity, and derive the corresponding correction factor(s).

3. Return the P-setting to zero to check that the electrometer again indicates zero, and hence that no charge has leaked on or off of the input circuit during the preceding sequence.

4. Close S, set the electrometer to the next charge range, and repeat steps 1 through 4, until all ranges have been calibrated.

Such a calibration should be repeated periodically (say, yearly), although significant capacitance changes are uncommon.

C. Current Measurement

The classical electrometer circuit for measuring current by a "null" method (i.e., using the electrometer only as a null-detecting voltmeter) is shown in Fig. 12.17b. Before discussing the operating procedure, the resistor R will be described.

1. HIGH-MEGOHM RESISTORS

The resistor R in Fig. 12.17b must of course be large compared to the internal resistance of the series potentiometer, and small compared to the input resistance of the electrometer. Since these two limits are usually at least ten orders of magnitude apart, they allow R to be selected simply to generate a convenient IR drop across it when the input current I passes through. For example, to obtain IR-drop values

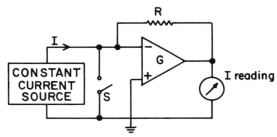

FIGURE 12.19b. Calibration method for a current-measuring feedback-controlled electrometer. The output impedance of the current source must be large compared to R.

between 0.1 and 2 V for all currents ranging from 10^{-6} to 10^{-14} A would require R-values of 10^6, 10^7, 10^8, 10^9, 10^{10}, 10^{11}, 10^{12}, and 10^{13} Ω.

Conventional carbon resistors are available in values up to 10^8 Ω; with higher values one must use so-called "high-megohm" resistors.* These are usually sealed in glass or plastic envelopes to protect them, and coated with silicone varnish to resist humidity-induced surface leakage. The silicone must be kept clean; only the metal leads may be handled.

Carbon-film-type high-megohm resistors tend to be unstable, electrically noisy, and to have high negative coefficients with respect to voltage and temperature. All of these tendencies increase with the nominal resistance value: at 10^{13} Ω the voltage coefficient is $\cong -0.1\%/V$, the temperature coefficient is $\cong -0.2\%/°C$, and calibration changes of $\sim 1\%$ are sometimes seen over short time intervals.

Metal oxide types of high-megohm resistors are generally better in all these respects, but are presently available only up to 10^{11} Ω. Resistances greater than this value are not used in most commercial electrometer circuits. Instead the IR drop of <0.1 V is amplified to provide a full-scale reading even on the 10^{-14}-A range. Another disadvantage of using larger resistances that is thereby avoided is the sluggish response that results from long RC time constants, where C is the distributed capacitance of the input circuit, including the ion chamber and cable.

2. OPERATING PROCEDURE

The sequence of steps involved in a current measurement by the circuit shown in Fig. 12.17b is as follows:

1. Select the value of R and the range of P to accommodate the current being measured. For example if a current of $\cong 3 \times 10^{-10}$ A is expected, the 10^9-Ω resistor will generate an IR drop of $\cong 0.3$ V, calling for the potentiometer to be set accordingly.

2. Select the electrometer voltage-sensitivity scale that will provide the largest

---

*Victoreen, Inc., Cleveland, Ohio; or K & M Electronics, West Springfield, Massachusetts.

possible on-scale reading when the current is flowing through R, and P is set at zero.

3. With the radiation beam turned off and P set at zero, open the input shorting switch S and set the electrometer's zero adjustment to give a zero reading, which will be taken as the null point. This compensates for any background current. (If it is desired to know the value of the background current, it can be observed separately by setting the null with S closed, then opening S and measuring the current with the radiation source turned off.)

4. Turn on the radiation source. For a constant ionization current I, a constant voltage IR will be developed across R, resulting in a constant electrometer reading. (Some random noise may be present in the signal, probably due to instability of the high-megohm resistor.) Now the potentiometer is to be adjusted to a value $P = -IR$, which brings the electrometer reading back to its null position again, since the input circuit is thus restored to the same potential it had just before the radiation was turned on. In the presence of a noisy signal this null adjustment must be a best estimate by eye, which decreases the precision possible. (Charge measurement with a capacitor is to be preferred in determining the time-averaged current with greater precision as well as accuracy.)

3. AUTOMATIC FEEDBACK OPERATION

As in the case of charge measurement with a capacitor, current measurement with a resistor can be done automatically by means of a feedback loop as in Fig. 12.18b. With negative current I flowing from the ion chamber and through R, the IR drop equals $P_i + P_0$. For an open-loop gain $G = 10^5$, $P_o = 10^5 P_i$; hence $IR = (1 + 10^{-5}) P_o \cong P_o$. The input potential P_i remains practically equal to zero.

Because R is usually a built-in resistor in the electrometer, it requires calibration *in situ*. There are usually several resistors of different orders of magnitude that can be switched into the circuit to change ranges, and each needs calibration. The output voltmeter in Fig. 12.18b is usually readable directly on a scale calibrated in amperes in place of volts when current is being measured. Thus a convenient method of calibration is to flow a known current into the electrometer input (see Fig. 12.19b) and compare it with the resulting current reading of the electrometer. This requires a constant-current source having an output impedance that is very large compared with R. The Keithley Model 261 current source is suitable for this purpose, providing currents in multiple ranges from 10^{-4} to 10^{-14} A.

As a cross-check between the current and charge calibration of a multifunction electrometer, it is advisable also to use the constant-current source to feed known currents into the electrometer input for accurately measured time intervals, with the electrometer set on the appropriate charge range. Assuming that the charge range has been correctly calibrated by the method shown in Fig. 12.19a, this current-integration check should give a charge reading in close agreement. Of the two methods the one shown in Fig. 12.19a is capable of greater accuracy, however, in case a discrepancy is observed. In fact the current source itself may be recalibrated by means of this cross-check. One should be suspicious, however, on finding serious ($>1\%$) calibration errors in the Keithley Model 261, especially on more than one range, unless it has been damaged.

If such a high-impedance current source is not available, one may simply use an ion chamber under constant irradiation to replace it in Fig. 12.19b. The correct value of its output current is first established by a measurement of the charge collected in a known time interval, using the method in Fig. 12.18a. (We assume that the electrometer's charge ranges have already been calibrated by the capacitor method shown in Fig. 12.19a.) Different-sized chambers and/or exposure rates can be used to produce suitable current levels for calibrating the various electrometer current ranges. The constancy of the current of course depends on the ambient temperature and pressure, as well as the exposure rate.

D. Atmospheric Corrections

1. AIR DENSITY

The charge or current collected from an ion chamber in a given field of radiation depends on the mass and type of gas in the chamber. If, as is most often the case, the chamber volume is open to the ambient atmosphere and is allowed to reach temperature equilibrium with its surroundings, the air density inside can be calculated from the following equation:

$$\rho = \rho_{0,760} \left[\frac{273}{273 + T(^\circ C)} \cdot \frac{P - 0.3783\, P_w}{760} \right] \qquad (12.16)$$

where $\rho_{0,760}$ is the density of dry air at at $0°C$ and 760 torr (1 atm), having a value of 1.2929 kg/m^3 or 0.0012929 g/cm^3 (note that $22°C$ and 760 torr are commonly used as reference conditions for the calibration of ion chambers); T is the Celsius temperature; P is the atmospheric pressure (torr); and P_w is the partial pressure of water vapor in the air (torr). Here 1 torr $= 1$ mm Hg $= 133.32$ Pa.

At $22°C$ the vapor pressure of water is 19.827 torr, and it increases with temperature at a rate of approximately 1.21 torr/$°C$ near that temperature. *Relative humidity* (RH) is the fraction (or more usually, percentage) of the saturated value of vapor pressure that is present. Thus at $22°C$ and 100% RH, $P_w = 19.827$ torr; at 50% RH, $P_w = 9.914$ torr, and so on. If $P = 760$ torr and $P_w = 9.914$ torr, for example, the air density calculated from Eq. 12.16 is 0.5% less than that obtained when the air is assumed to be dry ($P_w = 0$). Each 10% increase in RH evidently decreases the air density by about 0.1% at 760 torr, $22°C$.

The barometric pressure P, temperature T, and water-vapor pressure P_w all should be measured by suitable instruments located in the same room as the ion chamber. T should be measured to within $\pm 0.2°C$ at a location near the chamber, allowing adequate time for temperature equilibrium to be reached after the chamber is placed in position. P should be measured to within ± 0.5 torr. P_w should be determined within about ± 1.3 torr, through a measurement of RH within $\pm 7\%$. Such measurements will provide values of T, P, and P_w such that each will influence ρ by less than $\pm 0.07\%$, and their combined effect as independent parameters will be $\cong \pm 0.1\%$.

Since any of these parameters may vary with time, they should be remeasured at frequent enough intervals to avoid significant errors from this cause.

In practical ionization measurements the presence of humidity in air is often ignored because of the extra nuisance it involves, and because the effect of humidity on $\overline{W}/e$ is such that it works in opposition to the density change when correcting the observed ionization to the value that would result if the chamber contained dry air at 22°C, 760 torr. The resulting net error (typically $< 0.3\%$) will be discussed after the humidity effect on $\overline{W}/e$ has been described in the next subsection.

2. EFFECT OF HUMIDITY ON $(\overline{W}/e)_{\text{air}}$

For dry air exposed to x-rays or other low-LET radiation, $\overline{W}/e$ may be taken to have the value

$$(\overline{W}/e)_a = 33.97 \text{ J/C}$$

$(\overline{W}/e)_h$ for humid air is less, and the ratio $(\overline{W}/e)_h/(\overline{W}/e)_a$ has been reported by Niatel (1969) to follow the lower curve shown in Fig. 12.20. A decrease in $\overline{W}/e$ of

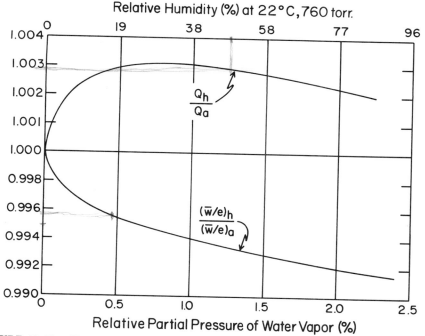

FIGURE 12.20. *Upper curve:* Ratio of the ionization Q_h produced in humid air to that (Q_a) produced in dry air, for a constant B–G cavity chamber volume, temperature, and total pressure, as a function of relative partial pressure of water vapor (bottom scale) or relative humidity (top scale). *Lower curve:* The ratio of $(\overline{W}/e)_h$ for humid air to $(\overline{W}/e)_a = 33.97$ J/C for dry air.

course means more ionization is produced by a given expenditure of energy. Evidently the effect is nonlinear, with the first 20% RH causing as much decrease in $(\overline{W}/e)_h$ as the RH change from 20% to 90%. This nonlinearity is probably related to the Jesse effect (see Section VI.F).

The upper curve in Fig. 12.20 (ICRU, 1979b) shows how the ionization Q_h produced in a B–G cavity ion chamber varies with the air humidity, assuming a constant chamber volume, temperature, and atmospheric pressure. Note that the density and mass of gas in the chamber under these conditions decrease with increasing humidity, as discussed in the preceding section. This decrease in mass tends to reduce Q_h, in opposition to the effect of $(\overline{W}/e)_h$ increasing Q_h as the humidity increases. However, the Q_h/Q_a curve in Fig. 12.20 is not simply the product $[(\overline{W}/e)_a/(\overline{W}/e)_h] \cdot (\rho_h/\rho_a)$. It will be shown as follows that the density ratio here should be replaced by a ratio of *linear* collision stopping powers.

Consider a B–G cavity chamber given identical x-irradiations when filled with (a) dry air or (b) humid air, at 22°C and 760 torr. The x-rays interact with the chamber wall to generate an electron fluence Φ crossing the cavity. In a B–G cavity these electrons are assumed to produce all the ionization observed in the cavity gas, and the gas is assumed not to perturb Φ.

The absorbed dose in the dry air is

$$D_a = \Phi\left(\frac{dT}{\rho dx}\right)_a = \frac{Q_a}{\rho_a V}\left(\frac{\overline{W}}{e}\right)_a \qquad (12.17)$$

where $(dT/\rho dx)_a$ = mass collision stopping power of the dry air with respect to the
    crossing electron fluence Φ,

$\qquad Q_a$ = charge of either sign produced in the cavity air,

$\qquad \rho_a$ = air density,

$\qquad V$ = chamber volume (constant), and

$\qquad (\overline{W}/e)_a$ = mean energy spent per unit charge produced in dry air.

The corresponding equation for absorbed dose in humid air is identical to Eq. (12.17), with subscript h replacing a. Solving both equations for Φ (which has the same value for both irradiations) and setting them equal gives

$$\Phi = \frac{Q_a}{\rho_a V}\left(\frac{\overline{W}}{e}\right)_a \frac{1}{(dT/\rho dx)_a} = \frac{Q_h}{\rho_h V}\left(\frac{\overline{W}}{e}\right)_h \frac{1}{(dT/\rho dx)_h} \qquad (12.18)$$

Cancellation of V and ρ_a simplifies this to

$$\frac{Q_h}{Q_a} = \frac{\left(\dfrac{\overline{W}}{e}\right)_a}{\left(\dfrac{\overline{W}}{e}\right)_h} \cdot \frac{\left(\dfrac{dT}{dx}\right)_h}{\left(\dfrac{dT}{dx}\right)_a} \qquad (12.19)$$

which provides the function plotted as the upper curve in Fig. 12.20. $(dT/dx)_h/(dT/$

$dx)_a$ decreases as a function of humidity only about two-thirds as fast as ρ_h/ρ_a, because the mass collision stopping power of water vapor is greater than that of air. As a result Q_h/Q_a is fortuitously flat, having a value 1.0028 ± 0.0003 over the range 15–75% RH.

3. ATMOSPHERIC CORRECTION OF AN EXPOSURE-CALIBRATED ION CHAMBER

The calibration of ion chambers in terms of x- and γ-ray exposure is a service provided by standardization laboratories such as the National Bureau of Standards and the Accredited Dosimetry Calibration Laboratories in the United States. Such calibrations are discussed generally in Chapter 13; we will only consider the atmospheric correction here.

The *exposure calibration factor* of a chamber for a specified quality of x or γ radiation is given as

$$N_X = \frac{X}{M} \tag{12.20}$$

in which X is the free-space exposure at the point occupied by the center of the chamber, and M is the charge collected from the chamber as a result of that exposure, normalized to 22°C and 760 torr. (We can ignore the effect of ionic recombination for present purposes; that will be considered in Section V).

At the time of this writing the standardization laboratories in the United States do *not* correct M for the humidity present in the air at the time of the calibration. The atmosphere in those air-conditioned laboratories is controlled to have a temperature in the neighborhood of 22°C, and the RH lies between 15% and 75%, usually around 50%. M is simply normalized to 760 torr and 22°C by the calibrating laboratory through application of the equation

$$M = M' \left(\frac{760}{P} \cdot \frac{273 + T(°C)}{273 + 22} \right) \tag{12.21}$$

where M' is the charge measured under the existing calibration conditions, and M is the corrected value to be divided into the exposure X to give the calibration factor N_X.

Since such a value of N_X is correct for typical laboratory humidity conditions, no humidity correction should be applied in using it. That is, when the chamber is used later to determine the x-ray exposure in a beam of similar quality, the measured charge M' should be corrected to 22°C, 760 torr through Eq. (12.21), then multiplied by N_X to obtain X according to Eq. (12.20). Assuming that the humidity effect is about the same ($\cong 0.3\%$) during calibration and application of the chamber (see Fig. 12.20, upper curve), its influence cancels and produces a negligible error.

In the event that a standardization laboratory is known to correct for atmospheric humidity in evaluating the factor N_X, then the user should do so also. This is done by replacing Eq. (12.21) with

$$M = M' \left(\frac{760}{P} \cdot \frac{273 + T(°C)}{273 + 22} \right) \cdot \left(\frac{Q_a}{Q_h} \right) \qquad (12.22)$$

where the value of (Q_a/Q_h) is either obtained from Fig. 12.20 if the user's air humidity is known, or estimated as $\cong 0.997$ for the typical range of humidities.

4. RELATIONSHIP OF IONIZATION TO ABSORBED DOSE IN AN ION CHAMBER

The ionization Q produced in any gas is related to the absorbed dose D in the gas by

$$D = \frac{Q}{\rho V} \cdot \frac{\overline{W}}{e} \qquad (12.23)$$

where each quantity refers to the gas under the actual conditions of the measurement. If humid air occupies the chamber, then Q is the charge (in coulombs) produced in the chamber, and ρ is the density (kg/m^3) of the humid air, as derived from Eq. (12.16). V is the chamber volume (m^3), which may usually be assumed to be independent of humidity; but for some wall materials (Nylon, A150 plastic) storage under humid conditions causes swelling, which increases V (Mijnheer et al., 1983). V is not an immediate function of the ambient humidity at the time of the measurement, however. $\overline{W}/e$ is the value appropriate for the air at the existing humidity level. From Fig. 12.20 (lower curve), it can be seen that for a relative partial vapor pressure of say, 1.0%, one has $(\overline{W}/e)_h/\overline{W}/e)_a = 0.994$. Since $(\overline{W}/e)_a = 33.97$ J/C, $(\overline{W}/e)_h = 33.8$ J/C in this case. D is the corresponding absorbed dose (J/kg) in the humid air.

Notice that in this case there are no standard conditions to which one is trying to normalize; hence only the existing conditions are relevant.

V. ION-CHAMBER SATURATION AND IONIC RECOMBINATION

A. Charge Produced vs. Charge Collected

The absorbed dose deposited in a gas by ionizing radiation is proportional to the charge Q *produced* in the gas, according to Eq. (12.23). In any practical case the charge Q' that is *collected* by the biased electrode in the chamber and measured by the electrometer circuit is less than Q, because of recombination of some positive and negative ions within the gas. An ion chamber is said to be *saturated* to the degree that such ionic recombination is absent. Increasing the ion-collecting potential applied to the chamber generally decreases recombination and asymptotically approaches saturation. Figure 12.21 illustrates the typical variation of the collected charge Q' as a function of applied potential.

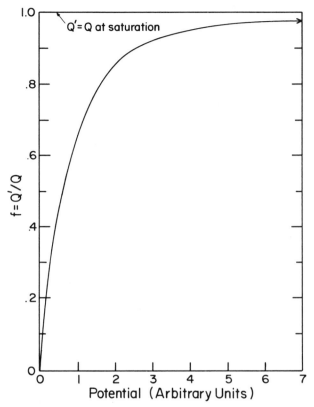

FIGURE 12.21. Variation of ionization charge Q' collected from an ion chamber vs. applied potential. Q is the charge produced by radiation.

It is not possible to increase the applied potential indefinitely to eliminate recombination altogether, because of the onset of either

a. electrical breakdown of insulators, or

b. gas multiplication, in which the free electrons gain enough kinetic energy from the electrical field within their mean free path in the gas to ionize the next atom they encounter. Thus extra ionization, not due to the ionizing radiation field, is produced. This is desired in proportional and Geiger–Müller counters, but not in ionization chambers.

Consequently it is necessary to estimate the magnitude of the charge deficiency $Q - Q'$, or of the *collection efficiency* $f = Q'/Q$, and make a correction to obtain the charge Q produced in an ion chamber. Fortunately this can be done simply in practice in most cases, assuming that the ion-chamber volume does not contain low-field ''pockets'' of persistent recombination as a result of poor geometry. For example, internal corners should be rounded, not sharp, and the ends of a cylindrical chamber should be hemispherical rather than flat.

B. Types of Recombination

1. INITIAL OR COLUMNAR RECOMBINATION

This process occurs when the $+$ and $-$ ions formed in the same charged-particle track meet and recombine. Therefore it is independent of dose or dose rate, since the number of tracks occurring per unit volume of gas does not influence the recombination within a given track, unless the space-charge density becomes so great that the electric field strength is weakened, or the tracks begin to overlap. Initial recombination is most likely to occur in densely ionized tracks, that is, for high-LET tracks such as those of α-particles. It may also be important for electron tracks in high-pressure gases, but is negligible for electrons at 1 atm or less with collecting fields > 100 V/cm.

The Jaffe–Zanstra theory (see Boag, 1966, 1986) treats this process mathematically in terms of cylindrical columns of ions; hence the alternative designation *columnar recombination*.

2. GENERAL OR VOLUME RECOMBINATION

This occurs when ions from different tracks encounter each other on their way to the collecting electrodes. Thus the amount of this type of recombination that occurs depends on how many ions are created per unit volume and per unit time. Consequently general recombination is dose-rate-dependent, since a greater density of ions of both signs moving past each other increases the probability that they will recombine.

C. Types of Gases

A free electron produced in an ionizing event may become attached to a neutral gas atom, thus making a negative *ion*. This is likely to happen in *electronegative* gases, for example, O_2, air, SF_6, Freon 12, and other gases containing even small amounts of O_2, H_2O, NH_3, HCl, SiF_4, or the halogens. It is difficult in practice to be certain that a gas is free enough of unwanted impurities to allow nonelectronegative behavior (no electron attachment). However in pure form N_2, CO_2, H_2, Ar, He, methane, ethylene, BF_3, butane, and methane-based TE gas are nonelectronegative.

In general it is much easier to saturate an ion chamber containing a nonelectronegative gas. This is because the drift velocity of a free electron under normal ambient conditions is $\sim 10^3$ cm/s per V/cm, while that of a negative ion is only about 1 cm/s per V/cm. Thus free electrons can be cleared out of the ion chamber so rapidly that they have little chance to recombine with the positive ions, even with usual applied potentials ($\sim 10^2$–10^3 V/cm). The following discussions of recombination deal with the electronegative case, which includes air.

D. Electric Field Strength vs. Chamber Geometry

1. Plane-parallel chambers have uniform field strength $\mathfrak{X} = P/d$ throughout the chamber volume (neglecting edge effects, which can be controlled by guard electrodes). Hence in the example shown in Fig. 12.22a, a potential of 100 V across a gap of $d = 2$ cm produces a homogeneous field strength of $\mathfrak{X} = 50$ V/cm.

2. Cylindrical chamber geometry can be characterized in terms of a, the radius of the outer electrode; b, the radius of the inner electrode; $\mathfrak{X}(r)$, the field strength at radius r; and the applied potential P, as indicated in Fig. 12.22b. $\mathfrak{X}(r)$ is related to the other parameters by

$$\mathfrak{X}(r) = \frac{P}{r \ln (a/b)} \tag{12.24}$$

In the example shown, if $a = 3$ cm and $b = 1$ cm, giving a separation d of 2 cm (the same as for the parallel case), a potential $P = 100$ V would result in a field strength of

$$\mathfrak{X}(r) = \frac{100}{r \ln (3/1)} = \frac{91}{r}$$

Thus $\mathfrak{X} = 91$ V/cm at $r = 1$ cm, i.e., at the inner electrode surface, 45.5 V/cm at $r = 2$ cm, and 30.3 V/cm at $r = 3$ cm, the outer wall.

3. Spherical chamber geometry is also illustrated by Fig. 12.22b. In that case the field at radius r is given by

$$\mathfrak{X}(r) = \frac{Pab}{r^2 (a - b)} \tag{12.25}$$

Hence for the same example

$$\mathfrak{X}(r) = \frac{100 \times 3 \times 1}{r^2 (3 - 1)} = \frac{150}{r^2}$$

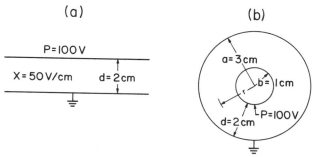

(a)   **(b)**

FIGURE 12.22.   Comparing electric field strengths in plane-parallel vs. cylindrical vs. spherical ion chambers: (a) plane-parallel geometry, (b) cylindrical or spherical geometry. P is taken as 100 V, d = 2 cm, a = 3 cm, and b = 1 cm for the examples considered.

and the field strengths are

$$\mathfrak{X}(1 \text{ cm}) = 150 \text{ V/cm} \qquad \text{(at the inner electrode)}$$

$$\mathfrak{X}(2 \text{ cm}) = 37.5 \text{ V/cm} \qquad \text{(midway between electrodes)}$$

and

$$\mathfrak{X}(3 \text{ cm}) = 16.7 \text{ V/cm} \qquad \text{(at the outer wall)}$$

The weakening of the electric field throughout a large part of the volume in cylindrical and spherical chambers, compared to plane chambers of the same electrode separation, requires a higher value of P to produce the same ion-collection efficiency, as will be discussed in the next section.

E. Boag's Treatment of Mie's Theory of General or Volume Recombination for Constant Dose Rate in an Electronegative Gas such as Air

The general equation for the charge-collection efficiency $f = Q'/Q$ for constant dose-rate in a continuous radiation field is

$$f = \frac{1}{1 + \frac{1}{6}\xi^2} \tag{12.26}$$

in any ion chamber containing electronegative gas (e.g., air), and where $f \gtrsim 0.7$.

For plane-parallel chambers, the dimensionless quantity ξ is given by

$$\xi = \sqrt{\frac{\alpha}{ek_1k_2}} \cdot \frac{d^2\sqrt{q}}{P} \equiv m\,\frac{d^2\sqrt{q}}{P} \tag{12.27}$$

where m = a gas constant, $36.7 \text{ V s}^{1/2} \text{ cm}^{-1/2} \text{ esu}^{-1/2}$ for air at STP,

d = plate separation (cm),

q = Q/vt (esu/cm^3 s),

P = applied potential (V),

α = recombination coefficient (cm^3/s),

e = electron charge = 4.8032×10^{-10} esu,

k_1 = mobility of positive ions (cm^2/Vs),

k_2 = mobility of negative ions (cm^2/Vs),

v = volume of ion chamber (cm^3), and

t = irradiation duration, assumed to be long compared to the ion-transit time of ~ 1 ms.

Here the electrostatic unit of charge (esu) is 3.3357×10^{-10} C.

Equation (12.26) for f easily reduces to

$$\frac{1}{Q'} = \frac{1}{Q} + \frac{m^2d^4}{6vt} \cdot \frac{1}{P^2} = \frac{1}{Q} + \frac{c}{P^2} \tag{12.28}$$

where $c = m^2 d^4/6vt$ is a constant. This equation predicts that $1/Q'$ values measured at several values of P can be extrapolated to $1/P^2 = 0$ to obtain $1/Q$, that is, to correct for general recombination in the case of continuous irradiation. Figure 12.23 illustrates this. Note that if Q_1' is the charge collected at a potential P_1, and Q_2' is that for potential $P_2 = P_1/2$, then $1/P_2^2 = 4/P_1^2$ and $(1/Q_1') - (1/Q) = [(1/Q_2') - (1/Q_1')]/3$; hence

$$Q = \frac{3Q_1'Q_2'}{4Q_2' - Q_1'} \quad \text{and} \quad A_{\text{ion}} \equiv \frac{Q_1'}{Q} = \frac{4}{3} - \frac{Q_1'}{3Q_2'} \qquad (\text{for} \quad P_1 = 2P_2) \quad (12.29)$$

That is, the change in reciprocal charge collected in going from P_1 to P_2 is 3 times that in going from P_1 to $P = \infty$, $(1/P = 0)$. A_{ion} is defined here in advance of its application in Chapter 13.

For cylindrical chambers Eq. (12.26) still gives the ion-collection efficiency for volume recombination, but ξ is given by

$$\xi_{\text{cyl}} = m \frac{[(a - b)K_{\text{cyl}}]^2 \sqrt{q}}{P} \qquad (12.30)$$

where a and b are the outer and inner electrode radii, respectively, as in Fig. 12.22b, and K_{cyl} is given by

$$K_{\text{cyl}} = \left\{ \frac{(a/b) + 1}{(a/b) - 1} \cdot \frac{\ln (a/b)}{2} \right\}^{1/2} \qquad (12.31)$$

For spherical-geometry chambers the corresponding ξ is given by

$$\xi_{\text{sph}} = m \frac{[(a - b) K_{\text{sph}}]^2 \sqrt{q}}{P} \qquad (12.32)$$

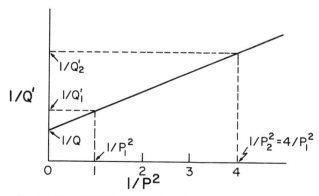

FIGURE 12.23.   Graph of Eq. (12.28), illustrating the extrapolation of $1/Q'$ vs. $1/P^2$ to $1/P^2 = 0$, yielding $1/Q$. Thus the charge Q produced can be determined for the case of continuous radiation with general recombination occurring in an electronegative gas.

in which K_{sph} is defined as

$$K_{sph} = \left\{ \frac{1}{3} \left(\frac{a}{b} + 1 + \frac{b}{a} \right) \right\}^{1/2} \tag{12.33}$$

In cylindrical and spherical geometries, increasing the applied potential to a value of $K_{cyl}^2 P$ or $K_{sph}^2 P$, respectively, produces the same collection efficiency as for a plane chamber with $d = a - b$ and potential P. For the example in Section D, where $a = 3$ cm, $b = 1$ cm, and $P = 100$ V, $K_{cyl}^2 P = 110$ V and $K_{sph}^2 P = 144$ V.

F. Extrapolation for Initial Recombination

In case volume recombination is negligible and only initial recombination remains, the Jaffe–Zanstra theory predicts for an electronegative gas that

$$\frac{1}{Q'} = \frac{1}{Q} + \frac{c'}{P} \tag{12.34}$$

where c' is a constant and P is the applied potential. Thus in this case the type of plot shown in Fig. 12.24 is used in obtaining Q. Note that for $P_2 = P_1/2$,

$$\frac{1}{Q_1'} - \frac{1}{Q} = \frac{1}{Q_2'} - \frac{1}{Q_1'} \tag{12.35}$$

That is, the change in reciprocal charge collected in going from P_2 to P_1 is the same as that from P_1 to $P = \infty$ in this case. Note that a straight-line region of $1/Q'$ vs. $1/P$ occurs when the potential gets large enough to virtually eliminate volume recombination, leaving some initial recombination. As mentioned before, this is only significant for high-LET radiation, high-pressure gas, or both.

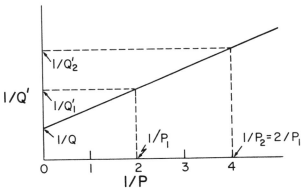

FIGURE 12.24. Graph of Eq. (12.34), illustrating the extrapolation of $1/Q'$ vs. $1/P$ to $1/P = 0$, yielding $1/Q$. Thus the charge Q can be determined for initial recombination with either pulsed or continuous radiation, or for general recombination with pulsed radiation only, in an electronegative gas.

G. Pulsed Radiation

Boag and Currant (1980) have recently updated Boag's earlier (1966) treatment of ionic recombination for pulsed radiation in electronegative gases. The pulses are assumed to be short compared to the ion transit time ($\sim 10^{-3}$ s), and the repetition rate must be slow enough so ions can clear out between pulses. Boag (1986) has discussed the problems of overlapping pulses and long pulses. For the case where many pulses occur during the ion transit time, one can approximate by using the continuous radiation theory of ionic recombination, referred to the *time-averaged* value for q in Eq. (12.27), or extrapolating according to Fig. 12.23. If pulses are very long compared to the transit time, continuous radiation theory obviously applies, where q is the value existing *during* the pulse or pulses.

In Boag's treatment of short pulses,

$$f = \frac{1}{u} \ln (1 + u) \qquad (12.36)$$

where

$$u = \frac{\alpha/e}{k_1 + k_2} \cdot \frac{\rho d^2}{P} \qquad (12.37)$$

in which ρ is the initial charge density of positive or negative ions created by a pulse of radiation (esu/cm^3), d is the electrode spacing (cm), and the other quantities are as previously defined. For cylindrical or spherical chambers, d is to be replaced by $(a - b)K_{cyl}$ or $(a - b)K_{sph}$, respectively.

Boag and Currant have shown that simply measuring the charges collected (Q_1', Q_2') at two different applied potentials (P_1, P_2) can yield an accurate value of f for pulsed radiation, as follows:

Assuming n pulses of fixed size ρ are measured in each run, the charge generated, of either sign is $Q = nv\rho$; hence

$$f_1 = \frac{Q_1'}{Q} = \frac{1}{u_1} \ln (1 + u_1), \qquad (12.38)$$

$$f_2 = \frac{Q_2'}{Q} = \frac{1}{u_2} \ln (1 + u_2) \qquad (12.39)$$

The ratio of Eq. (12.38) to Eq. (12.39) is

$$\frac{f_1}{f_2} = \frac{Q_1'}{Q_2'} = \frac{u_2 \ln (1 + u_1)}{u_1 \ln (1 + u_2)} \qquad (12.40)$$

or

$$\frac{Q_1'}{Q_2'} = \frac{P_1}{P_2} \frac{\ln (1 + u_1)}{\ln (1 + u_1 P_1/P_2)} \qquad (12.41)$$

since from Eq. (12.37)

$$u_1 = \frac{k}{P_1} \quad \text{and} \quad u_2 = \frac{k}{P_2} \tag{12.42}$$

where k is a constant. u_1 can then be solved for in Eq. (12.41) and employed in Eq. (12.38) to obtain f_1, the ion collection efficiency for voltage P_1; and Q, the charge produced in the gas.

For near-saturation conditions ($f > 0.96$), the simple $1/Q'$-vs.-$1/P$ graph shown in Fig. 12.24 is correct also for pulsed radiation. Furthermore, by using $P_2 = P_1/2$ one can again take advantage of the simple relationship in Eq. (12.35) to obtain the value of Q from the following equation:

$$Q \cong \frac{Q_1' Q_2'}{2Q_2' - Q_1'} \quad \text{(for } P_1 = 2P_2, f > 0.96) \tag{12.43}$$

The AAPM protocol (1983) has provided a graph of P_{ion}, the reciprocal of the ion-collection efficiency f at the given chamber voltage P_1, as a function of the charge ratio Q_1'/Q_2' observed when the voltage is halved to $P_2 = P_1/2$. Data are given for continuous radiation, pulsed radiation, and a pulsed *and* magnetically scanned electron beam (Boag, 1982). This figure is reproduced in Fig. 12.25. Simple mathematical statements of these curves have been provided elsewhere (Attix, 1984a).

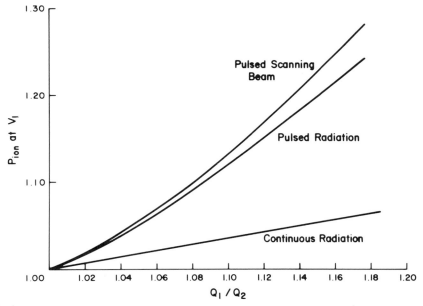

FIGURE 12.25. Ionization-recombination correction factors (P_{ion}) $\equiv Q/Q_1'$ for continuous radiation, pulsed radiation, and pulsed scanning electron beams. P_{ion}-values apply to the chamber potential P_1 when Q_1'/Q_2' is the collected charge ratio for potentials $P_1/P_2 = 2$. (AAPM, 1983. Reproduced with permission from R. J. Schulz and The American Institute of Physics.)

In conclusion, one should keep in mind that if saturation losses are excessive, the chamber may be malfunctioning (e.g., poor HV connection, or short to ground). Besides electrical continuity checks, a radiograph of the chamber may reveal a fault. If the chamber is found to be normal, the substitution of pure N_2 (or other non-electronegative gas) for air (e.g., by flowing) will greatly decrease the amount of recombination observed. Boag (1986) and Bielajew (1985) have discussed the effect of incomplete attachment of electrons in electronegative gases in small chambers, at low pressures and/or with high electric fields.

VI. IONIZATION, EXCITATION, AND *W*

A. Definition of *W* and $\overline{W}$

An atom can be ionized in a variety of ways, but collision by charged particles interacting with the atomic electrons through Coulomb forces is the most important in dosimetry, since the dose is deposited almost entirely by charged particles. Such collisions also produce excitation of atoms, in which an electron is raised to a higher energy level, and this energy is also part of the dose. The energy going into excitation decreases the ionization efficiency of a charged particle, so that one cannot compute the number of ions by dividing the initial kinetic energy T_0 by the ionization potential of an atom (i.e., minimum energy to ionize). Instead this efficiency is expressed in terms of *W*, the mean energy (in eV) spent by a charged particle of initial energy T_0 in producing each ion pair:

$$W = \frac{T_0}{\overline{N}} \tag{12.44}$$

where $\overline{N}$ is the expectation value of the number of ion pairs produced by such a particle stopping in the medium (usually a gas) to which *W* refers.

Alternatively *W* was also defined by the ICRU (1971) as

$$W = \frac{T_0(1 - g)}{N(1 - g')} \tag{12.45}$$

where *g* is the fraction of T_0 spent by the particle in bremsstrahlung production, and g' is the fractional number of ion pairs produced by the bremsstrahlung. This definition assumes the escape of the bremsstrahlung; therefore it is consistent with the definition of exposure in any dosimetry situation in which the bremsstrahlung energy is lost from the system.

For a large number *n* of charged particles having a multiplicity of starting energies, an average value of $\overline{W}$ may be defined as in Chapter 2, Section V.B, Eq. (2.21):

$$\overline{W} = \frac{\displaystyle\sum_{i=1}^{n} T_i(1 - g_i)}{\displaystyle\sum_{i=1}^{n} N_i(1 - g_i')} \tag{12.46}$$

where $T_i(1 - g_i)$ is the kinetic energy of the ith particle, exclusive of energy given to bremsstrahlung, and $N_i(1 - g_i')$ is the number of ion pairs created by the ith particle, exclusive of ionization resulting from the bremsstrahlung.

For charged particles heavier than electrons, g_i and g_i' in Eqs. (12.45) and (12.46) may be taken as zero. Furthermore $g_i \cong g_i'$ for electrons if T_i is high enough so that W is constant.

When one speaks of a $\overline{W}$-value for uncharged radiation (photons or neutrons), the definition in Eq. (12.46), applied to all the secondary charged particles that result from the interactions by the uncharged radiation in the medium in question, is what is commonly meant, assuming that bremsstrahlung escapes. If bremsstrahlung energy is to be included, Eq. (12.46) still applies, but with g_i and g_i' set equal to zero.

B. Calculation of *W*

In general W cannot be calculated for a gas, because of lack of knowledge of the relevant physical quantities. However, Robert Platzman (1961), who is responsible for much of our understanding of the role of excitation and ionization in dosimetry, was able to calculate W for helium. He wrote the following energy conservation equation for an electron stopping in He:

$$T_0 = \overline{N_i E_i} + \overline{N_{ex} E_{ex}} + \overline{N_i E_{se}} \qquad (12.47)$$

where T_0 = initial kinetic energy of the electron,

$\overline{N_i}$ = mean number of ion pairs (ionized atoms and free electrons) produced,

$\overline{E_i}$ = mean energy of an ionized atom,

$\overline{N_{ex}}$ = mean number of excited atoms produced,

$\overline{E_{ex}}$ = mean energy of an excited atom,

$\overline{E_{se}}$ = mean energy of subexcitation electrons (which degrades to heat through elastic collision in atomic gases, and also through rotational and vibrational modes in molecular gases).

The equation for W is

$$W = \frac{T_0}{\overline{N_i}} = \overline{E_i} + \frac{\overline{N_{ex}}}{\overline{N_i}} \overline{E}_{ex} + \overline{E}_{se} \qquad (12.48)$$

From theoretical atomic physics for helium Platzman derived the following values for the quantities on the right:

$$\overline{E}_i = 25.9 \text{ eV} \qquad\qquad = 62\% \text{ of } W$$

$$\overline{E}_{ex}\left(\frac{\overline{N_{ex}}}{\overline{N_i}}\right) = 20.8 \text{ eV} \times 0.40 = 20\% \text{ of } W$$

$$\overline{E}_{se} = 7.6 \text{ eV} \qquad\qquad = 18\% \text{ of } W$$

Hence $W = 41.8$ eV, which approximately equals the value (41.3 eV) obtained experimentally for pure He.

It will be seen that in this case about three-fifths of the energy spent goes into ionization, one-fifth into excitation, and a similar fraction is lost to subexcitation electrons, which heat the gas without creating further excitation or ionization. All three components are included in the energy imparted as absorbed dose. However, $\overline{E}_{se}$ has no biological consequences, and $\overline{E}_{ex}$ certainly has much less effect than $\overline{E}_i$ per unit energy spent.

Table 12.1 compares first ionization potentials (E_1) with measured values of W for several gases. It can be seen that the ratio of E_1 to W_e (for electrons) tends to have a value of about 0.58 ± 0.03 for the noble gases, and a somewhat lower value (0.43 ± 0.02) for the molecular gases. This is an indication that the ionization efficiency is lower in the molecular gases, which have more excitation modes than the noble gases.

C. Experimental Measurement of *W* or $\overline{W}$

In measuring W for a gas, charged particles of known kinetic energy T_0 are allowed to run their full range within an ion chamber containing the gas. The particles are counted (n), and simultaneously the ionization charge Q that they produce is measured. A typical apparatus is shown schematically in Fig. 12.26.

The value of W/e is given in J/C by

$$\frac{W}{e} = \frac{nT_0}{Q}$$

(12.49)

where T_0 is expressed in joules and Q in coulombs.

If the particles are not monoenergetic, their average energy $\overline{T}_0$ is substituted in Eq. (12.49) thus determining $\overline{W}/e$.

TABLE 12.1 First Atomic Ionization Potentials E_1 and W-Values in Several Gases for Electrons (W_e) and for 5-*MeV* α-Particles (W_α)

Gas	E_1 (eV)[b]	W_e (eV/i.p.)[a]	$\dfrac{E_1}{W_e}$	W_α (eV/i.p.)[a]	$\dfrac{W_\alpha}{W_e}$
He	24.6	41.3	0.60	42.7	1.034
Ne	21.6	35.4	0.61	36.8	1.040
Ar	15.8	26.4	0.60	26.4	1.000
Kr	14.0	24.4	0.57	24.1	0.988
Xe	12.1	22.1	0.55	21.9	0.991
H_2	15.4	36.5	0.42	36.43	0.998
N_2	15.6	34.8	0.45	36.39	1.046
O_2	12.1	30.8	0.39	36.39	1.047
CO_2	13.8	33.0	0.42	34.21	1.037

[a] Excerpted from ICRU (1979b). Reproduced with permission.
[b] Excerpted from the *Handbook of Chemistry and Physics*, 64th edition, CRC Press, Inc. (1983). Reproduced with permission.

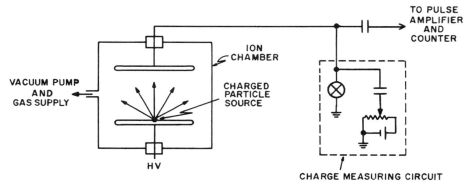

FIGURE 12.26. Schematic diagram of an experimental setup for measuring W/e.

In place of a simple ion chamber, a proportional counter of gas gain G may be required to give pulses large enough to count. The measured charge must then be divided by the gain factor G in determining W/e.

If the charged particles being employed in the experiment are electrons, the bremsstrahlung produced practically all escapes from the chamber, which is made just large enough to accommodate the electron ranges. Thus Q does not include a significant amount of ionization from bremsstrahlung, and T_0 alone must therefore be diminished accordingly:

$$\frac{W}{e} = \frac{nT_0(1 - g)}{Q/G} \tag{12.50}$$

where Q is shown also corrected for the gain factor, assuming that a proportional counter is used.

Typical values of g can be gotten for monoenergetic electrons from the "Radiation Yield" column in Appendix E. In air, $g = 0.004$ for $T_0 = 1$ MeV and 0.04 for $T_0 = 10$ MeV.

D. Energy Dependence of W

W is practically constant above energies for which the charged-particle velocity v is more than 10 times the velocity v_0 of an electron in the first Bohr orbit, where

$$v_0 \cong \frac{2\pi e^2}{h} \tag{12.51}$$

and h is Planck's constant. For lower values of v_0, W tends to increase because of the decreasing probability of ionizing reactions. This trend is most pronounced in non-noble gases.

Experimentally it is found that over the electron range above 1 keV, W varies by $\cong 2\%$ or less, and above 10 keV, W is found to be constant. That constancy is assumed in most cases involving photons or electrons, for which a low-LET radiation value is tabulated for a variety of gases in ICRU (1979b) and Myers (1968).

E. Dependence of *W* on Type of Radiation

Table 12.1 also lists W_α-values obtained with 5-MeV α-particles. These values tend to be approximately equal to, or 3–5% greater than, the low-LET values W_e. For most non-noble gases $W_\alpha > W_e$ by a few percent. Few W_p-values for protons have been obtained, and those are generally thought to be less reliable than the W_α-values. Consequently, where W_p is not reliably known for a gas, W_α is usually substituted.

Additional information can be found in ICRU (1979b).

F. *W* for Gas Mixtures

Approximately,

$$\left(\frac{1}{W}\right)_{mix} \cong \sum_i \left(\frac{P_i}{P} \cdot \frac{1}{W_i}\right) \tag{12.52}$$

where P_i is the partial pressure of the *i*th gas species, and P is the total pressure of the mixture. Hence P_i/P is the fractional number of molecules of each type present.

A more accurate mixing formula, including empirical weighting factors, is described in ICRU (1979b).

The noble gases have *W*-values that are very sensitive to the presence of impurity gases that have a lower first ionization potential E_i than an excitation energy level of the gas. The latter energy is channeled into additional ionization, and *W* is thus reduced in impure noble gases. For example, for helium $E_1 = 24.5$ eV, and this gas has a metastable excited level of 19.8 eV. For oxygen, $E_1 = 12.5$ eV, and for nitrogen $E_1 = 15.6$ eV. Both are below 19.8 eV. Thus if an excited He atom collides with an impurity molecule of O_2 or N_2 (or many other gases), the latter will be ionized. This extra ionization lowers the value of *W*. Jesse and Sadauskis (1952) first explained this effect.

G. "*W*" in Semiconductors

When a gas is condensed to a solid, the discrete energy levels of the isolated atoms broaden into conduction and valence energy bands in the solid. The energy gap E_g between valence and conduction bands is typically ~1 eV in semiconductors vs. ionization potentials of >10 eV in gases. Similarly to the situation in a gas, though, the energy spent by a charged particle is divided between electron–hole pairs (corresponding to ion pairs in a gas), phonon production (like excitation in a gas), and subexcitation electrons. The "*W*" value in Si at 300 K is 3.62 eV for α's and 3.68 for electrons, and in Ge at 77 K it is 2.97 eV for both.

PROBLEMS

1. A conventional standard free-air chamber has a diaphragm aperture 1.30 cm in diameter, and a collector plate 12.0 cm long, separated from the guard plates

by 0.5-mm gaps. The distance from the diaphragm to the front edge of the collector plate is 30 cm. The dry air in the chamber is at 23.1°C, 755 torr, and $(\mu/\rho)_{air} = 0.155$ cm^2/g. $f_e = 0.001$, and $f_s = 0.004$. Calculate the exposure at the diaphragm for a charge $Q = 6.17 \times 10^{-7}$ C (corrected for ionic recombination). Give the answer in C/kg and roentgens.

2. What is the effective atomic number of water, with respect to the photoelectric effect?

3. A condenser ion chamber is charged to $P_1 = 300$ V, then connected to the input of a high-gain charge-integrating electrometer such as that in Fig. 12.18a, giving a charge reading of $Q_1 = 3.70 \times 10^{-9}$ C. The procedure is repeated, this time giving the chamber an x-ray exposure of 10 R before reading out the charge at $Q_2 = 3.17 \times 10^{-9}$ C. Repeating again with an exposure of 20 R, the charge is $Q_3 = 2.65 \times 10^{-9}$ C. Repeating again with 40 R, the charge is $Q_4 = 1.71 \times 10^{-9}$ C.

    (a) Calculate the charge collected in the chamber per roentgen for each exposure.

    (b) What are the voltages corresponding to Q_2, Q_3, and Q_4?

    (c) What can you conclude about the collecting potential being used?

4. What are the capacitance and the collecting volume of a guarded flat chamber having a circular collecting region 2.5 cm in diameter, if an applied potential of 300 V is found to induce a charge of 5.21×10^{-10} C?

5. A 1-MV x-ray beam has a tissue dose rate of $\cong 1$ Gy/min at a point of interest where CPE exists. Employing a 0.1-cm^3 air-equivalent chamber at 760 torr and 22°C, what would be an appropriate high-megohm input-resistor value for exposure-rate measurements, assuming the balancing potential must remain below 2 V? For 1-min exposure periods, what would be an appropriate input-capacitor value for exposure measurements?

6. (a) What is the density of air at 650 torr, 23.5°C, 45% RH?

    (b) What is $(\overline{W}/e)_{air}$ for low-LET radiation at this humidity?

    (c) What is the percentage error in the density if the humidity is assumed to be zero?

    (d) Assume that a charge of 8.65×10^{-10} C is measured from a cavity chamber filled with the air in part (a). For the same irradiation, what charge would be measured if the chamber were filled with dry air at 760 torr, 22°C?

    (e) What is the absorbed dose in the humid air in (d) if the chamber volume is 3 cm^3 and recombination is nil?

7. (a) What potential should be applied to an air-filled cylindrical ion chamber, in which the collecting rod has a diameter of 3 mm and the wall an inside diameter of 1.5 cm, to obtain the same ion-collection efficiency as would exist in a flat chamber having the same interelectrode separation and an applied potential P? (Assume Mie-Boag theory).

(b) If the cylindrical chamber is air-equivalent, has a volume of 5 cm³ filled with air at STP, is operated with a collecting potential of 25 V, and is continuously exposed to x rays at 120 R/min, calculate the charge-collection efficiency f.

(c) Recalculate f if the potential is doubled.

(d) From the answers to (b) and (c), calculate the saturated charge (per unit time) from Eq. (12.29), and compare it with the value known from the exposure rate.

8. An ion chamber is exposed to pulsed radiation. A charge of 7.05×10^{-8} C is collected with an applied potential of 200 V, and 5.51×10^{-8} C at 90 V. Calculate the charge produced in the chamber. (*Hint:* You may solve for u_1 graphically or numerically.)

9. Another ion chamber is exposed to pulsed radiation. 6.65×10^{-9} C is collected at 400 V; 6.40×10^{-9} C at 200 V. Calculate the charge produced.

SOLUTIONS TO PROBLEMS

1. 3.27×10^{-2} C/kg, 126.7 R.
2. 7.5.
3. **(a)** 5.30×10^{-11}, 5.25×10^{-11}, 4.98×10^{-11} C/R.
   (b) P_2: 257 V; P_3: 215 V; P_4: 139 V.
   (c) Inadequate to approximate saturation over this exposure range; hence ΔQ vs. exposure is nonlinear.
4. 1.74 pF, 1.23 cm³.
5. 3×10^{10} Ω, 10^{-8} F.
6. **(a)** 1.012 kg/m³.
   (b) 33.7 J/C.
   (c) ρ is 0.6% too high.
   (d) 1.014×10^{-9} C.
   (e) 9.60×10^{-3} Gy.
7. **(a)** $1.21P$
   (b) 0.88.
   (c) 0.967.
   (d) 10 esu/s.
8. 9.61×10^{-8} C.
9. 6.92×10^{-9} C.

CHAPTER 13

Dosimetry and Calibration of Photon and Electron Beams with Cavity Ion Chambers

I. INTRODUCTION

The convenience, precision, and tissue relevance of low-Z cavity ion chambers makes them a natural choice for the calibration and routine dosimetry of radiation beams, especially for radiotherapy application. Their design and electrical characteristics were discussed in Chapter 12. In the present chapter the use of such chambers for photon- and electron-beam dosimetry will be considered. The special problems arising in neutron-beam dosimetry are best dealt with in a separate chapter (16).

Ion chambers can be employed as absolute or as calibrated dosimeters. Three approaches to their calibration are currently being used: exposure, "N_{gas}," and absorbed-dose calibrations. Finally, beam dosimetry can be done in free space as well as in a phantom, and in the latter case a correction must be made for field perturbation by the insertion of the chamber. All these cases will be discussed in this chapter.

II. ABSOLUTE CAVITY ION CHAMBERS

Cavity theory (see Chapter 10) provides a means of calculating the absorbed dose in the wall of a cavity chamber from a knowledge of the absorbed dose D_{gas} in the cavity gas. The value of D_{gas} (there called D_g) is given by Eq. (10.7). If the mass of gas, m_g, in the cavity is known without resorting to calibration in a known radiation field, then the ion chamber is regarded as an absolute dosimeter. We assume that electric charge can be measured absolutely.

To know m_g in this way requires evaluation of (a) the effective volume V_g from

346

which the ionization is collected, and (b) the gas density. V_g usually cannot be measured with sufficient accuracy except for large (e.g., > 10 cm^3) ion chambers that are machined to precise dimensions. The limitation on the accuracy of determining V_g depends upon the chamber design. If any of the generated charge is collected on the grounded guard ring or is allowed to recombine in a locally weak pocket of the electric field, the effective volume will be smaller than the physical volume. Nevertheless this absolute approach is feasible, and is used especially by the national laboratories in making instruments for calibrating their standard ^{60}Co and ^{137}Cs γ-ray beams. Graphite walls are used at these energies to approximate air equivalence, allowing calibrations to be expressed in terms of exposure rates or air kerma rates. Note also the close matching of wall and gas places little dependence on a knowledge of the wall–gas stopping-power ratio, which closely approximates unity in this case.

Ion chambers used in most dosimetry applications are manufactured commercially and are not constructed with exactly known effective volumes. Hence they require calibration by methods to be discussed.

An absolute cavity chamber can be employed in the same way as will be described for chambers calibrated in terms of "N_{gas}," except that N_{gas} for that case is simply equal to $(\overline{W}/e)_g m_g^{-1}$ [see Eq. (13.2a)].

III.   CALIBRATION OF ION CHAMBERS USING X-RAYS OR γ-RAYS

National laboratories, such as the National Bureau of Standards (NBS) in the United States, maintain standard ionization chambers and calibrated γ-ray beams. Regional calibration laboratories (such as the Accredited Dosimetry Calibration Laboratories in the United States) are closely linked to the national standards through frequent recalibrations of high-quality ion chambers. Routine instruments are generally calibrated for a fee at one of the regional laboratories, except in special cases when the facilities at a national laboratory are required. The addresses of the active ADCLs can be obtained either from the Center for Radiation Research of the NBS, or from the American Association of Physicists in Medicine (AAPM).

A.   Exposure Calibration of Ion Chambers

1.   WITH X-RAYS GENERATED AT 10–300 kV

In this energy range a cavity chamber is calibrated either by direct comparison with a standard free-air ionization chamber such as discussed in Chapter 12, or by indirect comparison through a secondary standard cavity chamber. Calibration laboratories make available a selection of beam qualities, specified in terms of kilovoltage and the first and second half-value layers in Al or Cu. Ion chambers should be calibrated for x-ray beam qualities simulating as closely as possible those for which the chamber will be used.

Chamber wall-thickness requirements were discussed in Chapter 12. For photon measurements the wall must always be made at least as thick as the maximum range of the electrons present, to provide CPE and keep out stray electrons. For x-rays below 300 keV the photoelectric effect is important enough so that wall thicknesses are chosen with that in mind. Conservatively one makes the thickness equal to the CSDA range of an electron having the same energy as the photon that produces it. For a 300-keV electron, for example, 0.086 g/cm^2 of polystyrene (or ~0.8 mm at $\rho = 1.06$ g/cm^3) is required. For ^{60}Co γ-rays, the maximum energy of a Compton electron is 1.116 MeV for the 1.33-MeV photons, and the wall of an ion chamber is customarily designed to provide CPE for those electrons. This would require 0.513 g/cm^2 (usually rounded upward to 0.52 g/cm^2) of polystyrene, or 4.9 mm.

Customarily cavity chambers are made with walls thick enough to provide CPE for x-rays up to 300 keV, requiring the addition of a slip-on plastic "buildup cap" to provide adequate wall thickness when the chamber is used for ^{60}Co γ-rays. Orthovoltage and lower x-ray calibrations are performed with the cap removed, unless otherwise specified. The attenuation of x-rays in common plastics such as Lucite and polystyrene increases sharply below 50 keV due to the photoelectric effect. Thus for dosimetry of x-ray beams having an appreciable component below that energy, such as x-rays used in mammography, thinner chamber walls are indicated. The CSDA range of a 50-keV electron in polystyrene is only about 42 μm.

The calibration procedure calls for the positioning of the ion chamber with its central point on the x-ray beam axis at a location P where the exposure rate in free space is known. That is, dX/dt is the exposure rate at P with the chamber removed. For cylindrical or spherical chambers the axis of the collecting electrode is oriented perpendicular to the beam, as in Fig. 13.1A. Flat chambers are placed perpendicular to the beam with the collecting electrode toward the rear (i.e., away from the source). The point P in that case is conventionally taken to be either midway between the chamber walls, as shown in Fig. 13.1B, or centered on the inner surface of the wall through which the beam enters.

The chamber is irradiated in this position for a measured time interval to deliver the free-space exposure X at the reference point P, in units of C/kg or roentgens. The measured charge reading (in coulombs or arbitrary scale divisions) is M, corrected to 22°C and one standard atmosphere for vented chambers according to Eq. (12.21) or (12.22).

Humidity effects on ion-chamber measurements have been discussed in Section IV.D of Chapter 12. The advice of the standardization laboratory, as indicated on the chamber calibration certificate, should be followed in this matter.

Naturally, no atmospheric correction is applied to sealed ion chambers, so long as the seal is intact.

The *exposure calibration factor* for an ion chamber is defined as

$$N_X = \frac{X}{M} \tag{13.1}$$

where N_X is stated in R/C, R/(scale division), kg^{-1}, or C kg^{-1}/(scale division). N_X applies specifically to the conditions under which it was obtained, including the voltage and polarity of the ion-collecting potential used. Note that neither M nor N_X

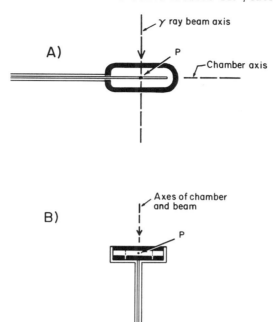

Figure 13.1. Ion-chamber calibration geometry in free space relative to beam axis and reference point *P*: (*A*) cylindrical or spherical chamber; (*B*) flat pillbox chamber, for which *P* may be alternatively located on the axis at the inner surface of the wall through which the beam passes instead of at the chamber center.

conventionally includes a correction for ion-recombination losses. So long as those losses are small (typically $<0.5\%$ for most $\sim 1\text{-cm}^3$ chambers with 300 V or more applied, at exposure rates <100 R/min), it will be satisfactory simply to use the chamber with the same voltage and polarity applied as used in its calibration. However, for best accuracy recombination losses should be corrected for. For that purpose the calibration should be obtained with at least two voltages and both polarities (say, ± 300 and ± 150 V). This will allow evaluation of the ion-collection efficiency $f = Q'/Q$ (as discussed in Chapter 12, Section V) as well as verifying that no unusual polarity differences exist due to ionization in cables, etc. It will be seen also in Section III.B of the present chapter that the ion-collection efficiency f, renamed A_{ion} in the AAPM (1983) protocol, must be evaluated to allow determination of the quantity N_{gas}. For this purpose it is recommended that the charge be measured at two applied potentials P_1 and P_2 such that $P_1 = 2P_2$, obtaining the corresponding collected charges Q'_1 and Q'_2, respectively. Then from Eq. (12.29), assuming that the calibration radiation is continuous, we have

$$A_{ion} = \frac{Q'_1}{Q} = \frac{4}{3} - \frac{Q'_1}{3Q'_2} \tag{13.1a}$$

This equation equals the reciprocal of the "continuous radiation" curve in Fig. 12.25, since $P_{ion} \equiv A_{ion}^{-1}$ for identical irradiations.

Another important consideration in the calibration is the electrometer. If the chamber, such as the Victoreen r-meter, is to be used with a "dedicated" electrometer that reads directly in roentgens, then the two are sent to the laboratory and calibrated together as a set. The value of N_X in that case would typically be a number near 1 R/(scale division). The calibration therefore belongs to the chamber + electrometer set, not to the ion chamber alone.

If an ion chamber is sent in alone for calibration, its charge output will be measured by means of a well-calibrated electrometer routinely used for that purpose by the calibration laboratory. The value of N_X for a ~ 1-cm^3 air-equivalent chamber would be typically $\sim 3 \times 10^9$ R/C or $\sim 8 \times 10^5$ kg^{-1}. The calibration is then effectively only as good as the accuracy of the electrometer to be used with the chamber at the field laboratory. If that accuracy is in doubt, it is advisable to have the electrometer electrically calibrated, which can usually be done also at the same calibration laboratory.

A less-important parameter of the calibration is the x-ray beam size used. For well-designed ion chambers with minimal radiation-induced insulator leakage (see Chapter 12, Section III.A.5) the beam size does not significantly influence N_X. Nevertheless, it is specified by calibration laboratories, and is usually 10 $\times$ 10 cm square or 10 cm in diameter; hence approximately 5 cm of the chamber connecting stem is in the beam during calibration under normal conditions.

2. EXPOSURE CALIBRATIONS OF ION CHAMBERS WITH ^{137}Cs AND ^{60}Co γ-RAYS

The preceding discussion of the exposure calibration of cavity chambers for x-rays at < 300 kV applies equally well for ^{137}Cs and ^{60}Co γ-rays, with the exception that the free-air chamber is replaced by the absolute graphite cavity chamber as a standard. ^{137}Cs γ-rays, having an energy of 0.662 MeV, are used much less frequently than ^{60}Co γ-rays (1.17 and 1.33 MeV) as a calibration source for ion chambers. ^{60}Co buildup caps are often used on chambers also for ^{137}Cs calibrations, even though they are thicker than necessary for that radiation.

^{60}Co γ-rays are commonly used not only to calibrate ion chambers for use in ^{60}Co γ-ray dosimetry, but also for higher-energy photon and electron beams, by methods to be described in Sections IV–VI. Moreover the exposure calibration factor of a B–G chamber can be estimated for ^{137}Cs γ-rays by applying a small correction to the ^{60}Co calibration factor, as described in Section IV.A.2.a.

B. N_{gas} Calibration of Ion Chambers

It was pointed out in Chapter 11, Section III.F.1.c, that one especially useful mode of calibrating dosimeters is in terms of the energy absorbed in the matter constituting the sensitive volume of the dosimeter itself. Thus a given dosimeter reading signifies a certain value of the average absorbed dose in the dosimeter's sensitive volume.

That can in turn be related to the dose in another medium that replaces the dosimeter at the same location, through application of cavity theory and/or through a ratio of mass energy-absorption coefficients. Such a calibration has the advantage of being directly applicable to all ionizing radiations for which the same dosimeter reading results from a given average absorbed dose in the sensitive volume.

This argument applies as well to the gas in cavity ion chambers, suggesting that a calibration of the charge produced as a result of a given average absorbed dose in the cavity gas would be applicable to all ionizing radiations for which $\overline{W}/e$ were constant, that is, all low-LET radiations, including photons and electrons above ~ 10 keV. The practical limitation of this approach is that relating the dose in the cavity gas to that in some other medium of interest requires application of cavity theory. As the photon energy is reduced below ~ 100 keV, the secondary-electron ranges become comparable with typical cavity dimensions, and simple cavity theory (e.g., B–G or Spencer) becomes inapplicable. Burlin theory may be employed, with some added complication. However, if the cavity chamber design includes significant amounts of more than one wall material (e.g., carbon walls and an aluminum collecting electrode), present cavity theories are invalid.

Such an approach to chamber calibration has been employed in a protocol for the determination of the absorbed dose delivered in phantoms by high-energy photon and electron beams. That protocol was developed for radiotherapy applications by the AAPM (1983) on the basis of a formalism by Loevinger (1981). The protocol defines a quantity called the *cavity-gas calibration factor*, which is symbolized by N_{gas} and given in units of Gy/C or Gy/(scale division). N_{gas} can be written as

$$N_{gas} = \frac{D_{gas} A_{ion}}{M} \tag{13.2}$$

where M is the electrometer reading at calibration, in coulombs or scale divisions, A_{ion} is the ion-collection efficiency at calibration, and D_{gas} is the corresponding mean absorbed dose in the cavity gas, in grays.

For an absolute cavity chamber Eq. (13.2) reduces to

$$N_{gas} = \frac{1}{m_g}\left(\frac{\overline{W}}{e}\right)_g \qquad \text{(Gy/C)} \tag{13.2a}$$

when Eq. (10.7), rewritten as $D_{gas} = M A_{ion}^{-1} m_g^{-1}\,(\overline{W}/e)_g$, is substituted for D_{gas}. For example, a 1-cm^3 chamber filled with dry air at 760 torr, 22°C, would have

$$N_{gas} = \frac{33.97 \text{ J/C}}{1.1965 \times 10^{-6} \text{ kg}} = 2.839 \times 10^7 \text{ Gy/C}$$

While air is certainly the most commonly used cavity gas, other gases may be substituted for special purposes, as noted in Chapter 12. Thus the more general term "N_{gas}" is used instead of "N_{air}."

The AAPM protocol recommends ^{60}Co γ-rays as a suitable and convenient calibration radiation to use in determining N_{gas} for low-LET applications, although in principle any other low-LET radiation could be used instead.

D_{gas} can be derived from the free-space exposure X employed in an exposure cal-ibration, as already described in Section III.A, through the following sequence of equations correlated with Fig. 13.2a–e. Identical γ-irradiations are assumed in each case.

The collision kerma (J/kg) in air at the calibration point P in free space (see Fig. 13.2a) is related to X by

$$(K_c)_a = X \left(\frac{\overline{W}}{e} \right)_a \tag{13.3}$$

where X is the free-space exposure (C/kg) at P, and $(\overline{W}/e)_a$ is the mean energy ex-pended per unit charge released, having the value 33.97 J/C in perfectly dry air. Imagining now an infinitesimal bit of the chamber's wall material w to be positioned at P in free space (see Fig. 13.2b), the collision kerma in it can be related to $(K_c)_a$ by

$$(K_c)_w = (K_c)_a \left(\frac{\overline{\mu_{\text{en}}}}{\rho} \right)_a^w \tag{13.4}$$

where $(\overline{\mu_{\text{en}}/\rho})_a^w$ is the ratio of mass energy-absorption coefficients for wall and air, averaged over the photon spectrum present [see Eq. (2.5a), substituting K_c for K and μ_{en} for μ_{tr}]. For ^{60}Co γ-rays one may simply assume a single photon energy, 1.25 MeV.

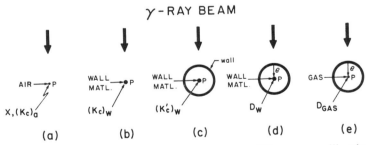

Figure 13.2.   The relation of D_{gas} to the free-space exposure X in a γ-ray calibration. Identical incident irradiations are assumed in each case. (*a*) Exposure at point P in free space is X; $(K_c)_a$ = $X(\overline{W}/e)_a$. (*b*) The collision kerma in an imaginary infinitesimal mass of wall material placed at P is $(K_c)_w = (K_c)_a(\overline{\mu_{\text{en}}/\rho})_a^w$. (*c*) The chamber is centered at P; wall attenuation reduces $(K_c)_w$ to $(K_c')_w = A_w(K_c)_w$. (*d*) The absorbed dose in the bit of wall material at P is $D_w = (K_c')_w (1 + \mu'\overline{x})$, delivered by electrons coming mostly out of the front wall. (*e*) The bit of wall material is removed from P; the dose in the cavity gas there is $D_{\text{gas}} = D_w(\overline{L}/\rho)_w^g$. After Attix (1984b). Reproduced with permission from the American Institute of Physics.

Now positioning the chamber with its center at P as in Fig. 15.2c, the broad-beam attenuation of the γ-rays in the wall reduces the collision kerma in the bit of wall material at P to

$$(K_c')_w = A_w(K_c)_w \qquad (13.5)$$

where A_w is the correction factor for photon attenuation in the wall, which can be approximated by

$$A_w = e^{-(\mu'/\rho)_w\rho t} \cong 1 - \left(\frac{\mu'}{\rho}\right)_w \rho t \cong 1 - \left(\frac{\mu_{en}}{\rho}\right)_w \rho t \qquad (13.6)$$

Here $(\mu'/\rho)_w$ is the effective mass attenuation coefficient under the broad-beam conditions applicable to the chamber wall. $(\mu'/\rho)_w$ may be replaced in the "straight-ahead approximation" by $(\mu_{en}/\rho)_w$, and ρt is the mass wall thickness including the buildup cap, if present. Note that A_w accounts for the attenuation of the photons in passing through the *entire* wall thickness ρt. No adjustment should be made for the secondary-electron range in the wall, since A_w applies to the collision kerma at P, as shown in Eq. (13.5), not to the absorbed dose. The electron-range effect will be included in a separate step in Eq. (13.7).

The coefficient $(\mu'/\rho)_w$ in Eq. (13.6) has been measured for ^{60}Co γ rays by Holt et al. (1979) for ion chambers with polystyrene walls; these same data will be adequate for other low-Z walls as well, since the Compton effect is dominant. Table 13.1 lists $(\mu'/\rho)_w$ values for several chamber radii, and μ_{en}/ρ for comparison. The apparent increase in $(\mu'/\rho)_w$ with increasing chamber radius is due to the larger effective wall thickness for rays passing obliquely through the wall. It makes no difference in Eq. (13.6) whether $(\mu'/\rho)_w$ or ρt is effectively increased to take account of this. In Table 13.1 Holt has chosen to leave ρt fixed at 0.52 g/cm^2, and increase $(\mu'/\rho)_w$ for the larger chamber radii.

The chamber length used by Holt et al. (1979) in obtaining these data was 5 mm. Longer chambers may be expected to have somewhat smaller $(\mu'/\rho)_w$ values because of additional photon scattering; thus A_w would be correspondingly closer to unity. However the results in Table 13.1 will be adequately correct for most small low-Z ion chambers.

It can be seen in the table that for an infinitesimal cavity size, $A_w = 0.988$. This may be taken as the best current value of the ^{60}Co equilibrium-thickness attenuation correction, called A_{eq} by Johns and Cunningham (1974), for which the conventional value was for many years taken as 0.985.* Table 13.1 shows that that value was consistent with the approximation $(\mu'/\rho)_w \cong (\mu_{en}/\rho)_w$ in Eq. (13.6).

The absorbed dose D_w in the imaginary bit of wall material at P is deposited by electrons that originate from Compton interactions in the chamber wall, mainly on the "upstream" side as indicated schematically in Fig. 13.2d. We will assume that the gas cavity is small enough, relative to the electron range, not to perturb the elec-

---

*See Section IV.B.1, Table 13.3, footnote b.

TABLE 13.1   **Effective Mass Attenuation Coefficients for Cylindrical Ion-Chamber Walls Irradiated by ^{60}Co γ-Rays^a**

Internal Radius (mm)	$(\mu'/\rho)_w$ (cm^2/g)			A_w
	Poly or Acrylic	Water	Graphite	
0	.0239	.0245	.0222	0.988
2.5	.0251	.0258	.0233	.987
5.0	.0261	.0268	.0242	.986
7.5	.0287	.0294	.0266	.985
	$(\mu_{en}/\rho)_w$ (cm^2/g)			
	.0288	.0296	.0267	.985
	ρt (g/cm^2)			
	.52	.50	.57	

^{a}$(\mu'/\rho)_w$ data for polystyrene were obtained with chambers 5 mm in length by Holt et al. (1979). Data for the other media were derived from the polystyrene data on the basis of $(\mu_{en}/\rho)_w$ ratios. A_w refers to Eq. (13.6), assuming $\rho t = 0.52$ g/cm^2 for polystyrene and acrylic plastic, 0.50 g/cm^2 for water, and 0.57 g/cm^2 for graphite to equal the maximum electron range for ^{60}Co γ-rays. Note that A_w has the same value for all these media. For a chamber radius of zero, $A_w = A_{eq}$ for ^{60}Co γ-rays. Reproduced with permission from R. L. Fleischer and The American Institute of Physics.

tron flux, i.e., to behave as a B–G cavity. Thus, since the chamber walls are thicker than the maximum electron range, transient charged-particle equilibrium (TCPE) may be assumed to exist in the wall material at P. We may therefore make use of Eq. (4.11) from Chapter 4, Section VII to relate D_w to $(K'_c)_w$:

$$D_w = \left(1 + \rho\bar{x}\,\frac{\mu'}{\rho}\right)_w (K'_c)_w \equiv \beta_w(K'_c)_w \tag{13.7}$$

where $(\rho\bar{x})_w \cong 0.14$ g/cm^2 (Roesch, 1967) is the mean distance the secondary electrons carry their kinetic energy through the wall material in the direction of the photon beam before depositing it as absorbed dose at P. The value of $(\mu'/\rho)_w$ may be taken from Table 13.1, giving a value of 1.003 or 1.004 for β_w with ^{60}Co γ-rays and typical small cavity chambers.

If now the bit of wall material is removed from P, letting the cavity gas replace it, one can calculate the absorbed dose in that gas from cavity theory. The electron fluence coming from the wall will be unchanged; thus the dose at P will be approximately proportional to the mass collision stopping power of the material occupying that position, according to B–G theory. However, δ-rays resulting from hard electron collisions can have ranges greater than the cavity radius. They will carry out their remaining energy, which is thus lost from D_{gas}. The application of Spencer's cavity theory (see Chapter 10), letting the cutoff energy Δ equal the cavity radius, will approximately compensate for this small error. $\Delta = 10$ keV applies to a gas cavity (at 1 atm) of roughly 2-mm radius, the order of magnitude of most small cavity chambers.

Using the terminology of the AAPM (1983) protocol, in which $(\overline{L}/\rho)^{gas}_{wall}$ is the ratio of the restricted mass collision stopping powers, D_{gas} can be written

$$D_{gas} = D_w(\overline{L}/\rho)^g_w \tag{13.8}$$

The difference between $(\overline{L}/\rho)^g_w$ and the corresponding average ratios of unrestricted mass collision stopping-powers, $[\overline{(dT/\rho dx)_c}]^g_w$, is small when the atomic numbers of the wall and gas are comparable, as in the case of typical cavity wall materials vs. $g = $ air. Table 13.2 illustrates this for ^{60}Co γ-rays.

Finally, we may combine the results of Eqs. (13.3) through (13.8) to obtain

$$D_{gas} = X\left(\frac{\overline{W}}{e}\right)_a \left(\frac{\overline{\mu_{en}}}{\rho}\right)^w_a A_w \beta_w \left(\frac{\overline{L}}{\rho}\right)^g_w \tag{13.9}$$

which can be substituted into Eq. (13.2) to give

$$N_{gas} = \frac{X(\overline{W}/e)_a(\overline{\mu_{en}/\rho})^w_a A_{ion} A_w \beta_w (\overline{L}/\rho)^g_w}{M} \tag{13.10}$$

Making use of Eq. (13.1) then produces the following relationship between N_{gas} (in Gy/C) and N_X (in kg^{-1}):

$$N_{gas} = N_X \left(\frac{\overline{W}}{e}\right)_a \left(\frac{\overline{\mu_{en}}}{\rho}\right)^w_a A_{ion} A_w \beta_w \left(\frac{\overline{L}}{\rho}\right)^g_w \tag{13.11}$$

In practice, the cavity gas g is usually air, but in some applications (e.g., neutron dosimetry) other gases may be flowed through the cavity. Note that g appears only as superscript to the last factor in Eq. (13.11); $(\overline{W}/e)_a$ and $(\overline{\mu_{en}/\rho})^w_a$ both refer to dry air and not necessarily to the gas in the cavity.

Equation (13.11) shows that N_{gas} can be determined from the value of the exposure calibration factor N_X, provided that the ion-collection efficiency (A_{ion}) is measured

TABLE 13.2.   Comparison of $[(\overline{L}/\rho)^g_w]_{\Delta = 10 \text{ keV}}$ and $[(dT/\rho dx)_c]^g_w$ for $g = $ Air and $w = $ Several Typical Cavity-Chamber Wall Materials and Water[a]

Wall	$[(\overline{L}/\rho)^g_w]_{\Delta = 10 \text{ keV}}$	$[(dt/\rho dx)_c]^g_w$
Polystyrene	0.899[b]	0.905[c]
Lucite	0.907	0.910
Graphite	0.990	0.991
C552 air-equiv. plastic	1.000	1.000
Water	0.883	0.886

[a] For ^{60}Co γ-rays.
[b] Data in this column are from AAPM (1983).
[c] Data in this column are from Johns & Cunningham (1983).

under the conditions of the calibration and the other terms can be evaluated. The AAPM (1983) protocol contains a great deal of specific information and tables of data to assist in this.

For the case where the chamber wall is enclosed within an equilibrium buildup cap of a different material (a complication to be avoided where possible) the AAPM (1983) protocol recommends that Eq. (13.11) be replaced by a semiempirical expression due to Almond and Svensson (1977):

$$N_{gas} = N_X \frac{(\overline{W/e})_a A_{ion} A_w \beta_w}{\alpha(\overline{L/\rho})_g^w (\overline{\mu_{en}/\rho})_w^a + (1 - \alpha)(\overline{L/\rho})_g^{cap}(\overline{\mu_{en}/\rho})_{cap}^a} \qquad (13.11a)$$

in which "cap" refers to the buildup cap material, α is the fraction of ionization due to electrons from the chamber wall, and $1 - \alpha$ is the fraction due to electrons from the cap, as given in Fig. 13.7a (Section V.B below).

C. Calibration of Ion Chambers in Terms of Absorbed Dose in Water

The National Bureau of Standards began recently to supply ion-chamber calibrations for ^{60}Co γ-rays on the basis of comparison with a graphite calorimeter (Pruitt et al., 1981). The comparison involves several steps: from a graphite calorimeter to a graphite-walled ion chamber (both in graphite phantoms), that chamber then being used to calibrate a point in a water phantom at which the user's chamber is to be placed for calibration. Corrections are applied for the differences between μ_{en}/ρ for water vs. the graphite wall w, and for the γ-ray attenuation and scattering in the phantom material (graphite or water) displaced by the chambers. The calibration is stated in terms of absorbed dose in water, D_{wat}, at the chamber midpoint location (in the absence of the chamber) per unit of corrected electrometer reading M:

$$N_D = \frac{D_{wat}}{M} \qquad (13.12)$$

N_{gas} may be derived from N_D as follows, assuming transient charged-particle equilibrium and a Bragg-Gray cavity:

a. $(K_c)_{wat} = D_{wat} \beta_{wat}^{-1}$ at P, the point of calibration in the water phantom.

b. Putting an infinitesimal piece of graphite wall w at P, the collision kerma in it is $(K_c)_w = (K_c)_{wat}(\overline{\mu_{en}/\rho})_{wat}^w$

c. Putting the chamber in the water phantom, centered at P, the presence of the void increases the collision kerma in w at P to $(K_c')_w = (K_c)_w/P_{repl}$, where P_{repl} is the *replacement correction*, which will be discussed in Section V.A.

d. The dose in the bit of graphite at P is $D_w = \beta_w(K_c')_w$.

e. Removing the bit of graphite from P, the dose there in the cavity gas g is $D_{gas} = (\overline{L/\rho})_w^g D_w$

Combining the relationships in steps a through e with Eq. (13.2) gives the following equation:

$$N_{\text{gas}} = \frac{D_{\text{gas}} A_{\text{ion}}}{M} = \frac{(\overline{L/\rho})^g_w \beta_w A_{\text{ion}}(\overline{\mu_{\text{en}}/\rho})^w_{\text{wat}} D_{\text{wat}}}{P_{\text{repl}} \beta_{\text{wat}} M} \tag{13.13}$$

Assuming $\beta_{\text{wat}} = \beta_w$ and substituting Eq. (13.12) simplifies this to

$$N_{\text{gas}} = \frac{N_D A_{\text{ion}}}{P_{\text{repl}}} \left(\frac{\overline{L}}{\rho} \right)^g_w \left(\frac{\overline{\mu_{\text{en}}}}{\rho} \right)^w_{\text{wat}} \tag{13.14}$$

IV. CALIBRATION OF PHOTON BEAMS WITH AN EXPOSURE-CALIBRATED ION CHAMBER

A. Calibrations in Free Space

1. FOR X-RAYS GENERATED AT 10–300 kV

To calibrate the free-space exposure rate at some point P in an x-ray beam below 300 kV, one may use an ion chamber for which the value of N_X is known for the quality of the radiation to be measured. In that case the ion chamber is to be centered at the point P and irradiated for a known time interval Δt. The exposure at P is

$$X = N_X M \tag{13.15}$$

assuming that the ion-collection efficiency in the chamber is the same as it was during the determination of N_X.

The average exposure rate during Δt is

$$\overline{\left(\frac{dX}{dt} \right)} = \frac{N_X M}{\Delta t} \tag{13.16}$$

where M is the electrometer reading in coulombs or scale divisions corrected to 22°C and 1 atm by Eq. (12.21), in which M' represents the "raw" electrometer reading, corrected only for positive or negative background charge collected during a like time interval Δt. This may be replaced by Eq. (12.22) if humidity is to be corrected for.

a. M–N_X Consistency

M and N_X should be instrumentally consistent with one another. If N_X for a chamber is given in roentgens (or C/kg) per scale division with respect to a certain electrometer and scale, then M should be measured with that electrometer and scale. If N_X is stated in R/C or in kg^{-1}, one may use any accurate electrometer to measure M.

b. Ionic Recombination

Since N_X has not been corrected for ionic recombination, the user should employ the same chamber voltage and polarity as were used at the time the chamber was calibrated. Assuming that the chamber is operated near saturation (e.g., 300–500 V on ~1-cm^3 chambers), remaining recombination losses are usually negligible. For best accuracy it is preferable to evaluate and correct for recombination losses by a procedure such as that described in Chapter 12. Equation (13.15) is then changed to

$$X = N_X A_{ion} MP_{ion} \tag{13.17}$$

where A_{ion} is the chamber's ion-collection efficiency during the calibration in which N_X was evaluated, and P_{ion} is the reciprocal of the ion-collection efficiency during measurement of the user's beam. Naturally, if the ionic recombination conditions are the same on both occasions, $A_{ion}P_{ion} = 1$. Otherwise Eq. (13.17) offers a more accurate value of X than Eq. (13.15).

c. Shutter Timing Error

$\overline{(dX/dt)}$ may be measured by timing a change ΔM in the electrometer reading, without interrupting the x-ray beam. In that case Eq. (13.16) is modified to

$$\overline{\left(\frac{dX}{dt}\right)} = \frac{N_X \, \Delta M}{\Delta t} \tag{13.18}$$

If a beam shutter is used with a timer that closes the shutter when a preset time has elapsed, the Δt measured by the timer may not agree exactly with the $\Delta t'$ representing the shutter-open period, due to shutter timing error. This can be easily detected by making two measurements for different timer settings, Δt_1 and Δt_2. The corresponding corrected electrometer readings are M_1 and M_2 [see Eq. (12.21)], and Eq. (13.18) is altered to

$$\frac{dX}{dt} = N_X \frac{M_2 - M_1}{\Delta t_2 - \Delta t_1} \tag{13.19}$$

where dX/dt must remain constant during the period that includes both measurements.

Figure 13.3 helps in understanding the shutter timing error and Eq. (13.19). The shutter is open for a time $\Delta t'$ that is shorter by the amount δ (here assumed to be

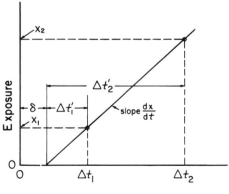

FIGURE 13.3. The effect of x-ray beam-shutter timing error. δ as shown is the amount of time by which the shutter-open interval $\Delta t'$ is less than the set timer interval Δt: $\delta = \Delta t - \Delta t'$.

positive) than the timer setting Δt. The exposure X_1, resulting from timer setting Δt_1, is given by

$$X_1 = (\Delta t_1 - \delta) \frac{dX}{dt} \tag{13.20}$$

Likewise, for timer setting Δt_2 the exposure is

$$X_2 = (\Delta t_2 - \delta) \frac{dX}{dt} \tag{13.21}$$

Combining Eqs. (13.20) and (13.21) produces an equation that can be solved for δ, the shutter timing error:

$$\frac{dX}{dt} = \frac{X_1}{\Delta t_1 - \delta} = \frac{X_2}{\Delta t_2 - \delta} \tag{13.22}$$

Thence

$$\delta = \frac{X_2 \, \Delta t_1 - X_1 \, \Delta t_2}{X_2 - X_1} = \frac{M_2 \, \Delta t_1 - M_1 \, \Delta t_2}{M_2 - M_1} \tag{13.23}$$

Example 13.1. An x-ray beam is measured by an ion chamber for which N_X is 4.09×10^9 R/C. For a shutter-timer setting of 5 s, a charge of 7.30×10^{-10} C is measured, and for 30 s, 4.60×10^{-9} C. The background drift of the chamber and electrometer circuit is measured on the same scale and found to be $\cong 3 \times 10^{-14}$ C/min. The atmospheric pressure is 733 torr (or mm Hg), and the chamber temperature is 24.3°C. What is the shutter error? Calculate the exposure rate in free space at the point of measurement. What exposure results from a timer setting of 12 s?

Solution: From Eq. (12.21), ignoring humidity,

$$M_1 = M_1' \left(\frac{760}{733} \times \frac{273 + 24.3}{273 + 22.0} \right) = 7.30 \times 10^{-10} \, (1.045)$$

$$= 7.63 \times 10^{-10} \, C$$

$$M_2 = 4.60 \times 10^{-9} \times 1.045 = 4.81 \times 10^{-9} \, C$$

Background is negligible. From Eq. (13.15), assuming $A_{ion} P_{ion} = 1$,

$$X_1 = N_X M_1 = 3.12 \, R$$

$$X_2 = N_X M_2 = 19.66 \, R$$

From Eq. (13.23),

$$\delta = \frac{19.66 \times 5 - 3.12 \times 30}{19.66 - 3.12} = 0.28 \, s$$

From Eq. (13.22),

$$\frac{dX}{dt} = \frac{19.66}{30 - 0.28} = 0.662 \text{ R/s}$$

For $\Delta t = 12$ s the true exposure duration

$$\Delta t' = 12 - 0.28 = 11.72 \text{ s}$$

Hence

$$X = 11.72 \text{ s} \times 0.662 \text{ R/s} = 7.76 \text{ R}$$

d. Beam Monitor-Chamber Calibration

If a continuous x-ray generator is not well enough stabilized to give a sufficiently reproducible output rate, there will be no point in calibrating the beam without a monitor chamber. A transmission-type monitor (e.g. Fig. 12.15), through which the x-ray beam passes on its way to the calibration ion chamber or other object to be irradiated, is probably the most satisfactory. However, a conventional cavity chamber placed at some fixed position in the beam can serve the purpose of a monitor if the spatial distribution of x-ray flux density within the beam is uniform. Note that if the spatial stability of the beam is a problem, a transmission chamber should be designed to sample only the partial solid angle of the beam that is to be employed; thus, the monitor should be positioned in the beam after it passes through its limiting collimator.

Most monitor chambers are open to the atmosphere, and therefore their charge output should be normalized to 22°C and 1 atm as in Eq. (12.21), not only during the beam calibration procedure but also during each subsequent use of the x-ray beam.

Using a monitor chamber requires a second electrometer, and HV supply (e.g., battery). A single HV supply should not be used for both the monitor and calibration chamber, as the latter should be adjustable in polarity and voltage without affecting the former.

It is essential that the monitor measure the x-ray beam for the identical time interval during which the calibrated chamber is exposed. Although this can be accomplished electronically by simultaneous ungrounding of the two electrometer inputs, followed by simultaneous readings of the electrometers after an arbitrary time interval, a shutter-controlled beam is more straightforward. The electrometers are ungrounded and zeroed just before the shutter is opened, and both are read immediately after completion of the exposure. If M is the electrometer reading of the calibrated chamber, corrected for background and normalized to 22°C and 1 atm by Eq. (12.21), and M_M is the correspondingly corrected monitor reading, then the free-space exposure X is given by Eq. (13.15) or (13.17), and the exposure per monitor electrometer-scale division (or per ''monitor unit'') is

$$N_M = \frac{X}{M_M} \tag{13.24}$$

Thus, so long as this monitor calibration remains unchanged, the free-space exposure at the point of calibration can be gotten as the product of N_M and the corrected monitor reading M_M obtained in any later irradiation:

$$X = N_M M_M \tag{13.25}$$

For purposes of estimating the exposure to be expected from a given shutter timer setting Δt (ignoring timing errors), the approximate exposure rate can also be obtained during the beam calibration as

$$\overline{\left(\frac{dX}{dt} \right)} \cong \frac{N_X M}{\Delta t} = \frac{X}{\Delta t} \tag{13.26}$$

from which the exposure can be estimated for a given timer setting Δt as

$$X \cong \overline{\left(\frac{dX}{dt} \right)} \Delta t \tag{13.27}$$

while the actual exposure delivered is calculated from Eq. (13.25) on the basis of the monitor reading upon completion.

A similar monitor-calibration procedure can be followed for a pulsed x-ray generator for which the output is not constant from pulse to pulse. Equation (13.24) provides the value of the monitor calibration, N_M, based on some given number of pulses n. For estimation purposes the mean exposure per pulse is X/n. The actual exposure corresponding to the monitor reading M_M in any later irradiation is given by Eq. (13.25).

e. Beam Calibration in Terms of Free-Space Collision Kerma or Absorbed Dose

Having calibrated the x-ray beam to allow the controlled delivery of a free-space exposure X at the point of calibration P, one may wish to relate X to K_c and D at the same point, in some material of interest.

The free-space collision kerma in the air at P for an exposure X is (From Eq. 2.23) simply

$$(K_c)_a = X \left(\frac{\overline{W}}{e} \right)_a \tag{13.28}$$

where $(K_c)_a$ is in grays if X is in C/kg, and $(\overline{W}/e)_a = 33.97$ J/C for dry air.

The collision kerma in an infinitesimal mass of any other material x placed at P and similarly irradiated is

$$(K_c)_x = (K_c)_a \left(\frac{\overline{\mu_{en}}}{\rho} \right)_a^x \tag{13.29}$$

where $(\overline{\mu_{en}/\rho})_a^x$ is the ratio of the spectrum-averaged mass energy-absorption coefficients for x and air, as in Eq. (13.4).

The absorbed dose at P is in general indeterminate without knowing the secondary-electron flux-density distribution there, since the electrons deliver the dose. However, under CPE conditions one can write that $D = K_c$ without further knowledge of the electron field, as discussed in Chapter 4.

By centering an imaginary spherical mass of the material of interest x at point P, and making the sphere's radius equal to the maximum secondary-electron range, CPE can be theoretically well approximated. Taking x to be water, the customary tissue-simulating reference material, and assuming only Compton interactions by 300-kV photons, the maximum recoil electron energy would be 162 keV, for which the CSDA range is about 0.32 mm.

Now centering the water sphere at P, the collision kerma $(K_c)'_{\text{wat}}$ at its center will be less than $(K_c)_{\text{wat}}$ in an infinitesimal mass of water at P in free space, by the amount of the broad-beam attenuation that the x rays undergo in penetrating to the center of the sphere:

$$(K_c)'_{\text{wat}} = A_{\text{eq}} \, (K_c)_{\text{wat}} \tag{13.30}$$

The *equilibrium-thickness attenuation correction* A_{eq} can be estimated for this case:

$$A_{\text{eq}} \cong 1 - \left(\frac{\overline{\mu_{\text{en}}}}{\rho} \right)_{\text{wat}} (\rho t)_{\text{wat}}$$

$$= 1 - (0.03 \text{ cm}^2/\text{g})(0.032 \text{ g/cm}^2) = 0.999 \tag{13.31}$$

Hence the absorbed dose D_w (in grays) to water at P under CPE conditions, for an exposure X (C/kg), is given by

$$D_{\text{wat}} \overset{\text{CPE}}{=} (K_c')_{\text{wat}} = A_{\text{eq}}(K_c)_{\text{wat}} = A_{\text{eq}} \, X \left(\frac{\overline{W}}{e} \right)_a \left(\frac{\overline{\mu_{\text{en}}}}{\rho} \right)_a^{\text{wat}} \tag{13.32}$$

or, according to Eq. (4.10), if D_w is instead expressed in rads and X in roentgens,

$$D_{\text{wat}} \overset{\text{CPE}}{=} 0.876 \, A_{\text{eq}} \, X \left(\frac{\overline{\mu_{\text{en}}}}{\rho} \right)_a^{\text{wat}} \tag{13.32a}$$

where $A_{\text{eq}} = 0.999$ for a water sphere just large enough to achieve CPE for 300-keV photons. For the still-smaller equilibrium spheres required for x-rays of lower energies, A_{eq} is even closer to unity. Hence for x-rays generated at 300 kV or lower, A_{eq} may be taken as 1.000, and Eq. (13.32) may be simplified to

$$D_{\text{wat}} \overset{\text{CPE}}{=} (K_c)_{\text{wat}} = X \left(\frac{\overline{W}}{e} \right)_a \left(\frac{\overline{\mu_{\text{en}}}}{\rho} \right)_a^{\text{wat}} \tag{13.33}$$

and Eq. (13.32a) to

$$D_{\text{wat}} \overset{\text{CPE}}{=} 0.876 \, X \left(\frac{\overline{\mu_{\text{en}}}}{\rho} \right)_a^{\text{wat}} \tag{13.33a}$$

D_{wat} in Eqs. (13.32) to (13.33a) is often referred to as the "absorbed dose to water in free space" in the x-ray beam at P. In other words, D_{wat} is the dose at the center of the smallest sphere of water that will produce CPE at its center.

One method of determining the dose at some depth d in a water phantom is to measure D_{wat} at a point P in free space and multiply it by a quantity called the *tissue–air ratio* to get the corresponding dose at the same point immersed at depth d in the phantom. This topic properly belongs in radiotherapy physics, and has been fully discussed by Johns and Cunningham (1983). Muscle tissue is sometimes substituted for water as the reference material x in the above discussion.

2. FREE-SPACE PHOTON-BEAM EXPOSURE CALIBRATION FOR ENERGIES ABOVE 300 KeV

Everything that was said in the preceding Section IV.A.1 applies as well to higher-energy photon beams, with certain exceptions to be discussed next.

a. ^{60}Co and ^{137}Cs γ-Ray Beams

Exposure calibrations for ^{60}Co and ^{137}Cs γ-ray beams can be carried out by the preceding methods, assuming that N_X is known for the air-filled ion chamber and γ rays to be used.

If N_X is not available for ^{137}Cs, its value may be estimated from a ^{60}Co value of N_X by two applications of Eq. (13.11), once for each radiation. N_{gas} may be taken to be the same for both, allowing a solution for the ratio $(N_X)_{\text{Cs}}/(N_X)_{\text{Co}}$. $(\overline{W}/e)_a$ and A_{ion} may each be canceled. $\beta_w = 1.003$ for ^{60}Co and 1.001 for ^{137}Cs. Assuming a polystyrene chamber wall 0.52 g/cm^2 in thickness, we have $A_w \cong 0.985$ for ^{60}Co and 0.984 for ^{137}Cs, using μ_{en}/ρ as an approximate attenuation coefficient for both. $(\mu_{\text{en}}/\rho)_a^w = 1.081$ for ^{60}Co and 1.076 for ^{137}Cs. $(\overline{L}/\rho)_w^g \cong [\overline{(dt/\rho dx)_c}]_w^g \cong 0.904$ for ^{60}Co and 0.901 for ^{137}Cs. The result is that $(N_X)_{\text{Cs}} \cong 1.011\ (N_X)_{\text{Co}}$, for such a chamber.

Now, assuming that one knows the free-space exposure X at a point P in a ^{60}Co or ^{137}Cs γ-ray beam, Eqs. (13.28), (13.29), and (13.30) may be used to obtain $(K_c)_a$, $(K_c)_{\text{wat}}$, and $(K'_c)_{\text{wat}}$, respectively. In the latter equation $A_{\text{eq}} = 0.988$ for ^{60}Co (see Table 13.1), and for ^{137}Cs a reasonable value can be estimated as follows: In polystyrene,

$$\left(\frac{\mu'}{\rho}\right)_{\text{Cs}} \cong \left(\frac{\mu'}{\rho}\right)_{\text{Co}} \cdot \frac{(\mu_{\text{en}}/\rho)_{\text{Cs}}}{(\mu_{\text{en}}/\rho)_{\text{Co}}}$$

$$\cong 0.0239\ \frac{0.0316}{0.0287} = 0.0263\ \text{cm}^2/\text{g} \qquad (13.34)$$

Therefore,

$$(A_{\text{eq}})_{\text{Cs}} \cong 1 - \left(\frac{\mu'}{\rho}\right)_{\text{Cs}} \rho t = 1 - 0.0263 \times 0.170$$

$$= 0.996$$

where $\rho t = 0.170$ g/cm^2 is the CSDA range in polystyrene of a 0.48-MeV electron, the maximum produced by 0.662-MeV ^{137}Cs photons in Compton interactions. As noted in Table 13.1, this A_{eq}-value applies to water as well as polystyrene.

For ^{137}Cs and ^{60}Co γ-rays CPE cannot be rigorously achieved at the center of the water sphere at P, because of the range and forward projection of the secondary electrons. However, TCPE exists at P, so we may use the relationship (13.7) to relate D_{wat} to $(K'_c)_{wat}$ and thence to X as in Eq. (13.32):

$$D_{wat} = \beta_{wat}(K'_c)_{wat} = \beta_{wat}A_{eq} X \left(\frac{\overline{W}}{e}\right)_a \left(\frac{\mu_{en}}{\rho}\right)_a^{wat} \tag{13.35}$$

or, if D_w is in rads and X in roentgens,

$$D_{wat} = 0.876\beta_{wat}A_{eq} X \left(\frac{\mu_{en}}{\rho}\right)_a^{wat} \tag{13.35a}$$

where $\beta_{wat} = 1.003$ for ^{60}Co and 1.001 for ^{137}Cs in the equilibrium sphere of water. Now $A_{eq} = 0.988$ for ^{60}Co and 0.996 for ^{137}Cs, and $(\mu_{en}/\rho)_a^{wat} = 1.111$ for ^{60}Co and 1.114 for ^{137}Cs. Substituting these data in Eqs. (13.35) and (13.35a), we find that for ^{60}Co

$$D_{wat} = \begin{cases} 37.4\ X & \text{for} \quad \text{Gy and C/kg} \\ 0.964\ X & \text{for} \quad \text{rad and R} \end{cases} \tag{13.36}$$

and for ^{137}Cs

$$D_{wat} = \begin{cases} 37.7\ X & \text{for} \quad \text{Gy and C/kg} \\ 0.973\ X & \text{for} \quad \text{rad and R} \end{cases} \tag{13.36a}$$

D_{wat} is the free-space absorbed dose in an equilibrium sphere of water at a point where the free-space exposure X has been determined, for example, by means of an exposure-calibrated ion chamber.

b. Higher-Energy Photons

Calibration laboratories do not at this time offer ion-chamber calibrations for photon beams above ^{60}Co in energy. However, it is possible to deduce a value of N_X for a higher-energy beam of quality λ through the double application of the N_{gas} equation, as was done in the preceding section for ^{137}Cs. The main difference here is that a thicker equilibrium buildup cap must be used to provide a total chamber wall thickness at least equal to the maximum range of the electrons produced by the higher-energy photons. The same cap is used for the ^{60}Co calibration to obtain $(N_X)_{Co}$ in this case.

Then, from Eq. (13.11), we have

$$N_{gas} = (N_X)_{Co} \left(\frac{\overline{W}}{e}\right)_a \left[\left(\frac{\mu_{en}}{\rho}\right)_a^w A_{ion} A_w \beta_w \left(\frac{\overline{L}}{\rho}\right)_w^g\right]_{Co}$$

$$= (N_X)_\lambda \left(\frac{\overline{W}}{e}\right)_a \left[\left(\frac{\mu_{en}}{\rho}\right)_a^w A_{ion} A_w \beta_w \left(\frac{\overline{L}}{\rho}\right)_w^g\right]_\lambda$$

Therefore,

$$(N_X)_\lambda = (N_X)_{Co} \frac{[(\mu_{en}/\rho)_a^w \, A_{ion} \, A_w \, \beta_w \, (\overline{L}/\rho)_w^g]_{Co}}{[(\mu_{en}/\rho)_a^w \, A_{ion} \, A_w \, \beta_w \, (\overline{L}/\rho)_w^g]_\lambda} \qquad (13.37)$$

where the subscript Co refers to quantities to be evaluated for ^{60}Co γ-rays, and λ refers to the higher-energy beam. N_{gas} is independent of the photon energy, and hence can be equated for the two beams to obtain Eq. (13.37).

The practical limitation on this equation is the present lack of well-established data for β_w, which no doubt will be remedied. Figure 13.4 contains some data for β_w in graphite walls, using $\bar{x}$-values calculated by Roesch (1968) (see Attix, 1979).

Notice that Eq. (13.37), in conjunction with Eq. (13.15), indicates that it is possible to measure with cavity ion chambers the free-space exposure X at higher photon

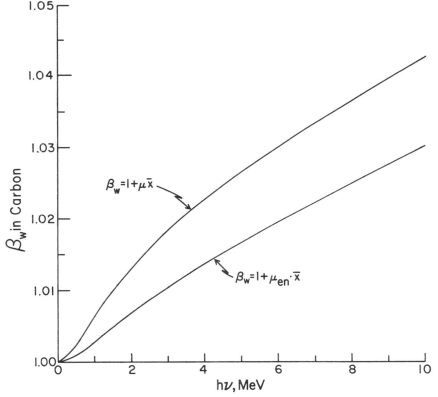

FIGURE 13.4. β_w in graphite, as a function of photon energy, from calculations of $\bar{x}$ by Roesch (1968) (see Attix, 1979). This $\bar{x}$ may be adequately approximated by 0.54 $\Re_{CSDA}$ for the average secondary-electron energy $\overline{T} = E_\gamma (\sigma_{en}/\sigma)$. The lower curve gives values of $\beta_w \cong 1 + \mu_{en} \bar{x}$; the upper curve is $\beta_w \cong 1 + \mu\bar{x}$. For chamber-wall applications, or at shallow depths in a phantom penetrated by a broad γ-ray beam, values of β_w approximate the lower limit. At greater depths in the phantom, β_w lies between the limiting values, tending to increase with increasing depth and with decreasing beam diameter. These results apply also to β_w for other low-Z media.

energies than the conventional limit of 3 MeV. That limit (see, e.g., ICRU, 1980) is based on CPE failure. However, if TCPE is achieved instead and β_w is known, then the physical reason for the limitation is removed. One may argue as to the need for exposure measurements with higher-energy photons, but that is a separate matter from the possibility of doing such measurements (see also Chapter 4, Sections VI.C and VII).

B. Calibration of Photon Beams in Phantoms by Means of an Exposure-Calibrated Ion Chamber

This has been the calibration method of choice in radiotherapy applications for many years. The N_{gas} method to be discussed in Section V is more elegant and is capable of greater accuracy if properly applied. However, the present method has the appeal of simplicity, and will no doubt continue to have its adherents for some time to come.

We need not discuss its use for photon energies below ^{60}Co, since the free-space beam calibration method, as already explained, is employed for those cases. For energies above ^{60}Co the secondary-electron range increases and requires a sizable imaginary sphere of water to produce TCPE at its center, and thus to allow the determination of the free-space absorbed dose. For example, the 4.76-MeV maximum Compton electrons resulting from 5-MeV photons would require a water sphere 4.9 cm in diameter. Thus even the concept of ''free-space'' absorbed dose tends to lose its meaning when such a large sphere of material is required at the point of interest in free space. Since the dose in a water phantom is what is wanted, it makes more sense to let the calibration be made at some point of reference within such a phantom, and relate the absorbed dose there to doses at other points of interest in the phantom.

The reference point must be chosen to be deep enough in the phantom to achieve TCPE. From ^{60}Co γ-rays to 15-MV x-rays, 5-cm depth in water is normally used, with the reference point located on the beam axis. From 16 to 25 MV, 7-cm depth should be used, and from 26 to 50 MV, 10 cm depth (AAPM, 1983). The phantom should be larger than the beam dimensions by at least 5 cm on all sides. At least 10 cm of water should remain behind the ion chamber at its deepest measurement position, to ensure adequate photon backscattering. Making measurements in a water phantom is best carried out with the photon beam horizontal, entering the phantom through one side, while the ion chamber (suitably waterproofed, e.g., by a rubber sheath), is lowered to the beam axis with the electrical connections remaining above water. The few millimeters of plastic (e.g., Lucite) entry wall through which the beam passes should be counted as equivalent to a layer of water having the same number of electrons per cm^2. For example, 3 mm of Lucite of density 1.17 g/cm^2 may be considered as equivalent to 3.4 mm of water in determining the depth of an ion chamber, since Lucite's electron concentration (cm^{-3}) is 1.137 times that in unit-density water.

1. FOR ^{60}Co γ RAYS

Assume now that a ^{60}Co-exposure-calibrated ion chamber is immersed in a water phantom, centered at the reference point P on the beam axis. The corrected electrometer reading M resulting from a given irradiation can be reduced to a free-space exposure X by the methods fully discussed in Section IV.A.1.a through d. Repeating Eq. (13.17), we have

$$X = N_X A_{ion} MP_{ion}$$

where N_X is the ^{60}Co exposure calibration factor and A_{ion} and P_{ion} are correction factors for ionic recombination during the calibration, and use, of the chamber, respectively.

The immediate question is: "What is the meaning of X within a phantom?" This can be best explained with reference to Fig. 13.5. In part a of that figure the ion chamber is shown centered at point P in the phantom, where it is irradiated to produce corrected reading M.

Imagine now (see Fig. 13.5b) that the chamber is removed, leaving behind a void just the size of the external chamber diameter (including the buildup cap, if present during the determination of N_X). X is the exposure at P at the center of the void, assuming that the N_X-value obtained in a free-space calibration still applies when the chamber is irradiated in the phantom. For this assumption to be satisfied requires that the chamber exhibit a constant response per roentgen for the scattered photons in the phantom, extending from ^{60}Co energy downward. In other words, the chamber must be air-equivalent within that energy range. Ion chambers approximating this response function reasonably well are commonly available; hence this assumption is not a serious obstacle to the application of this method.

If next the void is allowed to fill with water (Fig. 13.5c), the exposure at P is diminished to a value

$$X' = A_c X \qquad (13.38)$$

where A_c, called the *displacement correction*, is the fraction by which the exposure is decreased by broad-beam photon attenuation in the water occupying the former void. Holt et al. (1979) have measured A_c and A_{eq} (see Eq. (13.30)) for cylindrical polystyrene chambers in polystyrene or water phantoms, obtaining the values shown in Table 13.3.

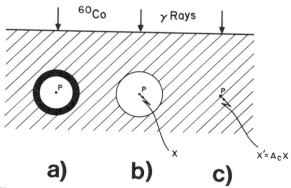

FIGURE 13.5. ^{60}Co γ-ray beam calibration in a water phantom, using an ion chamber calibrated in terms of free-space exposure with ^{60}Co γ-rays.

TABLE 13.3 A_c/A_{eq} and A_c for ^{60}Co γ-Rays and Cylindrical Polystyrene Ion Chambers[a]

D_o (cm)	A_c/A_{eq}	A_c
1.0 (0.9)	1.000 (1.000)	0.988[b] (0.988)
1.1 (1.0)	0.999 (0.999)	0.987 (0.987)
1.2 (1.1)	0.997 (0.997)	0.985 (0.985)
1.3 (1.2)	0.996 (0.995)	0.984 (0.983)
1.4 (1.3)	0.994 (0.993)	0.982 (0.981)
1.5 (1.4)	0.993 (0.992)	0.981 (0.980)
1.6 (1.5)	0.992 (0.991)	0.980 (0.979)
1.8 (1.7)	0.989 (0.987)	0.977 (0.975)
2.0 (1.9)	0.986 (0.984)	0.974 (0.972)
2.2 (2.1)	0.983 (0.981)	0.971 (0.969)
2.4 (2.3)	0.980 (0.977)	0.968 (0.965)

[a]Outside diameter D_o, wall thickness 0.5 cm, in water or polystyrene phantoms. A_{eq} is taken here to be 0.988, based on an equilibrium thickness of 0.52 g/cm^2. Figures in parentheses are estimated for a Lucite ion chamber in a Lucite phantom. The equilibrium thickness for Lucite of $\rho = 1.17$ g/cm^3 is 4.4 mm.
[b]Note that Holt et al. (1979), from whom the nonparenthetical data were taken, reported $A_{eq} = 0.9907$, which they rounded to 0.990. They included in A_{eq} a β_w-correction of 1.003 that we are accounting for separately. Thus their Table V data for A_c are higher by 0.002 for all D_o-values, since $0.9907/1.003 = 0.988$. Reproduced with permission from R. L. Fleischer and the American Institute of Physics.

Having obtained X' through application of Eq. (13.38), we can then derive the collision kerma in an imaginary infinitesimal mass of air placed at P in the water phantom, from the relation

$$(K_c)_a = X' \left(\frac{\overline{W}}{e} \right)_a \tag{13.39}$$

where $(K_c)_a$ is in J/kg, X' in C/kg, and $(\overline{W}/e)_a$ in J/C. The corresponding collision kerma in water at P is

$$(K_c)_{wat} = (K_c)_a \left(\frac{\mu_{en}}{\rho} \right)_a^{wat} \tag{13.40}$$

and the absorbed dose D_{wat} at point P in the unperturbed beam in the phantom, at a depth where TCPE is assumed to exist, is given in grays by

$$D_{wat} = \beta_{wat} (K_c)_{wat}$$
$$= \beta_{wat} A_c X \left(\frac{\overline{W}}{e} \right)_a \left(\frac{\mu_{en}}{\rho} \right)_a^{wat} \tag{13.41}$$

or, for D_{wat} in rads and X in roentgens,

$$D_{wat} = 0.876 \, \beta_{wat} A_c X \left(\frac{\mu_{en}}{\rho} \right)_a^{wat} \tag{13.41a}$$

These equations are identical to (13.35) and (13.35a) except for the replacement of A_{eq} by A_c.

Taking $\beta_{wat} \cong 1.005$ (for, say, a 5-cm depth and a 10 × 10-cm^2 beam), $(\overline{W}/e)_a$

= 33.97 J/C, and $(\mu_{en}/\rho)_a^{wat} = 1.111$ simplifies Eq. (13.41) to

$$D_{wat} = 37.9 \, A_c X \tag{13.42}$$

for D_{wat} in grays and X in C/kg, or

$$D_{wat} = 0.978 \, A_c X \tag{13.42a}$$

for D in rads and X in roentgens.

The value of the displacement correction A_c depends on the outer diameter of the chamber + buildup cap, according to Table 13.3; hence a single value cannot be assigned to further simplify Eqs. (13.42) and (13.42a).

2. FOR X-RAY BEAMS HIGHER IN ENERGY THAN ^{60}Co: THE C_λ CONCEPT

In-phantom dosimetry of high-energy x-ray beams has been done on the basis of ^{60}Co γ-ray-calibrated ion chambers for a number of years through application of the C_λ concept, originated by Greene (1962). C_λ is a conversion coefficient (rad/R) to derive the dose $[D_{wat}]_\lambda$ in rads at the point of reference in the water phantom from the reading M of an ion chamber irradiated by high-energy x-rays in that location. Simply, one can write that

$$[D_{wat}]_\lambda = C_\lambda \, N_X \, A_{ion} \, MP_{ion} \tag{13.43}$$

where N_X is the ^{60}Co exposure calibration factor (R/C), and M the atmosphere-corrected reading of the charge collected.

The following derivation of C_λ will clarify its meaning. Let us suppose that the ion chamber is a B–G cavity with water-equivalent walls (assuming it is located in a water phantom). That is, we ask that the same flux of secondary electrons cross the cavity as would be the case if the wall (and buildup cap, if present) were made of water. The wall material does not have to be identically water, provided that the errors in collision stopping power and mass energy-absorption coefficient cancel each other. For example, for ^{60}Co and polystyrene walls $(\mu_{en}/\rho)_{poly}^{water} = 1.028$ while $[(dT/\rho dx)_c]_{water}^{poly} \cong 0.979$, giving a product of 1.006. For the case of Lucite walls the corresponding product is 0.999. Unity indicates a close match to water-equivalent walls. These typical plastics evidently provide reasonably good approximations.

Leaving off the ^{60}Co buildup cap for measurements in the phantom, thereby allowing actual water to replace it around the relatively thin chamber wall, tends to further minimize any error due to non-water-equivalence. Note that the A_c value to be used in this case is unchanged, being determined by the outer diameter of the buildup cap employed in the ^{60}Co γ-ray calibration to determine N_X.

The alert reader will have noticed that now we are asking that the chamber wall be water-equivalent for ^{60}Co γ-rays and higher-energy x-rays, while in Section IV.B.1 we asked for its *air*-equivalence below ^{60}Co in energy. Actually air and water equivalence are not very different, as one may verify in Fig. 2.2a, which shows close tracking between the μ_{en}/ρ values for these media over a wide energy range. More to the point, however, plastics like polystyrene or Lucite are too low in atomic number to imitate either water or air at low energies where the photoelectric effect becomes important, requiring the addition of some higher-Z element. The use of an aluminum rod as the central collecting electrode is a familiar method for adjusting the low-energy air equivalence of an ion chamber, which has a negligible effect on the approximate water equivalence of its walls at higher energies where the Compton effect dominates. It has been suggested (Nahum and Greening, 1976, 1978; Kutcher et al., 1977; AAPM, 1983) that the inexact phantom-medium equivalence of chamber walls and buildup caps may cause significant dosimetry errors. Further developments may be expected in this area of research—for example, specifically water-equivalent plastic chamber walls for use in phantoms of water or water-equivalent plastic (Constantinou et al., 1982).

Returning now to our derivation of C_λ, we next imagine two irradiations with the chamber positioned at point P in the phantom: one with ^{60}Co γ-rays, and a second with the higher-energy x-ray beam that will be identified by the subscript λ. The two irradiations are adjusted to produce identical absorbed doses D_{gas} in the cavity gas, which we may take to be air. Since $(\overline{W}/e)_a$ is the same for ^{60}Co and the x-ray beam, the charge Q produced in the gas is also the same for both irradiations. Assuming equal ion-collection efficiencies, the atmosphere-corrected electrometer readings M are also identical.

D_{gas} can be related to the dose D_{wat} at P in the undisturbed water phantom through application of the B–G relation, Eq. (10.6):

$$[D_{wat}]_{Co} = D_{gas} \left[\overline{\left(\frac{dT}{\rho dx} \right)}_{c,Co} \right]_a^{wat} \tag{13.44a}$$

and

$$[D_{wat}]_\lambda = D_{gas} \left[\overline{\left(\frac{dT}{\rho dx} \right)}_{c,\lambda} \right]_a^{wat} \tag{13.44b}$$

where any perturbation of the radiation field by the presence of the cavity at P during the measurements is neglected by assuming it to be the same for the two radiations. Thus we can write an equation for $(D_{wat})_\lambda$ in terms of $(D_{wat})_{Co}$ as

$$[D_{wat}]_\lambda = [D_{wat}]_{Co} \frac{[\overline{(dT/\rho dx)}_{c,\lambda}]_a^{wat}}{[\overline{(dT/\rho dx)}_{c,Co}]_a^{wat}} \tag{13.45}$$

Combining this with Eqs. (13.17) and (13.41a), one can write for the x-ray dose in water, in rads,

$$[D_{wat}]_\lambda = \left[0.876\, \beta_{wat}\, A_c \left(\frac{\mu_{en}}{\rho} \right)_a^{wat} \right]_{Co} \frac{\left[\overline{\left(\frac{dT}{\rho dx} \right)}_{c,\lambda} \right]_a^{wat}}{\left[\overline{\left(\frac{dT}{\rho dx} \right)}_{c,Co} \right]_a^{wat}} N_X\, A_{ion}\, MP_{ion} \tag{13.46}$$

where $N_X M$ is expressed in roentgens. Comparing with Eq. (13.43), we see that

$$C_\lambda = \left[0.876 \, \beta_{\text{wat}} \, A_c \left(\frac{\mu_{\text{en}}}{\rho} \right)_a^{\text{wat}} \right]_{\text{Co}} \frac{\left[\overline{\left(\dfrac{dT}{\rho dx} \right)_{c,\lambda}} \right]_a^{\text{wat}}}{\left[\overline{\left(\dfrac{dT}{\rho dx} \right)_{c,\text{Co}}} \right]_a^{\text{wat}}} \qquad \text{(rad/R)} \qquad (13.47)$$

Hence

$$(D_{\text{wat}})_\lambda = C_\lambda N_X A_{\text{ion}} \, M P_{\text{ion}} \qquad \text{(rad)} \qquad (13.48)$$

The quantity C_λ has been evaluated by Greene and Massey (1968) under the assumption that $\beta_{\text{wat}} = 1$ (in place of the value $\cong 1.005$), and by letting $A_c = 0.985$ for an assumed outer chamber diameter of 1.6 cm for a Farmer chamber with a ^{60}Co buildup cap. (Note that Table 13.3 gives $A_c = 0.980$). Table 13.4 lists, in the second column, these values of C_λ for water phantoms and various photon energies, as quoted by the AAPM (1971). Columns 3 and 4 pertain to other phantom media, and will be discussed in the next section.

TABLE 13.4. Factors[a] C_λ for Water and $(C_\lambda)_p$ for Polystyrene and Acrylic[b]

Radiation	C_λ in Water (rad/R)	$(C_\lambda)_p$ in	
		Polystyrene (rad/R)	Acrylic[b] (rad/R)
γ-Rays:			
^{137}Cs	.95	.94	.95
^{60}Co	.95	.94	.95
x-Rays (MV):			
2	.95	.94	.95
4	.94	.93	.94
6	.94	.93	.93
8	.93	.93	.92
10	.93	.92	.92
12	.92	.92	.91
14	.92	.92	.91
16	.91	.92	.91
18	.91	.92	.91
20	.90	.92	.90
25	.90	.92	.90
30	.89	.91	.89
35	.88	.90	.89
40	.88	.90	.88
45	.87	.91	.89
50	.87	.91	.89

[a] AAPM (1971). Reproduced with permission from The Institute of Physics, U.K.
[b] Lucite, Plexiglas, and Perspex are acrylics.

The tendency of C_λ to decrease with increasing x-ray energy is attributable to the polarization effect (see Chapter 8), which causes the stopping power in (condensed) water to decrease relative to that in (gaseous) air. The numerator of the final factor in Eq. (13.47) controls the energy dependence of C_λ.

An improved calculation of C_λ for chamber diameters like that of the Farmer chamber (O.D. = 1.6 cm) can be performed by applying $A_c = 0.980$ and $\beta_{wat} \cong 1.005$ in Eq. (13.47), but the net change in Table 13.4 would be nil. For chambers of other outer diameters than 1.6 cm, the actual A_c from Table 13.3 should be used, along with $\beta_w \cong 1.005$. For example, if a water-equivalent-walled chamber with an outer diameter of 2.4 cm were used in a water phantom with 35-MV x-rays, then $C_\lambda = 0.88(1.005)(0.968/0.985) = 0.869 \cong 0.87$. Clearly it would be advantageous to tabulate C_λ/A_c with three significant figures if the C_λ formalism is retained.

Nahum and Greening (1976, 1978) have concluded that the C_λ tabulations in Table 13.4 are significantly in error when applied to practical ion chambers such as the Farmer chamber, which has either a Tufnol or a graphite wall that is more nearly air-equivalent than water-equivalent. This provided some of the motivation for the AAPM's preparing a new protocol based on the N_{gas} concept in place of C_λ. If the C_λ concept continues to be used, however, one may expect to see improved chamber-specific tabulations of C_λ that take into account the criticisms of Nahum and Greening and of others. Otherwise the N_{gas} approach in the new AAPM (1983) protocol and other comparable protocols (e.g., NACP, 1980) may be expected to replace the C_λ method altogether.

C. Substitution of Plastics for Water in Photon-Beam Phantoms

Solid plastic phantoms are frequently substituted for water as a matter of convenience. When that is done the following procedure should be used:

1.

The center of the chamber should be positioned at the same distance from the source as if a water phantom were used. Also the same beam collimator setting should be employed.

2.

The chamber walls (and ^{60}Co buildup cap, if present) should preferably be made of the same plastic as the phantom (but see Section V.B if not). The chamber should fit the receiving hole in the phantom snugly; any void around the connecting stem should be filled in with the same plastic.

3.

The depth d_p of the chamber center from the front of the plastic phantom should be adjusted to give the same photon attenuation as would occur with the chamber at depth d_{wat} in a water phantom. This will be closely approximated for photons below

10 MeV if the number of atomic electrons per cm^2 in a plastic layer of thickness d_p is the same as that in a water layer d_{wat}. That is,

$$d_p N_A \rho_p \overline{\left(\frac{Z}{A}\right)}_p = d_{wat} N_A \rho_{wat} \overline{\left(\frac{Z}{A}\right)}_{wat} \tag{13.49}$$

where N_A = Avogadro's constant,

$\rho_{p,\,wat}$ = density of plastic and water, respectively,

$$\overline{\left(\frac{Z}{A}\right)}_p = f_1 \left(\frac{Z}{A}\right)_1 + f_2 \left(\frac{Z}{A}\right)_2 + \cdots$$

and, for water,

$$\overline{\left(\frac{Z}{A}\right)}_{wat} = f_H \left(\frac{Z}{A}\right)_H + f_O \left(\frac{Z}{A}\right)_O$$

$$= 0.1119(0.9921) + 0.8881(0.5000)$$

$$= 0.5551$$

f_1, f_2, etc. are the elemental weight fractions in the plastic. For acrylic ($C_5H_8O_2$), $(Z/A)_p = 0.5394$, and for polystyrene (C_8H_8), $(Z/A)_p = 0.5377$.

The plastic density varies somewhat from piece to piece, and should be determined by weighing and measuring each sample. The density of pure water at 22°C is ρ_w = 0.9978 g/cm^3.

Equation (13.49) can be simplified to obtain the chamber depth in the plastic phantom as

$$d_p = \frac{\rho_{wat}}{\rho_p} \cdot \frac{\overline{(Z/A)}_{wat}}{\overline{(Z/A)}_p} d_{wat}$$

$$= \left[\frac{0.5538}{\rho_p \overline{(Z/A)}_p} \right] d_{wat} \tag{13.49a}$$

For example, if a polystyrene phantom of density 1.04 g/cm^3 were used in place of water, a 7-cm calibration depth in water would translate to d_p = 6.93 cm in the polystyrene. With a Lucite phantom of density ρ = 1.17 g/cm^3, a 7-cm depth in water would translate to 6.14 cm in the Lucite. Note that in the latter case the distance (the SSD) from the source to the phantom surface would be greater for the Lucite phantom than for a water phantom by $7 - 6.14 = 0.86$ cm, since the chamber remains at the same distance from the source in both phantoms.

For x-rays generated at 10 MV and above, pair production in plastics becomes significantly less than in water because of the substitution of carbon for oxygen. Thus Eq. (13.49a), based on the electron content of those media assuming only Compton interactions to attenuate the beam, becomes inaccurate. Table 13.5 lists values of

TABLE 13.5. Ratios d_w/d_p for Polystyrene of Density 1.04 g/cm^2 and Acrylic of Density 1.17 g/cm^3 [a]

Radiation	d_w/d_p	
	Polystyrene	Acrylic
γ-Rays:		
^{60}Co	0.99	0.88
X-Rays (MV):		
2–8	0.99	0.88
10–35	1.00	0.88
40–50	1.01	0.89

[a] AAPM (1983). Reproduced with permission from R. J. Schulz and The American Institute of Physics.

the ratio (d_{wat}/d_p) for polystyrene and acrylic, as provided by the AAPM (1983), that may be used in place of Eq. (13.49a) to evaluate d_p, especially at 10 MV and higher energies.

4.
Equation (13.48) can be rewritten for the absorbed dose D_p to the phantom of plastic instead of water, for a photon beam of quality λ, as

$$(D_p)_\lambda = (C_\lambda)_p \, N_X A_{\mathrm{ion}} M P_{\mathrm{ion}} \qquad (\mathrm{rad}) \qquad (13.50)$$

where N_X is the ^{60}Co exposure calibration factor, M is the atmosphere-corrected electrometer reading taken with the chamber in the plastic phantom irradiated by the x-ray beam of quality λ, and

$$(C_\lambda)_p = \left[0.876 \, \beta_p A_c \left(\frac{\mu_{\mathrm{en}}}{\rho} \right)_a^p \right]_{\mathrm{Co}} \frac{\left[\overline{\left(\frac{dT}{\rho dx} \right)}_{c,\,\lambda} \right]_a^p}{\left[\overline{\left(\frac{dT}{\rho dx} \right)}_{c,\,\mathrm{Co}} \right]_a^p} \qquad (13.51)$$

which is seen to be identical to Eq. (13.47) except for the replacement of the superscript wat (representing water) by p (for plastic). C_λ itself is always assumed to refer to water unless it has a subscript p. $\beta_p \cong \beta_w \cong 1.005$ for ^{60}Co at depth in a phantom. A_c is the same for polystyrene and water, but slightly less for the more dense Lucite, as indicated in parentheses in Table 13.3.

The values of $(C_\lambda)_p$ in Table 13.4 were provided by the AAPM (1971) for use where the chamber and phantom are both polystyrene, or both acrylic plastic. These data assume $\beta = 1.000$ and $A_c = 0.985$ as previously mentioned.

5.
Having obtained [from Eq. (13.50)] the absorbed dose $(D_p)_\lambda$ in the plastic phantom irradiated by an x-ray beam of quality λ, one can then derive the absorbed dose to

TABLE 13.6. **Ratios of Mean Energy-Absorption Coefficients for Water and Plastic**[a]

Radiation	$\left(\dfrac{\overline{\mu_{en}}}{\rho}\right)^{\text{water}}_{\text{acrylic}}$	$\left(\dfrac{\overline{\mu_{en}}}{\rho}\right)^{\text{water}}_{\text{polystyrene}}$
2–6-MV x rays, ^{60}Co γ rays	1.031	1.036
x rays (MV):		
8	1.032	1.038
10	1.033	1.039
15	1.040	1.049
20	1.041	1.054
35	1.049	1.068
45	1.064	1.096

[a] AAPM (1983). Reproduced with permission from R. J. Schulz and The American Institute of Physics.

water that would have occurred at the corresponding location in a water phantom. Since TCPE is present in both phantoms we can write that in the water phantom

$$(D_{\text{wat}})_\lambda = \beta_{\text{wat}}(K_c)_{\text{wat}} = \beta_{\text{wat}}\Psi\left(\frac{\overline{\mu_{en}}}{\rho}\right)_{\text{wat}} \tag{13.52}$$

and in the plastic phantom

$$(D_p)_\lambda = \beta_p(K_c)_p = \beta_p\Psi\left(\frac{\overline{\mu_{en}}}{\rho}\right)_p \tag{13.53}$$

For the case of an acrylic phantom (but not for polystyrene) one more correction factor is needed to obtain the dose to water in a water phantom. This is the *excess-*

TABLE 13.7. **Excess-Scatter Correction (ESC) Factors for Measurements in Acrylic Phantoms**[a]

Photon	Depth in Phantom (cm)	ESC			
		Size[b] = 5 × 5	10 × 10	20 × 20	30 × 30
γ-Ray:	0.5	.997	.996	.995	.996
^{60}Co	5.0	.986	.987	.989	.991
x-Ray (MV):					
2	0.4	.998	.994	.997	—
	5.0	.984	.982	.989	—
4	1.0	.998	.997	.998	—
	5.0	.994	.993	.993	—
6	1.5	.999	.998	.998	—
	5.0	.994	.994	.996	—

[a] Reproduced with permission from R. J. Schulz and The American Institute of Physics.
[b] Field size at depth (cm^2).

scatter correction (ESC) due to Casson (1978) and discussed in the 1983 AAPM protocol. For a given beam size the dose is thereby elevated in acrylic relative to water because the greater density of the acrylic gives rise to more scattered photons. Thus the equation for the dose to the water phantom at the point of measurement is gotten from Eqs. (13.52) and (13.53), assuming $\beta_p = \beta_{\text{wat}}$:

$$(D_{\text{wat}})_\lambda = (D_p)_\lambda \left(\overline{\frac{\mu_{\text{en}}}{\rho}}\right)_p^{\text{wat}} \cdot \text{ESC} \qquad (13.54)$$

for which the $\overline{(\mu_{\text{en}}/\rho)}_p^{\text{wat}}$ factor is given in Table 13.6. ESC = 1 for polystyrene phantoms, and for acrylic phantoms its value may be obtained from Table 13.7 (AAPM, 1983).

Clearly the calibration procedure requires fewer corrections in a water phantom, but this is partially offset by the relative inconvenience of working with a liquid vs. a solid medium.

V. CALIBRATION OF PHOTON BEAMS IN PHANTOMS BY THE N_{gas} METHOD

A. Chamber Wall Material Same as Phantom

Section III.B described the procedure for calibrating an ion chamber with ^{60}Co γ-rays in terms of the quantity N_{gas}. In the present section the use of such a chamber for calibrating a photon beam in a phantom will be described. A water phantom will be assumed unless otherwise specified, and the chamber wall and buildup cap (if present) are taken to be water-equivalent. The main photon application of this method is for x-ray beams generated at potentials of 2 MV or greater.

Consider an ion chamber, with or without its buildup cap, immersed in a water phantom and centered at a reference point P on the beam axis. The beam quality will be characterized by λ. An electrometer reading M'_λ is obtained, and corrected to atmospheric conditions at 22°C and 1 atm by Eq. (12.21) to obtain M_λ. This is to be corrected for ionic recombination losses by multiplying it by P_{ion} (see Fig. 12.25).

The absorbed dose to the cavity gas can be obtained from Eq. (13.2), substituting P_{ion} for A_{ion}^{-1}:

$$(D_{\text{gas}})_\lambda = M_\lambda P_{\text{ion}} N_{\text{gas}} \qquad (13.55)$$

This value of D_{gas} is typically larger than it would have been for a very small cavity located at P, due to lack of photon-beam attenuation in the actual gas-filled cavity. AAPM (1983) employs a multiplicative "replacement correction" P_{repl}, which depends on the photon gradient vs. depth and on the diameter of the *cavity*, to compensate for this error. Figure 13.6 gives values of P_{repl} in a water phantom for various x-ray beam energies and chamber inner diameters. Note that P_{repl} for ^{60}Co is approximately equal to A_c/A_{eq} for water in Table 13.3, for corresponding chamber sizes and a wall thickness of 5 mm.

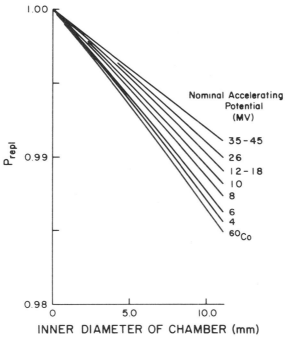

FIGURE 13.6. Replacement correction P_{repl} in water for ^{60}Co γ-rays and for x-rays generated at various energies (AAPM, 1983). Reproduced with permission from R. J. Schulz and The American Institute of Physics.

The absorbed dose $(D_{\text{wat}})_\lambda$ in the water at point P in the absence of the chamber can be gotten from application of the cavity relation:

$$(D_{\text{wat}})_\lambda = (D_{\text{gas}})_\lambda P_{\text{repl}} \left[\left(\frac{\overline{L}}{\rho} \right)_{\text{gas}}^{\text{wat}} \right]_\lambda$$

$$= N_{\text{gas}} M_\lambda P_{\text{ion}} P_{\text{repl}} \left[\left(\frac{\overline{L}}{\rho} \right)_{\text{gas}}^{\text{wat}} \right]_\lambda \qquad (13.56)$$

where $[(\overline{L}/\rho)_{\text{gas}}^{\text{wat}}]_\lambda$ for gas = air is tabulated for various photon energies in column 2 of Table 13.8. For the other phantom media acrylic and polystyrene Table 13.8 also gives values of $[(\overline{L}/\rho)_{\text{air}}^{p}]$. If the phantom, chamber wall, and buildup cap (if present) are all homogeneously made of polystyrene or acrylic plastic in place of water, the procedure for beam calibration is modified according to Section IV.C. The absorbed dose to the phantom medium may be gotten from Eq. 13.56 by replacing "wat" by "p" for plastic. Equation (13.54) then gives the dose to water.

TABLE 13.8. **Ratios of Average Restricted Stopping Powers, $[(\overline{L}/\rho)_{\text{air}}^{\text{wat}}]_\lambda$ and $[(\overline{L}/\rho)_{\text{air}}^{p}]_\lambda$ for Various Photon Spectra**[a]

Radiation	$[(\overline{L}/\rho)_{\text{air}}^{\text{wat}}]_\lambda$ Medium = Water	$[(\overline{L}/\rho)_{\text{air}}^{p}]_\lambda$ Acrylic	Polystyrene
γ-Rays:			
^{60}Co	1.134	1.103	1.113
x-Rays (MV):			
2	1.135	1.104	1.114
4	1.131	1.099	1.108
6	1.127	1.093	1.103
8	1.121	1.088	1.097
10	1.117	1.085	1.094
15	1.106	1.074	1.083
20	1.096	1.065	1.074
25	1.093	1.062	1.071
35	1.084	1.053	1.062
45	1.071	1.041	1.048

[a]Assuming $\Delta = 10$ keV (AAPM, 1983). Reproduced with permission from R. J. Schulz and The American Institute of Physics.

B.   Chamber Wall Material Different from Phantom

In case the ion chamber wall and cap (if present) are the same material, but it differs from the phantom medium, AAPM (1983) has provided a semiempirical formula for $(D_p)_\lambda$, the dose in the phantom medium p, as proposed by Almond and Svensson (1977):

$$(D_p)_\lambda = N_{\text{gas}} M_\lambda P_{\text{ion}} P_{\text{repl}}$$

$$\times \left[\alpha \left(\frac{\overline{L}}{\rho} \right)_{\text{gas}}^{\text{wall}} \left(\frac{\overline{\mu_{\text{en}}}}{\rho} \right)_{\text{wall}}^{p} + (1 - \alpha) \left(\frac{\overline{L}}{\rho} \right)_{\text{gas}}^{p} \right]_\lambda \quad (13.57)$$

where α is the fraction of the total ionization produced the cavity gas by electrons arising in the chamber wall and cap (if present), and $1 - \alpha$ is the fraction due to electrons originating in p.

For a very thin chamber wall, $\alpha \to 0$ and Eq. (13.57) becomes the same as Eq. (13.56), adapted to phantom medium p. For a wall + cap thickness exceeding the maximum secondary-electron range, $\alpha \cong 1$ and Eq. (13.57) simplifies to

$$(D_p)_\lambda = N_{\text{gas}} M_\lambda P_{\text{ion}} P_{\text{repl}} \left(\frac{\overline{L}}{\rho} \right)_{\text{gas}}^{\text{wall}} \left(\frac{\overline{\mu_{\text{en}}}}{\rho} \right)_{\text{wall}}^{p} \quad (13.58)$$

Values of α for intermediate thicknesses of chamber wall (+ cap if present) are shown in Figs. 13.7 a,b [Lempert et al. (1983), as reproduced in the AAPM 1983 protocol].

Additional complications arise if the buildup cap is made of a different material

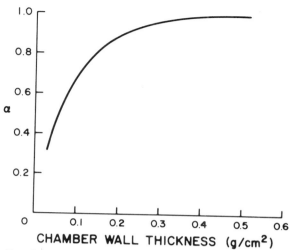

FIGURE 13.7 a. Fraction α of ionization due to electrons arising in the chamber wall, as a function of mass wall thickness, for ^{60}Co γ-rays [Lempert et al. (1983), as adapted by AAPM (1983)]. Reproduced with permission from R. J. Schulz and The American Institute of Physics.

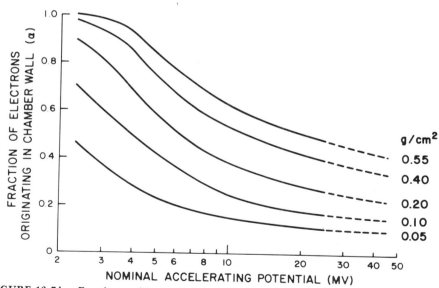

FIGURE 13.7 b. Fraction α of ionization due to electrons from the chamber wall irradiated by x-rays with nominal acceleration potentials of 2 to 50 MV. The dashed portions of the curves are extrapolations of the experimental data. [Lempert et al. (1983), as adapted by AAPM (1983). Reproduced with permission from R. J. Schulz and The American Institute of Physics.]

than either the chamber wall or the phantom during beam measurement (AAPM, 1983). That situation can and should be avoided. The AAPM (1983) recommends leaving off the buildup cap in the phantom, in which case the value of α should be selected for the remaining chamber wall thickness.

VI. CALIBRATION OF ELECTRON BEAMS IN PHANTOMS

A. Absolute Cavity-Chamber Measurements

The problem of calculating the absorbed dose deposited by an electron beam at a depth in a phantom where the electron fluence is known was discussed in the last section of Chapter 8.

Measurement of this dose may be done by inserting a suitable dosimeter, for example a B–G cavity ion chamber, at the point P in question. The B–G theory can then be applied to derive a value of the dose D_p in the phantom medium p from the value of the dose in the cavity gas, D_{gas}:

$$D_p = D_{\text{gas}} \left[\overline{\left(\frac{dT}{\rho dx} \right)_c} \right]_{\text{gas}}^p P_{\text{fl}} \qquad (13.59)$$

where $D_{\text{gas}} = (M_E P_{\text{ion}}/m)(\overline{W/e})_{\text{gas}}$, in which M_E is the charge collected and m is the mass of gas in the cavity, and where P_{fl} is a correction factor for perturbation of the electron fluence by the cavity in the phantom. Or, on the basis of Spencer's theory accounting for δ-ray escape from the cavity of energy-cutoff size Δ,

$$D_p = D_{\text{gas}} \left[\overline{\left(\frac{L}{\rho} \right)_\Delta} \right]_{\text{gas}}^p P_{\text{fl}} \qquad (13.60)$$

P_{fl} will be discussed in the following section. Note that the phantom medium p may be either a plastic or water in Eqs. (13.59) and (13.60).

B. Electron-Beam Perturbation Corrections for Cavity Chambers in Phantoms

We have already seen that photon-beam perturbation by a cavity chamber in a phantom is easily corrected for through either the displacement correction factor A_c [see Eq. (13.38)] or the replacement correction factor P_{repl} (see Fig. 13.6), depending upon the calibration procedure used. In either case the point in the phantom where the dose is being determined is the location of the geometric center of the cavity. The AAPM (1983) protocol names this a "gradient correction" because it depends upon the slope of the absorbed dose vs. depth, as well as the chamber size.

The electron-beam case is somewhat more complicated, requiring two different corrections to account for chamber perturbation. These are: (1) an electron-fluence scattering correction, and (2) positioning of the chamber with its geometric center deeper in the phantom than the point P at which the dose is being determined. These two corrections will be discussed separately in the next two sections.

1. ELECTRON-FLUENCE SCATTERING CORRECTION

It was pointed out by Harder (1968) that a cavity in a phantom is traversed by a somewhat greater number of electrons than the same volume filled by phantom material would be. This is because an electron is more likely to be scattered into the cavity by the surrounding higher-density medium than to be scattered out by the low-density cavity gas. This is illustrated by Fig. 13.8a. The average absorbed dose in the cavity gas is consequently greater than that in the same volume filled with phantom medium, assuming equal stopping powers.

A second effect noted by Harder is illustrated in Fig. 13.8b. This "obliquity" or pathlength effect results from the greater pathlength of an electron traversing the cavity when it is filled with phantom medium than when filled with gas. This is because of the greater probability of electron scattering in the denser material. The average absorbed dose in the cavity gas is less than that in the phantom-filled cavity on account of this.

The importance of each of these two effects depends on cavity shape and orientation, as discussed by Harder. For a thin (1–2 mm) flat coin-shaped cavity oriented perpendicular to the electron beam direction these effects are said to be negligible (AAPM, 1983). Thus P_{fl} may be taken as unity in Eqs. (13.59) and (13.60) for such chambers.

For a cylindrical cavity oriented with its axis perpendicular to the electron-beam direction, Harder found that the in-scattering effect dominated, and that the re-

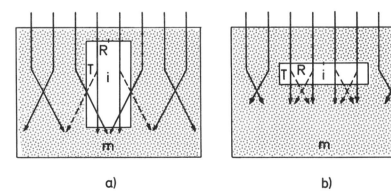

a) b)

FIGURE 13.8. The electron-beam perturbation effects caused by a gas-filled cavity in a solid or liquid phantom, as discussed by Harder (1968). Electron paths are idealized to emphasize the effects being shown. (*a*) *The in-scattering effect.* Electrons are more likely to be scattered into the cavity by the condensed medium *m* than to be scattered out by the gas (see dashed arrows). The dose in the gas is thereby *increased* relative to the dose in the medium. This effect predominates in chambers that are elongated in the beam direction. (*b*) *The obliquity or pathlength effect.* The electron paths through the cavity gas are straighter than those present (see dashed paths) when the phantom medium fills the cavity, because of the additional scattering in the condensed medium *m*. The dose in the gas is thus *decreased* relative to the dose in the medium, tending to counter the effect of side in-scattering as the chamber length is reduced. Reproduced with permission from D. Harder and Springer-Verlag.

TABLE 13.9.   Electron Fluence Correction Factor P_{fl} for Cylindrical Ion Chambers[a]

$\overline{T}^{b}$ (MeV)	P_{fl}					
	I.D.[c] = 3 mm	5 mm	6 mm	7 mm	10 mm	16 mm
1	—	— (.947)	—	—	—	—
2	.977	.962 (.970)	.956	.949	(.958)	—
3	.978	.966 (.978)	.959	.952	(.970)	(.962)
4	—	— (.984)	—	—	(.977)	(.972)
5	.982	.971 (.986)	.965	.960	(.981)	(.977)
7	.986	.977 —	.972	.967	—	—
10	.990	.985 (.992)	.981	.978	(.989)	(.987)
15	.995	.992 —	.991	.990	—	—
20	.997	.996 (.997)	.995	.995	(.995)	(.993)

[a] Data in parentheses are for an air cavity in a water phantom, due to Harder (1968) as given in ICRU (1972). Other data are from acrylic-phantom measurements of Johansson et al. (1977), as given in AAPM (1983).
[b] The mean electron energy $\overline{T}$ can be estimated for this purpose at the depth d of the effective chamber center by the equation $\overline{T} \cong T_o [1 - d/(\text{CSDA range})]$, where T_o is the incident energy of the electron beam, and the CSDA range of electrons of that energy is listed in Appendix E, column 5.
[c] Inner diameter.

sulting enhancement of cavity ionization was significant, as shown in Table 13.9. Values of the electron-fluence correction factor P_{fl} are listed there for several air-cavity inner diameters, and mean electron energies $\overline{T}$. Harder's calculated values for a water phantom are shown in parentheses. The other data were measured with air cavities in an acrylic phantom by Johansson et al. (1977). The data for the only cavity diameter (5 mm) in common between the two show some differences between them which remain to be resolved.

2.   CHAMBER-SHIFT CORRECTION

Accounting for the decrease in electron-beam attenuation in a phantom due to the finite size of the cavity could, in principle, be accomplished with a gradient-type correction factor, as was done for photon beams. The typical depth–dose shape of an electron beam, as shown in Fig. 8.14a, discourages that approach, however, because of the steep and rapidly changing slopes. Dutreix and Dutreix (1966) indicated an alternative method that is more satisfactory for electron-beam dosimetry. Those authors refer to it as a "displacement correction," in the sense that the geometric center of the chamber is displaced from the "effective center" of the chamber, i.e., the point at which the dose is determined in the phantom. Here we will describe this as a *chamber-shift correction* to avoid confusion, since A_c is usually referred to as a displacement correction in the sense that it corrects for photon-beam attenuation in the phantom medium displaced by the ion chamber.

The idea underlying the chamber-shift correction is that the ionization produced in a gas-filled cavity is generated by the electrons entering the cavity. For a monodirectional beam, this means the electrons entering through the cavity wall on the upstream side. The depth of the inner surface of that wall in the phantom determines how many electrons come in. Thus, for example, the ionization per unit mass of gas in a flat chamber will be the same for two different chamber thicknesses, so long as (a) the front cavity surface remains at the same depth in the phantom, (b) the chamber remains much smaller than the electron range, and (c) the electron-fluence correction factor P_{fl} remains at unity. This is illustrated in Fig. 13.9a. Clearly in that case the chamber geometric center is a distance s deeper than the effective center at point P on the front wall, at which the dose is determined. $2s$ is the chamber plate separation.

For cylindrical and spherical cavities of radius r (see Fig. 13.9b and c) the distance s of the front wall from the plane at the depth of the geometric center varies with the point of entry of each electron, unlike the case of the flat cavity. The average

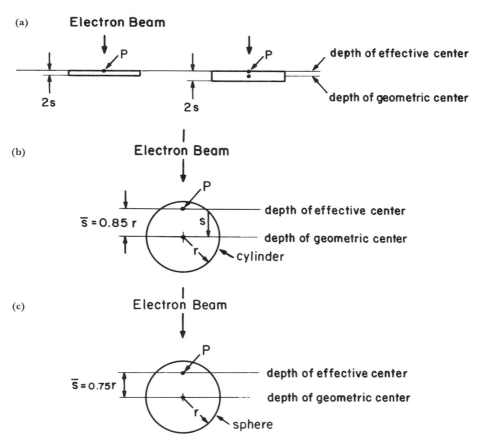

FIGURE 13.9. Illustrating the chamber-shift correction $\bar{s}$ for a monodirectional electron beam in a phantom. P indicates the effective center of the cavity, that is, the point where the absorbed dose is determined in the phantom. (a) *Flat cavities:* Shift correction $\bar{s} = s$. (b) *Cylinders:* Shift correction $\bar{s} = 8r/3\pi \cong 0.85r$. (c) *Spheres:* Shift correction $\bar{s} = 3r/4 = 0.75r$.

distance $\bar{s}$ can be obtained by integrating over the cross section of the cavity (as viewed by the beam) to obtain the mean distance from the front wall to the midplane of the chamber, weighted by the track length of each electron (assumed straight). This takes into account the relative ionization contributed by each electron. Thus for a cylindrical chamber of radius r irradiated perpendicular to its axis, one finds the value of $\bar{s}$ from

$$\bar{s} = \frac{\int_0^r (r^2 - x^2)\, dx}{\int_0^r (r^2 - x^2)^{1/2}\, dx} = \frac{8r}{3\pi} \cong 0.85r \qquad (13.61)$$

and for a sphere,

$$\bar{s} = \frac{\int_0^r x(r^2 - x^2)\, dx}{\int_0^r x(r^2 - x^2)^{1/2}\, dx} = \frac{3r}{4} = 0.75r \qquad (13.62)$$

For the Farmer chamber, having a radius of 3.25 mm, a value $\bar{s} \cong 2.5$ mm is appropriate.

Notice that the electron-fluence correction factor P_{fl} is used as a multiplier for the measured ionization or D_{gas} [for example, in Eq. (13.59) or (13.60)], and the chamber-shift correction $\bar{s}$ then locates the depth at which the dose measurement D_p applies, at point P in the phantom medium p. If the dose is to be measured at a depth d in the phantom, then the cavity chamber must be located with its effective center at that depth, and its geometric center at a depth $d + \bar{s}$. If two chambers of different shapes are to be compared in a phantom irradiated by an electron beam, they should be positioned with their effective centers at the same point P (see Fig. 13.9). Their geometrical centers will therefore be separated in depth by the difference in their $\bar{s}$-values.

Figure 13.10 shows the effect of the chamber-shift correction in the case of an imaginary chamber for which $\bar{s} = 5$ mm. It is seen that this simple leftward shift brings the dashed (dose vs. chamber-center) curve into coincidence with the solid (dose vs. effective depth) curve, which is the true depth–dose curve. To accomplish this through a multiplicative correction would require factors differing strongly from unity, and having a different value at every depth.

Thin, flat cavity chambers offer the advantage of requiring no electron-fluence correction, in addition to which their dose results can be accurately plotted at the depth of the inner surface of the front wall. Cylindrical and spherical chambers require both electron-fluence corrections and chamber-shift corrections, neither of which are as accurately known. On the other hand, flat chambers are more difficult to construct, especially while avoiding materials that are not phantom-equivalent.

The foregoing considerations of electron-beam perturbation corrections apply equally well to absolute cavities (Section VI.A), the C_E method (Section VI.C), and the N_{gas} method (Section VI.D). In every case it will be advantageous in calibrating

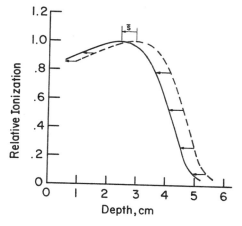

FIGURE 13.10. Illustrating the chamber shift correction, $\bar{s}$, assumed here equal to 5 mm, the length of the arrows. The dashed curve is the dose D_p, already corrected for electron-fluence error, but plotted vs. the depth of the geometric chamber center. The solid curve shows D_p vs. effecive-center depth in phantom, and is the correct depth–dose curve.

electron beams in a phantom to locate the effective center of the ion-chamber cavity at or near the depth where the absorbed dose reaches a maximum, since depth positioning will be least critical at that depth.

C. The C_E Method

If the sensitive volume of the cavity is not known, calibration of the chamber becomes necessary, analogous to the case already considered for photon beams. A procedure similar to the C_λ method described in Section IV.B.2 was suggested by Almond (1967, 1970) and Svensson and Pettersson (1967) for electron beams, using a corresponding factor C_E in place of C_λ. This approach was formalized by the ICRU (1972, 1984b) and more details will be found in those reports about electron-beam dosimetry in general, as well as this method in particular.

The value of C_E is obtained through a ^{60}Co γ-ray calibration in which the free-space exposure is X (C/kg). The ion-chamber wall and buildup cap are made of material w, and the cavity contains air. The dose in the cavity air, D_a, can be expressed in grays from Eqs. (13.9) and (13.17) as

$$D_a = X \left(\overline{\frac{W}{e}}\right)_a \left(\frac{\mu_{en}}{\rho}\right)_a^w A_w \beta_w \left(\frac{\overline{L}}{\rho}\right)_w^a$$

$$= M P_{ion} N_X A_{ion} \left(\overline{\frac{W}{e}}\right)_a \left(\frac{\mu_{en}}{\rho}\right)_a^w A_w \beta_w \left(\frac{\overline{L}}{\rho}\right)_w^a \qquad (13.63)$$

The ICRU (1972) made the implicit assumptions that the chamber wall and buildup cap were exactly air-equivalent for ^{60}Co γ rays [i.e., $(\mu_{en}/\rho)_a^w = (\overline{L}/\rho)_w^a = 1.000$], that $\beta_w = 1.000$, and $P_{ion} A_{ion} = 1$. Under these simplifying assumptions, Eq. (13.63) reduces to

$$D_a = M N_X \left(\overline{\frac{W}{e}}\right)_a A_w \qquad (13.64)$$

N_X and A_w apply to the ^{60}Co calibration, and $(\overline{W/e})_a = 33.97$ J/C, assuming dry air. Hence D_a/M has the same value in electron beams as for ^{60}Co γ-rays, assuming equal ion-collection efficiencies.

The chamber is next placed in a phantom of medium p (preferably water) with the effective center of the cavity at the point P where the absorbed dose D_p is to be determined in the phantom medium. For electron-beam calibration the ICRU recommends that the effective center be placed at the depth where D_p reaches a maximum, to minimize the influence of depth-positioning error.

The electron beam produces an electrometer reading M_E, which is related to a dose $(D_a)_E$ in the cavity by Eq. (13.64). The B–G relation (13.59) then allows the calculation of the absorbed dose D_p in the unperturbed phantom at the point P as

$$D_p = (D_a)_E \left[\overline{\left(\frac{dT}{\rho dx}\right)_c} \right]_a^p P_{\text{fl}}$$

$$= M_E P_{\text{ion}} N_X A_{\text{ion}} \left(\frac{\overline{W}}{e}\right)_a A_w \left[\overline{\left(\frac{dT}{\rho dx}\right)_c} \right]_a^p P_{\text{fl}} \qquad (13.65)$$

where D_p and $(D_a)_E$ are given in grays, N_X is the ^{60}Co exposure calibration factor in kg^{-1}, $(\overline{W/e})_a = 33.97$ J/C independent of beam quality, $[\overline{(dT/\rho dx)_c}]_a^p$ is the mean value of the ratio of mass collision stopping powers for phantom medium and air. evaluated for the spectrum of the electron beam crossing the cavity, and P_{fl} was defined with Eq. (13.59). If N_X is given instead in R/C and D_p is desired in rad, we have in place of Eq. (13.65)

$$D_p = 0.876 M_E P_{\text{ion}} N_X A_{\text{ion}} A_w \left[\overline{\left(\frac{dT}{\rho dx}\right)_c} \right]_a^p P_{\text{fl}}$$

$$= M_E P_{\text{ion}} N_X A_{\text{ion}} C_E \qquad (13.66)$$

where

$$C_E = 0.876 A_w \left[\overline{\left(\frac{dT}{\rho dx}\right)_c} \right]_a^p P_{\text{fl}} \text{ rad/R} \qquad (13.67)$$

in its customary units.

Notice in this case that the ionization in the cavity air is produced by the electrons in the primary beam. Any δ rays they create in the cavity that have long enough range to carry energy into the wall will be replaced by other δ-rays originating in the air-equivalent wall. Thus the mass collision stopping-power ratio is preferable

TABLE 13.10. Values of C_E for Electron Beams in Water[a]

Depth in water, z (cm)	C_E (rad/R)									
	$E_a^b = 5$	10	15	20	25	30	35	40	45	50
1	.922	.877	.843	.823	.808	.795	.784	.775	.768	.762
2		.893	.858	.835	.819	.806	.795	.786	.778	.771
3		.915	.871	.848	.830	.816	.804	.794	.786	.778
4		.947	.886	.859	.840	.824	.812	.801	.792	.785
5		.963	.901	.871	.847	.831	.819	.809	.799	.791
6			.933	.885	.856	.839	.825	.815	.806	.798
7			.965	.902	.867	.846	.832	.821	.812	.803
8				.941	.882	.854	.839	.827	.816	.808
9				.959	.898	.865	.847	.832	.820	.814
10				.926	.917	.878	.856	.840	.827	.819
11					.946	.890	.866	.848	.834	.823
12					.939	.906	.879	.857	.841	.829
13						.926	.890	.867	.818	.835
14						.959	.907	.877	.857	.842
15						.933	.924	.890	.866	.849
16							.954	.903	.876	.857
17							.929	.919	.887	.864
18								.940	.900	.874
19								.936	.915	.883
20									.935	.895
21									.943	.908
22									.921	.924
23										.945
24										.918

[a] A_w was assumed to be 0.985; the remaining factors within the Co bracket and P_{f1} in Eq. (13.68) were each taken as unity. [Kessaris (1970), as quoted in ICRU (1972).] Reproduced with permission from N. D. Kessaris and the International Commission on Radiation Units and Measurements.

[b] Initial electron energy (MeV).

to the restricted stopping-power ratio for use in Eqs. (13.65)–(13.67), because of the resulting δ-ray equilibrium.

Table 13.10 contains an array of C_E-values from ICRU (1972), computed by Kessaris (1970) by assuming p = water, A_w = 0.985 and P_{fl} = 1.000 in Eq. (13.67). One may ask what the combined error in C_E would be as a result of the several assumptions mentioned above, if the chamber wall were, say, graphite in place of perfectly air-equivalent material. A more complete equation for C_E for a non-air-equivalent walled chamber can be expressed as

$$C_E = 0.876 \left[\overline{\left(\frac{dT}{\rho\,dx} \right)_{c}^{\,p}} P_{fl} \left[A_w \left(\frac{\mu_{en}}{\rho} \right)_{a}^{w} \beta_w \left(\frac{\overline{L}}{\rho} \right)_{w}^{a} \right]_{Co} \right] \tag{13.68}$$

where the subscript Co indicates the factors that were evaluated in the ^{60}Co γ-ray chamber calibration. δ-ray equilibrium is still assumed between air and wall. The data in Table 13.10 were computed on the assumption that the entire Co bracket has the value 0.985 ($=A_w$), while a more correct evaluation for an equilibrium-thickness graphite wall would result from inserting the values A_w = 0.988, $(\mu_{en}/\rho)_a^w$ = 1.001, β_w = 1.003, and $(\overline{L}/\rho)_w^a$ = 0.990, yielding a product of 0.982 for the bracket value in Eq. (13.68). Thus we may conclude that Table 13.10 appears to be only about 0.3% too low for the case of a nonperturbing graphite-walled cavity chamber.

It can be seen in the table that the value of C_E decreases with decreasing depth in the phantom and with increasing incident beam energy T_0. These trends are controlled by the polarization effect, through the mass collision stopping-power factor in Eq. (13.67).

D. The N_{gas} Method

An ion chamber calibrated in terms of N_{gas} can be used for electron-beam calibrations in a phantom. The chamber wall need not exactly match the phantom medium, p, (preferably water) so long as the wall is fairly thin (e.g., ≤ 0.1 g/cm^2) and of low-atomic-number plastic. A matching buildup cap, increasing the wall thickness to provide TCPE, must be added during the ^{60}Co calibration. The following equation can be used to calculate the dose D_p in the unperturbed phantom medium at the location of the effective center of the chamber:

$$D_p = N_{gas} M_E P_{ion} P_{fl} [(L/\rho)_{gas}^p]_{\overline{T}} \tag{13.69}$$

where M_E is the atmosphere-corrected electrometer reading due to the electron irradiation, N_{gas} is obtained from the ^{60}Co chamber calibration, P_{ion} is the ionic recombination correction factor during the electron exposure, P_{fl} is the electron-fluence correction (see Table 13.9), and $[(L/\rho)_{gas}^p]_{\overline{T}}$ is the ratio of restricted stopping powers for phantom medium and cavity gas, evaluated at the mean electron energy $\overline{T}$ crossing the cavity.

Tables 13.11, 13.12, and 13.13 contain values of $[(L/\rho)_{air}^p]_{\overline{T}}$ for the media water, polystyrene, and acrylic plastic, respectively. Values are tabulated for depths in the phantom from 0 to 30 cm and incident electron energies T_0 from 5 to 60 MeV.

TABLE 13.11. $[(L/\rho)^p_{air}]_{\overline{T}}$ for Use in Eq. (13.69); Phantom Medium = Water[a]

Depth (g/cm²)	T_o^b = 60.0	50.0	40.0	30.0	25.0	20.0	18.0	16.0	14.0	12.0	10.0	9.0	8.0	7.0	6.0	5.0
							$[(L/\rho)^p_{air}]_{\overline{T}}$, Δ = 10 keV									
0.0	0.902	0.904	0.912	0.928	0.940	0.955	0.961	0.969	0.977	0.986	0.997	1.003	1.011	1.019	1.029	1.040
0.1	0.902	0.905	0.913	0.929	0.941	0.955	0.962	0.969	0.978	0.987	0.998	1.005	1.012	1.020	1.030	1.042
0.2	0.903	0.906	0.914	0.930	0.942	0.956	0.963	0.970	0.978	0.988	0.999	1.006	1.013	1.022	1.032	1.044
0.3	0.904	0.907	0.915	0.931	0.943	0.957	0.964	0.971	0.979	0.989	1.000	1.007	1.015	1.024	1.034	1.046
0.4	0.904	0.908	0.916	0.932	0.944	0.958	0.965	0.972	0.980	0.990	1.002	1.009	1.017	1.026	1.036	1.050
0.5	0.905	0.909	0.917	0.933	0.945	0.959	0.966	0.973	0.982	0.991	1.003	1.010	1.019	1.028	1.039	1.054
0.6	0.906	0.909	0.918	0.934	0.946	0.960	0.967	0.974	0.983	0.993	1.005	1.012	1.021	1.031	1.043	1.058
0.8	0.907	0.911	0.920	0.936	0.948	0.962	0.969	0.976	0.985	0.996	1.009	1.016	1.026	1.037	1.050	1.067
1.0	0.908	0.913	0.922	0.938	0.950	0.964	0.971	0.979	0.988	0.999	1.013	1.021	1.031	1.043	1.058	1.076
1.2	0.909	0.914	0.924	0.940	0.952	0.966	0.973	0.981	0.991	1.002	1.017	1.026	1.037	1.050	1.066	1.085
1.4	0.910	0.916	0.925	0.942	0.954	0.968	0.976	0.984	0.994	1.006	1.022	1.032	1.044	1.058	1.075	1.095
1.6	0.912	0.917	0.927	0.944	0.956	0.971	0.978	0.987	0.997	1.010	1.027	1.038	1.050	1.066	1.084	1.104
1.8	0.913	0.918	0.929	0.945	0.957	0.973	0.981	0.990	1.001	1.014	1.032	1.044	1.057	1.074	1.093	1.112
2.0	0.914	0.920	0.930	0.947	0.959	0.975	0.983	0.993	1.004	1.018	1.038	1.050	1.065	1.082	1.101	1.120
2.5	0.917	0.923	0.934	0.952	0.964	0.981	0.990	1.000	1.013	1.030	1.053	1.067	1.083	1.102	1.120	1.131
3.0	0.919	0.926	0.938	0.956	0.969	0.987	0.997	1.008	1.023	1.042	1.069	1.084	1.102	1.119	1.129	
3.5	0.922	0.929	0.941	0.960	0.971	0.994	1.004	1.017	1.034	1.056	1.085	1.102	1.118	1.128		
4.0	0.924	0.932	0.944	0.964	0.979	1.001	1.012	1.027	1.046	1.071	1.101	1.116	1.126			
4.5	0.927	0.935	0.948	0.969	0.985	1.008	1.021	1.037	1.059	1.086	1.115	1.125	1.127			
5.0	0.929	0.938	0.951	0.973	0.990	1.016	1.030	1.049	1.072	1.101	1.123	1.126				
5.5	0.931	0.940	0.954	0.978	0.996	1.024	1.040	1.061	1.086	1.113	1.125					
6.0	0.934	0.943	0.958	0.983	1.002	1.033	1.051	1.074	1.100	1.121						
7.0	0.938	0.948	0.965	0.993	1.017	1.054	1.075	1.099	1.118	1.122						
8.0	0.943	0.954	0.972	1.005	1.032	1.076	1.098	1.116								
9.0	0.947	0.960	0.981	1.018	1.049	1.098	1.114	1.118								
10.0	0.952	0.966	0.990	1.032	1.068	1.112	1.116									
12.0	0.962	0.980	1.009	1.062	1.103											
14.0	0.973	0.996	1.031	1.095	1.103											
16.0	0.986	1.013	1.056	1.103	1.107											
18.0	1.000	1.031	1.080													
20.0	1.016	1.051	1.094													
22.0	1.032	1.070														
24.0	1.048	1.082														
26.0	1.062	1.085														
28.0	1.071															
30.0	1.075															

[a] AAPM (1983). Reproduced with permission from R. J. Schulz and The American Institute of Physics.
[b] Electron-beam energies T_o (MeV) are those at phantom entry.

TABLE 13.12. $[(L/\rho)^p_{air}]_{\overline{T}}$ for Use in Eq. (13.69); Phantom Medium = Polystyrene[a]

$[(L/\rho)^p_{air}]_{\overline{T}}$, Δ = 10 keV

Depth (g/cm²)	T_o^b = 60.0	50.0	40.0	30.0	25.0	20.0	18.0	16.0	14.0	12.0	10.0	9.0	8.0	7.0	6.0	5.0
0.0	0.875	0.878	0.887	0.903	0.915	0.929	0.936	0.943	0.950	0.959	0.970	0.975	0.982	0.990	0.999	1.010
0.1	0.876	0.879	0.888	0.904	0.916	0.930	0.936	0.943	0.951	0.960	0.970	0.977	0.983	0.991	1.000	1.011
0.2	0.876	0.880	0.889	0.905	0.917	0.931	0.937	0.944	0.952	0.961	0.972	0.978	0.985	0.993	1.002	1.013
0.3	0.877	0.881	0.890	0.906	0.918	0.931	0.938	0.945	0.953	0.962	0.973	0.979	0.986	0.994	1.004	1.016
0.4	0.878	0.882	0.891	0.907	0.919	0.932	0.939	0.946	0.954	0.963	0.974	0.980	0.988	0.996	1.007	1.019
0.5	0.878	0.883	0.892	0.908	0.919	0.933	0.940	0.947	0.955	0.964	0.975	0.982	0.990	0.999	1.009	1.023
0.6	0.879	0.883	0.893	0.909	0.920	0.934	0.941	0.948	0.956	0.965	0.977	0.984	0.992	1.001	1.012	1.027
0.8	0.881	0.885	0.894	0.911	0.922	0.936	0.943	0.950	0.959	0.968	0.980	0.988	0.996	1.006	1.019	1.035
1.0	0.882	0.887	0.896	0.912	0.924	0.938	0.945	0.952	0.961	0.971	0.984	0.992	1.001	1.012	1.026	1.044
1.2	0.883	0.888	0.898	0.914	0.926	0.940	0.947	0.955	0.963	0.974	0.988	0.996	1.006	1.019	1.034	1.054
1.4	0.884	0.889	0.900	0.916	0.927	0.942	0.949	0.957	0.965	0.978	0.992	1.001	1.012	1.026	1.043	1.064
1.6	0.886	0.891	0.901	0.918	0.929	0.944	0.951	0.959	0.969	0.981	0.997	1.007	1.019	1.033	1.052	1.073
1.8	0.887	0.892	0.903	0.919	0.931	0.946	0.954	0.962	0.972	0.985	1.002	1.012	1.025	1.041	1.060	1.083
2.0	0.888	0.894	0.904	0.921	0.933	0.948	0.956	0.965	0.975	0.989	1.007	1.018	1.032	1.049	1.069	1.092
2.5	0.891	0.897	0.908	0.925	0.937	0.954	0.962	0.972	0.984	0.999	1.020	1.034	1.050	1.070	1.091	1.108
3.0	0.893	0.900	0.911	0.929	0.942	0.959	0.969	0.979	0.992	1.010	1.035	1.051	1.069	1.090	1.105	
3.5	0.896	0.903	0.914	0.933	0.947	0.965	0.975	0.987	1.002	1.023	1.051	1.069	1.088	1.103		
4.0	0.898	0.905	0.917	0.937	0.951	0.971	0.982	0.995	1.013	1.036	1.068	1.086	1.101			
4.5	0.900	0.908	0.920	0.941	0.956	0.978	0.990	1.005	1.024	1.051	1.085	1.099	1.105			
5.0	0.902	0.910	0.923	0.945	0.961	0.985	0.998	1.015	1.037	1.067	1.097	1.103				
5.5	0.904	0.913	0.927	0.949	0.966	0.992	1.008	1.026	1.051	1.081	1.102					
6.0	0.906	0.915	0.930	0.954	0.972	1.000	1.017	1.038	1.065	1.093						
7.0	0.910	0.920	0.936	0.963	0.984	1.018	1.040	1.063	1.089							
8.0	0.914	0.925	0.943	0.973	0.998	1.039	1.063	1.086								
9.0	0.918	0.930	0.949	0.985	1.013	1.061	1.084									
10.0	0.922	0.936	0.958	0.997	1.030	1.081										
12.0	0.931	0.949	0.976	1.024	1.067											
14.0	0.942	0.963	0.995	1.056	1.085											
16.0	0.953	0.978	1.016	1.078												
18.0	0.965	0.994	1.041													
20.0	0.979	1.011	1.061													
22.0	0.994	1.030														
24.0	1.008	1.047														
26.0	1.023	1.057														
28.0	1.036															
30.0	1.045															

[a] AAPM (1983). Reproduced with permission from R. J. Schulz and the American Institute of Physics.
[b] Electron-beam energies T_o (MeV) are those at phantom entry.

TABLE 13.13. $[(L/\rho)^p_{air}]_{\overline{T}}$ for Use in Eq. (13.69); Phantom Medium = Acrylic Plastic[a]

Depth (g/cm²)	$[(L/\rho)^p_{air}]_{\overline{T}}$, $\Delta = 10$ keV															
	$T_o^b = 60.0$	50.0	40.0	30.0	25.0	20.0	18.0	16.0	14.0	12.0	10.0	9.0	8.0	7.0	6.0	5.0
0.0	0.870	0.874	0.882	0.898	0.909	0.923	0.929	0.936	0.944	0.953	0.963	0.969	0.975	0.983	0.992	1.003
0.1	0.871	0.875	0.883	0.899	0.910	0.924	0.930	0.937	0.945	0.953	0.964	0.970	0.976	0.984	0.993	1.005
0.2	0.872	0.875	0.884	0.900	0.911	0.925	0.931	0.938	0.945	0.954	0.965	0.971	0.978	0.986	0.995	1.007
0.3	0.872	0.876	0.885	0.901	0.912	0.925	0.932	0.939	0.946	0.955	0.966	0.972	0.979	0.988	0.997	1.010
0.4	0.873	0.877	0.886	0.902	0.913	0.926	0.933	0.939	0.947	0.956	0.967	0.974	0.981	0.990	1.000	1.013
0.5	0.874	0.878	0.887	0.902	0.914	0.927	0.933	0.940	0.948	0.958	0.969	0.975	0.983	0.992	1.003	1.016
0.6	0.875	0.879	0.888	0.903	0.915	0.928	0.934	0.941	0.949	0.959	0.970	0.977	0.985	0.994	1.006	1.020
0.8	0.876	0.880	0.889	0.905	0.916	0.930	0.936	0.944	0.952	0.962	0.974	0.981	0.989	1.000	1.012	1.029
1.0	0.877	0.882	0.891	0.907	0.918	0.932	0.938	0.946	0.954	0.964	0.977	0.985	0.994	1.006	1.020	1.038
1.2	0.878	0.883	0.893	0.909	0.920	0.934	0.940	0.948	0.957	0.968	0.981	0.990	1.000	1.012	1.028	1.048
1.4	0.880	0.885	0.894	0.910	0.922	0.936	0.943	0.951	0.960	0.971	0.986	0.995	1.005	1.020	1.037	1.057
1.6	0.881	0.886	0.896	0.912	0.924	0.938	0.945	0.953	0.963	0.975	0.990	1.000	1.012	1.027	1.045	1.067
1.8	0.882	0.887	0.897	0.914	0.926	0.940	0.947	0.956	0.966	0.978	0.995	1.006	1.019	1.035	1.054	1.076
2.0	0.883	0.889	0.899	0.915	0.927	0.942	0.950	0.958	0.969	0.982	1.000	1.012	1.026	1.043	1.063	1.085
2.5	0.886	0.892	0.902	0.919	0.932	0.948	0.956	0.965	0.977	0.992	1.014	1.028	1.044	1.063	1.085	1.101
3.0	0.888	0.895	0.906	0.923	0.937	0.953	0.962	0.973	0.986	1.004	1.029	1.045	1.063	1.083	1.098	
3.5	0.891	0.898	0.909	0.927	0.941	0.959	0.968	0.980	0.996	1.016	1.045	1.063	1.082	1.096		
4.0	0.893	0.900	0.912	0.931	0.946	0.965	0.975	0.989	1.006	1.030	1.052	1.080	1.094			
4.5	0.895	0.903	0.915	0.935	0.951	0.971	0.983	0.998	1.018	1.045	1.079	1.092	1.097			
5.0	0.897	0.905	0.918	0.939	0.956	0.978	0.991	1.008	1.031	1.061	1.090	1.096				
5.5	0.900	0.908	0.921	0.943	0.962	0.986	1.000	1.020	1.045	1.075	1.095					
6.0	0.902	0.910	0.924	0.947	0.968	0.994	1.010	1.032	1.059	1.086						
7.0	0.905	0.915	0.930	0.957	0.981	1.012	1.033	1.058	1.083	1.092						
8.0	0.909	0.920	0.937	0.967	0.995	1.033	1.056	1.080	1.090							
9.0	0.913	0.925	0.945	0.979	1.011	1.055	1.077	1.088								
10.0	0.917	0.931	0.953	0.991	1.029	1.075	1.086									
12.0	0.926	0.943	0.970	1.018	1.067											
14.0	0.937	0.957	0.989	1.051	1.076											
16.0	0.948	0.973	1.011	1.071												
18.0	0.961	0.989	1.036													
20.0	0.974	1.006	1.055													
22.0	0.989	1.025														
24.0	1.004	1.042														
26.0	1.019	1.050														
28.0	1.031															
30.0	1.039															

[a] AAPM (1983). Reproduced with permission from R. J. Schulz and The American Institute of Physics.

[b] Electron-beam energies T_o (MeV) are those at phantom entry.

PROBLEMS

1. Show that the value of N_X for a fully saturated 1-cm^3 air-equivalent cavity ion chamber is 3.24×10^9 R/C or 8.36×10^5 kg^{-1}. (CPE, no attenuation).

2. What is the value of N_{gas} in Gy/C for an ion chamber containing 12.93 mg of air in its sensitive volume?

3. Calculate N_{gas} for an air-filled polystyrene ion chamber for which $N_X A_{ion} = 1.67 \times 10^5$ kg^{-1} for ^{60}Co γ-rays. The chamber's internal diameter is 1.5 cm, and the wall mass thickness is 1.00 g/cm^2.

4. The chamber in problem 3 is used to calibrate a ^{60}Co γ-ray beam. When the shutter is set at 10.0 s, the electrometer measures 2.47×10^{-8} C; at 100.0 s, 2.60×10^{-7} C. The air temperature is 23.2°C, $p = 749$ torr; the ion collection efficiency is 0.996. Background is negligible.

    (a) What is the exposure rate in free space at the chamber-center location?

    (b) What is the shutter timing error?

    (c) What is the free-space dose in water at the same location, for a shutter setting of 24.0 s?

5. An x-ray beam with a monitor chamber is calibrated at a point of reference by means of an ion chamber for which $N_X A_{ion}$ is 7.32×10^9 R/C for the beam quality used. The air temperature is 19.3°C at the (vented) calibrating chamber, and 19.8°C at the (vented) monitor chamber. The pressure is 709 torr. For a shutter-timer setting of 100 s the calibrated chamber yields a charge of 1.14×10^{-8} C at saturation, while the monitor chamber gives 4.26×10^{-6} C. What is the monitor calibration factor N_M, in roentgens at the reference point per coulomb collected from the monitor at 22°C, 760 torr? (Take shutter timing error = 0.)

6. At a later time the x-ray beam in problem 5 is to be used to deliver an exposure of 200 R at the same location. The monitor temperature is 21.4°C; the pressure is 720 torr.

    (a) Assuming N_M to be constant, and that the beam is automatically turned off at a preset monitor charge, what should that setting be?

    (b) Approximately what would be the irradiation time if the exposure rate is roughly the same as it was when the beam was calibrated?

7. A cylindrical polystyrene ion chamber containing air, with 0.52-g/cm^2 wall thickness (5 mm), outside diameter 2.4 cm, and $N_X A_{ion} = 1.103 \times 10^9$ R/C for ^{60}Co γ-rays, is used to calibrate a beam of 25-MV x-rays in a polystyrene phantom of density 1.04 g/cm^3. A saturation charge $M'_\lambda P_{ion} = 7.69 \times 10^{-8}$ C is measured for an exposure of exactly 1 min at 7-cm depth on the beam axis. $t = 20.0$°C, $p = 749$ torr.

    (a) Use the C_λ method to calculate the absorbed dose rate in polystyrene.

    (b) From (a), what would be the absorbed dose rate in water at approximately the same depth in a water phantom?

(c) Calculate N_{gas} for the chamber.

(d) Calculate the absorbed dose rate in polystyrene by the N_{gas} method. (Note: You may estimate P_{repl} by extrapolation of the 26-MV curve in Fig. 13.6.)

(e) From (d), what would be the absorbed dose rate in water at approximately the same depth in a water phantom?

(f) Assuming that (e) is correct, by what percentage is (b) in error?

8. Suppose the same x-ray beam as in problem 7 were measured with the same chamber immersed at 7-cm depth in a water phantom.

(a) What is the value of α for the chamber wall?

(b) Assuming problem 7(e) gives the correct absorbed dose rate in water, what value of $M_\lambda P_{ion}$ should be measured by the chamber in 1 min, assuming the same atmospheric conditions?

9. A cylindrical acrylic-plastic ion chamber filled with air has a wall thickness of 0.52 g/cm^2 (4.4 mm), an outside diameter of 1.5 cm, and $N_X A_{ion} = 1.024 \times 10^{10}$ R/C for ^{60}Co γ-rays. It is inserted in a Lucite phantom to calibrate a 10-MV, 10 × 10-cm^2 x-ray beam.

(a) If the density of the phantom plastic is found to be 1.15 g/cm^3, at what depth should the chamber center be placed to simulate 5-cm depth in water? What value of SSD would apply to the plastic phantom if the SSD for a water phantom were 100 cm?

(b) Evaluate N_{gas} for the chamber.

(c) Calculate the absorbed dose in Lucite in the phantom at the depth found in (a) if the measured ion-chamber charge is 2.69×10^{-8} C, for $p = 750$ torr, $T = 22.9°C$, and an ion-collection efficiency of 0.992.

(d) What would be the corresponding absorbed dose in the water phantom at 5-cm depth?

10. A flat polystyrene–air ion chamber with 1-mm plate separation is positioned with the inner surface of its front wall at a depth of 2.0 g/cm^2 in a polystyrene phantom. A beam of 15-MeV electrons incident on the phantom makes a charge reading of 6.42×10^{-8} C, where $p = 765$ torr, $T = 25.2°C$, and the ion collection efficiency is 0.973.

(a) What is the absorbed dose in the cavity air, known to have a mass of 4.31×10^{-4} g?

(b) What is the absorbed dose in the polystyrene at 2-g/cm^2 depth?

SOLUTIONS TO PROBLEMS

2. 2.63×10^6 Gy/C.
3. 5.37×10^6 Gy/C.

4. **(a)** 4.47×10^{-4} C/kg s.
   (b) 0.55 s.
   (c) 0.392 Gy.
5. **(a)** 1.956×10^7 R/C.
6. **(a)** 9.71×10^{-6} C.
   (b) 226 s.
7. **(a)** 0.786 Gy/min.
   (b) 0.833 Gy/min.
   (c) 9.28×10^6 Gy/C.
   (d) 0.760 Gy/min.
   (e) 0.805 Gy/min.
   (f) (b) is 3.5% too high.
8. **(a)** 0.47.
   (b) 7.90×10^{-8} C.
9. **(a)** 4.5 cm, 100.5 cm.
   (b) 8.72×10^7 Gy/C.
   (c) 2.59 Gy.
   (d) 2.66 Gy.
10. **(a)** 5.20 Gy.
    (b) 5.04 Gy.

CHAPTER 14

Integrating Dosimeters

I. THERMOLUMINESCENCE DOSIMETRY

A. The Thermoluminescence Process

1. PHOSPHORS

The sensitive volume of a thermoluminescent dosimeter (TLD) consists of a small mass (~ 1–100 mg) of crystalline dielectric material containing suitable *activators* to make it perform as a thermoluminescent phosphor. The activators, which may be present only in trace amounts, provide two kinds of *centers*, or crystal-lattice imperfections:

a. *Traps* for the electrons and "holes" (i.e., carriers analogous to positive ions in gases), which can capture and hold the charge carriers in an electrical potential well for usefully long periods of time.

b. *Luminescence centers*, located at either the electron traps or the hole traps, which emit light when the electrons and holes are permitted to recombine at such a center.

Figure 14.1 is an energy-level diagram illustrating the thermoluminescence process. At left it shows an ionization event elevating an electron into the conduction band, where it migrates to an electron trap (e.g., a site in the crystal lattice where a negative ion is missing). The hole left behind migrates to a hole trap. At the temperature existing during irradiation, for example room temperture, these traps should be deep enough in terms of potential energy to prevent the escape of the electron or hole for

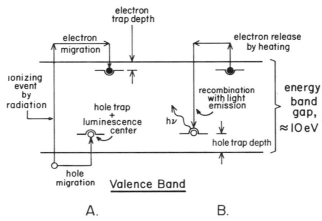

FIGURE 14.1. Energy-level diagram of the thermoluminescence process: (*A*) ionization by radiation, and trapping of electrons and holes; (*B*) heating to release electrons, allowing luminescence production.

extended periods of time, until deliberate heating releases either or both of them. At right in Fig. 14.1 the effect of such heating is shown. We will assume that the electron is released first, that is, that the electron trap in this phosphor is ''shallower'' than the hole trap. (The reverse might instead be true, so that the holes would be liberated first.) The electron again enters the conduction band and migrates to a hole trap, which may be assumed either to act as a luminescence center or to be closely coupled to one. In that case recombination is accompanied by the release of a light photon.

2. RANDALL–WILKINS THEORY

The simple first-order kinetics for the escape of such trapped charge carriers at a temperature $T(K)$ were first described for trapped electrons by Randall and Wilkins (1945) using the equation

$$p = \frac{1}{\tau} = \alpha e^{-E/kT} \tag{14.1}$$

where p is the probability of escape per unit time (s^{-1}), τ is the mean lifetime in the trap, α is called the *frequency factor*, E is the energy depth of the trap (eV), and k is Boltzman's constant ($k = 1.381 \times 10^{-23}$ J K^{-1} = 8.62×10^{-5} eV K^{-1}). A good discussion of this theory has been given by Becker (1973).

It is evident from Eq. (14.1) that, on the assumption of constant values for k, E, and α, increasing T causes p to increase and τ to decrease. Thus if the temperature T is scanned upward linearly vs. time, starting at room temperature, an increase in the rate of escape of trapped electrons will occur, reaching a maximum at some temperature T_m followed by a decrease as the supply of trapped electrons is gradually exhausted.

Assuming that the intensity of light emission is proportional to the rate of electron escape, a corresponding peak in thermoluminescence (TL) brightness will also be observed at T_m. This is called a *glow peak*, as shown in Fig. 14.2. The presence of more than one trap depth E gives rise to plural glow peaks, which may be unresolved or only partially resolved from one another in the *glow curve*.

The value of T_m is related to the linear heating rate q (K/s) by the following relation from Randall–Wilkins theory:

$$\frac{E}{kT_m^2} = \frac{\alpha}{q} e^{-E/kT_m} \tag{14.2}$$

which simplifies to the following approximate relationship on the assumption of $\alpha = 10^9/s$ and $q = 1$ K/s:

$$T_m = (489 \text{ K/eV}) \, E \tag{14.3}$$

hence $T_m = 216°C$ for $E = 1$ eV.

Although it is not obvious from Eq. (14.2), T_m increases gradually with q, so that $T_m = 248°C$ at $q = 5$ K/s, and $263°C$ at 10 K/s for the same values of α and E. The light-emission efficiency may be found to decrease with increasing temperature by a process called *thermal quenching*. Thus at higher heating rates some loss of total light

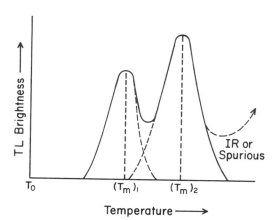

FIGURE 14.2. A thermoluminescence glow curve vs. temperature that results from the gradual heating of an irradiated thermoluminescent phosphor containing two trap depths. The phosphor temperature was T_0 at irradiation. The glow curve contains two glow peaks at $(T_m)_1$ and $(T_m)_2$, in this case not fully resolved. At temperatures above $\cong 300°C$ the infrared (IR) light from the heater begins to contribute to the detected brightness, possibly supplemented by spurious TL from triboluminescence and the like. Optical filters and/or flowing inert gas around the phosphor can reduce this spurious signal.

output may be noticed. Aside from this effect, varying the heating rate leaves total light output constant, preserving the area of glow curves in terms of brightness vs. time (but not brightness vs. temperature), given the same dose to the phosphor.

This is demonstrated very clearly in the remarkable results of Gorbics et al., shown in Fig. 14.3. They repeatedly irradiated a CaF_2 : Mn (manganese-activated calcium fluoride) TL dosimeter and read it out at eight linear heating rates ranging from q = 4 to 640°C/min. The TL brightness was simultaneously recorded vs. time and

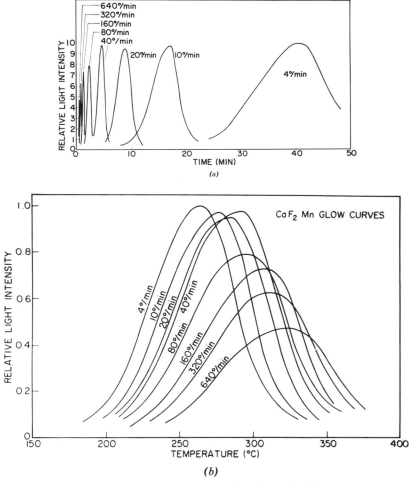

FIGURE 14.3.   (a) Glow curves vs. time obtained with a CaF_2 : Mn TL dosimeter at eight linear heating rates. The dose to the phosphor was adjusted to be inversely proportional to the heating rate in each case. (b) Glow curves vs. temperature recorded simultaneously with the curves in a. (Gorbics et al., 1969. Reproduced with permission from Pergamon Press, Ltd.)

vs. temperature. Instead of giving identical doses to the phosphor, the doses were adjusted to be *inversely proportional* to the heating rate employed in reading out the dosimeter. Thus the maximum TL brightness, which is *directly* proportional to the heating rate for a constant dose, should hold nearly constant, since CaF_2 : Mn responds linearly vs. dose over a wide range. This constancy is evident in Fig. 14.3 for heating rates up to 40°C/min, above which the influence of thermal quenching is seen to diminish the peak brightness down to about one-half at 640°C/min. Several other features of these curves should also be noticed:

a. The time to reach the glow peak is seen in Fig. 14.3a to be nearly inversely proportional to the heating rate.

b. For $q \leq 40$°C/min the glow curve areas are approximately constant in the TL brightness-vs.-temperature plot (Fig. 14.3b). However, the dose was 10 times larger for $q = 4$°C/min than for 40°C/min. In Fig. 14.3a it can be seen that the glow curve areas are approximately proportional to the dose in the absence of thermal quenching, as expected.

c. The temperature at which the glow peak occurs moves progressively higher with the heating rate; the onset of thermal quenching is around $T_m = 290$°C in this phosphor.

It can be seen that employing the light sum rather than the height of a glow peak as a measure of the absorbed dose is less subject to errors caused by fluctuations in the heating rate. However, the peak height may be used if the heating rate is very stable, and this may be advantageous in measuring small doses for which the upper limb of the glow curve rises due to IR and spurious effects, as shown in Fig. 14.2 and discussed in the next subsection.

3. TRAP STABILITY

The usefulness of a given phosphor trap (and its associated TL glow peak) for dosimetry applications depends on its independence of time and ambient conditions.

If the traps are not stable at room temperature before irradiation, but migrate through the crystal and combine with other traps to form different configurations, changes in radiation sensitivity and glow-curve shape will be observed. LiF (TLD-100) is such a phosphor, requiring special annealing (e.g., 400°C for 1 h, quick cooling, then 80°C for 24 h) to minimize sensitivity drift. In general TL phosphors give best performance as dosimeters if they receive uniform, reproducible, and optimal (depending on the phosphor) heat treatment before and after use.

The inability of traps to hold charge carriers at ambient temperature after irradiation is called *trap leakage*, and of course it becomes greater if the ambient temperature is increased. As a rule of thumb, in typical TLD phosphors a glow peak at $\cong 200$–225°C is ordinarily found to have small enough leakage for practical room-temperature dosimetry, having a half-life of trapped charge carriers measured in months or years. A glow peak at $\cong 150$°C usually has a half-life only of the order of a few days, while a 100°C peak decays in a matter of hours. Although short-term dosimetry may still be possible with rapidly leaking traps, careful timing control is required.

Higher-temperature traps than 200–225°C are usually even more stable, and would be advantageous for dosimetry except for the existence of two competing effects mentioned earlier:

1. *Heat (Infrared) Signal.* As the phosphor and its heating tray rise in temperature, the short-wavelength tail of the blackbody radiation begins to extend into the visible region and produce a non-dose-related response in the photomultiplier tube used for measuring the TL light output. A bandpass light filter in the TL spectral region (usually 400–500 nm) minimizes this effect, but above 300°C it still becomes a serious handicap in trying to measure small doses.

2. *Spurious Thermoluminescence Signal.* The combined effects of adsorbed gases, humidity, dirt, and mechanical abrasion of the phosphor surface tend to produce a spurious (i.e., not dose-related) TL emission, sometimes loosely called "triboluminescence." This light is believed to originate at the phosphor surface and in the adjacent gas. It tends to have wavelengths in the 500–600-nm range and is emitted mainly in the 300–400°C temperature region.

Flowing an oxygen-free inert gas such as N_2 or Ar through the space above the heater pan, thus surrounding the phosphor during the TL readout process, allows the stored energy due to these surface effects to be released without light emission. Thus N_2 flow is often used to reduce spurious background TL readings, especially when small doses (mrad) are to be measured.

4. INTRINSIC EFFICIENCY OF TLD PHOSPHORS

Only a small part of the energy deposited as absorbed dose in a TLD phosphor is emitted as light when the substance is heated, providing the dosimetric parameter to be measured. The ratio (TL light energy emitted per unit mass)/(absorbed dose) is called the intrinsic thermoluminescence efficiency. This has been measured by Lucke (1970) as 0.039% in LiF (TLD-100), 0.44% in CaF_2:Mn, and 1.2% in $CaSO_4$:Mn. The energy budget in LiF (TLD-100) has been estimated (Attix, 1975) to account for the loss of the missing 99.96% of the energy deposited by ionizing radiation that ultimately goes into heat production. It should not be surprising that TLDs must be used under reproducible conditions to obtain consistent results, considering that such a small fraction of the absorbed dose energy is relied upon as a measure of the entire dose.

B. TLD Readers

The instrument used to heat a TLD phosphor, and to measure the resulting thermoluminescence light emitted, is simply called a "TLD reader". Its design principle

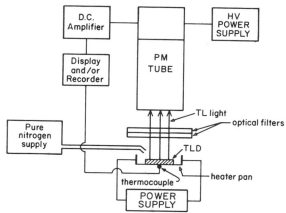

FIGURE 14.4. Schematic diagram of a typical TLD reader.

is shown schematically in Fig. 14.4. The TLD phosphor to be measured is placed in the heater pan at room temperature, and heated while the emitted light is measured with a photomultiplier.

Heating of the sample may be done by means of an ohmically heated pan as shown, or by preheated N_2 gas, or by an intense light spot from a projector lamp or a laser, or other suitable means. Often the heating program may be more complicated than simply linear vs. time. One typical scheme used in commercial TLD readers is to heat the phosphor rapidly through the unstable-trap region, ignoring light emission until some preset temperature is reached. Then the phosphor is either heated linearly or abruptly raised to a temperature sufficient to exhaust the glow peak of dosimetric interest, while measuring the emitted-light sum, which is displayed as a charge or dose reading. Finally, the phosphor may be heated further to (say) 400°C to release any remaining charges from deeper traps, while ignoring any additional light emitted, as it usually includes a significant contribution from spurious effects. Figure 14.5 illustrates such a heating program.

As noted before, heating-program reproducibility is vital in achieving reproducible TL dosimetry. In addition, one must provide constant light sensitivity so that a given TLD light output always gives the same reading. This requires constant PM-tube sensitivity (including a stable power supply and no PM-tube fatigue), and a clean optical system (filters, mirrors, lenses, light pipes, and heater-pan surface). Periodic cleaning may be required. A constant light source with an appropriate spectrum (e.g., a phosphor "button" excited by a small internal radioactive α- or β-source) may be built into the reader to substitute for a TLD as a check on the constancy of light sensitivity. This says nothing about heating constancy, however.

TLD readers for large-scale personnel monitoring may be equipped with magazine feed for automatic readout of large numbers of dosimeters, automatic iden-

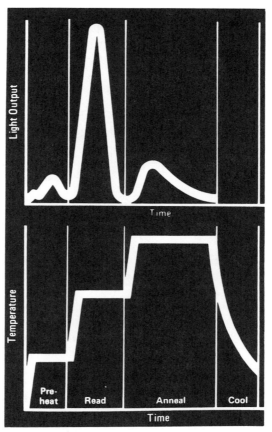

FIGURE 14.5. Typical programmed readout cycle in a modern TLD reader, consisting of a "preheat" period without light integration to discriminate against unstable low-temperature traps, a "read" period spanning the emission of the part of the glow curve to be used as a measure of the dose, an "anneal" period during which the remainder of the stored energy is "dumped" without light integration, and the cooling-down period after the heater-pan power is turned off. (Reproduced with permission from Victoreen, Inc., Cleveland, OH.)

tification of dosimeters from digital codes, and computer processing and storage of identity and dose information.

TLD readers are manufactured by a number of companies, including Eberline, Harshaw, Panasonic, Scanditronix, Teledyne Isotopes, and Victoreen.*

---

*Eberline, Santa Fe, NM 87504; Harshaw-Filtrol Partnership, 6801 Cochran Rd., Solon, OH 44139; Panasonic Co., Secaucus, NJ 07094; Scanditronix, inc., 106 Western Ave., Essex, MA 01929; Teledyne Isotopes, 50 Van Buren Ave., Westwood, NJ 07675; Victoreen, Inc., 10101 Woodland Ave., Cleveland, OH 44104.

C. TLD Phosphors

TLD phosphors consist of a host crystalline material containing one or more activators that may be associated with the traps, luminescence centers, or both. Amounts of activators range from a few parts per million up to several percent in different phosphors. The host crystal almost entirely determines the radiation interactions, since the activators are usually present in such small amounts.

Many different TLD phosphors have been studied and reported in the literature. A few representative ones are listed in Table 14.1. Figure 14.6 shows their glow curves at a heating rate of 40°C/min. Figure 14.7 gives their approximate light output vs. ^{60}Co γ-ray exposure. The dashed lines indicate strictly linear TL response vs. exposure. All the phosphors show some degree of "supralinearity" of response, this effect being most pronounced in lithium borate. In CaF_2: Mn the rise is only $\cong 4\%$ in the neighborhood of 10^4 R, which is too small to be seen on this figure. Supralinearity is shown to some extent by most TL phosphors, and may be due to the increased availability of luminescence centers when the charged-particle tracks become closer together, or to radiation-induced trap formation, or to other causes. At large enough doses all TL phosphors either saturate in their output as all available traps become filled, or maximize and then decrease due to radiation damage of the phosphor.

Lithium fluoride (Harshaw) has been by far the most commonly used, partly because of its low effective atomic number, only slightly greater than that of tissue and air. It is also available in a variety of forms (described in the next section) and with three levels of ^{6}Li/Li ratio: $\cong 0$ for LiF (TLD-700), $\cong 7\%$ for LiF (TLD-100), and $\cong 96\%$ for LiF (TLD-600). ^{6}Li has a high (n, α) capture cross section for thermal neutrons, while ^{7}Li is low in this respect. Thus in a mixed field of neutrons and γ-rays a LiF (TLD-700) dosimeter primarily measures the γ-ray dose, while a TLD-100 or TLD-600 dosimeter responds strongly to any thermal neutrons present as well. Such pairs of LiF dosimeters are widely used in personnel neutron-dose monitoring, as will be described in Chapter 16.

D. TLD Forms

The most common forms of TLDs are:

1. Bulk granulated, sieved to 75–150-μm grain size. Usually dispensed volumetrically into an irradiation capsule (e.g., pharmaceutical gel capsule). After irradiation, the powder is poured onto the reader heating pan.

2. Compressed pellets or "chips", usually 3.2 mm square by 0.9 mm (or 0.4 mm) thick. For best accuracy, individual chips may be calibrated with ^{60}Co γ-rays. Otherwise the batch sensitivity statistics (typically $\cong 5\%$ S.D.) must be relied upon. Groups of three or four chips are often packaged and irradiated together to improve precision.

3. A Teflon matrix containing 5% or 30% by weight of <40-μm grain-size TLD powder (from Isotopes, Inc.). Usually made in the shape of discs, 6 or 12

TABLE 14.1. Characteristics of TL Phosphors

Phosphor	LiF:Mg, Ti	CaF$_2$:Mn	Li$_2$B$_4$O$_7$:Mn	CaSO$_4$:Mn
Density (g/cm^3)	2.64	3.18	2.3	2.61
Effective atomic number	8.2	16.3	7.4	15.3
TL emission spectra (nm):				
Range	350–600	440–600	530–630	450–600
Maximum at	400	500	605	500
Temperature of main TL glow peak at 40°C/min (°C)	215	290	180	100
Approximate relative TL output for ^{60}Co	1.0	$\cong 3$	$\cong 0.3$	$\cong 70$
Energy response without added filter (30 keV/^{60}Co)	1.25	$\cong 13$	$\cong 0.9$	$\cong 10$
Useful range	mR–10^5 R	mR–3 × 10^5 R	mR–10^6 R	μR–10^4 R
Fading	Small, <5%/(12 wk)	~10% in first month	~10% in first month	50–60% in first 24 h

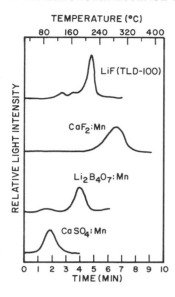

TEMPERATURE (°C)

LiF (TLD-100)

CaF$_2$:Mn

Li$_2$B$_4$O$_7$:Mn

CaSO$_4$:Mn

TIME (MIN)

FIGURE 14.6. Glow curves vs. temperature (upper scale) and time (lower scale) for four thermoluminescent dosimetry phosphors. Heating rate: 40°C/min. The amplitudes are arbitrary. (Gorbics et al., 1969. Reproduced with permission from Pergamon Press, Ltd.)

mm diam. by 0.1 or 0.3 mm thick. Film-badge-sized pieces are manufactured for personnel monitoring, to be used with filters to provide an estimate of the x-ray quality, as is usually done with photographic film badges. Ultrathin microtomed slices (6-mm-diam. discs) down to 25 μm thick are also available for approximating a B–G cavity.

4. A TLD pellet fastened on an ohmic heating element in an inert-gas-filled glass bulb, which plugs into a special reader. These are especially good for personnel monitoring in hostile environments (e.g., factories, shipyards, etc.), and for environmental γ-ray monitoring. Very small doses (~ 1 mrad) can be measured reproducibly.

5. Single-crystal plates, cleaved from a larger grown crystal boule. These are used only experimentally because of inconvenience, expense, and lack of reproducibility from one piece to another.

6. Powder enclosed in plastic tubing that can be heated, and through the wall of which the TL light passes to reach the PM tube (e.g., in the Scanditronix reader). This form is used mostly in clinical applications.

E. Calibration of Thermoluminescent Dosimeters

1. FORM

Solid TLD chips or Teflon–TLD discs are the preferred forms of the phosphor for most applications. They can be individually identified and calibrated, they do not require containment (which would attenuate low-energy radiation), and they are flat, so that they can be oriented perpendicular to a monodirectional radiation beam, thus presenting a known cross-sectional area.

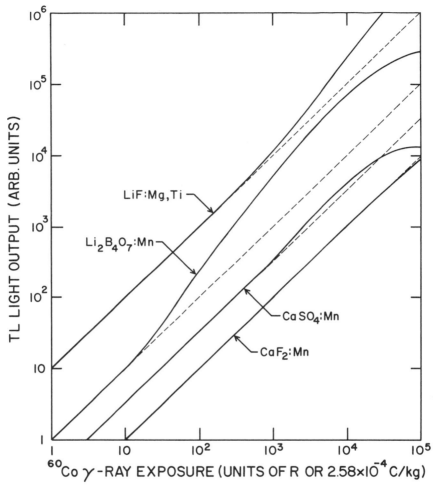

FIGURE 14.7. Glow-peak-area response vs. ^{60}Co γ-ray exposure for several TL phosphors. The relative TL output of the phosphors is arbitrary (see Table 14.1). The LiF:Mg, Ti curve was taken from Cameron et al. (1967); Li$_2$B$_4$:Mn, from Wilson and Cameron (1968); CaSO$_4$: Mn, from Bjarngard (1967); CaF$_2$: Mn, from Gorbics et al. (1973).

2. BASIS FOR CALIBRATION

Most TL phosphors have some threshold dose level below which the TL light output per unit mass is proportional to the absorbed dose in the phosphor, provided that: (a) the LET of the radiation remains low or practically constant, and (b) the phosphor sensitivity is kept constant by using reproducible annealing procedures.

Assuming TL-reader constancy, and negligible attenuation of light in escaping from the phosphor during heating, one can then say that the same TL reading will result from a given average phosphor dose in a TL dosimeter, regardless of the spatial distribution of absorbed dose within it, so long as the dose throughout remains in the linear range.

The practical consequence of this is that a ^{60}Co γ-ray calibration in terms of average phosphor dose in the TL dosimeter can then be used as an approximate calibration for all low-LET radiations, including x-rays, γ-rays, and electron beams of all energies above ~ 10 keV, even if they deposit dose nonuniformly in the dosimeter.

Relating the phosphor dose so measured to the dose in a similar mass of tissue hypothetically substituted for the TLD requires a separate step based on cavity theory. For the simplest (B–G) case of a thin TLD and very penetrating electrons, the dose ratio $D_{\mathrm{tiss}}/D_{\mathrm{TLD}}$ is proportional to the mass collision stopping-power ratio, $(dT/\rho dx)_{c,\,\mathrm{tiss}}/(dT/\rho dx)_{c,\,\mathrm{TLD}}$ evaluated at the mean electron kinetic energy.

If the incident radiation beam is completely stopped by the TLD, then the incident energy fluence can be derived (correcting for backscattering losses if necessary). The ^{60}Co calibration (under TCPE conditions) gives the TL reading per unit of average phosphor dose. Multiplying that dose by the mass of the TLD chip allows relating the TL reading to a given integral dose, or energy spent in the chip. If the chip area presented to the beam is A (m^2), its mass is m (kg), and the ^{60}Co γ-ray calibration factor is $k_{\mathrm{Co}} = (\overline{D}_{\mathrm{TLD}}/r)_{\mathrm{Co}}$ [Gy/(scale division)], where r is the TLD reading, then the energy fluence of a stopped beam is given by

$$\Psi = \frac{k_{\mathrm{Co}}\, rm}{A} \qquad (\mathrm{J/m^2}) \qquad (14.4)$$

3. ^{60}Co γ-RAY CALIBRATION

For a free-space ^{60}Co γ-ray exposure X (C/kg) at the point to be occupied by the center of the TLD in its capsule, the average absorbed dose in the TLD, in grays, under TCPE conditions is given by

$$\overline{D}_{\mathrm{TLD}} = 33.97 a\beta X \left[\frac{(\mu_{\mathrm{en}}/\rho)_{\mathrm{TLD}}}{(\mu_{\mathrm{en}}/\rho)_{\mathrm{air}}} \right]_{C_0} \qquad (14.5)$$

where a is a correction for broad-beam γ-ray attenuation in the capsule wall plus the half thickness of the TLD. For a LiF TLD chip in a Teflon capsule 2.8 mm in thickness, (for TCPE) the average absorbed dose calculated from Eq. (14.5) is approximately

$$\overline{D}_{\mathrm{LiF}} = 31.1 X \qquad (\mathrm{Gy}) \qquad (14.6)$$

If the resulting TLD reading is r scale divisions, then the calibration factor is k_{Co} $= (\overline{D}_{\mathrm{TLD}}/r)_{\mathrm{Co}}$, which applies at the dose value used in calibration and throughout the linear response-vs.-dose range. For all low-LET radiations, the average absorbed dose in the TLD can then be obtained from the observed TLD reading r by

$$\overline{D}_{\mathrm{TLD}} = k_{\mathrm{Co}} r \qquad (14.7)$$

For higher-LET radiations than ^{60}Co γ-rays, TLDs typically show some variation in efficiency, and consequently a reciprocal change in the low-LET calibration factor k_{Co}. Figure 14.8 gives the results of measurements by Tochilin et al. (1968) for lithium fluoride, lithium borate, and another phosphor, beryllium oxide. Their LET dependence is seen to be quite different, with lithium borate coming closest to constancy. All three, however, tend to rise somewhat in TL efficiency as the LET increases from about 0.25 keV/μm for ^{60}Co to about 1 keV/μm.

Figures 14.9 and 14.10 show the photon energy dependence of lithium fluoride and lithium borate. Curves A were obtained from the right side of Eq. (11.23), showing the CPE dose in the phosphors per unit of exposure, normalized to 1.25 MeV (^{60}Co). Curves B show the TL response per unit exposure, and curves C the TL response per unit of absorbed dose in the phosphors. Thus curves C represent the LET-dependence of the TL efficiency relative to ^{60}Co, or k_{Co}/k_{LET}. Equation (14.7) can be improved upon by using k_{LET} in place of k_{Co} where curve C diverges significantly from unity.

In the case of CaF$_2$:Mn, the results of Ehrlich and Placious (1968) indicate that approximately the same amount of TL light is emitted for a given energy imparted by ^{60}Co γ rays or electrons over the full range studied, that is, 20 to 400 keV incident on, and stopping in, the phosphor powder dispersed in Teflon.

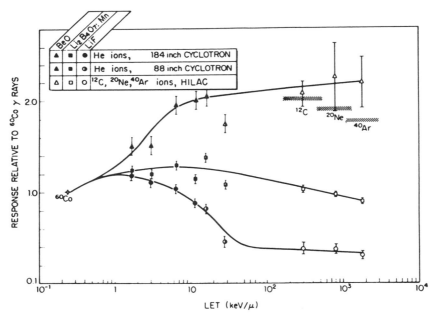

FIGURE 14.8.   LET response of BeO, Li$_2$B$_4$O$_7$:Mn, and LiF. The curves give values of $k_{Co}/$ k_{LET} as a function of LET in water, in keV/μm. The inset indicates the types of radiation sources and particles used. (Tochilin et al., 1968. Reproduced with permission from E. Tochilin.)

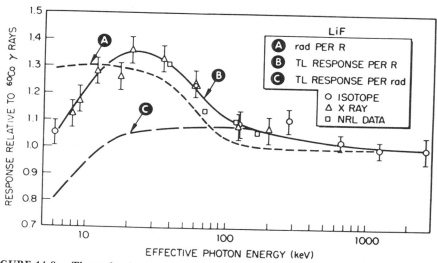

FIGURE 14.9.   Thermoluminescent response of LiF per roentgen and per rad for photon energies from 6 to 2800 keV. (Tochilin et al., 1968. Reproduced with permission from E. Tochilin.)

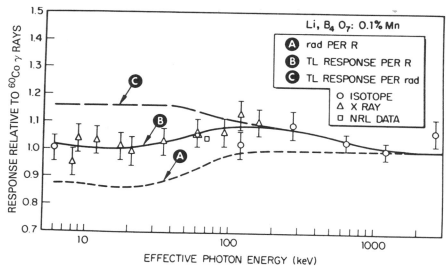

FIGURE 14.10.   Thermoluminescent response of $Li_2B_4O_7:Mn$ per roentgen and per rad for
photon energies from 6 to 2800 keV. Tochilin et al., 1968. Reproduced with permission from E.
Tochilin.)

F. Advantages and Disadvantages

1. ADVANTAGES

Specific characteristics vary from phosphor to phosphor, and are available from the manufacturer. We will describe the most widely used, LiF (TLD-100), where specifics are referred to.

   a. *Wide useful dose range*, from a few millirads to $\sim 10^3$ rad linearly, plus another decade (10^3–10^4) of supralinear response vs. dose.

   b. *Dose-rate independence*, 0–10^{11} rad/s.

   c. *Small size; passive energy storage.* Small TLDs can be used as dose probes with little disturbance of the radiation field in the medium (e.g., phantom or *in vivo*). They can be made thin enough to approach B–G conditions at high energies, but TCPE is easier to achieve because of their condensed state.

   d. *Commercial availability.* TLDs and readers are available from a number of suppliers, including those in the footnote in Section I.B.

   e. *Reusability.* By employing appropriate annealing procedures to release all the prior stored energy, and checking for possible alteration in radiation sensitivity, TLD phosphors can normally be reused many times until they finally become permanently damaged by radiation, heat or environment. Thus it is feasible to calibrate individual dosimeters.

   f. *Readout convenience.* TLD readout is fairly rapid (<30 s) and requires no wet chemistry.

   g. *Economy.* Reusability usually reduces the cost per reading.

   h. *Availability of different types with different sensitivities to thermal neutrons.* TLD-700 (^{7}LiF), TLD-100 (93% ^{7}LiF + 7% ^{6}LiF); TLD-600 (96% ^{6}LiF).

   i. *Automation compatibility.* For large personnel-monitoring operations automatic readers, capable of being interfaced with computers, are available.

   j. *Accuracy and precision.* Reading reproducibility of 1–2% can be achieved with care. Comparable accuracy may be obtained through individual calibration and averaging of several dosimeters in a cluster, since their volume is small.

2. DISADVANTAGES

   a. *Lack of uniformity.* Different dosimeters made from a given batch of phosphors still show a distribution of sensitivities, and different batches of phosphor generally have different average sensitivities. Thus individual dosimeter calibration, or at least batch calibration, is necessary for acceptable accuracy and precision.

   b. *Storage instability.* TLD sensitivity can vary with time before irradiation in some phosphors, as a result, for example, of gradual room-temperature migration of trapping centers in the crystals. Controlled annealing of the TLDs can usually restore them to some reference condition again.

   c. *Fading.* Irradiated dosimeters do not permanently retain 100% of their trapped charge carriers. This results in a gradual loss of the latent TLD signal. This must be corrected for, especially in applications (e.g., personnel monitoring) that involve long time delays.

   d. *Light sensitivity.* TLDs all show some sensitivity to light—especially UV, sunlight, or fluorescent light. This can cause accelerated ''fading'', or leakage of filled traps. Or it can produce ionization and the filling of traps, thus giving rise to spurious TL readings.

   e. *Spurious TL.* Scraping or chipping of TLD crystals (e.g., by rough tweezer handling) or surface contamination by dirt or humidity also can cause spurious TL readings. However, the presence of an oxygen-free inert gas during readout suppresses these signals.

   f. *''Memory'' of radiation and thermal history.* The sensitivity can be either increased or decreased after receiving a large dose of radiation and undergoing readout. Additional annealing procedures are needed to restore the original sensitivity, if possible. It may be more economical to throw away the phosphor after a single use, especially for large doses.

   g. *Reader instability.* TLD readings depend on the light sensitivity of the reader as well as on the heating rate of the phosphor. Thus reader constancy is difficult to maintain over long time periods.

   h. *Loss of a reading.* The measurement of the light out of a TLD (i.e., by heating it) erases the stored information. Unless special provision is made (e.g., a spare TLD), there is no second chance at getting a reading. Reader malfunction can lose a reading.

G. References

A very extensive literature has been generated for TL dosimetry in the last three decades. The following will be found particularly useful as general references: Proceedings of the International Conferences on Luminescence Dosimetry, from the 1965 conference at Stanford University (published in 1967) onward (1968, Gatlinburg, TN, U.S.A.; 1971, Risø, Denmark; 1974, Krakow, Poland; 1977, São Paulo, Brazil), Fowler and Attix (1966), Cameron et al. (1968), Holm and Berry (1970), Becker (1973), McKinlay (1981), and Horowitz (1984).

II. PHOTOGRAPHIC DOSIMETRY

A. Photographic Process

1. PHOTOGRAPHIC EMULSION

The emulsion consists of microscopic grains of silver bromide (AgBr), dispersed in a gelatin layer on either one or both sides of a supporting film. Incident charged particles produce ion pairs in or near the grains, and their effect is to convert Ag^+ ions to Ag atoms. A few such Ag atoms on a grain (containing typically 10^{10} Ag^+

ions) constitute a *latent image*, which renders the grain developable by a chemical process. In that process all of the Ag^+ ions are converted to Ag atoms and the bromine is removed, leaving behind an opaque microscopic grain of silver. The presence of this elemental silver may be detected optically and quantitatively related to the absorbed dose.

Two basic types of emulsions are used in dosimetry:

a. X-ray emulsions have a silver bromide content of 30–40% by weight. The grain size is 1–2 μm diameter. Each emulsion layer is 10–25 μm thick, with a typical density of 2 g/cm^3 and an average mass thickness of 2–5 mg/cm^2. A gel layer of 0.5 μm covers the emulsion to protect the surface grains from abrasion.

b. *Nuclear emulsions* have about 70–80% AgBr by weight, with a grain diameter of $\cong 0.3$ μm. The emulsion thickness ranges from a few micrometers up to $\cong 0.6$ mm, or about 1 to 200 mg/cm^2 for $\rho \cong 3.3$ g/cm^3.

2. CHEMICAL PROCESSING

This usually comprises three steps:

1. *Developing.* The developer molecules would reduce the Ag^+ ions to Ag atoms in all grains eventually, whether ionized or not. Those having a latent image are reduced much more rapidly, however, and the developing process can then be terminated. Thorough agitation of developing fluid and close temperature constancy are important for homogeneous and reproducible development.

2. *Stop Bath.* Immersion of the emulsion in a dilute acetic acid "stop bath" terminates development quickly. This is necessary for quantitative photographic dosimetry, since the optical density depends on the developing time as well as temperature, agitation, and developer characteristics.

3. *Hypo.* Sodium thiosulfate ("hypo") solution then is used to dissolve out the remaining undeveloped grains of AgBr, that is, those that did not contain a latent image. The film is finally washed in pure water and air-dried.

B. Optical Density of Film

In x-ray emulsions the radiation effect is measured in terms of the *light opacity* of the film, as measured by a densitometer.

Opacity is defined as I_0/I, where I_0 is the light intensity measured in the absence of the film, and I the intensity transmitted through the film in a direction perpendicular to its plane.

The *optical density* (OD) is defined as $\log_{10}(I_0/I)$.

If a is the average area (cm^2/grain) obscured by a single developed grain of silver, and n is the number of developed grains per cm^2 of film, then

$$\frac{I_0}{I} \cong e^{an} \tag{14.8}$$

and

$$\text{OD} = \log_{10}\left(\frac{I_0}{I}\right) = an \log_{10} e = 0.4343\, an \qquad (14.9)$$

so long as $n \ll N$, where N is the number of AgBr grains per unit area (cm^2) in the unexposed film.

Making the following additional assumptions leads to a simple but useful model:

a. Incoming x-rays give rise to a secondary-electron fluence of Φ (e/cm^2) passing perpendicularly through the film.

b. A single electron hit renders a grain developable.

c. All grains have the same projected area a, which is assumed not to change during development. That is, the target area for electron hits is the same as the light-stopping area of a silver grain.

For this case we can write for the fraction of grains struck and made developable

$$\frac{n}{N} \cong a\Phi \qquad (14.10)$$

which can be substituted into Eq. (14.9) to give

$$\text{OD} = 0.4343a^2 N\, \Phi \qquad (14.11)$$

From this relation we can see that, for a small fluence Φ (i.e., where $n \ll N$), the OD is proportional to Φ (and consequently also to the dose) in the emulsion. The OD is also proportional to the emulsion thickness, since $N \propto$ thickness. Furthermore, the OD is proportional to the square of the grain area, or the fourth power of the grain diameter.

Film-density measurements are often expressed in terms of the *standard density* (SD), defined as:

$$\text{SD} = \frac{(\text{OD}) - (\text{OD})_f}{(\text{OD})_m - (\text{OD})_f} \qquad (14.12)$$

where (OD) is the optical density of the exposed film, $(\text{OD})_f$ is that of the unexposed film (for which the OD level is referred to as "fog"; $(\text{OD})_f \cong 0.1\text{–}0.2$, usually), and $(\text{OD})_m$ is the maximum optical density measured if all the grains are developed, that is, if $n = N$. In practice $(\text{OD})_m$ is taken as the maximum OD detectable on the densitometer used.

It is evident that the SD of a film ranges from 0 for no exposure to unity for a nearly saturated film.

As an example, consider the case where $(\text{OD})_f = 0.1$, $(\text{OD})_m = 4$. An OD of 1 would give an SD of 0.23, OD $= 2$ would give SD $= 0.49$, and OD $= 4$ would give SD $= 1.00$.

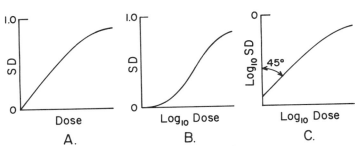

FIGURE 14.11. Three common types of plots of film dosimeter response: (A) standard density (SD) vs. dose (D) in tissue or water; (B) SD vs. $\log_{10} D$, and (C) $\log_{10}$ SD vs. $\log_{10} D$.

Three types of film-density plots vs. dose are commonly used, as shown in Fig. 14.11. Graphs like A and C are most useful for dosimetry, since they are linear at low doses for the case where the single-hit response dominates, as is usually found. The second plot (B) is called the "H and D" curve, after its originators Hurter and Driffield. It is of greater use in photography or radiography, since its slope $d(\text{SD})/d(\log_{10} \text{ dose})$, called the *contrast*, measures the ability of the film to distinguish between two nearly equal exposures by OD difference.

Densitometers used in photographic dosimetry are usually capable of measuring OD values from 0 to 4 (0.01% transmission) or, in some models, 0 to 6 (10^{-6} transmission). A number of commercial makes are available; some can scan film to obtain a spatial density profile.

C. Practical Exposure Range for X-Ray Film

Typical dosimetry film (Kodak Type 2) shows an OD increase of about 0.15 for an x-ray exposure of 100 mR at quantum energies above the photoelectric region (> 0.3 MeV). This roughly doubles the OD observed in unexposed film, depending upon the temperature and humidity conditions to which the film has been subjected and how long the film has been worn by personnel being monitored. In practice the lower limit for the useful personnel-monitoring range is $\cong 25$ mR with well-controlled processing. The upper useful OD limit of such a film is about 3, at an exposure of about 3 R. This range can be extended by stripping off the high-sensitivity side of the emulsion, after developing. The remaining low-sensitivity side then goes up to 300 R for OD $\cong 3$.

D. X-Ray Energy Dependence

Photoelectric effect in the AgBr grains causes the film to absorb x-ray energy 10–50 times more readily for $h\nu < 0.1$ MeV than does tissue or air, as exemplified by Fig. 14.12. This overresponse can either be compensated for by enclosing the film in a high-Z filter, as shown, or by making the film badge into a crude energy spectrometer by using different metal-foil filters over different segments of the film's area. Measuring the OD in the different film areas (at least two), accompanied by suitable

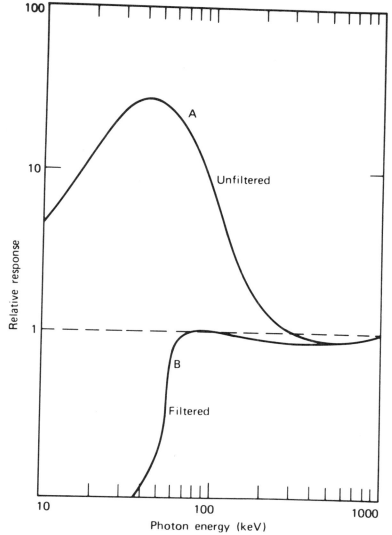

FIGURE 14.12. Relative response per unit of x-ray exposure, normalized to ^{60}Co γ-rays, for a typical film-badge dosimeter with and without a compensating filter (R. H. Herz, 1969).

calibration with x-ray beams of known energy spectra, allows the film badge to yield useful spectral information about the x-rays in addition to the dose reading.

E. Nuclear Track Emulsions

Aside from use of nuclear track emulsions in cosmic ray research, their main application is in the dosimetry of fast neutrons for personnel monitoring.

Fast neutrons deposit energy in an emulsion (or in tissue) mainly by elastic scattering interactions with hydrogen nuclei (protons). The absorbed dose from these (n, p) reactions in emulsion is proportional to the number of recoil protons produced per gram, and their average energy. The proton's energy can be determined from microscopic measurement of the length of its track in the emulsion, and reference to range-energy tables such as those of Barkas and Berger (1964). It will be seen that such a procedure is absolute inasmuch as calibration in a known neutron field is not needed. However, neutrons below $\cong 0.7$ MeV do not make recognizable proton tracks because they are too short; hence the nuclear emulsion is "blind" to lower-energy neutrons. This is an important failing, as the neutrons that penetrate through shielding are often below this threshold, yet are energetic enough to deposit significant dose in tissue.

The above procedure, requiring track-length measurement for each proton, is much too time-consuming and tedious for routine personnel monitoring. What is ordinarily done is simply to count the tracks in the sampled areas, usually by means of an enlarged projected display of the microscope view. It has been found empirically that Kodak Personal Neutron Monitoring Film Type A, for example, gives $\cong 1000$–2000 measurable tracks per cm^2 for a fast (>0.7 MeV) neutron dose-equivalent of 1 mSv, assuming 1 Sv = a dose of 0.1 Gy in tissue, i.e., that the quality factor is 10, independent of neutron energy (but see Fig. 16.6).

F. Advantages and Disadvantages of Photographic Dosimetry

1. ADVANTAGES

a. Spatial Resolution

Photographic film is unrivaled in allowing the observation of spatial distribution of dose or energy imparted. In practice it is limited mainly by the capabilities of the optical "probe" used to analyze the film. In the case of nuclear emulsions observed by microscope, single tracks can be located within $\cong 1$ μm.

b. Reading Permanence

The act of measuring the optical density (i.e., opacity) of a film, or of counting tracks in a nuclear emulsion, does not disturb the developed silver grains. Thus the record is permanent and can be remeasured for verification if desired (unlike TLD). However if developing is carried out improperly, the resulting dose measurement will be permanently incorrect.

c. Commercial Availability

Films are available from several manufacturers (in particular, Eastman Kodak in the United States) in a variety of types that have been made for many years, and have been extensively studied in a number of laboratories. Quality control in manufacturing is usually good, although individual film batches require calibration with respect to radiation response.

d. Geometry

The thinness and flat shape of photographic film, with large areas available, allows its simple use in field mapping, especially for electron beams, where overresponse due to the photoelectric effect is irrelevant. The physical flexibility of the film also allows it to follow cylindrical curvature if desired. For high-energy radiation the thickness of the emulsion can approach B–G cavity dimensions.

e. Linearity vs. Dose

Over useful dose ranges, the standard density is proportional to the dose. The upper useful range limit of linearity usually depends on depletion of the supply of un-developed grains, resulting in saturation and reduction in the slope of SD vs. dose. Lack of linearity at low doses usually indicates multiple-hit production of developable grains, which depends on the type of film (e.g., grain size) and type of radiation. In most dosimetry applications this problem is not encountered.

f. Dose-Rate Independence

Again depending on film type and radiation species, film usually shows *reciprocity*, or equality of SD as exposure time and dose rate are varied reciprocally. At low dose rates it fails because of gradual ion recombination that repairs partial radiation dam-age in grains where multiple hits are required to produce a latent image. This process is pronounced for light exposure, and may also occur in some emulsions for low-LET radiations. Fading of latent images (i.e., developable grains) may also occur during very long exposure times, such as occur in personnel monitoring.

2. DISADVANTAGES

a. Wet Chemical Processing

Photographic dosimetry requires careful control of the wet-chemical development process to obtain adequate reproducibility of optical density for a given dose to the film. This involves extra time, expense, space, and opportunity for error. Variations of $1\,°C$ in the developer bath can affect the OD (and thus the dose reading) by a few percent.

b. Energy Dependence for X Rays

The high Z of the silver bromide grains that constitute 30–80% of the emulsion mass gives rise to photoelectric effect with x rays below 300 keV. Thus the response (OD) per roentgen, or per rad in tissue, is strongly dependent upon $h\nu$, as shown in Fig. 14.12.

c. Sensitivity to Hostile Environments

Fading of developable grains is greatly exaggerated by high temperature–humidity combinations. Both optical density and track recognition (in nuclear track emul-sions) are reduced by this effect, especially in personnel monitoring.

d. Double-Valued Response Functions

The optical density is usually observed to maximize and decrease again at very large doses, due to a reversal of the process of formation of developable grains, called *solarization*. Interpretation of a given OD in terms of dose thus may require other information about the general dose level to be expected.

e. "Blindness" to Low-Energy Neutrons

In nuclear emulsions, fast neutrons less than $\cong 0.7 \mathrm{MeV}$ in energy cannot be detected, because their recoil proton tracks are too short to be recognized as such.

G. References

The following references can provide additional details about the photographic method of dosimetry: Dudley (1966), Becker (1966, 1973), Herz (1969), and McLaughlin (1970a, c).

III. CHEMICAL DOSIMETRY

A. Introduction

In chemical dosimetry, the dose is determined from quantitative chemical change in an appropriate medium, which may be liquid, solid, or gaseous. We will consider primarily aqueous liquid systems, especially the Fricke dosimeter, which is the most common and generally most relevant to the measurement of dose in tissue or other biological material. References will be given for information about some other useful chemical dosimeters.

B. Basic Principles

Since aqueous dosimeters usually consist of dilute solutions, one can generally assume that radiation interacts with the water, producing chemically active primary products in about 10^{-10} s or less. These products—including free radicals like H and OH which have an unpaired electron, and molecular products such as H_2 and H_2O_2 (hydrogen peroxide)—are distributed heterogeneously, close to the charged-particle tracks.

By 10^{-6} s after the initial interaction, the spatial distribution of these primary products tends to homogenize due to diffusion, simultaneous with their chemical interactions with the solutes present. The LET dependence (if any) of the dosimeter depends on the reaction rates during this interval, that is, before the initial spatial distribution is obliterated. Dense tracks (high LET) usually encourage competing reactions or back reactions (corresponding to initial recombination in gases), thus reducing the yield of the desired product to be measured.

The yield of the measured product is expressed as a *G-value*, or more recently (ICRU, 1980) in terms of the *radiation chemical yield*, $G(X)$, with respect to the product X. The G-value is the number of chemical entities (e.g., molecules) produced, destroyed, or changed by the expenditure of 100 eV of radiation energy. $G(X)$ is expressed in units of moles/J, and can be obtained from the corresponding G-value by multiplying it by 1.037×10^{-7}.

As an example, for a given value of $G(X)$ in moles/J, an average dose of 1 Gy spent in N liters of unit-density (1.00 g/cm^3) solution gives an integral dose (or total energy spent) of N joules. The amount of product X would thus be $NG(X)$ moles, or $G(X)$ moles per liter. That is, *a $G(X)$-molar solution of radiation product X always results from the deposition of an average dose of 1 Gy in $\rho = 1$ g/cm^3 solution, regardless of the volume.*

Since $G(X)$ is usually of the order of 10^{-6}–10^{-7} moles/J in aqueous chemical do-simeters, a dose of 10 Gy then requires measurement of $\sim 10^{-5}$–10^{-6} M solutions of the product with acceptable accuracy. This requires sensitive detection methods and careful procedures, and rules out the measurement of small doses by this means.

C. General Procedures

1. PREPARATION OF VESSELS FOR IRRADIATION OR STORAGE

To minimize errors due to chemical interference by impurities on the inner surface of storage or irradiation vessels, Vycor (fused silica) is preferred. After thoroughly washing and rinsing in triple-distilled water, vessels are heated at 550°C for 1 h to burn out any remaining organic impurities. Irradiation vessels are then filled with dosimeter solution for storage until use, when the old solution is discarded and replaced with fresh solution.

As an alternative to heat cleaning, the cells can be filled with triple-distilled water and irradiated to 10^3–10^4 Gy, then rinsed out with dosimeter solution and stored with that solution, as above. This method can also be used with plastic cells, (polystyrene or Lucite), which are preferable to Vycor (SiO$_2$) from the viewpoint of matching the atomic number of solution and cell material, as discussed generally in Chapter 11 and more specifically in the following subsection.

2. CAVITY-THEORY CONSIDERATIONS OF THE IRRADIATION VESSEL

Since it is impractical to make irradiation vessels for aqueous dosimeters small enough to behave as B–G cavities, it may be advantageous instead to make their diameter large compared with the range of secondary charged particles, so that wall effects become negligible and CPE or TCPE is achieved in the dosimeter solution itself for photon or neutron irradiations.

Alternative to using large vessels, the use of polystyrene (C$_8$H$_8$) or Lucite (C$_5$H$_8$O$_2$) vessels, "cleaned" by preirradiation, provides close enough matching of atomic numbers to water so that cavity wall effects are minimized. Burlin theory predicts that if the ratio $[(\mu_{en}/\rho)/(dT/\rho dx)]_c$ is the same for the wall material and the cavity material, cavity size no longer affects the dose in the cavity. Considering this criterion for ^{60}Co γ-rays (1.25 MeV, for which the average secondary-electron energy in an equilibrium spectrum is $\cong 0.3$ MeV), the above ratio has the values given in the last column of Table 14.2. It will be seen that both Lucite and polystyrene match water

TABLE 14.2.   Matching of Vessel Walls to Aqueous Dosimeters for ^{60}Co γ-Rays

Material	μ_{en}/ρ (cm^2/g)	$(dT/\rho dx)_c$ (MeV cm^2/g)	$[(\mu_{en}/\rho)/(dT/\rho dx)_c]$ (MeV^{-1})
Water	0.0296	2.355	0.0126
Vycor (SiO$_2$)	0.0266	1.961	0.0136
Lucite	0.0288	2.292	0.0126
Polystyrene	0.0288	2.305	0.0125

closely in this case, Lucite being exact, while SiO$_2$ shows an 8% mismatch. Thus irradiation vessels of either plastic would be expected to show no wall effects for ^{60}Co γ-rays, from cavity-theory considerations, and the solution inside can be assumed to be in transient charged-particle equilibrium if γ-ray attenuation can be neglected. This balance of stopping-power and energy-absorption-coefficient errors changes only very slowly with photon energy so long as the Compton effect dominates (i.e., the mass energy-absorption coefficient is proportional to the electron density in the material).

For electron beams, wall matching to the solution in the irradiation vessel is controlled by stopping-power and electron-scattering considerations. Again the choice of polystyrene or Lucite for the vessel is to be preferred, to minimize perturbation of the electrons passing through. $(dT/\rho dx)_c$ for these plastics is only about 3% less than that in water throughout the electron energy range 10 keV–50 Mev. Electron scattering is also slightly less than that in water. These differences are negligible for thin-walled vessels.

3.   ATTENUATION IN VESSEL WALLS

Polystyrene has a density $\cong 1.04$ g/cm^3, which is so close to that of water that the difference in radiation attenuation is negligible when such a thin-walled vessel is immersed in a water phantom.

For Lucite $\rho \cong 1.18$ g/cm^3; even in this case a 1-mm vessel wall immersed in a water phantom would only attenuate a photon beam by $\cong 0.04\%$ more than the water it displaces.

For SiO$_2$ vessels, $\rho \cong 2.2$ g/cm^3, hence an attenuation correction is called for when such a vessel is immersed in a water phantom. For photons, $(\mu_{en}/\rho)_{SiO_2} - (\mu_{en}/\rho)_{H_2O}$ may be used as an approximate net mass attenuation coefficient, assuming the "straight-ahead" approximation to broad-beam attenuation. For electron beams, SiO$_2$ irradiation vessels should be avoided because of scattering perturbations.

4.   REAGENTS AND WATER SUPPLY

The highest-purity reagents available should be used to minimize unwanted reactions, and triple-distilled water stored in heat-cleaned fused-silica (Vycor) containers should be used for all rinsing and solution mixing.

5. CALCULATION OF ABSORBED DOSE

The average absorbed dose in the dosimeter solution is given by

$$\overline{D} = \frac{\Delta M}{\rho G(X)} \tag{14.13}$$

where ΔM (mole/liter) is the change in molar concentration of product X due to the irradiation, and ρ (g/cm^3 or kg/liter) is the solution density. This assumes that $G(X)$ (mole/J) applies to the production of X throughout the molar range ΔM.

D. The Fricke Ferrous Sulfate Dosimeter

This is the chemical dosimeter of choice for most applications calling for a linear dose range from 40 to 400 Gy. Suitable special procedures are available for extending this range downward to $\cong 4$ Gy or upward to 4×10^3 Gy, as discussed by Fricke and Hart (1966). The following discussion pertains to the normal dose range, however, unless otherwise noted.

1. COMPOSITION

The standard Fricke dosimeter solution is composed of 0.001 M FeSO$_4$ or Fe(NH$_4$)$_2$(SO$_4$)$_2$ and 0.8 N H$_2$SO$_4$, prepared from high-purity reagents and triple-distilled water. A 0.1 M or 0.01 M stock solution of ferrous sulfate may be added to 0.8 N H$_2$SO$_4$ to complete the mixture. Stock solutions of ferrous sulfate (FeSO$_4$) gradually oxidize to ferric sulfate [Fe$_2$(SO$_4$)$_3$] over time. This process can be slowed by dark storage in a refrigerator. Since it simulates the effect of radiation, a background control reading from the same batch of solution is essential, and fresh solution should be prepared just before use for optimal results.

Adding 0.001 M NaCl to the above mixture desensitizes the system to organic impurities, and is therefore beneficial except where very high dose rates (e.g., pulsed electron beams) are to be measured, in which case the NaCl reduces the ferric ion yield, and should be avoided. Adding 0.001 M NaCl to the dosimeter solution provides a test for the presence of organic impurities; in their absence the NaCl has no effect on Fe^{3+} production at usual dose rates.

2. MEASUREMENT OF FERRIC ION (Fe^{3+}) PRODUCTION

This can be done by chemical titration of the irradiated and unirradiated samples to obtain ΔM of ferric ion, whence the dose is obtained from Eq. (14.13). Absorption spectroscopy is more convenient and sensitive, and requires only a small sample (~ 1 cm^3). Usually an absorption cell of 1-cm pathlength is used, at a wavelength of 304 nm in a constant-temperature chamber to control the effect of the 0.69%/°C temperature variation of the molar extinction coefficient for Fe^{3+}, which is ϵ(Fe^{3+}) = 2187 liter/mole cm at 25°C (Svensson and Brahme, 1979).

The ratio of the transmitted light intensity through the irradiated sample to that through the unirradiated sample is

$$\frac{I}{I_0} = 10^{-\Delta(OD)} \tag{14.14}$$

where $\Delta(OD)$ is the corresponding increase in optical density, given by

$$\Delta(OD) = \epsilon l\, \Delta M \tag{14.15}$$

Substituting for ΔM in Eq. (14.13), we have

$$\overline{D} = \frac{\Delta(OD)}{\epsilon l G(Fe^{3+})\rho} \tag{14.16}$$

where ϵ = 2187 liter/mole cm at 304 nm and 25°C,
      l = 1 cm (usually, but use the actual light pathlength through the cell),
$G(Fe^{3+})$ = 1.607 × 10^{-6} mole/J for low-LET radiations such as ^{60}Co γ rays,
      ρ = 1.024 kg/liter for standard Fricke solution at 25°C.
Hence

$$\overline{D} = 278\Delta(OD) \text{ Gy} \tag{14.17}$$

Thus the normal dose range of the Fricke dosimeter (40–400 Gy) corresponds to $\Delta(OD)$ values of $\cong 0.14$ to 1.4 for a 1-cm spectrophotometer cell at 304 nm. Figure 14.13 gives the approximate variation of G for Fe^{3+} production as a function of photon energy. The best value for ^{60}Co γ-rays is 15.5 molecules per 100 eV, or 1.607 × 10^{-6} mole/J (Svensson and Brahme, 1979).

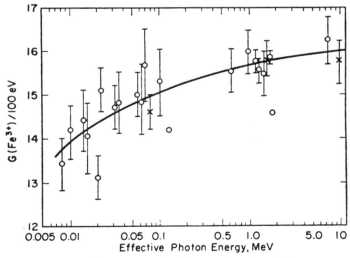

FIGURE 14.13. *G* value for ferric ion production as a function of photon energy. (Shalek et al., 1962. Reproduced with permission from R. J. Shalek and Academic Press.)

3. IRRADIATION CONDITIONS

The solution must be *air-saturated* during irradiation for the $Fe^{2+} \rightarrow Fe^{3+}$ oxidation reaction to proceed with the expected G value. Stirring the sample or bubbling air through it during irradiation may be necessary to avoid local oxygen depletion in case of inhomogeneous irradiation. The system is dose-rate-independent at least up to 2×10^6 Gy/s. $G(Fe^{3+})$ has a temperature coefficient probably lying between 0 and $0.1\%/°C$; hence this can be ignored in air-conditioned places where the solution is allowed to reach room temperature before irradiation.

4. EXTENDING THE DOSE RANGE OF THE FRICKE DOSIMETER

The upper dose limit of the Fricke system can be extended at least from 400 to 4000 Gy by raising the ferrous sulfate content from the usual 0.001 M to 0.05 M, and bubbling oxygen through the solution during irradiation. The same $G(Fe^{3+})$ still applies as for the standard solution (Fig. 14.13). However, the photoelectric effect in the iron and sulfur raises the energy-absorption coefficient above that for water by 4% at 0.1 MeV and 21% at 0.01 MeV. For the standard Fricke solution the μ_{en}/ρ differences from water are only about half as great.

The lower dose-range limit of the standard Fricke system can be reduced to $\cong 4$ Gy simply by increasing the spectrophotometric light path to 10 cm. Further dose-limit reductions are possible through use of a ^{59}Fe tracer and chemical separation of the ferric ion from the solution, a less convenient procedure.

Additional details concerning the Fricke dosimeter are discussed by Fricke and Hart (1966).

E. Other Chemical Dosimeters

A variety of other chemical dosimeters have been described by Fricke and Hart (1966) and by various authors in the book by Holm and Berry (1970). Most are limited to dose ranges still higher than the upper limit of the extended Fricke system ($>4 \times 10^3$ Gy). McLaughlin (1970a) exhaustively reviewed the literature and compiled an extensive table of dosimetry systems based on plastic films, polymer solutions, dye systems, gels, glasses, and a variety of other types. One especially versatile dosimeter is the radiochromic dye-cyanide system (Chalkley, 1952; McLaughlin, 1970b), which is commercially available in some forms.* Figure 14.14 gives typical response curves for that and some other dye dosimetry systems exposed to ^{60}Co γ-rays.

A sensitive aqueous dosimeter, covering the dose range from 0.2 to 50 Gy, is the benzoic acid fluorescence system, (see Fricke and Hart, 1966). An aerated solution of 0.001 M calcium benzoate, $Ca(C_7H_5O_2)_2 \cdot 3H_2O$, at a pH $\cong$ 6, produces hydroxybenzoates under ionizing irradiation in proportion to the absorbed dose. The product molecules fluoresce at about 400 nm under UV excitation at 290 nm. The fluorescence intensity under constant UV excitation can be calibrated (e.g., with the Fricke dosimeter) against absorbed dose. This system is reported to be practically

*Far West Technologies, Goleta, CA 93017.

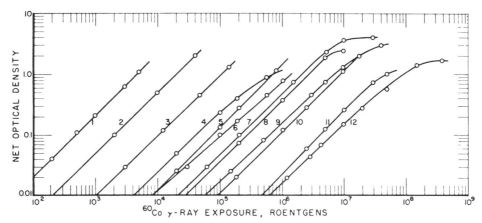

FIGURE 14.14.   Typical optical-density response curves of various dye-type dosimeters exposed to ^{60}Co γ-rays. Curve 1: 0.086 M pararosaniline–CN in methylcellosolve (1-cm optical path-length); 2: 3.0 g/cm^2 pararosaniline–CN in gelatin; 3: 0.002 M pararosaniline–CN in methyl cellusolve (1-cm pathlength); 4: cobalt glass; 5: 0.14 g/cm^2 pararosaniline–CN in gelatin; 6: leuco crystal violet, CBr$_4$, diphenylamine; 7: 0.075 g/cm^2 pararosaniline-CN in gelatin; 8: 0.019 g/cm^2 hexahydroxyethyl violet-CN in Nylon; 9: heavy pararosaniline–CN gelatin coating on triacetate; 10: 0.0075 g/cm^2 pararosaniline-CN in gelatin; 11: medium pararosaniline–CN gelatin coating on triacetate; 12: thin pararosaniline–CN gelatin coating on triacetate. (McLaughlin, 1970b. Reproduced with permission from W. L. McLaughlin and Marcel Dekker, Inc.)

independent of benzoate concentration, temperature near 25°C, and dose rate at least up to 1000 rad/min. Dosimeter solutions are stable before and after irradiation for at least a few days. This system appears to be potentially useful for in-phantom radiotherapy dosimetry.

F.   General Advantages and Disadvantages of Aqueous Chemical Dosimetry Systems

1.   Dilute aqueous solutions have an effective Z and μ_{en}/ρ that are close to those of water, which in turn is fairly similar to muscle tissue for photon energies over the entire range of practical interest. The density of dilute aqueous solutions approximates $\rho = 1.00$ g/cm^3, like water. Thus a dosimeter cell immersed in a water phantom does not require a polarization-effect correction, such as is needed for applying cavity theory to gaseous ion chambers for high energies (> 1 MeV). This is especially advantageous for in-phantom measurements with electron beams where the electron spectrum is not well known.

2.   Liquid dosimeters can, if desired, be irradiated in a container similar in shape and volume to the object being studied. Mixing the dosimeter solution irradiated in this manner, before taking a sample in which to determine the amount of the dosimetric radiation product, gives a measure of the average dose throughout the sensitive volume (i.e., the solution), provided that the response function is linear vs. dose. The average dose in an organ located within a phantom can thus be measured, for example.

3. In the unit-density solution it is relatively easy to achieve a large-size dosimeter, in the Burlin-theory sense (i.e., to achieve CPE or TCPE in the sensitive volume). However, it is correspondingly difficult to satisfy the B–G conditions.

4. Absolute dosimetry is possible, at least for the Fricke ferrous sulfate system.

5. Different chemical dosimeters can be used to cover various dose ranges within the limits $10–10^{10}$ rad.

6. Linear response vs. dose is found in some chemical dosimeters over limited but useful ranges.

7. Liquid dosimeters can be used to measure the energy fluence of relatively nonpenetrating beams (e.g., electron beams), as shown in Fig. 14.15. In the example shown, small positive corrections would be needed for energy losses due to electron backscattering and x-ray production. If $\overline{D}$ is the average dose (Gy) in the m kilograms of dosimeter solution, then the energy spent is $m\overline{D}$ and the electron energy fluence $\Psi = m\overline{D}/A$ (J/m^2) at the collimator of area A (m^2).

8. Lack of storage stability prevents commercial availability, requiring careful wet chemistry in the user's laboratory, a pronounced disadvantage.

9. Useful dose ranges tend to be too high for personnel monitoring or small-source measurements.

10. Individual systems usually show some degree of dose-rate and LET dependence, as well as dependence on the temperature of the solution during irradiation and during the readout procedure.

G. References

Shalek et al. (1962), Fricke and Hart (1966), Holm and Zagorski (1970), McLaughlin (1970a, b), Sehested (1970), Bjergbakke (1970a, b), Hart (1970), Hart and Fielden (1970), Holm (1970), Johnson (1970), Dvornik (1970), Artandi (1970), Orton (1970), Whittaker (1970), Goldstein (1970), and Sheldon (1970).

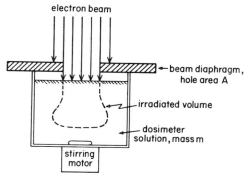

FIGURE 14.15.   Energy-fluence measurement by a liquid chemical dosimeter.

IV. CALORIMETRIC DOSIMETRY

The measurement of the temperature rise in calorimetric dosimeters comes closest of any method to providing a direct measurement of the full energy imparted to matter by radiation. Only relatively small corrections for thermal leakage and for chemical reactions are necessary.

A. Temperature Measurement

In principle any kind of thermometer can be applied in a calorimeter if the temperature change is large enough to measure with sufficient accuracy and precison. In practice only *thermocouples* and *thermistors* are sufficiently sensitive and small; thermistors are usually preferable because of their greater sensitivity.

The temperature increase per unit of absorbed dose to the material in the calorimeter's sensitive volume depends on its *thermal capacity*, which is usually expressed in cal/g °C or J/kg °C. The exact value of the calorie (i.e., the energy required to raise 1 g of water 1°C) depends upon the temperature of the water to which it refers. Usually thermal-capacity (or specific-heat) tables assume the value of the calorie for water at 15°C; hence 1 cal $= 4.185$ J $= 4.185 \times 10^7$ erg, and 1 cal/g °C $= 4185$ J/kg °C.

For a sensitive volume containing a material of thermal capacity h (J/kg °C), mass m (kg), and thermal defect δ, and that absorbs E joules of energy, the temperature increase is given by

$$\Delta T = \frac{E(1 - \delta)}{hm} = \frac{\overline{D}(1 - \delta)}{h} \qquad (°C) \qquad (14.18)$$

where $\overline{D}$ is the average absorbed dose (Gy) in the sensitive volume. Thus a measurement of $\overline{D}$ does not require explicit knowledge of m if h is known. The *thermal defect* δ is the fraction of E that does not appear as heat, due to competing chemical reactions, if any. δ is negative for exothermic reactions.

A few typical values of h are given in Table 14.3.

For example, in Al a dose of 1 Gy causes a temperature increase of 1.12×10^{-3} °C. To measure this temperature rise with 1% precision would require a thermometer capable of detecting temperature changes of the order of 10 μ°C.

TABLE 14.3. Thermal Capacity of Several Calorimetric Media

Material (at $\cong 20°C$)	h (cal g^{-1} °C^{-1})[a]	h (J kg^{-1} °C^{-1})
Aluminum	.214	896
Mercury	.03325	139.2
Copper	.0921	385.4
Graphite	.17	7.1×10^2
Gold (at 18°C)	.0312	130.6
Silicon (at 25°C)	.1706	714
Water	.999	4181

[a] The calorie is referred to water at 15°C

1. THERMOCOUPLES

Thermocouples typically have temperature coefficients of 40–70 μV/°C. A temperature change of 10 μ°C would then give a potential change of $(4-7) \times 10^{-10}$ V. This is too small to detect with available instruments, such as the Keithley nanovoltmeter.* Increasing the dose to 100 Gy would cause a temperature rise of 0.112°C, requiring detection of $(4-7) \times 10^{-8}$ V for 1% precision, which can be accomplished with a nanovoltmeter.

Thermocouples are generally found to be most useful in calorimeters where large doses (> 10 Gy) are given, usually in a short enough time period for thermal leakage to be negligible (i.e., under *adiabatic conditions*). Thermocouples have been applied, for example, to the calorimetry of intense pulsed beams of electrons, where the thermocouple may be spot-welded to a small metal foil or disc to be placed in the beam in vacuum to measure the dose delivered per pulse.

Thermocouple sensitivity can be multiplied by constructing a *thermopile*, consisting of a number of thermocouples in series, but this is usually not practical for calorimetric dosimetry because of the increase in perturbation of the medium in the sensitive volume by the thermocouples, and the number of thermal leakage paths provided by the two wires connected to each thermocouple.

Thermocouples are available with lead-wire diameters as small as 0.025 mm and an overall diameter of <0.25 mm.†

2. THERMISTORS

Thermistors can be obtained in sizes comparable to thermocouples. They are semiconductors made of metallic oxides and other constituents that are usually not specified by the manufacturer. They exhibit negative temperature coefficients of the order of several percent per °C at room temperatures, increasing in negative coefficient with decreasing temperature, as shown in Fig. 14.16.

The resistance of a thermistor at room temperature is typically 10^3–10^5 Ω, which can be conveniently measured with great precision and accuracy by a Wheatstone bridge as shown in Fig. 14.17. The bridge null detector must be sensitive enough so that the power dissipated in the thermistor is negligible compared to the radiation heating. A Keithley Model 520 nanowatt-dissipation resistance bridge is convenient and adequate for most cases. An example of its thermistor application has been described by Murray and Attix (1973).

B. Calorimeter Design

We will consider three general types of radiometric calorimeter designs, depending on whether absorbed dose in a reference medium, energy fluence in a radiation beam, or power output of a radioactive source is to be measured. Gunn (1964, 1970) also lists a fourth type, "in-reactor calorimeters", which are characterized by com-

*Keithley Instrument Co., Cleveland, OH, 44139 U.S.A.
†Omega Engineering, Inc., Box 47, Springdale, CT 06879, U.S.A.

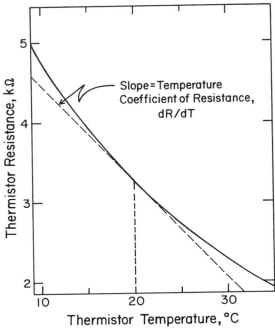

FIGURE 14.16. A typical resistance-vs.-temperature curve for a thermistor. The slope is the temperature coefficient of resistance at any temperature. For example, the slope dR/dT at 20°C, shown by the dashed line, is $\cong -120 \ \Omega/°C$ or $-3.7\%/°C$.

pactness, ability to operate in a remote, hostile environment, and large temperature range. These will not be discussed here.

1. ABSORBED-DOSE CALORIMETERS

An absorbed-dose calorimeter must have a sensitive volume that is small compared to the penetrating ability of the radiation and is thermally insulated from its surroundings to the extent necessary to attain acceptably small levels of thermal leakage. The sensitive volume (often called the *core*) is made of a thermally conductive material identical to, or simulating, a medium of dosimetric interest (e.g., graphite, tissue-equivalent plastic, or silicon), and contains a temperature sensor of negligible mass, usually a thermistor. The core is surrounded by a shell (''jacket'' or ''mantle'') of the same material to provide charged-particle as well as thermal equilibrium. If the thermal capacity and thermal defect of the core material are known, if the temperature sensor is correct, and if the thermal leakage is negligible, then the calorimeter can be operated adiabatically, without any energy calibration, to measure the average absorbed dose in the core by application of Eq. (14.18). The mass of the core need not be known in that case.

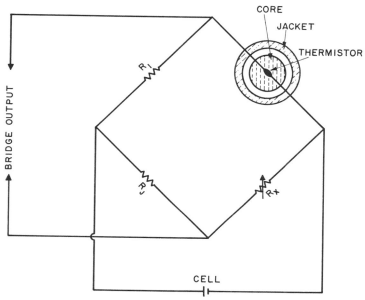

FIGURE 14.17. A Wheatstone bridge circuit for measuring the resistance of a thermistor in the sensitive volume (or "core") of a calorimetric dosimeter. R_c is the thermistor's resistance, R_x is an adjustable known resistor, and R_1 and R_J are known fixed resistors. All are chosen to be similar in resistance, and large enough so that the electrical power dissipated in R_c is negligible. When R_x is set to produce a null current reading, $R_c/R_x = R_1/R_J$, from which R_c can be determined. (Domen and Lamperti, 1974. Reproduced with permission from S. R. Domen.)

An example of such a calorimetric dosimeter that does not require calibration is shown in Fig. 14.18. This was designed to measure the dose deposited in silicon by intense single pulses of penetrating x rays. The core was a pea-sized sphere of high-purity silicon of known thermal capacity, enclosed in an equilibrium-thickness shell of the same material, which was insulated from the surrounding air by a shell of styrofoam. The core, containing a very small calibrated thermistor, was centered in a spherical void by four conical points of silicon projecting from the inside of the shell. Since the radiation pulse raises the temperature of the shell almost instantaneously ($\sim 10^{-7}$ s) by the same amount as the core, the heat-loss rate from the core was found to be initially negligible even without evacuating the surrounding gap, thus permitting the very simple design shown. Note that the spherical shape provides isotropic response as well.

It can be argued that, to avoid the complication of including an ohmic heater in the core and the necessity for knowing the mass of the core, one should whenever possible build the core and surrounding shell from a material that has an accurately known thermal capacity, as was the case for the silicon in the preceding design. Clas-

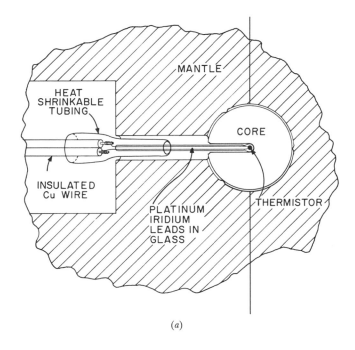

(a)

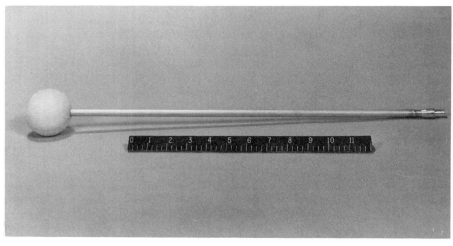

(b)

FIGURE 14.18.   An absolute adiabatic silicon calorimetric dosimeter of simple spherical design for measuring the absorbed dose to silicon from intense single pulses of penetrating x-rays. (a) Cross-sectional diagram; the diameter of the thermistor assembly is exaggerated ×3. (b) Photograph of the complete dosimeter, with scale in inches. (Murray and Attix, 1973. Reproduced with permission from the Health Physics Society.)

sical methods are available for measuring the thermal capacity of any given sample of material before it is incorporated into a calorimetric dosimeter.

However, the conventional practice has been to design an ohmic heater into the core, which can then be made of a material (or materials) for which the thermal capacity is only approximately known in advance. Again referring to Eq. (14.18), electrical energy E results in a temperature rise ΔT in the core, thus allowing the average value of h for the materials making up the core to be determined if its total mass is known.

Figure 14.19 is a schematic representation of this kind of absorbed dose calorimeter. The core is surrounded by two or more thermally insulated layers of the same material as the core, and the entire assembly is usually surrounded by a constant-temperature environment. Each layer may contain a thermistor and/or an ohmic heater, thus allowing measurement and control of the temperature environment of the core.

Dosimetry by means of such an apparatus is generally complicated and time-consuming. However, some clever simplifications have been devised to shorten the time necessary to reach thermal equilibrium before an exposure run (Domen, 1983) and automatically correct for heat leakage from the core to the jacket (Domen, 1969; Domen and Lamperti, 1974). Figure 14.20 illustrates the simple modification in the Wheatstone bridge that results in the measurement of the ΔT that *would have* occurred in the core due to electrical heating if none of the heat had leaked into the jacket. This requires, however, that the jacket have the same mass and be made of the same material as the core, and that their two thermistors must be virtually identical with respect to dR/dT as well as resistance. When the bridge is initially balanced,

$$R_1 R_x = R_j' R_c \qquad (14.19)$$

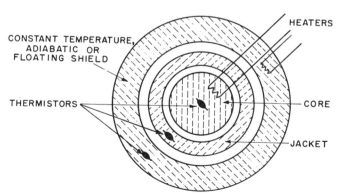

FIGURE 14.19. Schematic arrangement of a typical absorbed-dose calorimeter containing several concentric thermal bodies. Each may include thermistors and/or ohmic heaters for temperature measurement and control. (Domen and Lamperti, 1974. Reproduced with permission from S. R. Domen.)

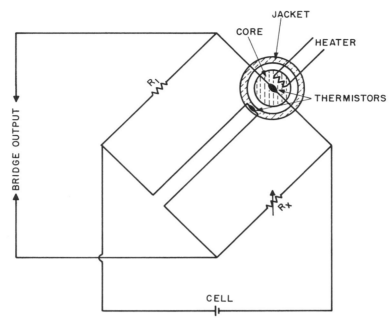

FIGURE 14.20. Modified Wheatstone bridge for measuring the core + jacket temperature rise, assuming that the two thermistors are identical in characteristics, and that the jacket has the same mass and is made of the same material as the core. (Domen and Lamperti, 1974. Reproduced with permission from S.R. Domen.)

where R'_J is the resistance of the thermistor in the jacket, and the other resistances are identified as in Fig. 14.17.

After electrical heating of the core and readjusting of R_x by the small amount ΔR_x necessary to balance the bridge again, Eq. (14.19) becomes

$$R_1(R_x - \Delta R_x) = (R'_J - \Delta R'_J)(R_c - \Delta R_c)$$

or

$$R_1 R_x - R_1 \, \Delta R_x = R'_J R_c - R_c \, \Delta R'_J - R'_J \, \Delta R_c + \Delta R'_J \, \Delta R_c$$

Using the equality in Eq. (14.19), and assuming that $R_1 = R_x = R'_J = R_c$, we have

$$\Delta R_x = \Delta R'_J + \Delta R_c - \frac{\Delta R'_J \, \Delta R_c}{R_1} \tag{14.20}$$

in which for small changes $\Delta R'_J$ and ΔR_c, the last term is vanishingly small.

Equation (14.20) means that ΔR_x has the same value whether all the electrical energy stays in the core ($\Delta R_c = \Delta R_x$, $\Delta R'_J = 0$) or some leaks to the surrounding jacket ($|\Delta R_c| < |\Delta R_x|$, $|\Delta R'_J| > 0$). Thus heat leakage out of the core during the electrical calibration is automatically corrected for, provided that thermal leakage from the jacket into the shield (see Fig. 14.19) is negligible. That can be assured by feedback control of the shield to maintain it at the same temperature as the jacket.

Before exposing the calorimeter to radiation, the Wheatstone bridge circuit is to be switched back to the circuit shown in Fig. 14.17, with $R_J = R'_J$. If the radiation is sufficiently penetrating, the core, jacket, and shield will be heated equally by the uniform dose. Supplementary electrical energy can be supplied to the shield to compensate for its thermal losses. Thus heat losses from the core can again be made negligible, so that the ΔT measured in the core can be correctly interpreted in terms of the core + jacket ΔT that was observed during the electrical calibration.

Several other absorbed-dose calorimeters deserve mention here:

1. Domen (1980) has found that it is possible to do calorimetry in a water phantom by sandwiching a thermistor between thin plastic films positioned horizontally at the desired measurement depth, thus preventing convection currents in the vicinity of the temperature sensor. There is no separate sensitive volume in this case; the thermistor simply measures the local temperature change as an indication of the local absorbed dose. Dose rates must be high enough to provide measurable temperature changes before heat can diffuse and radiate away from the dosed region. There are substantial thermal-defect problems in the water that depend on its purity and absorbed gases. This complication diminishes the convenience of the system, but its direct relevance to radiotherapy dosimetry will encourage its further study and development.

2. Holm (1969) has described the calorimetric dosimetry of an intense electron beam by means of a Petri dish full of water, enclosed in a Styrofoam insulating box. A thermocouple is immersed in the water with a connector outside of the box so that the apparatus can pass through the radiation beam on a conveyor belt while disconnected from the voltage-measuring instrument. The thermal-defect problem no doubt arises in this case also.

3. Calorimetric dosimeters operating at liquid-N_2 (Goldstein et al., 1967) or liquid-He (Mitacek and Frigerio, 1965) temperatures offer significant advantages that offset the inconvenience of cryogenic operation: Thermal capacities and radiative heat transfer are both greatly reduced, while the sensitivity of a thermistor is considerably increased. The design of Goldstein et al. is calibrated by means of a ^{60}Co γ-ray beam to eliminate the need for an ohmic heater, and was mechanically designed to rapidly achieve thermal equilibrium before starting an exposure. A precision of $\pm$ 1–2% S.D. was reported at 0.03 Gy/min.

2. ENERGY-FLUENCE CALORIMETERS

An energy-fluence calorimeter contains a core, usually consisting of a cylindrical piece of dense material such as lead or gold, large enough to stop an incident beam of radiation. The geometry is shown schematically in Fig. 14.21. The core is suspended by nylon strings in an insulated vacuum chamber, sometimes adjacent to

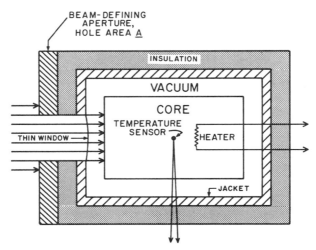

FIGURE 14.21.   Schematic arrangement of an energy-fluence calorimeter.

a twin core that serves as a control to determine thermal leakage. Because of the size of the core, more than one thermistor may be necessary to sample the temperature adequately, and the heater should be designed to distribute the heat uniformly. The high-Z core may require a significant backscattering correction.

Again referring to Eq. (14.18), h can be determined through electrical calibration as discussed before. The energy fluence of the radiation beam passing through the aperture of area A is given (neglecting δ) by

$$\Psi = \frac{E}{A} = \frac{\Delta T \, hm}{A} \qquad (14.21)$$

3. CALORIMETERS FOR MEASURING THE POWER OUTPUT OF A RADIOACTIVE SOURCE

A power-output calorimeter has a cup-shaped core into which a radioactive source can be inserted for measurement. The walls of the core are made thick enough to stop all the radiation to be measured from escaping. The usual method for electrical calibration can be used to determine h. Then the power output (W) is given by

$$P = \frac{dE}{dt} = hm \, \frac{\Delta T}{\Delta t} \qquad (14.22)$$

where temperature rise ΔT (°C) occurs in the core of mass m (kg) during the time interval Δt (s), and δ has been neglected.

Mann (1954) has described such a measurement, making use of a novel electrical heating and cooling arrangement based on the Peltier effect.

C. Advantages and Disadvantages of Calorimetric Dosimetry

Calorimeters offer several advantages for dosimetry:

1. They can be made absolute, either intrinsically or by means of electrical-heating calibration.

2. The measurement of temperature rise comes closest of any dosimetric technique to being a direct measurement of the energy involved in the absorbed dose. Only relatively small exothermic or endothermic chemical reactions, and thermal leakage, must be corrected for, and these are often negligible.

3. Almost any absorbing material, solid or liquid, can be employed in the calorimeter sensitive volume, so long as it is reasonably conductive thermally and has a known thermal defect.

4. Calorimeters are inherently dose-rate-independent under adiabatic conditions, and become more convenient to use as the dose-rate increases because thermal leakage during dose delivery becomes negligible. At high dose rates, where other dosimeters show saturation effects, calorimeters are at their best.

5. Calorimeters add up the energy contributions in the sensitive volume from different types of radiations (e.g., neutrons and γ rays) with weighting factors of unity, neglecting differences in thermal defect.

6. Calorimeters have no LET dependence (neglecting minor differences in thermal defect, if any), since ionic recombination is irrelevant to the temperature rise.

7. Calorimeters are relatively stable against radiation damage at high doses; the thermistor (if used as the temperature sensor) is usually the limiting factor in this respect.

The foregoing advantages are offset by certain disadvantages:

1. Temperature rises to be measured are typically very small, usually only a minute fraction of a degree, which limits calorimetry to relatively large doses.

2. Thermal insulation, and instrumentation for thermal control and measurement, often make the calorimeter apparatus bulky and difficult to transport and set up. This limits the kinds of situations to which calorimetry is usually applied to calibration of other dosimeters.

3. For low dose rates, thermal leakage in and out of the calorimeter sensitive volume limits the accuracy and precision achievable.

4. Some materials (e.g., tissue-equivalent plastic) undergo radiation-induced endothermic or exothermic reactions which cause a difference (thermal defect) between the integral dose and the energy available to heat the sensitive volume. In A150-type TE plastic about 4% of the absorbed dose goes to an endothermic reaction instead of heat.

D. Conclusions

The present brief introduction to calorimetric dosimetry deliberately errs on the side of simplicity, for two reasons. The first is that, in the simplest applications at high dose or fluence rates, especially for intense single pulses, adiabatic operation is well approximated, ΔT is large, and calorimetry becomes the dosimetry method of choice. Its reputation for difficulty is undeserved in those cases. Secondly, in the difficult applications of calorimetry (i.e., at low dose rates), the problems of heat leakage and temperature drift are too complicated to be dealt with adequately in an introductory text. The reader should thus be encouraged to consider calorimetry more readily than has been customary heretofore, while being wary that more detailed information should be sought in other references if needed. Gunn (1964, 1970) gives an exhaustive two-part review with hundreds of references; Laughlin and Genna (1966), Radak and Markovic (1970), Domen and Lamperti (1974), and Domen (1986) are also helpful.

PROBLEMS

1. What are the dosimeters of choice for
    (a) determining the response saturation of another dosimeter at its high-dose-rate limit,
    (b) measuring the average absorbed dose in an irregular volume, and
    (c) mapping the relative dose in an electron beam in a steep-gradient region?

2. Is the total light output from a TL dosimeter independent of heating rate? If not, what effect limits it?

3. A particular TL phosphor is known to exhibit thermal quenching when its glow peak occurs above 200°C.
    (a) Assuming $\alpha = 1 \times 10^9$/s and $E = 0.85$ eV, what is the maximum heating rate that can be used while obtaining a constant light sum?
    (b) What is the glow-peak temperature for a heating rate of 40°C/min?

4. A CaF_2: Mn TLD chip is enclosed in a capsule made of CaF_2: Mn, 0.5 g/cm^2 thick, and is given a free-space ^{60}Co γ-ray exposure of 2.58×10^{-2} C/kg. The chip thickness is 0.90 mm in the radiation direction. You may assume that $\beta \, (\equiv D/K_c) = 1.003$. Calculate the average absorbed dose in the TLD chip.

5. Redo problem 4 with the CaF_2: Mn capsule replaced by an aluminum capsule having the same mass wall thickness. (Hint: Use Eq. (14.5) to calculate the dose in Al under TCPE conditions, then Burlin cavity theory to relate the average dose in the CaF_2: Mn chip to the TCPE Al dose.)

6. If the TLD chip in problem 4 gave a TL reading of 3.49×10^{-8} C after the exposure described, what was the value of the dose calibration factor k_{Co}?

7. The same TLD chip as in problems 4 and 6 is exposed to a beam of 100-keV electrons, resulting in a TL reading of 2.36×10^{-7} C.
    (a) What is the average absorbed dose in the whole chip?
    (b) Assuming that the electrons strike the chip perpendicular to its 3.2 × 3.2-mm flat surface, what is the average dose within only the surface layer of thickness equal to the CSDA range of the electrons?

(c)   Is this dose still in the linear-response range for $CaF_2 : Mn$?

(d)   What was the fluence of electrons that struck the chip, assuming back-scattering to be negligible? (Chip mass = 29.3 mg.)

8. γ rays of 35 keV from ^{125}I are absorbed in Fricke dosimeter solution to produce an average dose of 17 Gy. Using the data of Shalek et al. (1962), what increase in optical density would result at 304 mm in a 1-cm cell? What is the easiest way to increase Δ(OD) into a range where the accuracy of this method is optimal?

9.   One liter of stirred Fricke solution at 25°C is irradiated by a 1-MeV electron beam passing through an aperture 2 cm in diameter, for a period of 1 min. If Δ(OD) = 1.20 at 304 nm in a 1-cm cell, what was the energy flux density at the aperture? (Neglect backscattering.)

10.   An absorbed-dose calorimeter contains a 30-g core of graphite with a heater of resistance 10 Ω. A current of 0.3 A is passed through it for 10 s under adiabatic conditions. A temperature increase of 0.42°C is measured. What is the value of the thermal capacity of the core material? What absorbed dose would cause a ΔT of 0.1°C under adiabatic conditions?

SOLUTIONS TO PROBLEMS

1.   (a)   Calorimetric dosimeter.

(b)   Liquid chemical dosimeter.

(c)   Photographic or chemical film dosimeter.

2.   No, thermal quenching limits it.

3.   (a)   q = 20°/s.

(b)   138°C.

4.   0.840 Gy.

5.   0.842 Gy.

6. 2.41×10^7 Gy/C.

7.   (a)   5.69 Gy.

(b)   87.9 Gy.

(c)   Yes.

(d) 1.016×10^{15} e/m^2

8.   (a)   0.058.

(b)   Use a 10-cm cell.

9. 1.81×10^4 J/m^2 s.

10.   714 J/kg °C, 71.4 Gy.

CHAPTER 15

Dosimetry by Pulse-Mode Detectors

I. INTRODUCTION

This chapter deals with dosimetry by means of gas proportional counters, Geiger–Müller counters, scintillators, and semiconductor detectors. Much has been written elsewhere about these devices, more commonly referred to as "radiation detectors" than as dosimeters. Excellent references, notably Knoll's textbook (1979) have provided a wealth of information about their design and operation, circuit electronics, and electrical pulse processing. The primary emphasis in those references is on pulse counting and radiation spectroscopy. While these techniques are also relevant to the use of radiation detectors as dosimeters, it would be needless duplication to cover that material in depth here. The reader is referred to Knoll's text for supplementary information.

The objective of the present chapter is to discuss the characteristics of these devices that make them useful for dosimetry, and how their output signals can be interpreted in relation to the absorbed dose. Principles of operation will be introduced only to the extent necessary to achieve that goal.

II. GEIGER–MÜLLER AND PROPORTIONAL COUNTERS

A. Gas Multiplication

Any ionization chamber with sufficiently good electrical insulation can in principle be operated at an applied potential great enough to cause *gas multiplication*, also called "gas amplication" or "gas gain." This is a condition in which free electrons from ionizing events can derive enough kinetic energy from the applied electric field, within a distance equal to the electrons' mean free path σ_e, to ionize other gas molecules with which they collide. Thus a single electron can give rise to an "avalanche," as the number of free electrons doubles repeatedly in their flight toward the anode. At atmospheric pressure the minimum field strength required for the onset of gas multiplication is $\sim 10^3$ V/mm.

Cylindrical counter geometry, with a thin axial wire serving as the anode and a cylindrical shell as the cathode, is often employed. This provides a sheathlike gas volume immediately surrounding the wire, in which the electric field strength $\mathfrak{X}$ is much larger than the average value obtained by dividing the applied potential P by the cathode-anode separation. Referring to Eq. (12.24), the electrical field strength $\mathfrak{X}(r)$ at radius r from the cylindrical axis is given by $\mathfrak{X}(r) = P/r \ln(a/b)$, where b is the radius of the wire anode and a that of the coaxial cylindrical cathode. Thus the maximum electric field, $\mathfrak{X}(r)_{\max}$, occurs at the surface of the wire, where it reaches a value of $\mathfrak{X}(b) = P/b \ln(a/b)$. For example, if $a = 1$ cm and $b = 10^{-3}$ cm, then $\mathfrak{X}(b) = 1.4 \times 10^5$ V/cm when $P = 1000$ V. $\mathfrak{X}(b)$ is approximately proportional to the reciprocal of the wire radius for constant a and P.

The gain factor **G** for cylindrical geometry is given approximately (Knoll, 1979) by:

$$\mathbf{G} \cong \exp\left\{ \frac{0.693P}{\Delta V \ln(a/b)} \ln \frac{P}{Kpb \ln(a/b)} \right\} \qquad (15.1)$$

where **G** is the number of electrons that arrive at the wire anode per electron released by ionizing radiation in the gas volume outside of the gas-multiplication "sheath" surrounding the wire; ΔV is the average potential difference (eV) through which an electron moves between successive ionizing events, which is greater than the ionization potential V_i because of energy "wasted" in atomic excitations; K is the minimum value of the electric field strength per atmosphere of gas pressure, below which multiplication cannot occur in a given gas; p is the gas pressure in atmospheres (1 atm = 760 torr); and P, a, and b are defined as before.

Some typical values of K and ΔV in gases that are often employed to achieve useful gas multiplication in proportional counters are given in Table 15.1.

For example, a cylindrical proportional counter with $a = 1$ cm, $b = 10^{-3}$ cm, $P = 1000$ V, and containing P-10 gas at 1 atm would have a gain factor of about 100, while reducing the gas pressure to 0.5 atm would increase **G** to $\cong 2000$. Substitution of the He–isobutane mixture at 1 atm would provide an even higher **G** of about 4000.

Although Eq. (15.2) predicts that very large gas gain factors are attainable for some combinations of parameters, the upper **G** limit for *proportional* gas multiplication is $\sim 10^4$. Above that value, space-charge effects cause **G** to be less for large groups of initiating electrons traveling together (as might result from an α-particle traversing the counter) than for the few initial electrons that might result from the passage of a low-LET particle. It is important in proportional counters that the gain factor be

TABLE 15.1.   Characteristics of Typical Proportional-Counting Gases

Gas	K (V/cm atm)	ΔV (eV)
90% Ar + 10% methane ("P-10")	4.8×10^4	23.6
Methane	6.9×10^4	36.5
96% He + 4% isobutane	1.48×10^4	27.6

the same for all sizes of primary ionizing events, so that the gas-amplified pulse size will properly represent the relative contributions of such events to the absorbed dose in the gas.

To obtain useful levels of gas gain, a nonelectronegative gas or gas mixture must be used (see Chapter 12, Section V.C, and Table 15.1), so that the free electrons do not become attached to atoms. A few percent of a polyatomic gas such as methane or isobutane is added to the noble gases for proportional counting to absorb secondary UV photons that are emitted from excited gas atoms. The energy of such photons is thus dissipated in vibrational and rotational motion, instead of causing new ionizing events in the gas or at the cathode. Such events can cause new electron avalanches that do not represent dose deposition by the original ionizing radiation.

In Geiger–Müller (G–M) counters the gaseous UV absorber is omitted because these photons are essential to the process of propagating the discharge throughout the tube. Certain "quenching" gases (the halogens Cl or Br, or organics like ethyl alcohol) are added (5–10%) to the filling gas instead, to prevent repeated or continuous gas discharge from occurring. When a positive gas ion arrives at the cathode, it is neutralized by an electron taken from that surface. If the ionization potential of the gas is more than twice the surface work function, there is a chance that two electrons instead of one may be released. Since the second electron is then free, it will be drawn to the anode and hence will trigger another G–M discharge. A quenching-gas molecule has a small enough ionization potential that it can serve as the positive charge carrier without releasing more than the one electron needed to neutralize its own charge. Thus additional spontaneous G–M counts do not occur. Organic quenching-gas molecules (not the halogens) are broken apart in dissipating the excess energy in this process, however, limiting the lifetime of an organic-quenched G–M tube to ~ 10^9 counts.

It should be obvious that the central wire must serve as the *anode* (i.e., be connected to the + polarity of the voltage source), since otherwise the free electrons produced by radiation in the counter filling gas would travel outward, away from the high-field sheath around the wire where the gas multiplication occurs. This sheath is very thin, as can be seen from the following considerations. At a pressure p (atm) the field strength $\mathfrak{X}(r)$ must equal or exceed pK for gas multiplication to occur. That is,

$$pK \leq \mathfrak{X}(r) = \frac{P}{r \ln(a/b)} \tag{15.2}$$

Hence the radius r_s of the outer boundary of the amplifying sheath region is

$$r_s = \frac{P}{pK \ln(a/b)} \tag{15.3}$$

For example in a cylindrical counter containing P-10 gas at 1 atm, with $b = 10^{-3}$ cm, $a = 1$ cm, and $P = 1000$ V, one has $r_s = 3 \times 10^{-3}$ cm. The sheath thickness is therefore equal to 2×10^{-3} cm or 20 μm, occupying only about 0.001% of the chamber's gas volume. The probability that the radiation field will produce primary ion pairs within the sheath volume, thus giving rise to electron avalanches of lesser gain, is nil. Electrons originating anywhere else in the gas undergo the same gain factor in an ideal cylindrical counter without end effects.

For a chamber operating with a fixed gain **G**, the total charge collected at the wire during a given exposure to ionizing radiation will be just **G** times that collected if the device had been operated as a saturated ion chamber. An ion chamber operating with **G** > 1 is called an *amplifying ion chamber*. Its advantages over a simple ion chamber are: (a) greater sensitivity, since the charge collected is **G**-fold larger, and (b) that the gas-filled cavity comes closer to satisfying the B–G conditions if reduced pressure is employed.

B. Proportional Counters

1. OPERATION

A proportional counter is just an amplifying ion chamber with its output measured in terms of numbers and amplitudes of individual pulses, instead of the charge collected. The electrometer circuit is usually replaced by a preamplifier, a linear amplifier, and a pulse-height analyzer, although specific requirements of an experiment may also call for coincidence circuits, pulse-shape discriminators, and other pulse-processing electronics, as discussed by Knoll (1979).

An "ionizing event" in the present context includes all of the ionization that is produced in the counter gas by the passage of a single charged particle and its δ-rays. All of the resulting free electrons reach the anode wire within ~ 1 μs. The measured electrical pulse, however, is primarily due to the motion of positive ions away from the wire, since they move greater distances within the amplifying sheath than the electrons do, on the average. About half of the electrons (and positive ions) originate in the innermost mean-free-path layer (typically 1–2 μm) surrounding the wire.

Although the positive ions are much slower than the electrons, they virtually all originate simultaneously within the amplifying sheath and move outward "in unison." Since the electric field near the wire is so strong, the positive-ion motion there gives rise to a sharply defined fast-rising electrical pulse that can be clipped electronically to eliminate the later slow component contributed as the ions progress outward toward the cathode. The cloud of positive ions is small in volume, and does not interfere with the ions resulting from other ionizing events taking place elsewhere in the counter. The amount of positive charge in a given ion cloud is proportional to the number of electrons in the associated avalanche, which in turn is proportional to the number of ion pairs created in the original ionizing event. Thus the size (i.e., height) of the electrical pulse generated by the positive ions is proportional to the energy imparted to the gas in the initial event, provided that $\overline{W}/e$ is constant. In fact, as noted in Chapter 12, Section VI, $\overline{W}/e$ differs by as much as a few percent between electrons and α-particles, depending on the gas employed in an ion chamber or counter. Although this effect usually has been ignored in the application of proportional counters because of the unavailability of reliable $\overline{W}/e$ values as a function of LET, one should be aware of this source of error in correlating pulse height with energy imparted.

Proportional counters can operate with pulse resolving times of about a microsecond where only gross pulse counting is required. If pulse heights are to be measured also, the average interval between pulses should be greater, approaching the transit times for the positive ions ($\sim 100~\mu s$) for greatest accuracy. Reducing the gas gain by lowering the applied voltage and replacing that gain by an adjustment of the linear amplifier can provide a check on whether the pulse-height spectrum is being distorted by the proportional counter.

Figure 15.1 shows how the pulse height from a proportional counter (or the charge output from an ion chamber) increases as the applied potential P is raised. Two curves are shown, representing initial ionizing events releasing 10 and 10^3 electrons. Both curves rise steeply at low voltages to reach the ion-chamber region, in which the voltage is great enough to closely approach complete collection of charge without causing gas multiplication. That is, at saturation all 10 or 10^3 electrons, respectively (and their corresponding positive ions) would be collected, but no more. A similar saturation curve is shown in Fig. 12.21 in Chapter 12, Section V, where ionic recombination is discussed.

At still higher voltages the gas-multiplication threshold is passed and the proportional-counting region begins. The factor-of-100 difference between the two

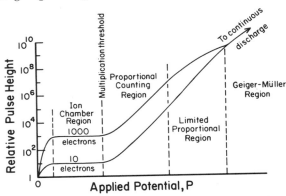

FIGURE 15.1.   Pulse height from a proportional counter as a function of applied potential. The upper curve represents an initial event in which 1000 electrons are released; the lower curve one in which 10 electrons are released. For an amplifying ion chamber the ordinate would be labeled "Relative Charge Collected".

curves in the ion-chamber region extends throughout the proportional-counting region as well, while **G** rises from 1 to $\sim 10^4$.

Further increase in the applied potential results in gain factors that are so large that space-charge effects limit the growth of the larger pulses, and strict proportionality of pulse height with the number of original electrons no longer obtains. This is called the region of limited proportionality.

Finally, at still higher voltages the two curves merge, indicating that initiating events of different sizes produce equal output pulses. This is the G–M region, to be discussed presently. Increasing the voltage beyond the G–M region results in spontaneously repeated or continuous electrical discharge in the gas.

2. USE WITH PULSE-HEIGHT ANALYSIS

If the amplified output from a proportional counter is connected to a multichannel analyzer, the number of pulses of each height (i.e., in each channel) can be counted to obtain a differential distribution of counts per channel vs. channel number, as shown in Fig. 15.2. To facilitate the calibration of the pulse height h in terms of absorbed dose to the counter gas, some proportional counters are equipped with a small α-particle source (see inset) with a gravity-controlled shutter. This source can send a narrow beam of α-particles through the counter along a known chord length ΔX. The expectation value of the dose contributed to the gas by each α-particle can be written as

$$\overline{D}_\alpha = \frac{1}{m} \left(\frac{dT}{\rho dx} \rho \Delta x \right) \tag{15.4}$$

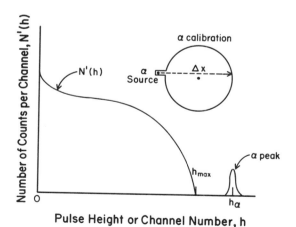

FIGURE 15.2. Differential distribution of counts per pulse-height channel vs. channel number for a proportional counter, as measured by a pulse-height analyzer. A built-in α-particle source is used to calibrate the channel number h in terms of absorbed dose to the counter gas. Assuming a constant $\overline{W}/e$ value for all events, the channel number is proportional to the absorbed dose contributed to the gas by each event. Thus the dose to the gas that is represented by a count in channel h is $D(h) = (h/h_\alpha)\overline{D}_\alpha$.

where $dT/\rho dx$ = mass collision stopping power of the gas for the α-particles,

ρ = gas density in the counter,

Δx = chord length,

m = mass of the gas,

and a suitable conversion factor can be applied to give desired dose units.

This value of dose is to be associated with the pulse height h_α at which the α-particle peak appears, as shown in Fig. 15.2. Since the h-scale is linear vs. event size, the dose contribution by a pulse of any size is thereby known, assuming $\overline{W}/e$ to be the same for all event sizes. The total dose D_g in the gas, represented by the distribution in Fig. 15.2, can then be obtained by summing all the counts, each weighted by its pulse height h expressed as dose:

$$D_g = \sum_{h=0}^{h_{max}} N'(h) \frac{h}{h_\alpha} \overline{D}_\alpha = \sum_{h=0}^{h_{max}} N'(h) \, D(h) \qquad (15.5)$$

where $N'(h)$ is the distribution of counts per channel vs. channel number h, h_α is the mean channel number where the α-counts appear, $\overline{D}_\alpha$ is the mean absorbed dose each α-particle deposits in the gas, and $D(h)$ is the dose per count in channel h.

Evidently such a proportional counter can be used as an absolute dosimeter, by virtue of the built-in α-source. D_g can of course be related to the dose in the counter wall by cavity theory.

Equation (15.5) can be restated in terms of linear energy transfer if one makes the obviously crude assumption that all of the incident particles traverse the counter along the same path that is followed by the calibrating α-particles, namely the diameter. If the particle ranges are also large compared to Δx, and if the ranges of their associated δ-rays are small compared to Δx, it can be seen that the pulse height produced by any crossing particle will be proportional to L_∞, the unrestricted linear energy transfer. Under these restrictive conditions Eq. (15.5) can be written in the form

$$D_g = \sum_{L=0}^{L_{max}} N'(L) \frac{L}{L_\alpha} \overline{D}_\alpha = \sum_{L=0}^{L_{max}} N'(L) \, D(L) \qquad (15.6)$$

where L represents L_∞ and is proportional to channel number h, $N'(L)$ is the number of counts in the channel corresponding to the linear energy-transfer value L, L_α is the L_∞-value for the α-particles in the calibration, and $D(L)$ is the dose per count in channel L.

Notice that the pulse-height scale can be calibrated in terms of L_∞ at the α-peak position by employing the value of $(dT/\rho dx)\rho$ from Eq. (15.4), since

$$L_\infty = \frac{(dT/\rho dx)\rho}{10} \qquad (15.7)$$

where L_∞ is in keV/μm, and $(dT/\rho dx)\rho$ is in MeV/cm.

The most important example of proportional counters that are used with pulse-height analyzers in dosimetry applications is the Rossi counter (Rossi and Rosen-

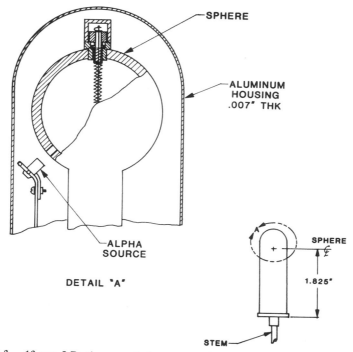

FIGURE 15.3. 13-mm-I.D. tissue-equivalent proportional counter, designed by EG&G, Santa Barbara Operations, now available from Far West Technology, Goleta, CA 93117. The original concept was due to Rossi and Rosenzwieg (1955). Figure reproduced with permission from W.M. Quam (FWT).

zweig, 1955; Rossi, 1968), a commercial model of which is illustrated in Fig. 15.3. These counters are usually made with spherical walls of A-150 tissue-equivalent plastic, and are operated while flowing a tissue-equivalent counting gas through at reduced pressure, typically $\sim 10^{-2}$ atm. The most common size is about 13 mm in inner diameter of the wall. Proper adjustment of the gas pressure allows simulation of biological target objects such as individual cells, in terms of the energy lost by a charged particle in crossing it. This is the primary experimental instrument used in *microdosimetry*, especially in characterizing neutron fields, as discussed in Chapter 16.

To provide a uniform field and thus uniform gas gain all along the central wire, in spite of the spherical shell, that wire is encircled by a helical spring that is typically operated at about 20% of the wire potential relative to the electrically grounded shell. Electrons from primary ionizing events occurring anywhere in the spherical volume are thus drawn toward the wire by the inhomogeneous electric field outside the helix, and they pass through the helical coil into the high-field region where they form uniform avalanches.

3. APPLICATIONS WITHOUT PULSE HEIGHT ANALYSIS

Proportional counters of various designs are also used for many applications in which pulse-height analysis is not used. The main advantages of proportional counters over G–M counters in this connection are (a) their short pulse length ($\sim 1 \mu s$) with practically no additional dead time, accommodating high count rates, and (b) the capability of discriminating by simple means against counting small pulses that might result, for example, from background noise, or γ-ray interactions in a mixed γ + neutron field. Some gases with large thermal-neutron interaction cross sections, notably BF_3 and ^3He, can be employed in proportional counters for neutron dosimetry, as discussed in Chapter 16. Windowless proportional counters through which the gas is continuously flowed at 1 atm are employed to determine the activity of thin α- or β-ray sources that can be inserted into the counter volume. Flat, multiwire position-sensitive proportional counters allow the (x, y) location of the initial ionizing event to be determined in a plane. The various types and capabilities of proportional counters are described by Knoll (1979) and the other references given in that text.

C. Geiger–Müller Counters

1. OPERATION

In Fig. 15.1 it was shown that as the voltage applied to a gas counting tube is increased beyond the upper limit for proportional gain, the pulse height begins to saturate for the larger events, gradually reaching the G–M region of operation. For any voltage in that region all the gas-amplified pulses come out approximately the same, regardless of the size of the initiating event. If the resulting pulse size is larger than the counter-circuit threshold h_t, then the pulses will be counted; if they are too small, they will not. As a result, since the pulse size gradually increases as a function of applied potential, one would expect to see a step function in the count-rate-vs.-voltage curve where the pulse height begins to exceed h_t.

Figure 15.4 shows that the step is actually S-shaped, due to the Gaussian dis-

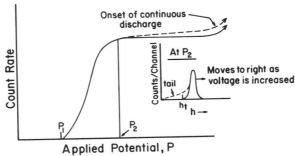

FIGURE 15.4. The counting plateau in a G–M tube. The solid curve is an "ideal" G–M plateau that would be seen for a narrow distribution of pulse heights. The dashed curve has a residual slope within the G–M region because of the presence of a low-amplitude "tail" on the pulse-height distribution (see inset).

tribution of pulse sizes produced in the counter even under ideal G-M conditions. At the applied potential P_1 no counts are obtained. At P_2 the pulses in the ideal G-M counter are all larger than h_t, as shown by the solid curve inset in Fig. 15.4. In that case a flat plateau would be observed, as indicated by the solid curve in the graph of count rate vs. P.

In actual G-M tubes there is a residual slope in the plateau region, as shown by the dashed curve in the inset of Fig. 15.4. This is caused by a small-pulse ''tail'' on the Gaussian distribution of pulse heights, as indicated by the dashed curve in the inset of Fig. 15.4. These small pulses are mostly produced by the ionizing events that occur during the period before the G-M tube has fully recovered from the preceding discharge. Figure 15.5 illustrates this effect.

2. DEAD TIME

Immediately after a discharge the positive space charge so weakens the electric field near the wire that gas multiplication cannot occur. Thus the tube does not respond to radiation at all until the positive-ion cloud starts arriving at the cathode and the electric field strength gradually builds up again. As that takes place, the tube becomes capable of responding to an ionizing event with a discharge of less than full size. The *true dead time* is the time from the start of the preceding pulse until the tube recovers to the point where a minimum-sized pulse can be generated. The *recovery time* is the time until a full-sized pulse is again possible, as shown in Fig. 15.5. The threshold peak size h_t necessary for counting by a G-M counter circuit is considerably less than the average pulse size that would be generated by a fully recovered G-M tube when it is being normally operated at a potential in the middle of the G-M plateau (see Fig. 15.4). Thus the *minimum time between detectable pulses* will be less than the recovery time. This is the *pulse resolving time*, but is more commonly referred to as the ''dead time'' in place of the narrower definition above.

It should be pointed out that if an ionizing event occurs during the true dead time, as defined above, the event causes no electron avalanche and hence has no effect on

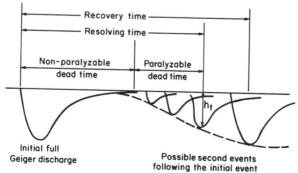

FIGURE 15.5. Dead time and recovery time of a G-M tube. Reproduced with permission from G. F. Knoll.

the tube. Thus an event that occurs during the true dead time is simply not counted, but does not influence the ability of the tube to respond to later events. This is called *nonparalyzable* dead-time behavior. If, however, an ionizing event occurs after the end of the true dead time, but before the resulting pulse is large enough to be counted (i.e., $> h_l$), not only will that event go uncounted but a new dead-time period will begin. Thus the tube will also fail to count any later event that happens before the end of the resolving time. This is called *paralyzable* dead-time behavior. Obviously a G–M counter exhibits dead-time behavior that is intermediate, being a mixture of the paralyzable and nonparalyzable cases. Reducing the detectable pulse-height threshold h_l tends to decrease the paralyzable component.

If m is the observed count rate, n is the true count rate, and τ is the pulse resolving time (commonly called "dead time"), then for the nonparalyzable case the correction for dead-time counting losses is

$$n = \frac{m}{1 - m\tau} \tag{15.8}$$

and for the paralyzable case

$$m = ne^{-n\tau} \tag{15.9}$$

which must be solved for n iteratively. In the limiting case of small dead-time counting losses, ($n \ll 1/\tau$), both types of behavior reduce to

$$m \cong n(1 - n\tau) \tag{15.10}$$

At high values of the true count rate n, the value of m approaches $1/\tau$ asymptotically in a nonparalyzable counter. However, in the paralyzable case m reaches a flat maximum at $n = 1/\tau$, then gradually *decreases* with further increases in n because of overlapping chains of dead-time periods. Thus a low reading of a G–M counter may result from a strong radiation field if the dead-time behavior is predominantly paralyzable. In that case reducing the field strength will cause the observed count rate to rise.

The value of τ in Eq. (15.8) or (15.9) can be measured by methods described by Knoll (1979). A very simple scheme for Eq. (15.8) uses a radioactive source that is large enough to produce significant dead-time counting losses, giving an observed count rate m_2 (c/s), and then reduces (e.g., attenuates) the *true* count rate by exactly $\frac{1}{2}$ to obtain an observed count rate m_1. The value of τ (in seconds) is given for the nonparalyzable case by

$$\tau = \frac{2}{m_2} - \frac{1}{m_1} \tag{15.11}$$

3. G–M COUNTER APPLICATIONS

Since G–M counters are only *triggered* by ionizing events, producing discharge pulses of more or less the same size regardless of the initiating event, the observed output conveys little information about the dose to the counter gas. Nevertheless G–M counters are used in some dosimetry applications because they offer several advantages: They require little if any further amplification, since pulses of 1–10 V can be obtained directly; they are also inexpensive and versatile in their construction and geometry. Thus they are often used in radiation survey meters to measure x- and γ-ray fields in radiation-protection applications. When equipped with a thin (∼ 1 mg/cm^2) window they can also be used to detect β-rays. In some designs the output current is measured in place of the pulse counting rate.

Scale calibrations of G–M counters, if given in terms other than the count rate, should always be suspect because of the aforementioned lack of dose response. Moreover, because most G–M tubes are constructed of materials that are higher in atomic number than tissue or air, they exhibit strong photoelectric-effect response below ∼ 100 keV. Figure 15.6 shows the typical response of a G–M counter per unit of tissue dose, as a function of photon energy. It can be seen from curve a that the counter responds about 5 times more strongly to 50-keV x rays producing a given absorbed dose (under CPE conditions) in tissue, than to 670-keV photons depositing the same tissue dose. Enclosing the G–M tube in a suitable high-Z filter tends to flatten the overresponse at low energies, as seen in curve b. Such an energy-compensated G–M tube can respond to photons over a limited range of energies in a way that is reasonably proportional to tissue dose, or to exposure. Thus with proper calibration it can be used as an approximate dose-rate or exposure-rate meter in spite of its inherent shortcomings as a dosimeter.

G–M counters respond to γ-rays by the action of the secondary electrons that are produced in the cathode wall and enter the gas. Thus a high-sensitivity counter can be designed for the energy region where the photoelectric effect is strong (≲ 100 keV) by using high-Z material for the cathode. The wall thickness should approximate the maximum projected range of the secondary electrons for maximum sensitivity.

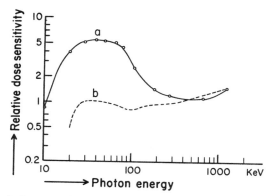

FIGURE 15.6. Typical energy-dependence curves of the response relative to tissue dose for survey meters containing G–M tubes of the following types: (a) uncompensated, and (b) compensated with metallic filters to produce flatter response. (Kiefer et al., 1969. Reproduced with permission from R. Maushart and Academic Press.)

The energy dependence of such a counter, in terms of exposure or tissue dose, would of course be more pronounced than that shown by curve *a* in Fig. 15.6.

Another dosimetry application of G–M counters is in measuring the γ-ray dose component in a mixed neutron + γ-ray field. Because the large ionizing events produced in the tube by the heavy secondary charged particles from neutron interactions give rise to the same-sized pulses as the smaller γ-ray secondary-electron events, the response per unit dose is much less for the neutrons than for the γ-rays. Thus the neutron dose is discriminated against. Further discussion of this application is given in Chapter 16.

III. SCINTILLATION DOSIMETRY

A Introduction

Many transparent substances, including certain solids, liquids, and gases, scintillate (i.e., emit flashes of visible light) as a result of the action of ionizing radiation. Through the application of a sensitive light detector such as a photomultiplier (PM) tube, the light emitted can be converted into an electrical signal. A light photon incident on the photocathode of a PM tube may release an electron, which is then numerically amplified as much as $\times 10^7$ in passing through the dynode chain in the tube. Either the output electrical pulses from numerous such events can be counted (with or without pulse-height analysis), or the output current can be measured. Figure 15.7 shows the schematic design of such a device.

Scintillators have been widely applied as detectors of ionizing radiation, especially in nuclear physics. Very fast decay times, down to $\sim 10^{-9}$ s, make organic liquid and plastic scintillators excellent choices for coincidence measurements with good time-resolution, and they can occupy whatever volume shape and size one wishes.

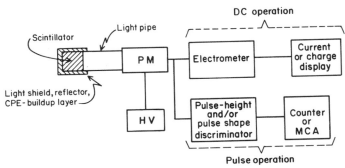

FIGURE 15.7.   General schematic design for a scintillation detector for dosimetry applications. A light pipe optically couples the scintillator to the photomultiplier tube. The scintillator is otherwise enclosed in an optically opaque and internally reflective envelope that may also filter out short-range radiation and may additionally serve as a CPE buildup layer for indirectly ionizing radiation.

Scintillators, especially NaI(Tl), also have been used extensively for x- and γ-ray energy spectrometry but have been largely replaced by Si(Li) and Ge(Li) semi-conductor detectors for best energy resolution. However, scintillators continue to be widely used for those γ-ray spectrometry applications in which resolution is less critical, because of lower cost and the greater convenience of operating the detector at room temperature instead of inside a cryostat.

In the present context we will focus on the dosimetry characteristics of scintillators.

B. Light Output Efficiency

Only a very small part of the energy imparted to a scintillator appears as light; the rest is dissipated as heat. In typical situations ~ 1 keV of energy is spent in the scintillator for the release of one electron from the PM tube's photocathode. However, the large gain available in the PM tube and external amplifiers still provides an adequate output signal. The light generated in a scintillator by a given imparted energy depends on the linear energy transfer (LET) of the charged particles delivering the energy. In typical organic scintillators such as the commercially available plastic NE-102, increasing the particle LET decreases the light output for a given energy imparted, as can be seen in Fig. 15.8. The light response from electrons that spend their full track length in the scintillator is found to be proportional to their starting energy

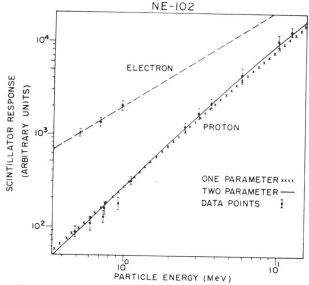

FIGURE 15.8. Light output vs. particle energy for electrons and protons stopped in the plastic scintillator NE-102. The light output is proportional to electron energy, but not to proton energy. Curves are based on Birks's theory (1964) that dense ionization tracks create damaged molecules, which lower the scintillation efficiency. (Craun and Smith, 1970. Reproduced with permission from North-Holland Physics Publishing.)

above about 125 keV. For protons, the light output is only about 15% as great as for electrons at 1 MeV, rising to about 40% as great at 10 MeV. That LET dependence must be taken into account and corrected for, in relating pulse-height distributions to distributions of dose per pulse, in cases where both low- and high-LET radiations are present. It does not affect the use of an organic scintillator for photon or electron dosimetry above about 125 keV, assuming that the signal output is correctly calibrated in terms of absorbed dose. Proportional counters (and, as we shall see, semiconductor detectors) do not require an LET correction even for heavy particles, which is one advantage they have over scintillators.

The technique of *pulse-shape discrimination* allows the separation of dose components on the basis of particle LET, so different calibration factors can be applied. This will be discussed in Section III.F.

It should be apparent that for dosimetry of γ-rays or electrons, either the PM-tube output should be measured as an electric current or the pulse-heights must be analyzed and calibrated in terms of dose, as discussed for proportional counters. Simple counting of pulses without regard to their size is not a measure of the dose in a scintillator.

C. Scintillator Types

For most dosimetry applications where soft tissue is the dose-relevant material, organic plastic scintillators such as NE-102,* organic liquids such as NE-213,* and the organic crystals stilbene and anthracene are the most useful because they are made mostly of the low-atomic-number elements C and H. Thus they do not overrespond to photons through the photoelectric effect, and the hydrogen content makes the (n, p) elastic-scattering interaction the main process for fast-neutron dose deposition, as it is in tissue.

Table 15.2 lists the principle characteristics of a few representative types of scintillators. Knoll (1979) gives a more comprehensive list. Notice that the liquid scintillator NE-226 contains no hydrogen, making it insensitive to fast neutrons, while NE-228 is rich in hydrogen, and thus is sensitive to neutrons.

D. Light Collection and Measurement

1. SCINTILLATOR ENCLOSURE

A light reflector, optimally a thin layer of MgO powder, is useful to maximize light-collection efficiency from a scintillator. If the scintillator has polished surfaces, all the light incident from the inside is reflected if the angle of incidence is greater than the critical angle. The MgO reflector will recapture most of the light that escapes at smaller angles.

For small or thin scintillators (plastic ones may be as thin as ~ 20 μm) one should keep in mind cavity-theory considerations. Simplest dosimetric interpretation for indirectly ionizing radiation calls for surrounding the scintillator by a nonscintil-

---

*Nuclear Enterprises, Ltd., Bath Rd, Beenham, Reading, Berkshire, RG7 5PR, U.K.

TABLE 15.2. Characteristics of Some Scintillators

Type	Specific Gravity	Refractive Index	Softening or Melting Point (°C)	Light Output Rel. to Anthracene (%)	Decay Const., Main Component (ns)	Maximum λ (nm)	Approx. Composition
Plastic NE-102	1.032	1.581	75	65	2.4	423	1.104[a]
Liquid NE-213	0.874	1.508	141	78	3.7	425	1.213[a]
Liquid NE-226	1.61	1.38	80	20	3.3	430	0[a]
Liquid NE-228	0.735	1.403	99	45	—	385	2.00[a]
Organic crystal:							
stilbene	1.16	1.626	125	50	4.5	410	$C_{14}H_{12}$
anthracene	1.25	1.62	217	100	30	447	$C_{14}H_{10}$
Inorganic crystal:							
NaI (Tl)	3.67	1.85	661	200	230	410	NaI
CsI (Tl)	4.51	1.80	626	90	10^3	565	CsI

[a] Ratio of H to C atoms.

lating layer of the same composition, thick enough to provide CPE (e.g., see Lawson and Watt, 1964). In the case of plastic scintillators a shell of Lucite will usually suffice, surrounding the thin reflector. Outside of this an opaque covering such as aluminum foil is required to exclude ambient light. NaI and CsI scintillators require hermetic seals, as they are hygroscopic.

The use of large-volume scintillators for dosimetry requires attention to the light-collection efficiency from different interior regions. Attenuation within the scintillator itself is not usually a problem; rather, the surface-reflection geometry differs from place to place. Improvement in uniformity may be obtained through varying the effectiveness of the surface reflector from one part of the surface to another, or by subdividing a large scintillator into a number of smaller volumes, each with its own PM tube.

2. LIGHT PIPE AND PM TUBE

The exit surface of a scintillator is optically coupled to the PM-tube photocathode through a light pipe, usually consisting of a solid cylinder of polished Lucite. The interfaces (scintillator, light pipe, tube face) are filled with an optical coupling agent such as high-viscosity silicone oil or transparent epoxy cement. Ideally all materials along the optical path should have nearly the same refractive index as the glass face of the PM tube, $\cong 1.5$. To the extent that this is not true, light is lost by reflection. For energy-spectrometry applications the spectral resolution may suffer on this account, but for dosimetry the penalty is simply a loss of radiation sensitivity. Except for very low-dose-rate applications this is usually not a serious problem.

The main purpose of the light pipe in dosimetry is to remove the PM tube from the radiation field that the scintillator is measuring. PM tubes are of course capable of responding to ionizing events occurring within their structure. This direct radiation response is undesirable because the interactions occur in different media than the scintillator, at different locations, and with variable gain factors. Moreover, large doses can so damage a PM tube (e.g., by discoloring the photocathode glass face) that its light sensitivity is permanently decreased.

A wide variety of PM tubes is available to satisfy many types of applications. Dosimetry does not place unusual demands on such tubes; relatively inexpensive models can be chosen. The main relevant characteristics of PM tubes are these:

1. *Spectral Sensitivity.* This should be adequately matched to the scintillator output spectrum, which is usually in the blue region (see Table 15.2).
2. *Size.* The photocathode diameter should be large enough to allow the light pipe to be optically coupled to it. Reducing the light pipe's cross-sectional area, however gradually, in going from the scintillator to the PM tube, loses light. On the other hand, minimizing the PM-tube size allows more compact and rugged instrument design.
3. *Voltage Requirements.* Different models require operating potentials from $P = 900$ to 2400 V. Great stability is required of the power supply, as the gain varies

in proportion to P^6–P^9 for a 10-dynode tube. A PM tube requiring only 1000 V may be satisfied by a high-quality supply that is relatively inexpensive and can be used alternatively for ion chambers.

4. *Gain Linearity.* The average gain of the dynode chain in a PM tube is independent of how many electrons are simultaneously ejected from the photocathode, from one to many thousands. The size of an electrical output pulse is thus proportional to the number of electrons in the originating pulse leaving the photocathode. Likewise the average current from the PM-tube anode is proportional to that ejected from the photocathode. The ultimate output limit occurs at the last gain step between the final dynode and the anode. This is either due to space-charge effect, or because the last dynode draws too much current from the resistor string that supplies its voltage, which consequently decreases and lowers the gain. Manufacturers' recommendations should be followed in limiting the PM-tube output.

5. *Photocathode Fatigue.* This results from exposing the tube to light while the HV is applied, or delivering too bright a scintillation signal to it. Until it recovers, which may take some time, the light sensitivity is reduced, and the dosimetric calibration changed accordingly.

6. *Magnetic Effects.* PM tubes are sensitive to magnetic fields, which deflect the electrons during their flight between dynodes and thereby affect the gain. Proximity to magnets (e.g., at linacs) or electrical conductors carrying large currents may require such remedial action as use of a Mu-metal magnetic shield or relocation of the PM tube by use of a longer light pipe.

7. *Temperature Dependence.* The gain of a PM tube may depend on its operating temperature by as much as $\cong 1\%\,°C$. Temperature-controlled housings that operate at reduced temperatures not only stabilize the gain, but also lower the tube's background current and random noise signal.

8. *Transit Time.* For high-dose-rate applications a short-decay-time scintillator may be used with a short-transit-time PM tube if the shape of a brief pulse of radiation is to be preserved. The fastest organic scintillators have decay constants around 1 ns. Continuous-channel-type PM tubes, or microchannel plates made of many such adjacent channels, offer the shortest electron transit times, a few nanoseconds. More importantly, the statistical spread in transit times, which would distort a measured pulse, is only ~0.1 ns. Thus the scintillator decay time is the limiting factor in such a measurement.

E. Comparison with an Ionization Chamber

Scintillators are often used as a more sensitive substitute for an ionization chamber in a γ-ray survey meter for health-physics applications. It is instructive to consider what factors are involved in estimating the difference in current output from a scintillator and an ion chamber of the same volume.

The analogue in a scintillator of $\overline{W}$ in a gas is the average energy spent by an electron per light photon produced. For plastic scintillators this is around 60 eV, or about twice $\overline{W}$ for gases, for low-LET radiation. For good optical coupling $\cong \frac{1}{3}$ of the photons reach the PM-tube photocathode. Typical photocathode efficiency is about 15%, and tube gain about 10^6. Thus for equal masses of chamber gas and plastic scintillator, the output current for the latter is $\cong 3 \times 10^4$ greater. Assuming 1 g/cm^3 for the scintillator and 0.001 g/cm^3 for the gas in the ion chamber, equal volumes would favor the scintillator by a factor of $\cong 3 \times 10^7$. This is comparable in sensitivity to a G–M tube of the same size. However, the plastic scintillator has an output current for electrons with energies over 125 keV that is proportional to the absorbed dose in the plastic medium, which approximates tissue.

F. Pulse-Shape Discrimination

In most scintillators, the promptly emitted light comprises nearly all of the observed scintillation. In some materials, notably stilbene and NE-213 liquid scintillator, a sizable longer-time-constant component exists that is LET-dependent. Particles with denser tracks thus have a more pronounced component of longer decay time constant, as shown in Fig. 15.9.

Suitable electronic discrimination can be provided to count pulses of differing lengths separately, correlated with the LET of the particles that produced them. Thus it becomes possible to apply different dose calibrations to the pulse heights for radiations having different LETs. As noted before, the efficiency of scintillators decreases with increasing LET, and this technique allows that defect to be compensated for. This feature is especially useful for dosimetry in combined neutron–γ-ray fields.

Combinations of two different scintillators coupled to the same PM tube, called "phoswiches," are useful for some dosimetry situations. The scintillators are chosen to have different decay times so pulse-shape discrimination can be applied to separate

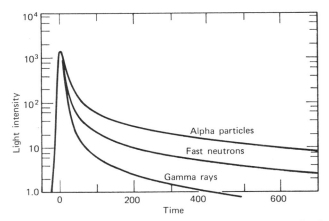

FIGURE 15.9. Time dependence of scintillation pulses in stilbene, normalized to equal heights at time zero, when excited by radiations of different LET. The curve labeled "neutrons" represents the protons generated by (n, p) interactions. (Bollinger and Thomas, 1961. Reproduced with permission from L. M. Bollinger and The American Institute of Physics.)

the signals. For example, one thin scintillator can be used to stop a relatively non-penetrating component of radiation, say β-rays, while a thicker scintillator behind the first interacts more strongly with more penetrating γ-rays.

G. Beta-Ray Dosimetry

A plastic scintillator covered by a thin opaque window and coupled to the PM tube face can be used to measure the planar energy-flux density due to incident β-rays, assuming that the scintillator is thick enough to stop them, and that the light output is proportional to β-ray energy. In other words, the light signal brightness (and PM-tube output current) will be proportional to the radiant energy carried into the scintillator by β-rays per unit time, irrespective of their angle of incidence, except for those that enter and then escape from the edge of the scintillator. That loss can be minimized by using a high-Z electron backscattering foil around the scintillator sides, and/or by making the scintillator in the shape of a truncated cone with the base against the PM tube. The distribution of dose vs. depth in tissue can be gotten from the reductions in light output observed when a series of tissue-equivalent plastic absorbing layers are placed over the front of the scintillator.

IV. SEMICONDUCTOR DETECTORS FOR DOSIMETRY

A. Introduction

Silicon and germanium detectors have been used mainly for energy spectrometry, and have largely replaced scintillators in this application where highest energy resolution is required.

However, semiconductor detectors have characteristics that also make them very attractive as dosimeters, for measuring either dose or dose rate, as a substitute for an ion chamber. Moreover, they can also serve as a solid-state analogue of a proportional counter, since the ionization produced by a charged particle in traversing the sensitive volume of the detector is proportional to the energy spent, irrespective of LET, for particles lighter than α's. Some internal amplification is even possible in the "avalanche detector" mode of operation, but external amplification is usually preferred. This broad lack of LET-dependence is an advantage over scintillation detectors, allowing simpler interpretation of pulse heights in terms of energy imparted.

In a totally different method of application, semiconductor detectors may be employed as neutron dosimeters by measuring the resulting radiation damage done by the neutrons.

In the following sections the various methods of dosimetry application will be outlined.

B. Basic Operation of Reverse-Biased Semiconductor Junction Detectors

Figure 15.10 illustrates the operation of a typical reverse-biased semiconductor detector, the silicon p–n junction.

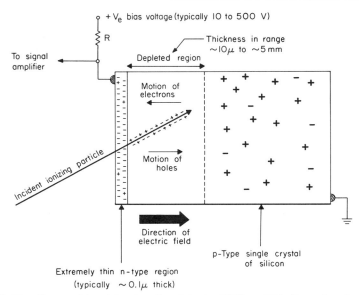

FIGURE 15.10. Reverse-biased p–n junction detector (Miller, 1961. Reproduced with permission from the Brookhaven National Laboratory. Drawing made available by courtesy of J. F. Fowler, 1966.)

We need not discuss here how such a device is prepared by "doping" an initially very pure silicon crystal. Suffice it to say that the bulk of the crystal consists of a "p" region having an excess of "holes", while a thin layer at the surface is an "n" region having an excess of electrons. Electrical conduction in each region occurs through motion of these majority charge carriers (holes or electrons).

When a positive potential (~ 10–10^3 V) is applied to the n-terminal relative to the opposite evaporated-metal surface contact, electrons and holes are pulled out of an intermediate region called the *depletion layer*, and current cannot then flow across the junction except for some leakage current. The thickness of the depletion layer is proportional to the square root of the applied potential, and usually ranges from micrometers to $\cong 5$ mm in thickness.

If a charged particle passes through the depletion layer while the junction is in this reverse-biased condition, it forms electron–hole pairs by the usual collision processes. The mean energy spent per electron–hole pair in Si at 300 K is 3.62 eV for α's and 3.68 for electrons, and in Ge at 77 K it is 2.97 eV for both. These figures are only about one-tenth of the analogous W-values for gas ion chambers; hence ~ 10 times as much ionization is formed in semiconductor detectors as in ion chambers for the same energy expenditure. This also helps account for the good energy resolution of Si and Ge detectors.

Electrons have mobilities of 1350 cm/s per V/cm in Si and 3900 in Ge, at 300 K. Hole mobilities are 480 cm/s per V/cm in Si and 1900 in Ge, at 300 K. Thus typically they can reach the boundary of the depletion layer in 10^{-7}–10^{-8} s, producing a comparable voltage-pulse rise time.

A charge-sensitive linear preamplifier and linear voltage amplifier comparable to those used for proportional counters, but with suitably shorter time constants, are used to amplify the charge pulses for charge measurement or pulse-height analysis and counting.

C. Silicon Diodes without Bias

Although the sensitivity is greater and the response time is less for Si diode detectors with reverse bias applied, for DC operation there is an advantage in operating without any external bias: As the bias voltage is reduced to zero, the DC leakage current decreases more rapidly than the radiation-induced current. Since this leakage current is strongly temperature-dependent, minimizing its magnitude is advantageous. The residual zero-bias radiation-induced current results from alteration of charge-carrier concentrations, and in turn gives rise to a potential difference between the electrodes. The measurement of the radiocurrent is done with a low-impedance circuit such as an operational amplifier as in Fig. 15.11b.

The ranges of dose rate that are measured in radiotherapy applications (0.03–3 Gy/min) produce adequate output currents from an unbiased silicon diode detector with a typical sensitivity of $\cong 2 \times 10^{-11}$ A per R/min. A commercial device of this type is marketed by Nuclear Associates, with a sensitive volume of 0.2 mm^3 (Model 30-490 with probe only; Model 05-595 including readout circuit).

Gager et al. (1977), designed a high-Z filter to surround the silicon detector shown in Fig. 15.11a, to flatten the energy dependence per roentgen or per tissue rad. Wright and Gager (1977) compared depth–dose measurements of linac x-ray beams taken with this detector and with a Farmer ion chamber. They found that the shielded Si detector agrees well with the ion chamber, but gives a better signal-to-noise ratio, allowing more rapid measurements to be made with equal precision.

D. Lithium-Drifted Si and Ge Detectors

The most common types of semiconductor detectors are the lithium-drifted type. These are prepared by diffusing Li$^+$ ions into high-purity (but slightly p-type) Si or Ge crystals. The Li$^+$ ions lodge at interstitial positions next to the electron-acceptor sites (trivalent impurity atoms), then capture electrons to become electron donor sites, which thereby neutralize the acceptor sites. The crystal is then said to be compensated, by having the same number of electrons in the conduction band as it has holes in the valence band. In this condition it acts like an intrinsic material, that is, one that is free of all donor and acceptor sites, being almost completely pure. Drifted regions up to almost 2 cm in thickness can be achieved in this way, and the entire intrinsic volume acts as the dosimeter's sensitive volume. Changing the applied potential varies the electric field strength across this volume, but doesn't change its depth. If the Li-drifted region extends completely through the crystal, it is said to be fully depleted.

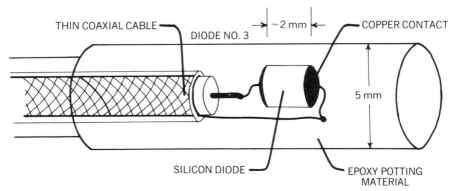

FIGURE 15.11a. Design of unbiased silicon $p-n$ junction (Gager et al., 1977. Reproduced with permission from L. D. Gager and the American Institute of Physics.)

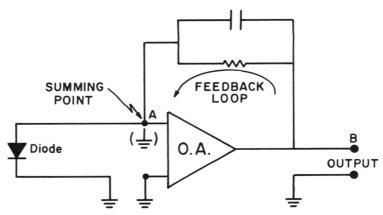

FIGURE 15.11b. Operation of unbiased silicon $p-n$ junction (Gager et al., 1977. Reproduced with permission from L. D. Gager and The American Institute of Physics.)

Si(Li) and Ge(Li) detectors can be made as thin as 10 μm to serve as "dE/dx" measuring devices for charged particles passing through, by which is meant that they respond proportionally to the collision stopping power of the material (ignoring δ-ray production). Likewise they can serve as thin dosimeters, or to measure LET distributions of charged-particle fields.

Ge(Li) detectors are preferred over Si(Li) for x- or γ-ray spectrometry above 50 keV, or for energy-fluence measurements, because the higher Z (32) of Ge gives it a greater photoelectric cross section than Si ($Z = 14$), so that Ge stops the beam more efficiently. Si(Li) detectors are preferred for lower-energy x rays and for β-ray dosimetry because their backscattering is much less. Detectors with areas as great as 15 cm^2 are available. Geometries of detectors available are not only planar, but also cylindrical and annular for special applications (e.g., "well" counting of radioactive sources).

One disadvantage of Ge(Li) and Si(Li) detectors is that, to maintain their energy resolution for spectrometry, they must be maintained and operated at liquid-N_2 temperature. Allowing Ge(Li) detectors ever to warm up to room temperature deteriorates them by allowing the Li ions to migrate, thus disturbing donor–acceptor compensation. Si(Li) detectors usually may be allowed to reach room temperature without damage, because of lower Li-ion mobility. The manufacturer's advice should be followed however.

Another type of germanium detector, intrinsic germanium (IG), has been developed in comparable sizes and other characteristics to Ge(Li), but may be stored at room temperature and only cooled to make measurements. It achieves donor–acceptor compensation through purity of manufacture instead of lithium drifting.

E. Use of Si(Li) as an Ion-Chamber Substitute

The density of Si is about 2.3 g/cm^3, or about 1800 times that of air. Thus, considering also the $\overline{W}$ difference, a Si(Li) detector will produce about 18,000 times as much charge as an ion chamber of the same volume, in the same x-ray field, at energies ($>$ 100 keV) where the photoelectric effect is unimportant.

F. Use of Si(Li) Junctions with Reverse Bias as Counting Dose-Rate Meters

Raju et al. (1969, 1971) have used Si(Li) detectors (e.g., 1 mm thick) as probes for measuring the depth dose due to heavy charged particles, including pions. The pulse height was found to be proportional to the energy spent by the particle in the sensitive volume of the detector. Pulses were stored in a computer and analyzed later. Scintillators were used in a time-of-flight method to separate the doses due to pions and electrons, which are faster than the pions.

Richman et al., (1978) extended the method for pion dosimetry to provide separation of dose components on the basis of the LET of the contributing radiation components. They used Si(Li) detectors from 10 μm to 5 mm thick to emphasize components of different penetrating power, and to study the perturbing effect of the detector on the radiation field. They were able to get results on dose vs. LET which were consistent with those of a Rossi proportional counter.

G. Fast-Neutron Dosimetry

Silicon detectors are damaged by very high doses ($> 10^4$ Gy) of electrons or x rays, but are much more sensitive to damage by fast neutrons. Doses of 0.1 to 10 Gy (tissue) cause permanent defects in the Si crystal lattice, which act as traps for charge carriers. As a result the resistance of the detector is effectively increased. The voltage drop across the detector when a constant test current ($\cong$ 25 mA) is passed through it in a forward direction increases gradually vs. dose from an initial value of about 1 V to 4 V. The damage is dose-rate-independent, and is influenced only very slightly by electron or γ-ray dose (McCall et al., 1978).

The response of these detectors per gray of neutron tissue kerma or (CPE) dose in free space is constant ($\pm 20\%$) from $\cong 300$ keV to 14 MeV. Below 200 keV the response decreases rapidly.

PROBLEMS

1. Calculate the gain factor for a cylindrical proportional counter having a central wire diameter of 2.54×10^{-3} cm and a cathode diameter of 1.50 cm, filled with methane at 76 torr, with 800 V applied potential.

2. Without changing the counter geometry or the gas in problem 1, give two parameter changes, each of which would raise the gain factor to 1×10^4.

3. How thick is the amplifying sheath surrounding the anode in problem 1?

4. What pressure of methane-based tissue-equivalent gas in a Rossi spherical proportional counter 13 mm in diameter would be used to simulate a water-density biological object 1 μm in diameter? You may assume that the density of the TE gas is 1.057 g/liter at 22°C, 760 torr.

5. A gas counter gives an observed count rate of 3.94×10^4 min^{-1} when the true count rate is 4.15×10^4 min^{-1}. What is the dead time if assumed to be (a) nonparalyzable, (b) paralyzable? (c) Why are these values so nearly equal? (d) What type of counter is this, assuming that the dead time is characteristic of the counter itself?

6. The counter in problem 5 is used to measure a γ-ray field in which the true count rate is 2×10^4 c/s. What would be the observed count-rate on the assumption of (a) nonparalyzability and (b) paralyzability? (c) What would you conclude about using a G–M counter where dead-time losses are large?

SOLUTIONS TO PROBLEMS

1. 560.

2. Apply $P = 1054$ V, or reduce pressure to 0.0298 atm.

3. 0.17 mm.

4. 55.3 torr.

5. (a) 77 μs.
   (b) 75 μs.
   (c) $n \ll 1/\tau$.
   (d) G–M counter.

6. (a) 7.87×10^3 c/s.
   (b) 4.46×10^3 c/s.
   (c) Not advisable because of uncertainty about paralyzability vs. nonparalyzability in G–M counters.

CHAPTER 16

Neutron Interactions and Dosimetry

I. INTRODUCTION

This chapter is intended to provide an introduction to neutron dosimetry that is relevant to the human body, from the viewpoint of either radiation hazard or neutron-beam radiotherapy. We will avoid the topic of neutron shielding, which more properly belongs in a health-physics or nuclear-engineering course. The reader may consult Profio (1979) and Lewis and Miller (1984) as useful references on that subject.

Dosimetry that is explicitly relevant to neutron damage in solid-state media is also avoided here. Such damage is only poorly correlated with absorbed dose, because of the existence of kinetic-energy thresholds below which the damage does not occur if it is associated with atomic displacements, for example. Thus the observed damage per unit of absorbed dose may be strongly dependent on neutron energy. The problem of dosimetry in such cases then becomes primarily a neutron spectrometry problem. The use of radioactivation threshold detectors (usually metal foils) has proved valuable in this application, as described by Moteff (1969).

In the present context we will be primarily concerned about neutron interactions with the majority tissue elements H, O, C, and N, and the resulting absorbed dose. Because of the short ranges of the heavy secondary charged particles that are produced in such interactions, CPE is usually well approximated. Thus, since no bremsstrahlung x-rays are generated, the absorbed dose can be assumed to be equal to the kerma at any point in neutron fields at least up to an energy $E \cong 20$ MeV.

II. NEUTRON KINETIC ENERGY

For dosimetry purposes it is convenient to divide neutron fields into the following energy categories.

A. Thermal Neutrons

Thermal neutrons have only the Maxwellian distribution of thermal motion that is characteristic of the temperature of the medium in which they exist. Their most probable kinetic energy at 20°C is $E = 0.025$ eV. However, all neutrons with energies below 0.5 eV are usually referred to as thermal because of a simple experimental

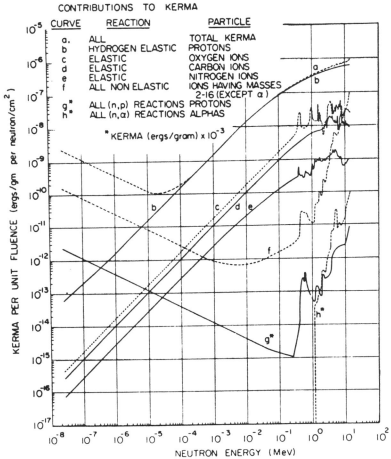

FIGURE 16.1. Kerma per unit fluence contributed by various interactions in a small mass of tissue in free space, as a function of incident neutron energy. Note that curves g and h are displaced downward by the factor 10^{-3}. (Auxier et al., 1968. Reproduced with permission from J. A. Auxier and Academic Press.)

test that can be applied to a neutron field to measure how completely it has been "thermalized" by passage through a moderator. A cadmium filter 1 mm thick absorbs practically all incident neutrons below about 0.5 eV, but readily passes those above that energy. A thermal-neutron detecting foil such as gold can be radioactivated by neutrons through the ^{197}Au(n, γ)^{198}Au interaction, with a cross section that is inversely dependent on the neutron velocity or $\sqrt{E}$. Exposing two such foils in the neutron field, one foil bare and the other enclosed in 1 mm of Cd, provides two activation readings. The ratio of the bare to the Cd reading is called the *cadmium ratio*; it is unity if no thermal neutrons are present, and rises toward infinity as the thermal-neutron component approaches 100%.

B. Intermediate-Energy Neutrons

Neutrons with energies above the thermal cutoff of 0.5 eV but below 10 keV are called intermediate-energy neutrons. Above 10 keV, the dose in the human body is dominated by the contribution of recoil protons resulting from elastic scattering of hydrogen nuclei. Below that energy the dose is mainly due to γ-rays resulting from thermal-neutron capture in hydrogen. Thus the neutron quality factor rises steeply above 10 keV, as will be seen in Fig. 16.6, because of the greater biological effectiveness of heavy charged particles.

C. Fast Neutrons

These neutrons cover the energy range from 10 keV upward.

III. NEUTRON INTERACTIONS IN TISSUE

A. Tissue Composition

Table 16.1 gives the atomic composition, in percentage by weight, of human muscle tissue and the whole body. The ICRU composition for muscle has been assumed in most cases for neutron-dose calculations (see ICRU, 1977), lumping the 1.1% of "other" minor elements together with oxygen to make a simple four-element (H,O,C,N) composition. Table 16.1 shows that the ICRP (1975) skeletal-muscle

TABLE 16.1.　Human Tissue Composition[a]

Element	ICRU (1977) Muscle	ICRP Skeletal Muscle	Whole Body
H	10.2	10.06	10.5
O	72.9	75.48	67.7
C	12.3	10.78	18.7
N	3.5	2.77	3.1
Other	1.1	0.91	—
Total	100.0	100.00	100.0

[a]Data are given in percent by weight.

composition (see also Appendix B.3) differs somewhat from the ICRU composition, and both are substantially different from the average whole-body composition in the last column, used by Auxier et al. (1968) in computing the data tabulated in Section V.

B. Kerma Calculations

For a single neutron energy, type of target atom, and kind of interaction, the kerma that results from a neutron fluence Φ (cm^{-2}) at a point in a medium is given by

$$K = 1.602 \times 10^{-8} \, \Phi \sigma N_t m^{-1} \, E_{tr} \tag{16.1}$$

where σ is the interaction cross section in cm^2/(target atom), N_t is the number of target atoms in the irradiated sample [see Eq. (6.38)], m is the sample mass in grams, and E_{tr} is the total kinetic energy (MeV) given to charged particles per interaction. K is thus given in rad (or centigrays), and its value is equal to the absorbed dose D at the same point under the usual CPE conditions. The product of $(1.602 \times 10^{-8} \sigma N_t m^{-1} E_{tr})$ is equal to the kerma factor F_n in rad cm^2/n, as discussed in Chapter 2, Section II.C. Thus Eq. (16.1) reduces to

$$D \overset{\text{CPE}}{=} K = \Phi F_n \tag{16.2}$$

Tables of F_n-values from Caswell et al., (1980) will be found in Appendix F for several elements, compounds, and mixtures. F_n is not generally a smooth function of Z and E, unlike the case of photon interaction coefficients. Thus interpolation vs. Z cannot be employed to obtain values of F_n for elements for which data are not listed, and interpolation vs. E is feasible only within energy regions where resonance peaks are absent. Figure 16.1 illustrates this lack of regularity of F_n-values for neutrons in muscle tissue (Auxier et al., 1968).

For a continuous neutron spectrum with a differential fluence distribution $\Phi'(E)$ (n/cm^2 MeV), the kerma contribution by j-type interactions with i-type target atoms is

$$K_{ij} = 1.602 \times 10^{-8} \, N_i m^{-1} \int_0^{E_{\max}} \Phi'(E) \, \sigma_{ij}(E) \, [E_{tr}(E)]_{ij} \, dE \tag{16.3}$$

where $N_i m^{-1}$ is the number of target atoms of type i per gram of the medium, $\sigma_{ij}(E)$ is the cross section for j-type interactions with i-type atoms by neutrons of energy E, and $[E_{tr}(E)]_{ij}$ is the total kinetic energy given to charged particles per type-j interaction with type-i atoms by neutrons of energy E. For the same units as in Eq. (16.1), K_{ij} is given in rads or centigrays. It can be summed over all i and j to obtain the kerma (or dose) due to all types of interactions and target atoms:

$$D \overset{\text{CPE}}{=} K = \sum_i \sum_j K_{ij} \tag{16.4}$$

C. Thermal-Neutron Interactions in Tissue

There are two important interctions of thermal neutrons with tissue: neutron capture by nitrogen, $^{14}N(n, p)^{14}C$, and neutron capture by hydrogen, $^{1}H(n, \gamma)^{2}H$.

The nitrogen interaction releases a kinetic energy of $E_{tr} = 0.62$ MeV that is shared by the proton (0.58 MeV) and the recoiling nucleus (0.04 MeV). The interaction cross section in this case is $\sigma = 1.84 \times 10^{-24}$ cm²/atom, and the number of nitrogen atoms per gram of muscle tissue is $N_t/m = 1.50 \times 10^{21}$.* Thus the kerma deposited in muscle per unit fluence of thermal neutrons is given by Eq. (16.1) as

$$F_n = 1.602 \times 10^{-8} \times 1.84 \times 10^{-24} \times 1.50 \times 10^{21} \times 0.62$$

$$= 2.74 \times 10^{-11} \text{ rad cm}^2/n.$$

Since the range of the secondary proton is ~ 10 μm in tissue, CPE exists and $K = D$ even in very small tissue samples.

Thermal neutrons have a larger probability of capture by hydrogen atoms in muscle, even though $\sigma_H = 3.32 \times 10^{-25}$ cm²/atom $< \sigma_N = 1.84 \times 10^{-24}$ cm²/atom, because there are 41 times more H atoms than N atoms in tissue. The energy given to γ-rays per unit mass of tissue and per unit fluence of thermal neutrons can be obtained from an equation similar to Eq. (16.1), but replacing E_{tr} by $E_\gamma = 2.2$ MeV (the γ-ray photon energy released in each neutron capture):

$$\frac{R_\gamma}{\Phi m} = 1.602 \times 10^{-6} \sigma N_t m^{-1} E_\gamma$$

$$= (1.602 \times 10^{-6} \text{ erg/MeV}) \times (3.32 \times 10^{-25} \text{ cm}^2/\text{atom})$$

$$\times (6.09 \times 10^{22} \text{ atoms/g}) \times (2.2 \text{ } \gamma\text{-MeV}/n)$$

$$= 7.13 \times 10^{-8} \text{ erg/g } n \text{ cm}^{-2}$$

$$= 7.13 \times 10^{-16} \text{ J/kg } n \text{ m}^{-2} \tag{16.5}$$

This of course does not contribute directly to the kerma, since the γ-rays must interact and transfer energy to charged particles to produce kerma. For that reason the result of Eq. (16.5) is expressed in terms of the radiant energy of γ-rays produced per unit mass and per neutron fluence. If the irradiated tissue mass is small enough to allow the γ-rays to escape, the kerma due to thermal neutrons is only that resulting from the nitrogen (n, p) interactions. In larger masses of tissue the γ-rays are increasingly reabsorbed before escaping, thus contributing to the kerma. In the center

---

*One gram of muscle contains approximately 0.102 g of H, 0.123 g of C, 0.740 g of O, and 0.035 g of N. Avogadro's constant (6.022×10^{23} atoms) is contained in 1 mole, or 1.008 g of H, 12.01 g of C, 16.00 g of O, or 14.01 g of N. Hence the number of H atoms per gram of muscle is 6.022×10^{23} (0.102/1.008) $= 6.09 \times 10^{22}$ atoms/g, and likewise there are 6.17×10^{21} (C atoms)/g, 2.79×10^{22} (O atoms)/g, and 1.50×10^{21} (N atoms)/g, totaling 9.65×10^{22} atoms/g.

of a 1-cm-diameter sphere of tissue the kerma contributions from the (n, p) and (n, γ) processes (the latter indirectly) are comparable in size. In a large tissue mass (radius > 5 times the γ-ray mean free path) where radiation equilibrium is approximated, the kerma due indirectly to the (n, γ) process is 26 times that of the nitrogen (n, p) interaction. The human body is intermediate in size, but large enough so the H(n, γ) ^{2}H process dominates in kerma (and dose) production, not only for thermal neutrons but for intermediate neutrons as well, as they become thermalized in the body.

D. Interaction by Intermediate and Fast Neutrons

Figure 16.1 summarizes the processes that contribute directly to kerma in a small mass of tissue in free space. The ordinate is the kerma factor in units of erg/g per n/cm^2, plotted vs. neutron energy from thermal (2.5×10^{-8} MeV) to 14 MeV. The dashed curve a is the sum of all the others. It is dominated below 10^{-4} MeV (100 eV) by curve g, which represents (n, p) reactions, mostly in nitrogen. Above 10^{-4} MeV elastic scattering of hydrogen nuclei (curve b) contributes nearly all of the kerma.

The average energy transferred by elastic scattering to a nucleus is closely approximated (i.e., assuming isotropic scattering in the center-of-mass system) by

$$\overline{E}_{tr} = E \frac{2 M_a M_n}{(M_a + M_n)^2} \tag{16.6}$$

where E = neutron energy,

$\quad M_a$ = mass of target nucleus,

$\quad M_n$ = neutron mass.

For hydrogen recoils $\overline{E}_{tr} = E/2$ with E_{tr}-values ranging from 0 (for protons recoiling at 90°) to $E_{tr} = E$ for protons recoiling straight ahead. For other tissue atoms, elastic scattering gives $\overline{E}_{tr} = 0.142E$ for C atoms, $0.124E$ for N atoms, and $0.083E$ for O atoms.

IV. NEUTRON SOURCES

The most widely available neutron sources are nuclear fission reactors, accelerators, and radioactive sources. Useful descriptive references have been provided by DePangher and Tochilin (1969), Moteff (1969), Tochilin and Shumway (1969), and ICRU (1977).

Fissionlike spectra have average neutron energies around 2 MeV, and are available from nuclear reactors (beam ports, not thermal columns, which moderate the neutrons to a thermal distribution), ^{252}Cf radioactive (spontaneous fission) sources, critical assemblies, and other ''mock'' fission sources such as that produced by 12-MeV cyclotron-accelerated protons on a thick Be target. Figure 16.2 shows several such spectra, the Watt spectrum being an idealized shape for unmoderated reactor neutrons.

By filtering a reactor spectrum, the National Bureau of Standards makes available

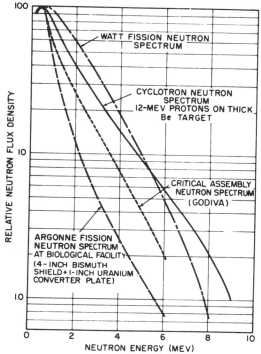

FIGURE 16.2. Fission-neutron spectra from reactors (Watt spectrum), the Godiva critical assembly, and the Argonne Biological Facility, as well as a "mock" fission spectrum generated by 12-MeV protons on a thick Be target. (Tochilin and Kohler, 1958. Reproduced with permission from E. Tochilin and the Health Physics Society.)

for calibration purposes neutron beams with narrow spectra having intermediate energies around 2, 24, and 144 keV (Schwartz and Grundl, 1978).

Several types of Be(α, n) radioactive sources are in common use, employing ^{210}Po, ^{239}Pu, ^{241}Am, or ^{226}Ra as the emitter. Neutron yields are of the order of 1 neutron per 10^4 α-particles. Figure 16.3 exemplifies the neutron spectra emitted, which have average energies $\cong$ 4 MeV.

The γ-ray background emitted by Be(α, n) sources depends on the α-source, being highest for ^{226}Ra in equilibrium with its daughter products (835 mR/h at 1 m from 1 Ci). A 1-Ci ^{239}Pu–Be neutron source was recently measured by Yang Yin et al. (1984) to have a γ-ray output of mostly 4.4-MeV γ rays that gave an exposure rate of 0.062 mR/h at 1 m, or about $\frac{1}{6}$ of the total $n + \gamma$ tissue dose rate there. For ^{252}Cf sources in free space, filtered by 0.7 mm of Pt–Ir, the γ-ray dose rate in tissue is about $\frac{1}{3}$ of the total dose rate (ICRU, 1977).

Low-energy neutron generators accelerate deuterium to 0.1–0.4 MeV and impinge them on targets containing either deuterium or tritium. The output neutrons,

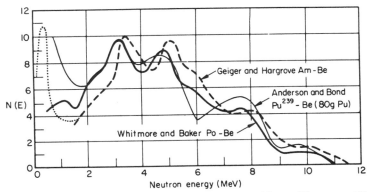

FIGURE 16.3. Neutron spectra for three Be(α, n) sources: ^{241}Am, ^{210}Po, and ^{239}Pu. (From DePangher and Tochilin, 1969. Sources of the data are given in that reference. Reproduced with permission from E. Tochilin and Academic Press.)

due to high-Q reactions, are in the range of 1.9–3.4 MeV for the D(d, n) ^{3}He reaction, and 12.9–15.6 MeV for $T(d$, $n)$ ^{4}He, depending on the angle of neutron emission, incoming particle energy, and target thickness, as shown in Figs. 16.4a and 16.4b. Outputs of the order of 10^{11} and 10^{13} n/s, respectively, can be achieved in this way.

Cyclotrons can be used to produce neutron beams by accelerating protons or deuterons into various targets, most commonly beryllium. Figure 16.5 shows the typical bell-shaped neutron spectra that result from deuteron bombardment. The neutron energies extend from zero to somewhat above the deuteron energy, and have an average of about 0.4 times that energy. The neutron outputs from this "stripping" reaction have been discussed by August et al. (1976). The neutron beam becomes narrower and more forward-directed as the deuteron energy is increased. Tissue dose

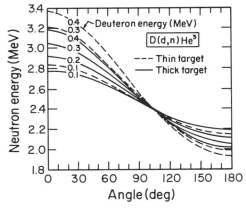

FIGURE 16.4a. Neutron energy vs. angle for the D(d, n) ^{3}He reaction. (Seagrave, 1958. Reproduced with permission from J. D. Seagrave and the Los Alamos National Laboratory.)

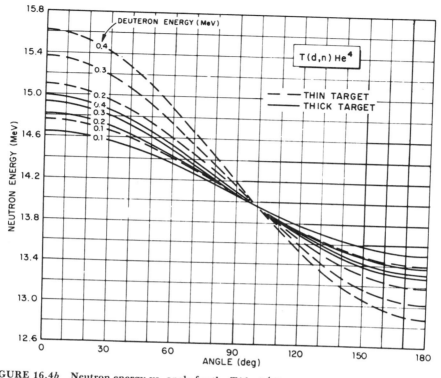

FIGURE 16.4b Neutron energy vs. angle for the T(d, n) ^{4}He reaction. (Seagrave, 1958. Reproduced with permission from J. D. Seagrave and the Los Alamos National Laboratory.)

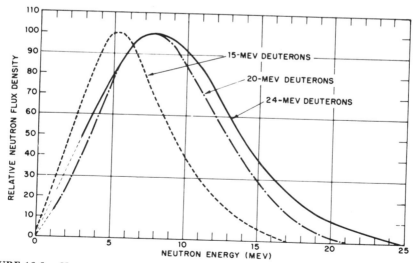

FIGURE 16.5. Neutron spectra on the beam axis generated by 15-, 20-, and 24-MeV deuterons striking a thick Be target. (Tochilin and Kohler, 1958. Reproduced with permission from E. Tochilin and the Health Physics Society.)

rates of tens of rads per minute on the beam axis are readily achievable at 1 m from the target, with γ-ray backgrounds of a few percent or less of the dose in tissue.

V. NEUTRON QUALITY FACTOR

For purposes of neutron radiation protection the dose equivalent H is equal to DQ, where Q is the quality factor, which depends on neutron energy according to the curve in Fig. 16.6 (ICRP, 1971). The quality factor for all γ-rays is taken to be unity for purposes of combining neutron and γ-ray dose equivalents.

ICRP quality factors are intended to apply to long-term occupational exposure situations, not to radiation accidents (e.g., reactor criticality) in which acute biological damage to blood cells, bone marrow, and gastrointestinal tract are predominant. In such cases the quality factor for neutrons lies between 1 and 2, and it has been common practice to simply sum the n and γ absorbed doses in such acute exposures (Kiefer et al., 1969).

VI. CALCULATION OF THE ABSORBED DOSE IN A CYLINDRICAL PHANTOM REPRESENTING THE HUMAN BODY

Auxier et al. (1968) have carried out a Monte Carlo calculation of the absorbed dose and dose equivalent in each of the volume segments of a cylindrical phantom 30 cm in diameter by 60 cm in height, as shown in Fig. 16.7. Monoenergetic neutrons of various energies from thermal to 14 MeV were incident perpendicularly to the cylindrical axis, covering the whole phantom homogeneously. Table 16.2 gives the values of quality factor that were assumed for evaluating the dose equivalent on the

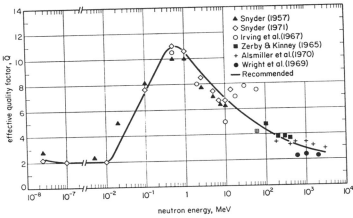

FIGURE 16.6. Quality factors for neutrons, that is, the maximum dose equivalent divided by the absorbed dose at the same depth in the body. The curve represents the recommendation of the ICRP. (ICRP, 1971. References in the figure are given in that report. Reproduced with permission from Pergamon Press, Ltd.)

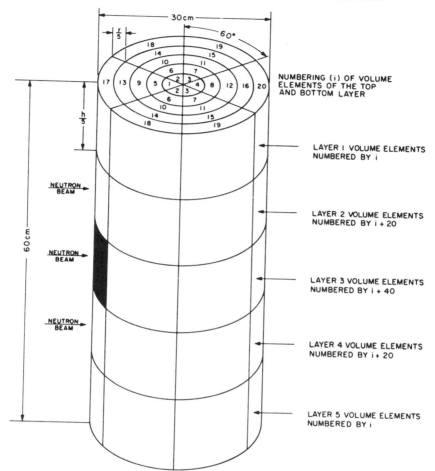

FIGURE 16.7. Cylindrical phantom employed for Monte Carlo calculation of D and H by Auxier et al. (1968). The black area indicates volume element 57, to which Table 16.3 refers. (Reproduced with permission from J. A. Auxier and Academic Press.)

basis of the secondary-charged-particle spectrum in each volume segment. Secondary electrons from the absorption of the 2.2-MeV capture γ-rays from the $^1H(n, \gamma)^2H$ reaction were included.

The resulting tables of Auxier et al. (1968) contain a wealth of information on the penetration of neutrons into the body and the resulting spatial distributions of D and H. Volume number 57, the front segment halfway up the phantom, is of special interest. It is 12 cm high, 3 cm thick, and about 15 cm wide. The data for that segment have been excerpted from the tables of Auxier et al. and are reproduced in Table 16.3. It should be noted that the absorbed doses in column 2 include the capture

TABLE 16.2. Quality Factor vs. Linear Energy Transfer Used by Auxier et al. (1968) in Monte Carlo Calculation[a]

L_∞ (keV/μm)	Q
0 – 3.5	1.00
3.5– 7.0	1.50
7.0– 15.0	2.82
15.0– 25.0	4.47
25.0– 35.0	6.18
35.0– 50.0	8.28
50.0– 62.5	10.3
62.5– 75.0	11.8
75.0– 87.5	13.6
87.5– 100	14.9
100 – 200	17.5
200 –1000	20.0

[a] Reproduced with permission from J. A. Auxier and Academic Press.

γ-ray contributions in the last column, and that the dose equivalent is based on the total dose including the γ-ray contribution.

Figure 16.8, based on the data in Table 16.3, clearly shows that the γ-rays deposit about 85% of the absorbed dose for neutrons below 10 keV. Above that energy the relative importance of the γ-rays decreases steadily, to become negligible for neu-

TABLE 16.3. Monte Carlo Calculation Results for Volume Segment 57[a]

Neutron Energy		Absorbed Dose [10^{-10} rad/(n/cm^2)]	Dose Equivalent [10^{-10} rem/(n/cm^2)]	Absorbed Dose from ^{1}H$(n, \gamma)^2$H [10^{-10} rad/(n/cm^2)]
0.025	eV	4.68	11.53	4.00
1	eV	5.89	13.42	5.14
10	eV	5.18	12.10	4.49
100	eV	4.45	10.05	3.89
1	keV	4.32	8.85	3.83
10	keV	4.34	9.92	3.42
100	keV	8.02	48.6	3.31
500	keV	18.11	188	2.80
1	MeV	30.1	326	2.23
2.5	MeV	39.9	349	1.84
5	MeV	57.2	441	1.48
7	MeV	57.0	403	1.68
10	MeV	72.5	431	3.79
14	MeV	83.1	615	7.21

[a] Reproduced with permission from J. A. Auxier and Academic Press.

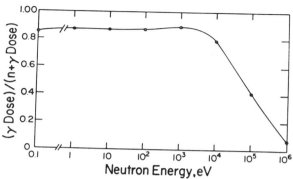

FIGURE 16.8. Ratio of capture γ-ray tissue dose to the total $n + \gamma$ dose in volume element 57, as a function of incident neutron energy. (From data of Auxier et al., 1968.)

trons above about 1 MeV. It is evident in Table 16.3 that both the absorbed dose (column 2) and dose equivalent rise abruptly above 10 keV, as the elastic scattering reaction with hydrogen takes over from the (n, γ) reaction as the principal dose contributor.

VII. $n + \gamma$ MIXED-FIELD DOSIMETRY

A. Occurrence of $n + \gamma$ Mixed Fields

Neutrons and γ-rays are both indirectly ionizing radiations that are attenuated more or less exponentially in passing through matter. Each is capable of generating secondary fields of the other radiation, by (n, γ) and (γ, n) reactions, respectively. (γ, n) reactions are only significant for high-energy γ-rays ($\gtrsim 10$ MeV), but (n, γ) reactions can proceed at all neutron energies and are especially important in the case of thermal-neutron capture, as discussed for ${}^1H(n, \gamma){}^2H$. As a result neutron fields are normally found to be "contaminated" by secondary γ-rays.

Since neutrons generally have more biological effectiveness per unit of absorbed dose than γ-rays, especially at low dose rates, it is usually desirable to perform dosimetry in a way that provides separate dose accounting of the γ and n components. Naturally this makes the measurement procedures more complicated.

It will be convenient to discuss three general categories of dosimeters for $n + \gamma$ applications:

a. Neutron dosimeters that are relatively insensitive to γ rays.

b. γ-ray dosimeters that are relatively insensitive to neutrons.

c. Dosimeters that are comparably sensitive to both radiations.

It is especially important in the case of neutron dosimeters to specify the reference material to which the dose reading is supposed to refer. For example, item **c** above is meaningless unless one specifies how the γ-ray and neutron fields are to be measured. Usually, because of the universal interest in radiation effects on the human body, kerma or absorbed dose in muscle tissue provides the reference basis for specifying dosimeter performance. That is, a dosimeter is said to be equally sensitive to a γ-ray field and a neutron field if the dosimeter gives identical readings when exposed to the two fields for times that would result in equal free-space tissue kermas (or doses under CPE conditions) in a small mass of muscle tissue at the dosimeter location.

It should be noted that water is not as close a substitute for muscle tissue for neutrons as it is for photons. Water is $\frac{1}{9}$ hydrogen by weight; muscle is $\frac{1}{10}$ hydrogen. Also, water contains no nitrogen, and hence can have no $^{14}N(n, p)^{14}C$ reactions by thermal neutrons. While $(\mu_{en}/\rho)_{muscle}$ is 99% of $(\mu_{en}/\rho)_{water}$ for 1-MeV γ-rays, $(F_n)_{muscle}$ is only 91% of $(F_n)_{water}$ for 1-MeV neutrons, for example. This difference emphasizes the importance of the elastic scattering of hydrogen as the principal kerma-producing interaction by fast neutrons in tissue.

B. Equation for $n + \gamma$ Dosimeter Response

The general equation for the response of a dosimeter to a mixed field of neutrons and γ-rays can be most simply written in the form

$$Q_{n,\gamma} = AD_\gamma + BD_n \tag{16.7}$$

or alternatively as

$$\frac{Q_{n,\gamma}}{A} = D_\gamma + \frac{B}{A} D_n \tag{16.8}$$

where $Q_{n,\gamma}$ = total response (i.e., reading—for example, the charge produced in an ion chamber or the light output measured from a TLD) due to the combined effects of the γ-rays and neutrons,

A = response per unit of absorbed dose in tissue for γ-rays,

B = response per unit of absorbed dose in tissue for neutrons,

D_γ = γ-ray absorbed dose in tissue, and

D_n = neutron absorbed dose in tissue.

By convention the absorbed dose referred to in these terms is assumed to be that under CPE conditions in a small imaginary sphere of muscle tissue, centered at the dosimeter midpoint with the dosimeter absent. Most commonly this tissue sphere is taken to be just large enough (0.52-g/cm^2 radius) to produce CPE at its center in a ^{60}Co γ-ray beam, the radiation usually employed in calibrating such dosimeters.

In protocols for neutron radiotherapy such as that given by the AAPM (1980) the foregoing convention is expressed somewhat differently for tissue-equivalent (TE) plastic ion chambers: The TE plastic wall, usually also 0.52 g/cm^2 in thickness for dosimetry of neutrons up to 20 MeV, is substituted for the imaginary tissue sphere, and the absorbed dose in tissue under CPE conditions is taken to be that at the center of the chamber. The amount of radiation attenuation in penetrating the chamber wall is practically the same as would occur in the radial distance to the center of the tissue sphere. Thus these two approaches to specifying the absorbed dose in tissue for purposes of Eqs. (16.7) and (16.8) are equivalent where the dosimeter is a TE ion chamber having an equilibrium-thickness wall. However, for a non-tissue-equivalent dosimeter type, such as a TLD or a miniature G–M tube, the dosimeter itself evidently can no longer serve as a proxy for the imaginary equilibrium tissue sphere. One must then recognize the necessity for this convenient fiction in order to be able to state the neutron dose under consistent conditions, independent of the kind of dosimeter to be employed.

Equation (16.8) is more commonly found in the literature written in terms of other symbols (e.g., ICRU, 1977):

$$R'_{n,\gamma} = kD_n + hD_\gamma \tag{16.9}$$

where $R'_{n,\gamma}$ is the total response $R_{n,\gamma}$ of a dosimeter exposed to a mixed $n + \gamma$ field, divided by its sensitivity to the γ-rays (usually ^{60}Co) used for dosimeter calibration; D_n and D_γ are defined to be the absorbed doses in tissue (i.e., muscle) from the neutrons and the photons, respectively, in the mixed field; k is the ratio of the dosimeter sensitivity for the neutrons in the mixed field to that for the γ-rays used in calibration; and h is the ratio of dosimeter sensitivity for the photons in the mixed field to that for the γ-rays used in the calibration. $h = 1$ is often assumed and is usually well approximated, especially for low-Z dosimeters where the photoelectric effect is unimportant.

The sensitivity $(1/\alpha)$ of a dosimeter, in the sense in which it is employed here, is defined by the same reference to be the quotient of the dosimeter response R to the absorbed dose in the material of interest (tissue). Multiplying Eq. (16.9) by the γ-ray sensitivity $1/\alpha_\gamma$ gives

$$\frac{R'_{n,\gamma}}{\alpha_\gamma} = R_{n,\gamma} = \frac{k}{\alpha_\gamma} D_n + \frac{h}{\alpha_\gamma} D_\gamma \tag{16.10}$$

and letting

$$A \equiv \frac{h}{\alpha_\gamma} \quad \text{and} \quad B \equiv \frac{k}{\alpha_\gamma} \tag{16.11}$$

allows Eq. (16.10) to be simplified to the more intuitively obvious forms (16.7) and (16.8), where the symbol $R_{n,\gamma}$ is defined the same as our $Q_{n,\gamma}$. Equation (16.11) relates the present A and B symbols to the more conventional h and k, respectively. For present purposes it will be preferable to use the simpler Equations (16.7) and (16.8).

C. Separate Measurement of Neutron and γ-Ray Dose Components by Paired Dosimeters

If a mixed $n + \gamma$ field is measured by means of two dosimeters having different values of B/A (i.e., neutron-to-γ-ray sensitivity ratio), Eq. (16.8) can then be applied to each one and solved simultaneously to obtain D_γ and D_n, so long as B and A have known values.

If A is zero (i.e., no γ-ray sensitivity) for either dosimeter, then its response equation (16.7) reduces to

$$Q_{n,\gamma} = B D_n \tag{16.12}$$

which can be directly solved for D_n. That can be substituted into the other dosimeter's response equation to solve for D_γ.

Consider the more general case where neither A nor B is zero. For example, let the first dosimeter be a tissue-equivalent ion chamber and the second one be a non-hydrogenous TLD with a relatively low value of B/A. We will consider later how to determine the A and B values for these dosimeters. Let $Q_{n,\gamma}^{TE}$ and $Q_{n,\gamma}^{TLD}$ be the readings (charge produced in the ion chamber, light-output reading in arbitrary units for the TLD) obtained for equal irradiation times at the same location in a constant $n + \gamma$ field. The two response equations, which must be solved simultaneously for D_γ and D_n, are

$$\frac{Q_{n,\gamma}^{TE}}{A_{TE}} = D_\gamma + \left(\frac{B}{A}\right)_{TE} D_n \tag{16.13}$$

and

$$\frac{Q_{n,\gamma}^{TLD}}{A_{TLD}} = D_\gamma + \left(\frac{B}{A}\right)_{TLD} D_n \tag{16.14}$$

Example 16.1.   To illustrate the procedure, we will assume the value $(B/A)_{TE} = 0.960$, $A_{TE} = 3.00 \times 10^{-7}$ C/Gy (tissue) for the γ-ray calibration of the ion chamber, $(B/A)_{TLD} = 0.110$, and $A_{TLD} = 6.20 \times 10^{-5}$ C/Gy (tissue). If the readings due to the (identical) mixed-field irradiations are $Q_{n,\gamma}^{TE} = 2.12 \times 10^{-7}$ C and $Q_{n,\gamma}^{TLD} = 9.73 \times 10^{-6}$ C, then Eqs. (16.13) and (16.14) become, respectively,

$$\frac{2.12 \times 10^{-7} \text{ C}}{3.00 \times 10^{-7} \text{ C/Gy}} = 0.707 \text{ Gy} = D_\gamma + 0.960 D_n$$

$$\frac{9.73 \times 10^{-6} \text{ C}}{6.20 \times 10^{-5} \text{ C/Gy}} = 0.157 \text{ Gy} = D_\gamma + 0.110 D_n$$

the solution to which is

$$D_\gamma = 0.086 \text{ Gy}$$

and

$$D_n = 0.647 \text{ Gy}$$

The total $n + \gamma$ dose in tissue is thus 0.733 Gy, of which about 88% is contributed by neutrons and the remainder by γ-rays.

Various combinations of dosimeters have been tried in this method to characterize mixed $n + \gamma$ fields, especially neutron beams that contain a γ-ray component capable of delivering a few percent of the dose in tissue. For this purpose the best dosimeter pair is a TE–plastic ion chamber containing TE gas (for which $B/A \cong 1$) to measure the total $n + \gamma$ dose, and a nonhydrogenous dosimeter having as little neutron sensitivity as possible (i.e., minimal B/A) to measure the γ-ray dose. Ideally this dosimeter should measure *only* γ-rays. The miniature G–M, counter comes closest to this ideal, having B/A values that increase gradually from 0.001 to 0.03 for neutron energies from 0.1 to 20 MeV (Mijnheer et al., 1982). Magnesium ion chambers with argon gas, ^{7}LiF TLDs, and CaF_2 : Mn TLDs all show fast-neutron B/A values roughly 7-fold greater, and graphite ion chambers with CO_2 filling have a B/A that is roughly 15 times greater than the miniature G–M counter.

The closer together the B/A values are for the dosimeter pair, the poorer becomes the accuracy with which γ-ray and neutron doses can be separately determined in a mixed field. Obviously, when the two values of B/A are the same, all ability of the pair to discriminate D_γ from D_n is lost. The use of a dosimeter pair in which the TE ion chamber is replaced by a neutron-only detector such as an activation foil ($A = 0$) suggests itself as a means of obtaining even stronger discrimination. However, the TE ion chamber is usually preferable because of the energy independence of its response per unit tissue dose for neutrons as well as γ-rays. That is, $B/A \cong$ 1 over a wide range of neutron energies, while activation foils exhibit energy thresholds below which B decreases rapidly. Thus having the TE ion chamber or calorimeter as one member of the dosimeter pair provides more accurate and reliable dosimetry in terms of dose to tissue.

D. Relative *n* vs. γ Sensitivity of Dosimeters

1. DOSIMETERS WITH COMPARABLE NEUTRON AND γ-RAY SENSITIVITIES ($B/A \cong$ 1)

a. A-150 TE Plastic Ion Chambers ($B/A \cong$ 1)

Any hydrogenous dosimeter that responds to the absorbed dose deposited by the protons set in motion by neutron elastic-scattering events will have comparable neutron and γ-ray sensitivities, that is, $B/A \sim 1$. However, the premier instrument of this type is the tissue-equivalent plastic ion chamber made of A-150 TE plastic. This plastic and several other tissue- and air-equivalent plastics were first devised by Shonka et al. (1959).

A-150 plastic is used to manufacture ion chambers of several sizes commercially by at least two companies.* It has a composition that closely matches muscle tissue in content of hydrogen (10.2% by weight) and nitrogen (3.5%), but the carbon content is 76.1% in place of 12.3%, and there is only 5.2% oxygen in the plastic instead of 72.9%. Fortunately, the kerma factors for C and O are sufficiently similar, and that of H is so much larger, that the kerma factor for A-150 plastic is only a few percent greater than that for muscle at most neutron energies (see Appendix F), in spite of

---

*Far West Technologies, Inc., 330 So. Kellogg Ave., Goleta, CA 93117; Exradin, Inc., Box Q, Warrenville, IL 60555.

this gross difference in composition. A correction is made for the resulting error, as will be shown presently.

The cavity gas is flowed through the chamber at a rate (typically $\cong 5$ cm^3/min) sufficient to flush out de-adsorbed gases and maintain flow-gas purity, while avoiding any significant pressure increase over ambient atmospheric pressure. An initial flushing at a much higher flow rate will hasten removal of air. The most common TE gas is a premixed, commercially available mixture of 64.4% CH_4 (methane), 32.4% CO_2, and 3.2% N by partial pressure, or 10.2% H, 45.6% C, 40.7% O, and 3.5% N by weight. Thus it has C and O proportions that are intermediate between muscle tissue and A-150 plastic.

The plastic wall is electrically conducting volumetrically by virtue of its graphite content, and thus need not be coated with a conducting layer. As mentioned before, a wall thickness of 0.52 g/cm^2 is usually employed, being adequate to provide TCPE for ^{60}Co γ rays and CPE for neutrons up to 20 MeV. The density of this plastic is typically 1.127 g/cm^3.

The γ-ray sensitivity value A is determined for a TE plastic chamber, and for other mixed-field dosimeters also, through a ^{60}Co γ-ray calibration. The ratio B/A is derived from that calibration by application of B–G theory in a method to be described in Section VII.E.

b. Rossi TE Proportional Counter ($B/A \cong 1$)

In principle this device, as usually constructed with tissue-equivalent plastic walls, can be operated as an ion chamber at full atmospheric or reduced pressure. However, it is usually operated as a proportional counter, as discussed in Chapter 15, Section II.B. The meaning of B in that usage is the value of Eq. (15.5) per unit of neutron absorbed dose in tissue, while A is the same quantity for γ-rays.

Weaver et al. (1977) and others have used Rossi proportional counters made of TE plastic to separate neutron and γ-ray doses on the basis of pulse-height analysis. August et al. (1978), and DeLuca et al. (1980) have shown that nonhydrogenous Rossi proportional counters with graphite or Mg walls respond very little to neutrons in comparison with γ-rays. The remaining neutron response, due to secondary charged particles heavier than protons, can be clearly separated from the small-pulse γ-ray response on the basis of pulse-height analysis. Such a counter can effectively achieve B/A values comparable to those of miniature G–M counters (see Section VII.D.3.d below).

c. Tissue-Equivalent Plastic Calorimeters ($B/A \cong 1$)

Calorimeters of A-150 TE plastic have been designed for neutron dosimetry, for example by McDonald et al. (1976). The thermal defect of A-150 plastic is about 4% for neutrons (Goodman and McDonald, 1980), which is about the same as its γ-ray value. The low dose rate in most neutron beams makes calorimetric dosimetry especially challenging. Nevertheless McDonald, et al. (1981) have reported calorimetric measurements of the neutron dose to A-150 plastic in cyclotron neutron beams with uncertainties of about 1.5%, considerably better than the 4.7% reported for TE ion chambers (AAPM, 1980). Both of these figures are increased substantially (a few percent) by the further uncertainty in the ratio $(F_n)_{\text{muscle}}/(F_n)_{\text{A-150}}$ that enters when the neutron dose in muscle is determined from its measured value in the plastic.

Figure 16.9 shows how this ratio of kerma factors varies with neutron energy, according to ICRU (1977) for the dashed curve and Caswell et al. (1980) for the solid curve. Uncertainties stem partly from the structured nature of the energy dependence itself, which calls for accurate knowledge of the incident neutron spectrum. Additional uncertainty results from lack of definitive data, as evidenced by the differences between the two curves in Fig. 16.9, both of which were calculated by Caswell et al. at different times. It is not clear at the time of this writing which of the curves is the more nearly correct (Awschalom et al., 1983; Mijnheer et al., 1986). The kerma factor for carbon is believed to be the most questionable among the tissue elements, especially at the higher energies where inelastic reactions (such as the breakup of the ^{12}C nucleus into three α-particles) become important.

d.   Aqueous Chemical Dosimeters ($B < A$)

Aqueous chemical dosimeters, such as the Fricke system described in Chapter 14, are generally LET-dependent in their G value. The higher-LET secondary charged particles that result from neutron interactions in matter thus produce a smaller radiochemical response per unit of absorbed dose than is the case for γ-ray secondaries. Hence B is usually less than A in Eqs. (16.7) and (16.8) for aqueous chemical dosimeters.

e.   Organic or Plastic Scintillators ($B < A$)

Although such scintillators can have a hydrogen content that is comparable to that in tissue, the value of B is LET-dependent. Moreover, B/A is a function of the size

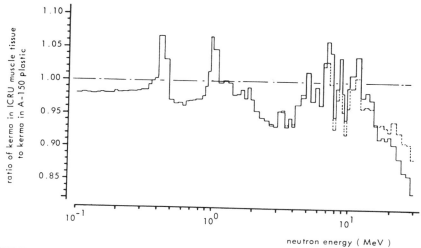

neutron energy (MeV)

FIGURE 16.9.   Ratio of kerma factors in ICRU muscle tissue to A-150 plastic, according to ICRU (1977, dashed curve) and Caswell et al. (1980, solid curve). (Broerse et al. 1985. Reproduced with permission from J. J. Broerse and Academic Press.)

of the scintillator relative to the charged-particle ranges. Thin scintillators favor CPE for neutron secondary charged particles, but let electrons from γ interactions escape, thus maximizing B/A. Larger scintillators allow the electrons also to produce light output, thus increasing A and reducing B/A.

Only a moderate degree of n–γ discrimination is possible in this way, but pulse-shape discrimination allows much stronger separation of neutron and γ-ray dose components, by a factor of up to ~ 1000.

2. NEUTRON DOSIMETERS INSENSITIVE TO γ-RAYS ($A \ll B$)

a. Activation of Metal Foils ($A \cong 0$)

Since significant levels of radioactivation by photonuclear reactions can occur only above the energy range of γ radiation ($h\nu \gtrsim 10$ MeV), metal foils are only activated by the neutrons in a mixed $n + \gamma$ field. The resulting activity of the foil is usually measured by counting the γ-rays emitted, using a G–M counter for example. A discussion of foil activation in relation to the half-life of the activation produced will be found in Chapter 6, Section VIII, and a general treatment of neutron-flux-density measurements by foil activation methods, focused primarily on reactor applications, has been given by Moteff (1969).

The observed γ-ray counting rate is related to the foil activity and the differential neutron flux density by

$$C(T, t) = \epsilon A'(T, t) = \epsilon N_t'(1 - e^{-\lambda t}) e^{-\lambda T} \int_0^\infty \sigma(E) \, \varphi'(E) \, dE \qquad (16.15)$$

where $C(T, t)$ = measured value of the specific γ-ray counting rate (c/s per gram of foil),

ϵ = overall counting efficiency (counts per disintegration) including geometric effects,

$A'(T, t)$ = specific activity of the target atoms in the foil (disintegrations s^{-1} per gram of foil),

t = duration of the neutron irradiation (s),

λ = decay constant (s^{-1}),

T = delay after irradiation before counting (s),

N_t' = number of target atoms per gram of foil,

$\sigma(E)$ = activation cross section of target atoms for neutrons of energy E (cm^2/atom), and

$\varphi'(E)$ = differential neutron flux density (cm^{-2} s^{-1} MeV^{-1}).

For thermal neutrons $\sigma(E)$ has a fixed value σ, and can be thus moved outside of the integral sign. Its value can be obtained from tables such as those found in the *Handbook of Chemistry and Physics* (CRC Press, Boca Raton, FL). Equation (16.15) can then be solved for the integral thermal neutron flux density φ.

Fast-neutron activation detectors exhibit energy thresholds below which their cross sections decrease to zero more or less steeply. The sulfur ^{32}S(n, p) ^{32}P reaction has such a threshold at 3.0 MeV, above which its average cross section $\bar{\sigma}$ is about 6.5×10^{-26} cm^2/atom (Moteff, 1969). (The ^{32}P atoms emit 1.71-MeV β rays instead of γ-rays for counting.) Equation (16.15) can then be solved with $\bar{\sigma}$ outside the integral for obtaining the value of the integral flux density φ of the neutrons above 3 MeV.

A set of foils with different thresholds allows determination of the spectrum of neutron flux density by an iterative computer program such as SAND II, as discussed by Moteff (1969).

b. Fission Foils (A = 0)

Fissionable activation foils were proposed by Hurst et al. (1956) for personnel monitoring in fission neutron fields, because of the low threshold energies of these foils, shown in Figs. 16.10a and 16.10b. This method makes use of foils of ^{239}Pu, ^{237}Np, and ^{238}U. The ^{239}Pu foil must be enclosed in a boron spherical shell 1–2 g/cm^2 thick to stop neutrons below about 10 keV, thus creating an artificial threshold. Measurements of γ-ray activity of the Pu, Np, and U foils, respectively, give a determination of the neutron fluence above threshold energies of approximately 10 keV, 0.6 MeV, and 1.5 MeV. β-ray counting of a sulfur pellet irradiated also (outside of the boron shell) provides yet another threshold, at 3 MeV. Thus, by taking differences, neutron fluences in the regions 10 keV–0.6 MeV, 0.6–1.5 MeV, 1.5–3 MeV, and above 3 MeV can be determined.

This method is seriously handicapped by requiring gram quantities of fissionable

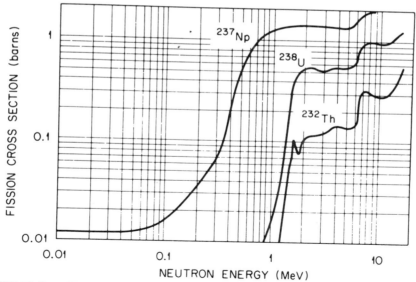

FIGURE 16.10a. Fission cross section of different fast-neutron threshold detectors as a function of neutron energy. (Becker, 1973. Reproduced with permission from CRC Press, Inc.)

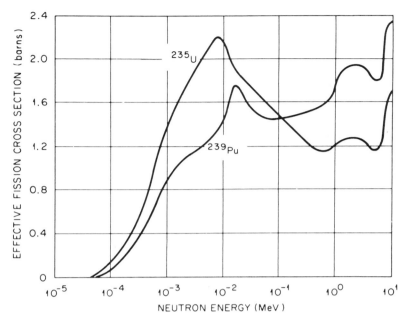

FIGURE 16.10b.   Effective fission cross section of ^{235}U and ^{239}Pu, encapsulated in 1.65 g/cm^2 of ^{10}B, as a function of neutron energy. (Rago et al., 1970. Reproduced with permission from E. Tochilin and the American Nuclear Society.)

materials that require licensing and careful control, in addition to the activity measurements requiring decay corrections. When this system is coupled with the track-etch method to be described next, however, the handicaps are greatly reduced.

c. Etchable Plastic Foils (A ≅ 0)

During the 1960s investigators in several laboratories became aware that dielectric materials (e.g., glass, mica, plastics) were rendered more chemically etchable by ionizing radiation. An avalanche of applications of this technique was triggered by Fleischer and Price (1963). There are several good reviews of different areas of interest. One by Becker (1973) focuses on dosimetry applications, and includes an extensive bibliography.

Although very high doses ($> 10^5$ Gy) by electrons or γ rays can produce bulk etchability in plastics, this has not been exploited in dosimetry applications and is probably not practically useful for that purpose. The important feature of the radiation induction of etchability is that the local imparting of comparably high levels of energy per unit mass along the tracks of densely ionizing (high-LET) heavy charged particles makes the dielectric chemically etchable within the volume where the "dose"* is sufficiently high. Later action by an etchant (e.g., HF, NaOH, etc.)

---

*Actually *specific energy imparted*, a stochastic quantity to be defined in Section VIII.

causes removal of the radiation-damaged volume, leaving a conical or cylindrical pit or hole large enough to see with low magnification, and to count and interpret dosimetrically.

Theories of nuclear-track registration differ for different kinds of dielectric materials (organic plastics vs. other media). However, it will suffice for present purposes to consider them all as being damaged to the point of etchability when the specific energy imparted in the particle track exceeds some threshold level that is characteristic of each dielectric (and of its ambient conditions to some extent). The threshold (minimum) specific energy, which is usually characterized simply in terms of the $dT/\rho dx$ or L_∞ of the charged particle for a given material, means that the kinetic energy of a given heavy charged particle should not be too high (see Fig. 8.2). Less-aggressive etching generally requires a higher specific energy threshold to produce a visible etch pit.

Inorganic materials have a threshold L_∞ mostly exceeding 15 MeV cm^2/mg, corresponding to 500 keV/μm in unit-density tissue. Plastics tend to have lower thresholds. One of the most radiation-vulnerable plastics commonly in use is cellulose nitrate, some samples of which have thresholds as low as 1 MeV cm^2/mg, or L_∞ = 100 keV/μm in tissue. Since protons have L_∞ around 10 keV/μm or less, they cannot be detected with cellulose nitrate. However, a plastic called CR-39 has been reported to have a low enough LET threshold to detect protons. This will be discussed presently.

A second limitation on detectability is imposed at the low-energy end. Even though a charged particle may be low enough in energy to have an L_∞ value exceeding the threshold of detectability, its kinetic energy may be too low for the particle to have sufficient range in the material to produce a recognizable track after chemical etching. This creates an energy "window" of detectability for each combination of charged particle, material, irradiation conditions, and etch processing. In many cases this window is closed and no detection is possible.

It should be noted that except for CR-39 plastic, the lowest threshold L_∞ in tissue ($=100$ keV/μm for cellulose nitrate) occurs around where the RBE reaches a maximum in many mammalian biological systems. The RBE range of greatest interest occurs from $L_\infty \cong 0.2$ keV/μm (minimum ionizing radiation) to $L_\infty \cong 100$ keV/μm, above which energy is wasted in the track of the charged particle due to "overkill" of cells.

The latent-damage track in plastics is reasonably stable against spontaneous repair at storage temperatures below 50°C. Approaching the softening temperature of a plastic results in rapid annealing and repair, thus removing etchability. Ultraviolet light also may have a similar effect. In general lower-L_∞ tracks tend to anneal first, higher-L_∞ tracks later, so that heat can be employed to remove lower-L_∞ events preferentially, if desired, to clear the field for viewing the denser tracks.

Becker has reviewed many details of various etching procedures, which can be quite complicated, and will not be dealt with here. The combination of an etchant with high-voltage AC across the film has been found to improve etching speed and reproducibility in some cases.

Two distinctly different approaches have been used in neutron dosimetry by the track-etch method: (1) with fission-foil converters, and (2) by direct interaction of neutrons in the etchable film and overlying plastic layer. These will be described separately.

(1) *Neutron dosimetry with fission-foil converters.* When a foil of fissionable material is struck by neutrons of energies above its fission threshold energy, very heavy energetic charged particles are generated. If the foil is adjacent to a plastic film, etchable damage tracks are efficiently produced.

The number of such etchable tracks has been found to be 1.16×10^{-5} per neutron barn (Becker, 1973). Here the fission cross section is expressed in barns (1 barn = 10^{-24} cm^2), and it is assumed that the thickness of the fission foil exceeds the maximum range ($\cong 10$ mg/cm^2) of the fission fragments. This simple relationship arises from the nearly constant detection efficiency of plastics for fission fragments, and the fact that the common fissile materials yield similar distributions of fragment species.

Figures 16.10a and 16.10b give the fission cross sections of several fissile foils having different energy thresholds. ^{235}U or ^{239}Pu foils, when used, are enclosed within a sphere of ^{10}B (1–2 g/cm^2 wall) to eliminate the effect of the large thermal-neutron cross section, and thus to create a synthetic threshold $\cong 10^{-2}$ MeV, as mentioned in the preceding section. The fission-foil neutron dosimeter of Hurst et al. (1956), also mentioned there, is improved in every way by being operated in conjunction with the track-etch method. The advantages of the track-etch procedure over the γ-counting method are overwhelming:

- Tracks are permanent and can be processed at any later time. γ-ray counting requires decay corrections.

- Latent tracks can be accumulated over practically limitless exposure times.

- 1 mg or less of fissionable materials is required, vs. 1 g or more for γ-ray counting.

- Moreover the track-etch method is at least 10 times as sensitive in neutron detection.

Although the energy thresholds for fission foils are not simple step functions, and the fission cross sections are not strictly constant above the thresholds, their average values $\bar{\sigma}$ above the nominal thresholds for a fission spectrum are taken to be 1.7 barns for ^{239}Pu, 1.6 barns for ^{237}Np, and 0.55 barn for ^{238}U. The (n, p) cross section for ^{32}S can be taken as 0.30 barns. Using these figures, the individual detector counts can be interpreted in terms of n/cm^2 above the threshold energy.

Subtracting the Φ (n/cm^2) obtained with a lower-threshold detector from that obtained with the next higher threshold detector, one can obtain the neutron fluence in the energy bins shown in Table 16.4. The average coefficients for converting these fluences of neutrons to tissue kerma are given in the last column, again assuming

TABLE 16.4

Neutron Energy Bins (MeV)	QF	Neutron Kerma Factors (Tissue) (Gy cm^2/(10^{11} n)]
0.01–0.6	$\cong 9$	0.63
0.6 –1.5	10.5	2.23
1.5 –3.0	9.5	3.07
>3	7	4.04

a fissionlike spectrum. The total tissue kerma (or absorbed dose under the usual CPE conditions) is then obtained in grays from the neutron fluence in each energy bin:

$$K = 0.63 \, (\Phi_{Pu} - \Phi_{Np}) + 2.23 \, (\Phi_{Np} - \Phi_{U})$$

$$+ 3.07 \, (\Phi_{U} - \Phi_{S}) + 4.04 \, \Phi_{S} \qquad (16.16)$$

where the neutron fluences are to be given in units of 10^{11} n/cm^2.

A typical chemical etching scheme, used with polycarbonate films, consists of a bath in 30% KOH solution at 60°C for times from 5 to 50 min, for track concentrations ranging from 10^6 to 10^3 tracks/cm^2 respectively, to optimize optical counting convenience. Many schemes for counting the etch pits have been devised, including an ingenious electrical-sparking method due to Cross and Tommasino (1970), which has been fully described by Becker (1973).

The remaining drawback of the fission-foil neutron dosimetry technique, even in conjunction with the track-etch method, is the use of controlled nuclear materials, which require special licensing and careful accounting, even though the quantities are small. In practice this prohibits their use in many personnel-monitoring situations outside of restricted government laboratories.

(2) *Neutron dosimetry by neutron interactions in plastic films: cellulose nitrate.* Fast neutrons striking cellulose nitrate films cause recoiling C, O, and N atoms, which make etchable tracks, $\cong 0.5 \times 10^{-5}$ to 3×10^{-5} tracks/neutron. The tracks are inconveniently small under ordinary etching procedures. Their size can be greatly enhanced by the application of an AC voltage ($\cong 2000$ V at 1 kHz) across the film in the etching bath, between Pt electrodes to avoid corrosion. This results in large enough pits for ready viewing with an ordinary microfiche projector and visual counting. At present neutrons with energies less than about 1 MeV cannot be detected by this method; in that respect it is not quite as good as the personnel neutron photographic emulsion, which goes down to $\cong 0.7$ MeV in neutron energy.

A commercial plastic called CR-39* (Cartwright et al., 1978) has a low enough L_∞ threshold to detect the protons resulting from elastic collisions with hydrogen nuclei either in the CR-39 itself or in an overlying polyethylene layer. Because the

---

*American Acrylics and Plastics, Inc., 25 Charles St., Stratford, CT 06497.

fast-neutron dose in tissue is mostly delivered through this interaction, such a dosimeter might be expected to be inherently capable of close correlation with dose in tissue as a function of neutron energy. However, this is not the case, because the recoiling protons cannot be detected if their energy is above a few MeV. The L_∞ threshold, below which the proton tracks are not dense enough to cause etchable damage, is reported to be $\cong 10^2$ MeV cm²/g, or 10 keV/μm in tissue (as compared to 100 keV/μm for cellulose nitrate). 10 keV/μm is approximately the L_∞ for a 4-MeV proton; hence protons of greater energy (that is, lesser L_∞) are not detected until they slow down to 4 MeV. Although an 8-MeV proton contributes twice as much energy to the absorbed dose as does a 4-MeV proton, they are each capable of producing only one etchable damage site. Thus the CR-39 film response per unit tissue dose decreases above a few MeV. The response instead tends to be constant per unit neutron fluence, provided that the overlying polyethylene layer in which the recoiling protons mostly originate is thick enough for CPE. Using several different polyethylene thicknesses over different areas of the CR-39 film will allow some neutron-energy spectrometry information to be obtained, which can assist in interpreting the readings of etch pits per unit area in terms of tissue dose or dose equivalent.

The lowest detectable neutron energy appears to be about 30 keV; below this the recoiling protons do not have enough range to make a visible track when optimally etched (Cross et al., 1985; Hankins et al., 1985).

The neutron-detecting sensitivity of CR-39 with a 1-mm-thick polyethylene overlayer is $\cong 8.6 \times 10^{-4}$ tracks/n or $\cong 2.3$ tracks/μSv for the AmBe source neutron spectrum $[\overline{E}_n = 4.4$ MeV; $(\overline{F}_n)_\text{tiss} = 3.8 \times 10^{-11}$ Gy/(n/cm²)]. This is 40 times greater than the corresponding sensitivity for cellulose nitrate.

d. Damage to Silicon Diodes (A $\cong$ 0)

Neutron damage causes a permanent increase in the forward resistance of a Si pn junction, as discussed in Chapter 15, Section IV.G, and in ICRU (1977, p. 36). Thus it can serve as an integrating dosimeter for fast neutrons.

e. Hurst Proportional Counter (A $\cong$ 0)

This counter (Hurst, 1954; Wagner and Hurst, 1959) has polyethylene walls and contains ethylene or cyclopropane gas at 1 atm. These gases have the same atomic composition as polyethylene, and since the polarization effect is negligible for protons, the Fano theorem applies and the neutron dose is the same in the wall and gas. Gamma-ray secondary electrons make much smaller charge pulses than do the denser tracks of recoiling protons, and can be discriminated against by a pulse-height threshold. This allows neutron tissue dose rates of about 10^{-5} Gy/h to be measured in the presence of 1 Gy/h of γ rays. This is a large (4 cm diam., 10 cm long) and sensitive counter and thus is only useful at low neutron dose rates. The pulse height is calibrated by a built-in α-particle source similar to that used in the Rossi counter.

f. Rem Meters

Nachtigall and Burger (1972) and Patterson and Thomas (1973) have provided thorough treatments of this subject, which requires much more space than can be devoted to it here.

An ideal *rem counter** or *rem meter** is an instrument that is designed to measure the neutron dose equivalent, H, evaluated at the depth in the body where it reaches a maximum for each incident neutron energy. The ICRP (1971) has provided the curve in Fig. 16.11 that relates the fluence-to-maximum dose-equivalent conversion factor $d(E)$ (mrem per n cm^{-2}) to the neutron energy incident on the body. The ordinate in the figure is equal to $[3600d(E)]^{-1}$. In terms of $d(E)$ the dose equivalent can be written as

$$H = \int_{E=0}^{E_{\max}} \Phi'(E)d(E)\, dE \tag{16.17}$$

in which $\Phi'(E)$ is the energy spectrum of the incident neutron fluence (n/cm^2 MeV). This equation can be modified as follows to take into account the response function $\epsilon(E)$ of the measuring instrument (i.e., the reading per n cm^{-2}):

$$H = \int_E \frac{d(E)}{\epsilon(E)}\, \epsilon(E)\Phi'(E)\, dE \tag{16.18}$$

If the response function is proportional to $d(E)$, that is, if

$$d(E) = k_1\epsilon(E) \tag{16.19}$$

where k_1 is an energy-independent constant, then Eq. (16.18) becomes

$$H = k_1 \int_E \epsilon(E)\Phi'(E)\, dE = k_1\, Q_n \tag{16.20}$$

Q_n is the reading that results from irradiating the instrument identically in free space with the same neutron field as strikes the body (or representative phantom). k_1 is the instrument calibration factor, in units of mrem (or 10^{-5} Sv) per unit reading. That can be determined for this ideal rem counter through any neutron irradiation for which the dose equivalent is known, and can be thus related to the instrument reading.

Practical rem meters are typically not ideal in their neutron-energy dependence. They generally consist of a massive cylinder or sphere of polyethylene that serves as a neutron moderator, surrounding a BF$_3$ thermal-neutron counter or other type of thermal-neutron detector. The Andersson–Braun counter shown in Fig. 16.12 exemplifies this type of device. The cylindrical mass of polyethylene (weighing 8.5

---

*It would be more appropriate to call them "dose-equivalent meters" or simply "H meters", to avoid the connection with the rem unit.

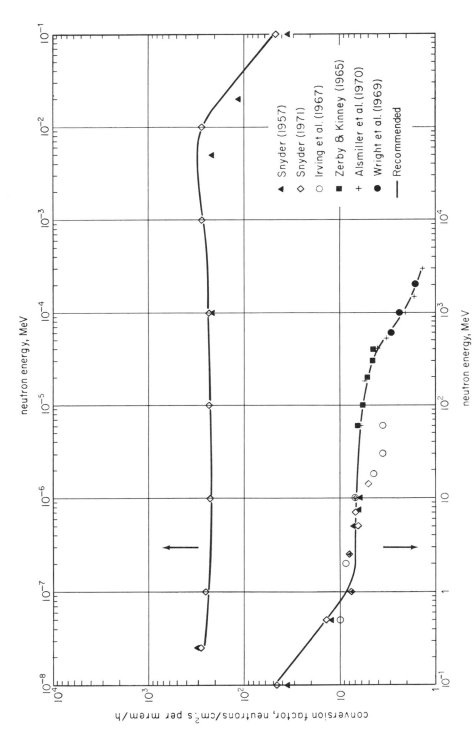

FIGURE 16.11 The quantity $[3600 \, d(E)]^{-1}$ in n/cm^2 s per mrem/h, relating the maximum value of the dose equivalent in the body to the energy of the perpendicularly incident neutrons. The body is represented by a unit-density tissue slab 30 cm in thickness. [From ICRP (1971), where the cited references are listed. Reproduced with permission from Pergamon Press, Ltd.]

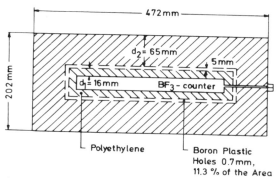

FIGURE 16.12 Sectional view through the axis of the cylindrical Andersson–Braun rem counter. (Andersson and Braun, 1964.) Reproduced with permission from J. Ö. Andersson, Studsvik, Sweden.)

kg) is interrupted by a 5-mm layer of perforated boron-loaded plastic to reduce the overresponse to intermediate-energy neutrons. The response to neutrons arriving perpendicularly to the cylindrical axis was reported to be within $\pm 25\%$ of ideal rem-meter response from about 20 keV to 10 MeV.

Another approach to dose-equivalent measurements is the *Bonner multisphere spectrometer*, also discussed in detail by Nachitgall and Burger (1972) and by Patterson and Thomas (1973). This requires measurement of the neutron field with thermal-neutron dosimeters (LiI scintillators or LiF TLDs) centered in polyethylene spheres of different diameters (5 through 30 cm). Each size produces a different dosimeter response function, and if those functions are known, the dose equivalent can be derived from the set of dosimeter readings. The group of response functions is called the *response matrix*; examples are given in the above references.

g. Long Counters

The *long counter* is a special type of moderating counter that approximates a constant $\epsilon(E)$, or response per unit fluence, over a wide range of fast-neutron energies. Thus its reading Q_n may be divided by ϵ to obtain the total incident neutron fluence Φ within that energy range. The dose equivalent is then given by

$$H = \bar{d}\Phi \tag{16.21}$$

where $\bar{d}$ is the average value of $d(E)$, defined as

$$\bar{d} \equiv \frac{1}{\Phi} \int_E d(E)\, \Phi'(E)\, dE \tag{16.22}$$

Thus the evaluation of $\bar{d}$ requires a knowledge or assumption about the neutron spectral shape.

The first shielded-type long counter was designed by Hanson and McKibben (1947). Many variations followed in attempts to further flatten the fluence response and extend the energy range. The precision long counter of DePangher and Nichols

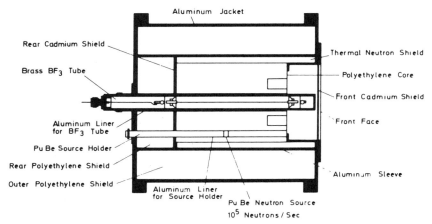

FIGURE 16.13. Precision long counter of DePangher and Nichols (1966). (Nachtigall and Burger, 1972. Reproduced with permission from G. Burger and Academic Press.)

(1966) is shown in Fig. 16.13. Such devices are to be irradiated along the cylindrical axis, from the right as shown in the figure.

3. GAMMA-RAY DOSIMETERS WITH RELATIVELY LOW NEUTRON SENSITIVITY ($B < A$)

There are no known dosimeters for which $B = 0$ while $A \neq 0$. The primary means available for minimizing the value of B is the avoidance of hydrogen in a dosimeter, including its CPE buildup layer, since elastic scattering of H nuclei accounts for most of the absorbed dose in the interaction of fast neutrons in tissue and other hydrogenous media. B/A is usually found to increase with fast-neutron energy for neutron-insensitive (low-B/A) dosimeters.

The paired-dosimeter method discussed in Section VII.C usually employs one of the dosimeters described in this section together with a TE-plastic ion chamber.

a. Non-hydrogenous Ion Chambers

Graphite-walled ion chambers through which CO_2 gas is flowed at 1 atm have the advantage of being low in atomic number, thus avoiding overresponse for low-energy γ rays due to photoelectric effect. However, the discrimination against neutrons is only moderate, with B/A approximately equal to 0.30 at 15 MeV for a 0.3 cm³ cylindrical chamber, decreasing gradually as the neutron energy is decreased (ICRU, 1977). The porosity of graphite allows air to leak into the chamber and dilute the CO_2 unless the chamber is enclosed in an impermeable barrier (Pearson et al., 1980).

Somewhat better neutron discrimination (i.e., lower B/A) can be achieved with a magnesium chamber containing argon, because of the decrease in the energy transferred to the heavier nuclei by neutron elastic scattering, as predicted by Eq. (16.6). For a 2.4-cm³ spherical Mg–Ar chamber the B/A value for 14.8-MeV neutrons is about 0.17 (Attix et al., 1979).

b. Thermoluminescent Dosimeters

[7]LiF (TLD-700) and CaF_2 : Mn thermoluminescent dosimeters both have B/A values comparable to that of the Mg–Ar ion chamber. Thus either of these TLDs can be employed as the neutron-insensitive member in the paired-dosimeter method. [7]LiF, at least, has been shown to have a B/A value that is nearly proportional to the energy of the fast neutrons below 15 MeV (McGinley, 1972; ICRU, 1977). As a rule of thumb, for fast neutrons up to 15 MeV the numerical value of B/A for [7]LiF TLDs is comparable to the neutron energy divided by 100 MeV.

A LiF (TLD-100) or [6]LiF (TLD-600) TLD can be employed as an indirect fast-neutron dosimeter by coupling it with a large moderating mass, for example, by wearing it in a personnel badge on the body. The incident fast neutrons become thermalized by multiple elastic collisions in the body and some of them diffuse back out to the dosimeter. There they undergo [6]Li(n, α)[3]H reactions, for which the cross section is 945×10^{-24} cm^2/atom. This is called an *albedo dosimeter* because its reading depends on the ability of the body to "reflect" the thermalized neutrons. (Albedo is a synonym for reflectance.)

Figure 16.14 shows the ratio of the number of thermal neutrons diffusing back out of the body to the number of fast neutrons of various incident energies. This is a gradually decreasing function, opposite to the trend of $d(E)$ in Fig. 16.11, especially for fast neutrons ($E > 10^{-2}$ MeV). Thus albedo dosimeters must be calibrated for the neutron spectrum to which they will be subjected, if a valid dose-equivalent measurement is to be obtained. In practice the calibration is often done with a fission spectrum (e.g., from [252]Cf), which means that the dose equivalent due to more degraded unknown neutron spectra will be overestimated by as much as severalfold. This disadvantage is accepted in many health-physics operations, however, in preference to photographic nuclear track emulsions which are blind to neutrons below about 0.7 MeV. Hoy (1972) and many other investigators (see Becker, 1973) have designed multiple-TLD albedo dosimeter packages which are intended to provide improved neutron-energy dependence.

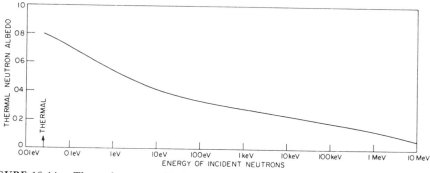

FIGURE 16.14. Thermal-neutron albedo from the human body, as a function of the energy of perpendicularly incident neutrons. (Harvey, 1967. Reproduced with permission from J. R. Harvey, Berkeley Nuclear Laboratories, U.K.)

Since ^{6}LiF and LiF (containing natural lithium with 7% ^{6}Li content) both are sensitive to γ rays also, it is usually necessary to provide a second TLD in the dosimeter package that is insensitive to thermal neutrons. ^{7}LiF is the common choice, as the thermal-neutron cross section for ^{7}Li$(n, γ)^8$Li is only 3.3×10^{-26} cm^2. Note that both dosimeters in the pair require γ-ray calibration, as their γ-ray sensitivities are seldom identical.

An alternative to using ^{7}LiF as a separate γ-ray dosimeter in the albedo package is offered by the fact that LiF and ^{6}LiF show an extra TLD glow peak at about 250–300°C, produced by the thermal-neutron dose deposited by the secondary α-particle and the triton. This peak is shown in Fig. 16.15. Nash and Johnson (1977) have exploited this feature of the glow curve to separate the γ-ray and neutron dose components, and have applied this method in personnel dosimetry at the Naval Research Laboratory. Johnson and Luerson (1980) found, however, that the high-temperature thermal-neutron glow peak fades more rapidly after irradiation than the 200°C glow peak, requiring a time-dependent correction.

^{6}LiF powder or hot-pressed solid material can serve a very useful purpose as a shield against thermal neutrons. Unlike other thermal-neutron shields such as a cadmium, ^{6}Li absorbs thermal neutrons by an $(n, α)$, rather than an $(n, γ)$ reaction. Thus it can be used to shield a γ-ray-sensitive dosimeter against thermal neutrons without generating a γ-ray response. ^{6}LiF powder can be packed between the walls of a double-walled vessel, or solid ^{6}LiF cups and lids can be obtained from TLD-phosphor manufacturers. This solid, having a density of about 2.6 g/cm^3 and being about 25.6% ^{6}Li, contains more ^{6}Li ($\cong 0.66$ g/cm^3) than does pure metallic ^{6}Li ($\cong 0.53$ g/cm^3), per unit volume. Metallic lithium is too unstable to be used for this purpose anyway.

c. X-Ray Film

Nuclear-track emulsions are thick enough to allow fast neutrons to scatter protons elastically, and to allow them to spend their energy internally in producing chemically developable tracks. An x-ray film has an emulsion thickness of 2–5 mg/cm^2, which is comparable to the range of a 1-MeV proton. Thus, if the film is sandwiched

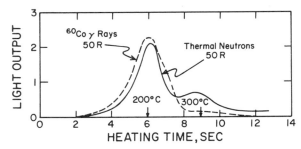

FIGURE 16.15.   Glow curves for LiF (TLD-100) irradiated by thermal neutrons and by ^{60}Co γ-rays. The thermal-neutron irradiation was adjusted to give approximately the same glow-curve area. (Wingate et al., 1967. Reproduced with permission from E. Tochilin.)

between Pb foils to keep out protons from the film's surroundings, B/A can be reduced to even lower levels than those exhibited by ^{7}LiF (Tochilin and Shumway, 1969; ICRU, 1977). The fast-neutron sensitivity of x-ray film can of course be enhanced if desired for neutron radiography by placing a sheet of polyethylene against the film on the neutron-source side.

Thermal neutrons interact with film either by the ^{14}N$(n, p)^{14}$C reaction with nitrogen in the gelatin, or by radioactivating the silver to ^{108}Ag (β^-, $\tau_{1/2} = 2.4$ min) and ^{110}Ag (β^-, $\tau_{1/2} = 24$ s).

d.   Miniature G–M Counters

A miniature stainless-steel G–M counter with a high-Z filter to flatten the energy dependence of the γ-ray response has been found to have the lowest B/A ratio of any known γ-ray dosimeter: approximately 0.02 for 15-MeV neutrons, decreasing gradually with decreasing neutron energy. This low value is due in part to the absence of hydrogen and the low efficiency for elastic scattering of iron nuclei. Another important factor is that only a single count is registered by the counter, either for a large primary ionizing event by a neutron secondary charged particle or for a small event by a γ-ray secondary electron. Thus the neutrons make fewer counts for a given amount of tissue dose deposited.

Counters of this type can be made small enough (e.g., the Philips No. 18529, $\cong$ 1 cm^3) to operate in a phantom with minimal perturbation of the radiation field. Units complete with shielding and waterproof housing can be obtained commercially.*

The miniature G–M counter was first designed to be applied for this purpose by Wagner and Hurst (1961). Operational details are well described in ICRU (1977). Thermal-neutron response is suppressed by a shield of ^{6}LiF in the Far West model.

E.   Calibration of a Tissue-Equivalent Ion Chamber for $n + \gamma$ Dosimetry

Tissue-equivalent ion chambers were described in Section VII. D.1.a. In the present section a method for calibrating such chambers will be outlined.

The γ-ray calibration factor A is first obtained from a ^{60}Co γ-ray beam for which the free-space exposure rate is known. The absorbed dose at the center of an equilibrium sphere of tissue, 0.52 g/cm^2 in radius, for a timed run that produces a free-space exposure X (C/kg) at the same location, is given (in grays) by

$$D_\gamma \overset{\text{TCPE}}{=} \beta(K_c)_\gamma = \beta A_{eq} X \left(\frac{\overline{W}}{e}\right)_{\text{air}} \left(\frac{\mu_{en}}{\rho}\right)_a^{\text{tiss}} \tag{16.23}$$

where $\beta \cong 1.003$,

A_{eq} = (attenuation of photons in penetrating to the center of the tissue sphere)
         $\cong 0.988$,

$(\overline{W}/e)_a = 33.97$ J/C, and

$(\mu_{en}/\rho)_a^{\text{tiss}}$ = the ratio of mass energy absorption coefficients for tissue/air, 0.0293/ 0.0266 = 1.102

*Far West Technologies, Inc., 330 S. Kellogg Ave., Goleta, CA 93117.

Equation (16.23) thus reduces to

$$D_\gamma = 37.1X \text{ Gy} \tag{16.24}$$

If $(Q_\gamma)_{\text{TE}}$ is the charge (C) produced in the TE ion chamber when it is given the same γ-irradiation that deposits D_γ (Gy) in the tissue sphere, then

$$A_{\text{TE}} \equiv \frac{(Q_\gamma)_{\text{TE}}}{D_\gamma} \quad \text{(C/Gy)} \tag{16.25}$$

The absorbed dose D_γ in muscle tissue can be related to the dose $(D_\gamma)_{\text{TE}}$ in the TE plastic chamber wall under TCPE conditions by the following expansion of Eq. (16.25):

$$A_{\text{TE}} \equiv \frac{(Q_\gamma)_{\text{TE}}}{D_\gamma} = \frac{(Q_\gamma)_{\text{TE}}}{(D_\gamma)_{\text{TE}}} \cdot \frac{(D_\gamma)_{\text{TE}}}{D_\gamma} \overset{\text{TCPE}}{=} \frac{(Q_\gamma)_{\text{TE}}}{(D_\gamma)_{\text{TE}}} \left(\frac{\mu_{\text{en}}}{\rho}\right)^{\text{TE}}_{\text{tiss}} \tag{16.26}$$

The B–G relation, assumed to be valid here, allows one to write

$$\frac{(Q_\gamma)_{\text{TE}}}{(D_\gamma)_{\text{TE}}} = \frac{V\rho}{(\overline{W}_\gamma/e)_g \, \overline{(S_\gamma/\rho)}_g^{\text{TE}}} \tag{16.27}$$

where $V =$ chamber sensitive volume (m^3),

$\rho =$ density of the filling gas g (kg/m^3), usually methane-based TE gas, for which $\rho = 1.046$ g/l or kg/m^3 at 25°C,

$(\overline{W}_\gamma/e)_g =$ value of $\overline{W}/e$ for γ rays and gas g [for methane-based TE gas it has the value 29.3 J/C (Goodman and Coyne, 1980)], and

$\overline{(S_\gamma/\rho)}_g^{\text{TE}} =$ mass collision stopping power ratio of TE plastic to TE gas for electrons.

Substituting Eq. (16.27) into (16.26) gives

$$A_{\text{TE}} = \left(\frac{\mu_{\text{en}}}{\rho}\right)^{\text{TE}}_{\text{tiss}} \frac{V\rho}{(\overline{W}_\gamma/e)_g \, \overline{(S_\gamma/\rho)}_g^{\text{TE}}} \tag{16.28}$$

The neutron calibration factor B_{TE} for the TE ion chamber can next be expressed in a form similar to Eq. (16.26):

$$B_{\text{TE}} \equiv \frac{(Q_n)_{\text{TE}}}{D_n} = \frac{(Q_n)_{\text{TE}}}{(D_n)_{\text{TE}}} \cdot \frac{(D_n)_{\text{TE}}}{D_n} \overset{\text{CPE}}{=} \frac{(Q_n)_{\text{TE}}}{(D_n)_{\text{TE}}} (F_n)^{\text{TE}}_{\text{tiss}} \tag{16.29}$$

where $(Q_n)_{\text{TE}} =$ charge produced in the TE chamber when it is given the same neutron irradiation that would deposit an absorbed dose D_n in the tissue sphere,

$(D_n)_{\text{TE}} =$ corresponding neutron absorbed dose in the TE chamber wall, and

$(F_n)^{\text{TE}}_{\text{tiss}} =$ relevant neutron kerma factor ratio of F_n for TE plastic to F_n for muscle tissue.

Applying the B–G relation to the neutron case, an equation corresponding to Eq. (16.27) can be obtained:

$$\frac{(Q_n)_{\mathrm{TE}}}{(D_n)_{\mathrm{TE}}} = \frac{V\rho}{\overline{(W_n/e)}_g\ \overline{(S_n/\rho)}_g^{\mathrm{TE}}} \qquad (16.30)$$

Now substituting Eq. (16.30) into (16.29) gives

$$B_{\mathrm{TE}} = (F_n)_{\mathrm{tiss}}^{\mathrm{TE}}\ \frac{V\rho}{\overline{(W_n/e)}_g\ \overline{(S_n/\rho)}_g^{\mathrm{TE}}} \qquad (16.31)$$

$(B/A)_{\mathrm{TE}}$ for the TE chamber is gotten as a ratio of Eq. (16.31) to (16.28):

$$\left(\frac{B}{A}\right)_{\mathrm{TE}} = (F_n)_{\mathrm{tiss}}^{\mathrm{TE}}\ \left(\frac{\mu_{\mathrm{en}}}{\rho}\right)_{\mathrm{TE}}^{\mathrm{tiss}}\ \frac{\overline{(W_\gamma/e)}_g\ \overline{(S_\gamma/\rho)}_g^{\mathrm{TE}}}{\overline{(W_n/e)}_g\ \overline{(S_n/\rho)}_g^{\mathrm{TE}}} \qquad (16.32)$$

The compositions of the TE gas and TE-plastic wall are sufficiently similar that $\overline{(S_\gamma/\rho)}_g^{\mathrm{TE}}$ and $\overline{(S_n/\rho)}_g^{\mathrm{TE}}$ are both close to unity, as is their ratio (Mijnheer et al., 1986). The ratio $(\mu_{\mathrm{en}}/\rho)_{\mathrm{TE}}^{\mathrm{tiss}}$ is also nearly unity, since differences in the carbon and oxygen content in the gas and wall have no effect. These elements have practically identical μ_{en}/ρ values over the wide range of γ-ray energies where the Compton effect dominates. Equation (16.32) therefore can be simplified to the following approximation for the TE-gas-filled TE-plastic chamber:

$$\left(\frac{B}{A}\right)_{\mathrm{TE}} \cong (F_n)_{\mathrm{tiss}}^{\mathrm{TE}}\ \frac{\overline{(W_\gamma/e)}_g}{\overline{(W_n/e)}_g} \qquad (16.33)$$

The value of the ratio $(F_n)_{\mathrm{tiss}}^{\mathrm{TE}}$ is obtained from tables such as those in Appendix F, entered at the appropriate neutron energy for A-150 plastic and ICRU muscle. For example, at a neutron energy of 14.5 MeV Appendix F gives a value $(F_n)_{\mathrm{tiss}}^{\mathrm{TE}} = 1.028$. If a neutron fluence spectrum $\Phi'(E)$ is present, the average kerma factors for TE plastic and for muscle tissue are each calculated from Appendix F, using an integration similar to that used to obtain $\bar{d}$ in Eq. (16.22). Then the ratio of these average values is taken to obtain $(\bar{F}_n)_{\mathrm{tiss}}^{\mathrm{TE}}$.

The reciprocal of the $\overline{W}$-ratio in Eq. (16.33) has been computed as a function of neutron energy by Goodman and Coyne (1980) for methane-based TE gas. Their curve is shown in Fig. 16.16. Its value is about 1.062 at 14–15 MeV.

Putting these values into Eq. (16.33) gives the following value for $(B/A)_{\mathrm{TE}}$ at 14–15 MeV, for example:

$$\left(\frac{B}{A}\right)_{\mathrm{TE}} \cong \frac{1.028}{1.062} = 0.97 \qquad (16.34)$$

At about 2 MeV this ratio has the value $1.04/1.07 = 0.97$, and at 0.2 MeV it is $1.02/1.10 = 0.93$. Evidently it stays in the neighborhood of unity, rolling off only very slowly as the neutron energy is decreased. For broad continuous spectra of neutrons the effect of the discontinuities due to interaction resonances (see Fig. 16.16) is smoothed out.

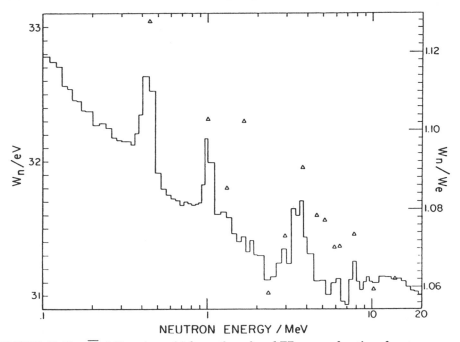

FIGURE 16.16. $\overline{W}_n$ (eV per ion pair) for methane-based TE gas as a function of neutron energy (left ordinate). The right-hand scale gives the corresponding ratios $\overline{W}_n/\overline{W}_e$, where $\overline{W}_e = \overline{W}_\gamma = 29.3$ eV per ion pair. The triangular points are evaluated at point energies of prominent resonances or minima. The step curve indicates values averaged over the indicated energy bins. (Goodman and Coyne, 1980. Reproduced with permission from L. J. Goodman and Academic Press.)

F. Calibration of the Low-Neutron-Sensitivity Dosimeter for Use in the Paired-Dosimeter Method

In principle one could use Eq. (16.32) to calculate B/A for a graphite–CO_2 or Mg–Ar ion chamber to be employed in the paired-dosimeter method. However the resulting B/A value so obtained is seldom accurate enough to be useful, especially where the γ-ray content is fairly low, say contributing only a few percent of the tissue dose.

The most practical approach to determining B/A is an experimental one employing a narrow neutron beam of the desired spectrum. Basically, the method makes use of a Pb filter to remove the γ-ray contamination from the beam, while passing most of the neutrons, which have a smaller attenuation coefficient. Secondary radiation produced in the filter escapes from the narrow beam, which is thus maintained purely primary. A previously calibrated TE chamber is used to calibrate the beam in terms of neutron tissue dose D_n. The low-neutron-sensitivity dosimeter (x) for which the value of $(B/A)_x$ is to be determined is given an identical irradiation (i.e., the same value of D_n), yielding the reading Q_x. B_x is simply equal to Q_x/D_n, assuming D_γ to be zero. A_x for that dosimeter is obtained from a ^{60}Co γ-ray exposure, thus completing the determination of $(B/A)_x$.

The foregoing method is somewhat oversimplified. In practice one does not know the degree to which the beam is initially contaminated with γ radiation, how much Pb filtration is needed to purify the beam adequately, or how much of the γ-ray contamination may come from elsewhere than the beam port. Gamma rays emitted from the face of the shield would, for example, not be removed by a beam filter.

A solution to this problem was first devised and applied by Attix et al. (1973, 1974) at the Naval Research Laboratory. That experiment illustrates the narrow-beam Pb-filtration method for determining $(B/A)_x$, as follows: The neutron beam was generated by 35-MeV deuterons on Be; its average energy was 15 MeV. It was collimated by a 2-cm hole through a large Benelex (pressed wood) shield, as shown in Fig. 16.17. The dosimeters in that measurement were a TE-plastic–TE-gas chamber and an air-filled graphite chamber. The three beam filtrations chosen were open beam, 7.6-cm Pb, and a steel plug 66 cm long filling the entire bore hole to block the γ-rays almost entirely.

The six measurements and response equations are listed in Table 16.5. $(Q/A)_{TE}$ is the ratio of the charge Q_{TE} produced in the TE chamber by a given irradiation time in the open beam, divided by the chamber's γ-ray calibration factor A_{TE}. $(Q'/A)_{TE}$ and $(Q''/A)_{TE}$ are the corresponding values obtained when the neutron beam is filtered or plugged, respectively. $(Q/A)_G$, $(Q'/A)_G$, and $(Q''/A)_G$ are the corresponding graphite-chamber data for the same situations. All irradiations are the same. The A-values for both chambers were measured in a ^{60}Co γ-ray beam.

D_γ^a was the absorbed dose at the measurement location in the open beam due to γ rays coming out of the beam port. 7.6 cm of Pb in narrow-beam geometry attenuates this to $0.0276D_\gamma^a$, assuming the minimum attenuation coefficient for lead. The steel plug reduces it practically to zero.

D_γ^s is the dose contributed by γ rays from elsewhere—mostly H-capture γ rays emitted from the face of the Benelex shield. D_γ^s is unaffected by the filter or plug.

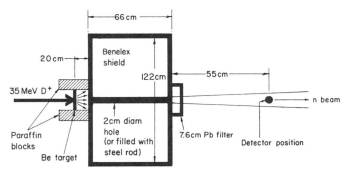

FIGURE 16.17. Experimental arrangement for measuring B/A for a low-neutron-sensitivity dosimeter by comparison with a TE chamber in a narrow beam of neutrons. (Attix et al., 1974.)

TABLE 16.5. Six Simultaneous Response Equations Applicable in Determining $(B/A)_G$ for a Graphite–Air Chamber in a Cyclotron Neutron Beam[a]

Beam	Ion Chamber	Response Equation		
Open	TE	$(Q/A)_{TE} =$	$D_\gamma^a + D_\gamma^s + (B/A)_{TE} D_n$	
Open	Graphite	$(Q/A)_G =$	$D_\gamma^a + D_\gamma^s + (B/A)_G D_n$	
7.6 cm Pb	TE	$(Q'/A)_{TE} =$	$0.0276\, D_\gamma^a + D_\gamma^s + (B/A)_{TE} D_n'$	
7.6 cm Pb	Graphite	$(Q'/A)_G =$	$0.0276\, D_\gamma^a + D_\gamma^s + (B/A)_G D_n'$	
Plug	TE	$(Q''/A)_{TE} = 0$	$+ D_\gamma^s + (B/A)_{TE} D_n''$	
Plug	Graphite	$(Q''/A)_G = 0$	$+ D_\gamma^s + (B/A)_G D_n''$	

[a] Attix et al. (1974).

D_n is the open-beam neutron dose, D_n' is that with the Pb filter, and D_n'' that with the plug in place.

The six equations in Table 16.5 can be solved simultaneously for the six unknowns D_n, D_n', D_n'', D_γ^a, D_γ^s, and $(B/A)_G$. Table 16.6 gives the numerical results that were obtained, normalized to a total $n+\gamma$ tissue-dose value of 100 units in the open beam. $(B/A)_G$ was simultaneously found to have a value of 0.318. $(B/A)_{TE}$ had been taken as 0.991, based on the ^{60}Co calibration and the application of B–G theory as described approximately in Section VII.E.

Later developments of this method made use of a number of graded-thickness Pb filters, simultaneous solutions being found for different combinations of three of them. This allows testing to see which of several assumptions about the aperture-photon energy gives the most consistent solutions for different sets of three filter thicknesses (Attix et al., 1977; Hough, 1979).

It can be seen that this experimental approach to determining $(B/A)_x$ for a low-neutron-sensitivity dosimeter provides a value that is consistent with the $(B/A)_{TE}$ of the tissue-equivalent chamber with which it is compared, and is relevant to the neutron spectrum of the beam used. The method works as well with TLDs, G–M counters or other nonhydrogenous dosimeters as it does with ion chambers.

Narrow-beam geometry is required for this calibration procedure. The beam must

TABLE 16.6 Solutions Found for Equations in Table 16.5 When Applied to NRL Cyclotron Neutron Beam[a]

Beam	Aperture γ-Rays	Other γ-Rays	Total γ-Rays	Neutrons	Total Dose
Open	0.75	0.32	1.07	98.92	100.00
7.6 cm Pb	0.02	0.32	0.34	25.21	25.55
Plug	0	0.32	0.32	0.40	0.72

[a] Attix et al. (1974). B/A value for graphite–air chamber, $(B/A)_G = 0.318$.

be narrow enough, and the measurement location distant enough from the filters, so that significant amounts of secondary radiation from the filters cannot reach the dosimeters. The method therefore requires a collimatable beam of neutrons.

VIII. MICRODOSIMETRY

Microdosimetry most generally means determination of absorbed dose on a microscopic scale of spatial distribution. More specifically, it is the science that deals with the spatial, temporal, and energy-spectral distributions of energy imparted in cellular and subcellular biological structures, and the relationship of such distributions to biological effects. Microdosimetry seeks to express the "quality" of radiation in terms of sufficiently subtle physical parameters to allow quantitative prediction of biological effects for different types of ionizing radiations. It has made considerable progress toward that goal.

As might be expected in dealing with this interface between dosimetry and radiobiology, a great deal more needs to be said than can be included in an introductory text on dosimetry. Only a brief outline of the subject will be given here. It is appended to the neutron-dosimetry chapter because practical interest in microdosimetry stems primarily from the differences in relative biological effectiveness (RBE) observed for neutrons vs. photons. There are excellent references on microdosimetry that, amongst them, provide the needed coverage (Rossi, 1968; Katz et al., 1972; ICRU, 1970, 1979a, 1983; Kellerer, 1985, Goodhead, 1987).

A. Track-Descriptive Approach: Linear Energy Transfer

The earliest approaches to microdosimetry focused on the rate of energy loss of the charged particles that deliver the absorbed dose in a medium. Initially the linear energy transfer (L_∞) was defined (Lea, 1946; Zirkle et al., 1952) and applied in various attempts at developing radiobiological target theories. Since a medium under irradiation contains a spectrum of charged-particle energies, and since L_∞ is energy-dependent, there is likewise a distribution of L_∞-values characterizing the radiation field. Thus even this simplest approach results in a very complex descriptive parameter. Attempts to compress this information into meaningful average values ($\overline{L_\infty}$) depend strongly on the method of averaging employed (track-weighted averaging vs. dose-weighted averaging; see ICRU, 1970). Neither method is satisfactory or clearly preferable.

There are several serious limitations on L_∞ as a means of specifying biologically relevant differences in radiations.

1. *Range Effect.* L_∞ says nothing about the range of the particle or whether it can traverse a given biological target volume. If the particle stops in it, L_∞ is obviously irrelevant. If the particle spends an appreciable part of its range in crossing the target volume, the value of L_∞ upon entering will change as it passes through. Obviously the range vs. target size is important.

2. *Delta-Ray Production* L_∞ does not describe the *diameter* of a charged-particle track, only the rate of energy loss along the track. Delta rays generated in a track can carry energy radially outward, thus distributing the dose laterally out to their maximum range. Different types and energies of charged particles can have different δ-ray energies and thus different track diameters, yet have the same value of L_∞. For example, a 10-MeV proton and a 167-MeV α-particle have the same L_∞, but the velocity ($\beta = v/c$) of the α-particle is twice that (0.145) of the proton. Thus, according to Eq. (8.4), the maximum energy of δ-rays generated by the α particle is 92 keV, while that for the proton is 21 keV. In water these δ-rays would have ranges of about 120 and 9 μm, respectively. The diameter of the α-track would therefore be 13 times as large as that of the proton track in this case, and the average energy density per unit volume in the α track would be less than 1% of that in the proton track.

Katz et al. (1972) developed a δ-ray theory of track structure that addressed itself to this specific problem. In that model, sensitive elements of the detector are grouped into sets that lie in volumes between cylindrical γ-ray isodose shells having the principal particle track as their common axis. By calibrating various types of dosimeters with ^{60}Co γ-rays and evaluating necessary parameters in Katz' theory, one can show that it has considerable capability of predicting the dosimeter response to other radiations. It is a marked improvement over the L_∞ approach for characterizing a radiation field.

3. *Random Variations (Energy-Loss Straggling).* L_∞ describes the expectation value of the rate of energy loss by a charged particle of a given type and energy. It does not address the random nature of energy losses along a track, which may leave zero energy in a small target volume or give it orders of magnitude more energy than would be predicted on the basis of L_∞. In other words, the stochastic nature of the energy deposition process becomes important and cannot be ignored for small target objects, e.g., of the order of a micrometer or less in diameter. Even the absorbed dose itself, being nonstochastic, fails as a quantity for describing energy imparted per unit mass, and must be replaced by a stochastic quantity (to be discussed later).

Figure 16.18, due to Kellerer and Chmelevsky (1975), shows the combinations of site diameter and particle energy for which energy delivery by protons (*a*) and electrons (*b*) is strongly influenced by the range effect, straggling, and/or the δ-ray effect. It can be seen in Fig. 16.18*a* that in region II the proton enjoys relative freedom from all three, and L_∞ adequately describes energy deposition. In region I range-effect errors are excessive ($> 15\%$) because the range is less than 6 times the site diameter. In regions III and IV energy-loss straggling can cause variations in energy deposition that exceed the track-length distribution due to different chord lengths through the site. In region IV more than 10% of the energy is dissipated by δ-rays at distances exceeding the site radius.

In Fig. 16.18*b* it will be seen that the range- and straggling-effect regions overlap for electrons, so that L_∞ has no region of validity for those particles.

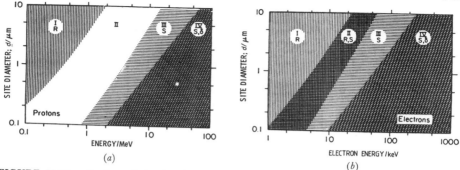

FIGURE 16.18. Regions of site diameter d and particle energy in which the energy deposition of individual events is influenced strongly by range (R), energy-loss straggling (S), and delta-ray (δ) effects for protons (a) and electrons (b). In the white region (II for protons) energy deposition is approximately proportional to L_∞. (Kellerer and Chmelevsky, 1975. Reproduced with permission from A. M. Kellerer and Academic Press.)

B. Site-Relevant Approach

In order to take into account all at once the range, δ-ray, and stochastic effects just described, a different approach was needed in which the energy spent by radiation in a defined site volume could be accounted for. Such an innovation was supplied by Rossi (1959), who defined new stochastic quantities in terms of which the energy dissipated in microscopic sites by individual ionizing events could be stated. Rossi and Rosenzweig (1955) also devised a spherical tissue-equivalent proportional counter (discussed in Chapter 15, Section II.B.2) that could measure the distribution of ionizing-event sizes that occur in the target site, simulated by the gas volume.

Although the name *microdosimetry* is most commonly associated with the Rossi approach, the review by Goodhead (1987) discusses others as well, emphasizing the importance of Monte Carlo simulation of track structure and spatial distributions of energy depositions.

C. Stochastic Quantities

ICRU (1983) defined the following stochastic quantities for use in microdosimetry:

1. *Energy Deposit ϵ_i.* This is the energy deposited in a single interaction i:

$$\epsilon_i = T_{in} - T_{out} + Q_{\Delta m} \qquad (16.35)$$

where T_{in} = energy of the incident ionizing particle (exclusive of rest mass),
T_{out} = sum of the energies of all ionizing particles leaving the interaction (exclusive of rest mass), and
$Q_{\Delta m}$ = changes of the rest mass energy of the atom and all particles involved in the interaction ($Q_{\Delta m} > 0$: decrease of rest mass; $Q_{\Delta m} < 0$: increase of rest mass).

ϵ_i may be considered as the energy deposited at the point of interaction, if quantum-mechanical uncertainties and collective effects (e.g., plasmons and phonons) are neglected. ϵ_i is to be expressed in joules or eV.

2. *Energy Imparted ϵ.* This quantity, defined already in Eq. (2.17), may be restated in terms of ϵ_i as

$$\epsilon = \sum_i \epsilon_i \tag{16.36}$$

ϵ is to be expressed in joules or eV. The ϵ_i may be due to more than one energy-deposition event, that is, statistically independent particle track.

3. *Specific Energy Imparted z.* This is the quotient of ϵ by m, where ϵ is the energy imparted by ionizing radiation to matter of mass m:

$$z = \frac{\epsilon}{m} \tag{16.37}$$

z is to be expressed in J/kg or grays.

4. *Lineal Energy y.* This is the quotient of ϵ by $\bar{l}$, where ϵ is the energy imparted to the matter in a volume by a *single energy-deposition event*, and $\bar{l}$ is the mean chord length in that volume:

$$y = \frac{\epsilon}{\bar{l}} \tag{16.38}$$

Note the special definition applied to ϵ in this case, limiting it to single events. y is to be expressed in J/m or keV/μm. $\bar{l}$ is the mean length of randomly oriented chords in the volume. For a convex body of volume V and surface area S,

$$\bar{l} = 4V/S \tag{16.39}$$

It is evident that the specific energy imparted functions as the stochastic replacement for absorbed dose in microdosimetry, and the lineal energy conceptually replaces L_∞.

PROBLEMS

1. A fluence of thermal neutrons is 6.5×10^{12} n/cm^2 in a layer of muscle-equivalent tissue 0.1 g/cm² thick. What is the absorbed dose at the middle of the layer?

2. Assume that the above neutron fluence is approximately uniform throughout a tissue sphere 5 cm in radius, due to thermalization of a field of intermediate-energy neutrons penetrating the sphere. What is the absorbed dose at the center resulting from thermal-neutron-capture γ rays? How does it compare with the total absorbed dose that results (directly or indirectly) from the thermal neutrons? (Assume unit-density tissue).

3. You have an A-150 tissue-equivalent plastic ion chamber with 0.52-g/cm² wall thickness and an $N_x A_{ion}$ value of 4.60×10^9 R/C for ^{60}Co γ-rays. Calculate A for use in the mixed-field response equation.

4. Calculate B/A for this chamber, assuming it contains TE gas and is irradiated by 4.2-MeV neutrons.

5. Pairing this chamber with a Mg–Ar chamber having $A = 3.60 \times 10^{-8}$ C/Gy and $B = 1.67 \times 10^{-9}$ C/Gy, a saturated charge of 4.23×10^{-8} C is measured with the TE plastic chamber and 6.79×10^{-9} C from the Mg–Ar chamber. Calculate the γ-ray and neutron doses.

SOLUTIONS TO PROBLEMS

1. 1.80 Gy.
2. 5.46 Gy, 75% of total.
3. 2.27×10^{-8} C/Gy.
4. 0.97.
5. $D_\gamma = 0.10$ Gy (5%); $D_n = 1.81$ Gy (95%).

References

AAPM (1971). Protocol for the dosimetry of x- and gamma-ray beams with maximum energies between 0.6 and 50 MeV. *Phys. Med. Biol.* **16,** 379.

AAPM (1980). Protocol for neutron beam dosimetry. Report 7, American Association of Physicists in Medicine, American Institute of Physics, New York.

AAPM (1983). A protocol for the determination of absorbed dose from high-energy photon and electron beams. *Med. Phys.* **10,** 741.

Almond, P. R. (1967). The physical measurement of electron beams from 6 to 8 MeV: Absorbed dose and energy calibrations. *Phys. Med. Biol.* **12,** 13.

Almond, P. R. (1970). The use of ionization chambers for the absorbed dose calibration of high energy electron beam therapy units. *Int. J. Appl. Rad.* **21,** 1.

Almond, P. R. and Svensson, H. (1977). Ionization chamber dosimetry for photon and electron beams. *Acta Radiol. Ther. Phys. Biol.* **16,** 177.

Anderson, D. W. (1984). *Absorption of Ionizing Radiation,* University Park Press, Baltimore, MD.

Anderson, H. H., and Ziegler, J. F. (1977). *Hydrogen Stopping Powers and Ranges in all Elements,* Pergamon Press, New York.

Andersson, I. O. and Braun, J. (1964). A neutron rem counter. Report E-132, Aktiebolaget Atomenergi Studsvik.

Artandi, C. (1970). Rigid vinyl-film dosimetry. In *Manual on Radiation Dosimetry* (N. W. Holm and R. J. Berry, eds.), Marcel Dekker, New York.

Attix, F. H. and De La Vergne, L. (1954). Plate separation requirements for standard free-air ionization chambers. *Radiology* **63,** 853.

Attix, F. H., De La Vergne, L., and Ritz, V. H. (1958). Cavity ionization as a function of wall material. *J. Res. NBS* **60**, 235.

Attix, F. H. (1961). Electronic equilibrium in free-air chambers and a proposed new chamber design. Report 5646, Naval Research Laboratory, Washington, DC 20375.

Attix, F. H., Roesch, W. C., and Tochilin, E. (1966–1969). *Radiation Dosimetry*, 2nd ed., Vols. I–III, Academic Press, New York.

Attix, F. H. and Gorbics, S. G. (1968). Guardring shielding to eliminate instability of collecting volume in ionization chambers. *Rev. Sci. Instr.* **39**, 1766.

Attix, F. H. (1970). Thermoluminescence dosimetry with calcium fluoride. In *Manual on Radiation Dosimetry* (N. W. Holm and R. J. Berry, eds.), Marcel Dekker, New York.

Attix, F. H., Theus, R. B., Bondelid, R. O., and Rogers, C. C. (1973). Neutron dosimetry for the MANTA facility at NRL (Proc. of 2nd Meeting on Fundamental and Practical Aspects of the Application of Fast Neutrons in Clinical Radiotherapy, The Hague, Netherlands). *Europ. J. Cancer* **10**, 314.

Attix, F. H., Theus, R. B., and Rogers, C. C. (1974). Measurement of dose components in air in an (n, γ) field. In *Proceedings of 2nd Symposium on Neutron Dosimetry in Biology and Medicine, Neuherberg, Germany*, EUR 5273d-e-f, Commission of the European Communities, Luxembourg.

Attix, F. H. (1975). Further consideration of the track-interaction model for thermoluminescence in LiF (TLD-100). *J. Appl. Phys.* **46**, 81.

Attix, F. H., Theus, R. B., and Miller, G. E. (1976). Attenuation measurements of a fast-neutron radiotherapy beam. *Phys. Med. Biol.* **21**, 530.

Attix, F. H., Pearson, D. W., Capestrain, R. R., Jr., and Theus, R. B. (1977). An improved method for measuring the (n/γ) response ratio of gamma-ray dosimeters. Report COO-1105-252, U.S.E.R.D.A., Dept. of Medical Physics, Univ. of Wisconsin, Madison, WI 53706.

Attix, F. H., DeLuca, P. M., Jr., Pearson, D. W., and Goetsch, S. J. (1979). Measurement of neutron/gamma sensitivity ratios for a GM counter and for CO_2-filled graphite and Ar-filled magnesium ion chambers, by the lead-filter method with 14.8 MeV neutrons. Report WMP-109, COO-1105-264, Dept. of Medical Physics, Univ. of Wisconsin, Madison, WI 53706.

Attix, F. H. (1979). The partition of kerma to account for bremsstrahlung. *Health Phys.* **36**, 347; **36**, 536.

Attix, F. H. (1983). Energy imparted, energy transferred, and net energy transferred. *Phys. Med. Biol.* **28**, 1385.

Attix, F. H., Lopez, F., Owolabi, S., and Paliwal, B. R. (1983). Electron contamination in Co-60 gamma-ray beams. *Med. Phys.* **10**, 301.

Attix, F. H. (1984a). Determination of A_{ion} and P_{ion} in the new AAPM radiotherapy dosimetry protocol. *Med. Phys.* **11**, 714.

Attix, F. H. (1984b). A simple derivation of N_{gas}, a correction in A_{wall}, and other comments on the AAPM Task Group 21 protocol. *Med. Phys.* **11**, 725.

August, L. S., Attix, F. H., Herling, G. H., Shapiro, P., and Theus, R. B. (1976). Stripping-theory analysis of thick-target neutron production for D + Be. *Phys. Med. Biol.* **21**, 931.

August, L. S., Theus, R. B., and Shapiro, P. (1978). Gamma measurements with a nonhydrogenous Rossi counter in a mixed field. In *Proceedings of Sixth Microdosimetry Symposium,* EURATOM, Luxembourg.

Auxier, J. A., Snyder, W. S., and Jones, T. D. (1968). Neutron interactions and penetration in tissue. in *Radiation Dosimetry,* Vol. I., 2nd ed. (F. H. Attix and W. C. Roesch, eds.), Chapter 6, Academic Press, New York.

Awschalom, M., Rosenberg, I., and Mravca, A. (1983). Kerma for various substances averaged over the energy spectra of fast neutron therapy beams: A study in uncertainties. *Med. Phys.* **10**, 395.

Baily, N. A. (1980). Electron backscattering. *Med. Phys.* **7**, 514.

Barkas, W. H. and Berger, M. J. (1964). Tables of energy losses and ranges of heavy charged particles. NASA Tech. Rept. SP-3013, National Aeronautics and Space Administration, Washington, DC.

Becker, K. (1966) *Photographic Film Dosimetry* (English translation), Focal Press, New York.

Becker, K. (1973). *Solid State Dosimetry,* CRC Press, 2000 Corporate Blvd., NW, Boca Raton, FL 33431.

Beers, Y. (1953). *Introduction to the Theory of Errors,* Addison-Wesley, Reading, Mass.

Berger, M. J. (1963). Monte Carlo calculation of the penetration and diffusion of fast charged particles. In *Methods in Computational Physics,* Academic Press, New York.

Berger, M. J., and Seltzer, S. M. (1964). Tables of Energy Losses and Ranges of Electrons and Positrons. NASA Tech. Rept. SP-3012, National Aeronautics and Space Administration, Washington, DC.

Berger, M. J. (1968). Energy deposition in water by photons from point isotropic sources. MIRD Pamphlet 2, Society of Nuclear Medicine, 475 Park Ave. South, New York, NY 10016.

Berger, M. J. (1981). *Theoretical Aspects of Electron Dosimetry* (AAPM Proceedings Series No. 2), American Assn. of Physicists in Medicine, American Institute of Physics, New York.

Berger, M. J. and Seltzer, S. M. (1983). Stopping powers and ranges of electrons and positrons. NBSIR 82-2550-A, National Bureau of Standards, Washington, DC, 20234.

Berger, R. T. (1961). The x- or gamma-ray energy absorption or transfer coefficient: Tabulations and discussion. *Rad. Res.* **15**, 1.

Bichsel, H. (1968). Charged particle interactions. Chap 4 in Radiation Dosimetry, 2nd ed., Vol. I (F. H. Attix and W. C. Roesch, eds.), Academic Press, New York.

Bielajew, A. F. (1985). The effect of free electrons in ionization chamber saturation curves. *Med. Phys.* **12**, 197.

Biggs, P. J. and Ling, C. C. (1979). Electrons as the cause of the observed d_{max} shift with field size in high energy photon beams. *Med. Phys.* **6**, 291.

Biggs, P. J. and Russell, M. D. (1983). An investigation into the presence of secondary electrons in megavoltage photon beams. *Phys. Med. Biol.* **28**, 1033.

Birkhoff, R. D. (1958). The passage of fast electrons through matter. In *Handbuch der Physik,* Vol. 34, p. 53, Springer-Verlag, Berlin.

Birks, J. B. (1964). *The Theory and Practice of Scintillation Counting,* Pergamon Press, Oxford, U.K.

Birks, L. S. (1970). Convex curved crystal x-ray spectrograph. *Rev. Sci. Instr.* **41**, 1129.

Bjarngard, B. (1967). Use of manganese- and samarium-activated calcium sulfate in thermoluminescence dosimetry. In *Proceedings of the First International Conference on Luminescence Dosimetry* (CONF-650637), p. 195, U.S. Atomic Energy Commission.

Bjergbakke, E. (1970a). The ferrous-cupric dosimeter. In *Manual on Radiation Dosimetry* (N. W. Holm and R. J. Berry, eds.), Marcel Dekker, New York.

Bjergbakke, E. (1970b). The ceric-sulfate dosimeter. In *Manual on Radiation Dosimetry* (N. W. Holm and R. J. Berry, eds.), Marcel Dekker, New York.

Boag, J. W. (1966). Ionization chambers. In *Radiation Dosimetry*, Vol. II (F. H. Attix and W. C. Roesch, eds.), Chapter 9, Academic Press, New York.

Boag, J. W. and Currant, J. (1980). Current collection and ionic recombination in small cylindrical ionization chambers exposed to pulsed radiation. *Brit. J. Radiol.* **53**, 471.

Boag, J. W. (1982). The recombination correction for an ionization chamber exposed to pulsed radiation in a "swept beam" technique. *Phys. Med. Biol.* **27**, 201.

Boag, J. W. (1986). Ionization chambers. In *Dosimetry of Ionizing Radiation*, Vol. 2 (K. R. Kase, B. Bjarngard, and F. H. Attix, eds.), Academic Press, New York.

Bollinger, L. M. and Thomas, G. E. (1961). Measurement of the time-dependence of scintillation intensity by a delayed-coincidence method. *Rev. Sci. Instr.* **32**, 1044.

Bothe, W. (1949). Zur Rückdiffusion schneller Elektronen. *Z. Naturforsch.* **4A**, 542.

Bothe, W. (1949). Einige einfache Überlegungen zur Rückdiffusion schneller Elektronen. *Ann. Physik* **6**, 44.

Boutillon, M., and Perroche, A.-M. (1985). Effect of a change of stopping-power values on the W value recommended by ICRU for electrons in dry air. Bureau International des Poids et Mesures, Sèvres, Rept. CCEMRI(I)/85-8.

Bragg, W. H. (1910). Consequences of the corpuscular hypothesis of the gamma and x rays, and the ranges of beta rays. *Phil. Mag.* **20**, 385.

Bragg, W. H. (1912). *Studies in Radioactivity*, Macmillan, New York.

Brahme, A. (1981). *Physics of Electron Beam Penetration: Fluence and Absorbed Dose* (AAPM Proceedings Series No. 2), American Assn. of Physicists in Medicine, American Institute of Physics, New York.

Broerse, J. J., Lyman, J. T., and Zoetelief, J. (1985). Dosimetry of external beams of nuclear particles. In *Dosimetry of Ionizing Radiations* (K. R. Kase, B. Bjarngard, and F. H. Attix, eds.), Chapter 4, Academic Press, New York.

Brownell, G. L., Ellett, W. H., and Reddy, A. R. (1968). Absorbed fractions for photon dosimetry. MIRD Pamphlet 3, Society of Nuclear Medicine, 475 Park Ave. South, New York, NY 10016.

Burch, P. R. J. (1955). Cavity ionization chamber theory. *Rad. Res.* **4**, 361.

Burhop, E. H. S. (1952). *The Auger Effect*, Cambridge Univ. Press, England.

Burlin, T. E. (1966). A general theory of cavity ionization. *Brit. J. Radiol.* **39**, 727.

Burlin, T. E. (1968). Cavity chamber theory. *Radiation Dosimetry*, Vol. I (F. H. Attix and W. C. Roesch, eds.), Chapter 8, Academic Press, New York.

Burlin, T. E., Snelling, R. J., and Owen, B. (1969). The application of general cavity ionization theory to the dosimetry of electron fields. In *Proceedings of the 2nd Symposium on Microdosimetry* (EUR 4452 d-f-e), pp. 455–473.

Cameron, J. R., Zimmerman, D. W., and Bland, R. W. (1967). Thermoluminescence vs. roentgens in lithium fluoride: A proposed mathematical model. In *Proceedings of the First International Conference on Luminescence Dosimetry* (CONF 650637), p. 47, U.S. Atomic Energy Commission.

Cameron, J. R., Suntharalingam, N., and Kenney, G. N. (1968). *Thermoluminescent Dosimetry.* Univ. of Wisconsin Press, Madison, WI.

Cameron, J. R. (1970a). Radiophotoluminescent and thermoluminescent dosimetry. In *Manual on Radiation Dosimetry* (N. W. Holm and R. J. Berry, eds.), Marcel Dekker, New York.

Cameron, J. R. (1970b). Lithium fluoride thermoluminescent dosimetry. In *Manual on Radiation Dosimetry* (N. W. Holm and R. J. Berry, eds.), Marcel Dekker, New York.

Cartwright, B. G., Shirk, E. K., and Price, P. B. (1978). CR-39: A nuclear track-recording polymer of unique sensitivity and resolution. *Nucl. Inst. Meth.* **153**, 457.

Casson, H. (1978). Correction of measurements in plastic phantoms to obtain dose in water (Abstract). *Med. Phys.* **5**, 321.

Caswell, R. S. (1966). Deposition of energy by neutrons in spherical cavities. *Rad. Res.* **27**, 92.

Caswell, R. S., Coyne, J. J., and Randolph, M. L. (1980). Kerma factors for neutron energies below 30 MeV. *Rad. Res.* **83**, 217.

Chalkley, L. (1952). *J. Opt. Soc. Am.* **42**, 387.

Chilton, A. B. (1978). A note on the fluence concept. *Health Phys.* **34**, 715.

Chilton, A. B. (1979). Further comments on an alternate definition of fluence. *Health Phys.* **36**, 637.

Cohen, M. (1976). The properties and dosimetry of radium substitutes. In *Proceedings of the Summer School on Radiation Dosimetry* (sponsored by the American Association of Physicists in Medicine), Univ. of Vermont, Burlington, VT.

Constantinou, C., Attix, F. H., and Paliwal, B. R. (1982). A solid phantom material for radiotherapy x-ray and gamma-ray beam calibrations. *Med. Phys.* **9**, 436.

Cowan, F. P. (1969). Ultrahigh-energy radiation and uncommon types of particles. In *Radiation Dosimetry*, 2nd ed., Vol. III, (F. H. Attix and E. Tochilin, eds.), Chapter 27, Academic Press, New York.

Craun, R. L. and Smith, D. L. (1970). Analysis of response data for several organic scintillators. *Nucl. Inst. and Meth.* **80**, 239.

Cross, W. G. and Tommasino, L. (1970). Rapid reading technique for nuclear particle damage tracks in thin foils. *Radiat. Eff.* **5**, 85.

Cross, W. G., Arneja, A., and Ing, H. (1985). The energy dependence of the response of electrochemically-etched CR-39 dosimeters to neutrons (abstract). *Health Phys.* **49**, 143.

Davisson, C. M. and Evans, R. D. (1952). Gamma-ray absorption coefficients. *Rev. Mod. Phys.* **24**, 79.

DeLuca, P. M., Jr., Higgins, P. D., Pearson, D. W., and Attix, F. H. (1980). Comparison of photon doses determined with a graphite-walled proportional counter and with paired dosimeters irradiated by 14.8 MeV neutrons. Report WMP-121, DOE/EV/01105-272, Dept. of Medical Physics, Univ. of Wisconsin, Madison, WI 53706.

DePangher, S. J. and Nichols, L. L. (1966). A precision long counter for measuring fast neutron flux density. Report BNWL-260, Battelle Memorial Institute, Pacific Northwest Lab., Richland, WA.

DePangher, S. J. and Tochilin, E. (1969). Neutrons from accelerators and radioactive sources. In *Radiation Dosimetry*, 2nd ed., Vol. III, (F. H. Attix and E. Tochilin, eds.), Chapter 23, Academic Press, New York.

Dick, C. E., Lucas, A. C., Motz, J. W., Placious, R. C., and Sparrow, J. H. (1973). Large-angle K x-ray production by electrons. *J. Appl. Phys.* **44**, 815.

Dillman, L. T. and Von der Lage, F. C. (1975), Radionuclide decay schemes and nuclear parameters for use in radiation dose estimation. MIRD Pamphlet 10, Society of Nuclear Medicine, 475 Park Ave. South, New York, NY 10016.

Domen, S. R. (1969). Heat-loss compensated calorimeter. *Nature* **222**, 1061.

Domen, S. R. and Lamperti, P. J. (1974). A heat-loss compensated calorimeter: Theory, design and performance. *J. Res. NBS* **78A**, 595.

Domen, S. R. (1980). Absorbed dose water calorimeter. *Med. Phys.* **7**, 157.

Domen, S. R. (1983). A temperature-drift balancer for calorimetry. *Int. J. Appl. Radiat. Isot.* **34**, 927.

Domen, S. R. (1986). Advances in calorimetry for radiation dosimetry. In *Dosimetry of Ionizating Radiation*, Vol. II, (K. R. Kase, B. Bjarngard, and F. H. Attix, eds.), Academic Press, New York.

Duane, W. and Hunt, F. L. (1915). On x-ray wavelengths. *Phys. Rev.*, Ser. II, **6**, 166.

Dudley, R. A., (1966). Dosimetry with photographic emulsions. In *Radiation Dosimetry*, Vol. II (F. H. Attix and W. C. Roesch, eds.), Chapter 15, Academic Press, New York.

Dutreix, J. and Bernard, M. (1966). Dosimetry at interfaces for high energy x and gamma rays. *Brit. J. Radiol.* **39**, 205.

Dutreix, J. and Dutreix, A. (1966). Etude comparée d'une série de chambres d'ionisation dans des faisceaux d'electrons de 20 et 10 MeV. *Biophysik* **3**, 249.

Dvornik, I. (1970). The ethanolchlorobenzene dosimeter. In *Manual on Radiation Dosimetry* (N. W. Holm and R. J. Berry, eds.), Marcel Dekker, New York.

Ehrlich, M. and Placious, R. C. (1968). Thermoluminescence response of CaF_2:Mn in polytetrafluoroethylene to electrons. *Health Physics* **15**, 341.

Ellett, W. H., Callahan, A. B., and Brownell, G. L. (1964). Gamma-ray dosimetry of internal emitters. I: Monte Carlo calculations of absorbed dose from point sources. *Brit. J. Radiol.* **37**, 45.

Ellett, W. H., Callahan, A. B., and Brownell, G. L. (1965). Gamma-ray dosimetry of internal emitters. II: Monte Carlo calculations of absorbed dose from uniform sources. *Brit. J. Radiol.* **38**, 541.

Ellett, W. H. (1968). Application of gamma-ray diffusion theory to radiation dosimetry, Thesis, Univ. of London.

Ellett, W. H. and Humes, R. M. (1971). Absorbed fractions for small volumes containing photon-emitting radioactivity. MIRD Pamphlet 8, Society of Nuclear Medicine, 475 Park Ave. South, New York, NY 10016.

Emery, E. W. (1966). Geiger-Mueller and proportional counters. In *Radiation Dosimetry*, Vol. II (F. H. Attix and W. C. Roesch, eds.), Chapter 10, Academic Press, New York.

Etter, L. E. (1965). *The Science of Ionizing Radiation*, C. C. Thomas, Springfield, IL.

Evans, R. D. (1955). *The Atomic Nucleus*, McGraw-Hill; reprinted (1982), R. E. Krieger, Malabar, FL.

Evans, R. D. (1968). X-ray and gamma-ray interactions. In *Radiation Dosimetry*, 2nd ed., Vol. I (F. H. Attix and W. C. Roesch, eds.), Chapter 3, Academic Press, New York.

Fano, U. (1953a), Gamma-ray attenuation; basic processes. *Nucleonics* **11**(8), 8.

Fano, U. (1953b). Gamma-ray attenuation; analysis of penetration. *Nucleonics* **11**(9), 55.

Fano, U. (1954). Note on the Bragg–Gray cavity principle for measuring energy dissipation. *Radiat. Res.* **1**, 237.

Fleischer, R. L. and Price, P. B. (1963). Tracks of charged particles in high polymers. *Science* **140**, 1221.

Ford, R. L. and Nelson, W. R. (1978). The EGS code system. Report 210, Stanford Linear Accelerator Center, Stanford, Calif.

Fowler, J. F. (1966). Solid state electrical conductivity dosimeters. In *Radiation Dosimetry*, Vol. II (F. H. Attix and W. C. Roesch, eds.), Chapter 14, Academic Press, New York.

Fowler, J. F. and Attix, F. H. (1966). Solid state integrating dosimeters. In *Radiation Dosimetry*, Vol. II (F. H. Attix and W. C. Roesch, eds.), Chapter 13, Academic Press, New York.

Fricke, H. and Hart, E. J. (1966). Chemical dosimetry. In *Radiation Dosimetry*, Vol. II (F. H. Attix and W. C. Roesch, eds.), Chapter 12, Academic Press, New York.

Gager, L. D., Wright, A. E., and Almond, P. R. (1977). Silicon diode detectors used in radiological physics measurements. Part I: Development of an energy compensating shield. *Med. Physics* **4**, 494.

Galbraith, D. M., Rawlinson, J. A., and Munro, P. (1984). Dose errors due to charge storage in electron-irradiated plastic phantoms. *Med. Physics* **11**, 197.

Gilfrich, J. V., Burkhalter, P. G., and Birks, L. S. (1973). X-ray spectrometry for particulate air pollution—a quantitative comparison of techniques. *Analytical Chemistry* **45**, 2002.

Goldstein, H. (1957). The attenuation of gamma rays and neutrons in reactor shields. Report, U.S. Atomic Energy Commission, Washington, DC.

Goldstein, N., Schleiger, E. R., and Tochilin, E. (1967). Absorbed dose measurements with a portable calorimeter. *Health Physics* **13**, 806.

Goldstein, N. (1970). Cinemoid color films. In *Manual on Radiation Dosimetry*, (N. W. Holm and R. J. Berry, eds.), Marcel Dekker, New York.

Goodhead, D. T. (1987). Relationship of microdosimetric techniques to applications in biological systems. In *The Dosimetry of Ionizing Radiation*, Vol. II (K. R. Kase, B. E. Bjarngard, and F. H. Attix, eds.), Academic Press, New York.

Goodman, L. J. and Coyne, J. J. (1980). W_n and neutron kerma for methane-based tissue-equivalent gas. *Radiat. Res.* **82**, 13.

Goodman, L. J. and McDonald, J. C. (1980). Measurement of the thermal defect of A-150 plastic. *Radiat. Res.* **83**, 491.

Gorbics, S. G., Nash, A. E., and Attix, F. H. (1969). Thermal quenching of luminescence in six thermoluminescent dosimetry phosphors—II: Quenching of thermoluminescence. *Int. J. Appl. Radiat. and Isotopes* **20**, 843.

Gorbics, S. G., Attix, F. H., and Kerris, K. (1973). Thermoluminescent dosimeters for high-dose applications. *Health Phys.* **25**, 499.

Gordon, B. M. and Kraner, H. W. (1971). Development of a system for trace element analysis in the environment by charged particle x-ray fluorescence. Report BNL-16182, Brookhaven National Laboratory, Upton, NY.

Gray, L. H. (1929). Absorption of penetrating radiation. *Proc. Roy. Soc. (London)* **A122**, 647.

Gray, L. H. (1936). Ionization method for the absolute measurement of gamma-ray energy. *Proc. Roy. Soc. (London)* **A156**, 578.

Greene, D. (1962). The use of an ethylene-filled polythene chamber for dosimetry of megavoltage x rays. *Phys. Med. Biol.* **7**, 213.

Greene, D. and Massey, J. B. (1968). The use of the Farmer–Baldwin and Victrometer ionization chambers for dosimetry of high-energy x radiation. *Phys. Med. Biol.* **13**, 287.

Greening, J. R. (1950). A determination of x-ray wavelength distributions from absorption data. *Proc. Phys. Soc. (London)* **A63**, 1227.

Greening, J. R. (1972). Dosimetry of low-energy x-rays. In *Topics in Radiation Dosimetry*, (F. H. Attix, ed.), Academic Press, New York.

Gross, B. and Nablo, S. V. (1967). High potentials in electron-irradiated dielectrics. *J. Appl. Phys.* **38**, 2272.

Gross, B. (1978). Compton currents—historical aspects and recollections. *IEEE Trans. Nuclear Sci.* **NS-25**(4), 1048.

Gunn, S. R. (1964). Radiometric calorimetry: A review. *Nucl. Instr. and Meth.* **29**, 1.

Gunn, S. R. (1970). Radiometric calorimetry: A review (1970 supplement). *Nucl. Instr. and Meth.* **85**, 285.

Hall, E. J. (1973). *Radiobiology for the Radiologist.* Harper and Rowe, Hagerstown, MD.

Hankins, D. E., Homann, S. G., and Davis, M. D. (1985). Personnel neutron dosimetry using an improved technique for electrochemical etching of CR-39 plastic (abstract). *Health Phys.* **49**, 141.

Hanson, A. O. and McKibbin, J. L. (1947). A neutron detector having uniform sensitivity from 10 keV to 3 MeV. *Phys. Rev.* **72**, 673.

Harder, D. (1968). Einfluss der Vielfachstreuung von Elektronen auf die Ionisation in gasgefüllten Hohlräumen. *Biophysik* **5**, 157.

Harder, D. (1974). Fano's theorem and multiple scattering correction. In *Proceedings of 4th Symposium on Microdosimetry*, EUR 5122 d-e-f, Luxembourg.

Hart, E. J. (1970). The water dosimeter. In *Manual on Radiation Dosimetry* (N. W. Holm and R. J. Berry, eds.), Marcel Dekker, New York.

Hart, E. J. and Fielden, E. M. (1970). The hydrated electron dosimeter. In *Manual on Radiation Dosimetry* (N. W. Holm and R. J. Berry, eds.), Marcel Dekker, New York.

Harvey, J. R. (1967). The energy dependence of a personal neutron dosimeter which utilizes a thermal neutron detector at the body surface. Rept. RD/B/N827, Berkeley Nuclear Lab., Berkeley, England.

Hebbard, D. F. and Wilson, P. R. (1955). The effect of multiple scattering on electron energy loss distributions. *Austral. J. Phys.* **8**, 90.

Hendee, W. R. (1970). *Medical Radiation Physics.* Year Book Medical Publishers, Chicago.

Herz, R. H. (1969). *The Photographic Action of Ionizing Radiations.* Wiley, New York.

Hine, G. J. (1951). Scattering of secondary electrons produced by gamma-rays in materials of various atomic numbers. *Phys. Rev.* **82**, 755.

Holm, N. W. (1969). Dosimetry in industrial processing. In *Radiation Dosimetry*, 2nd ed., Vol. III (F. H. Attix and E. Tochilin, eds.), Academic Press, New York.

Holm, N. W. (1970). The oxalic acid dosimeter. In *Manual on Radiation Dosimetry* (N. W. Holm and R. J. Berry, eds.), Marcel Dekker, New York.

Holm, N. W. and Berry, R. J. (1970). *Manual on Radiation Dosimetry.* Marcel Dekker, Inc., New York.

Holm, N. W. and Zagorski, Z. P. (1970). Aqueous chemical dosimetry. In *Manual on Radiation Dosimetry* (N. W. Holm and R. J. Berry, eds.), Marcel Dekker, New York.

Holt, J. G., Fleischman, R. C., Perry, D. J., and Buffa, A. (1979). Examination of the factors A_c and A_{eq} for cylindrical ion chambers used in Co-60 beams. *Med. Phys.* **6**, 280.

Horowitz, Y. S. and Dubi, A. (1982). A proposed modification of Burlin's general cavity theory for photons. *Phys. Med. Biol.* **27**, 867 (1982).

Horowitz, Y. S., Moscovitch, M., and Dubi, A. (1983). Modified general cavity theory applied to the calculation of gamma dose in Co-60 thermoluminescence dosimetry. *Phys. Med. Biol.* **28**, 829.

Horowitz, Y. S. (1984). *Thermoluminescence and Thermoluminescent Dosimetry* (3 vols.). CRC Press, Orlando, FL.

Hough, J. H. (1979). A modified lead attenuation method to determine the fast neutron sensitivity k_u of a photon dosimeter. *Phys. Med. Biol.* **24**, 734.

Hoy, J. E. (1972). An albedo-type personnel neutron dosimeter. *Health Phys.* **23**, 385.

Hubbell, J. H. (1969). Photon cross sections, attenuation coefficients, and energy absorption coefficients from 10 keV to 100 GeV. Report NSRDS-NBS29, U.S. National Bureau of Standards. See also *Radiation Dosimetry*, Vol. I (F. H. Attix and W. C. Roesch, eds.), Chapter 3, tables by R. D. Evans in Academic Press, New York, 1968.

Hubbell, J. H., Gimm, H. A., and Øverbø, I. (1980). Pair, triplet and total cross sections for 1 MeV–100 GeV photons in elements $Z = 1$–100. *J. Phys. Chem. Ref. Data* **9**, 1023.

Hubbell, J. H. (1982). Photon mass attenuation and energy-absorption coefficients from 1 keV to 20 MeV. *Int. J. Appl. Rad. Isot.* **33**, 1269.

Hurst, G. S. (1954). An absolute dosimeter for fast neutrons. *Brit. J. Radiol.* **27**, 353.

Hurst, G. S., Harter, J. A., Hensley, P. N., Mills, W. A., Slater, M., and Reinhardt, P. W. (1956). Techniques of measuring neutron spectra with threshold detectors; tissue dose determination. *Rev. Sci. Instr.* **27**, 153.

Hurst, G. S. and Ritchie, R. H. (1962). A generalized concept of radiation dosimetry. *Health Phys.* **8**, 117.

ICRP (1971). Data for protection against ionizing radiation from external sources: Supplement to ICRP Publication 15. Publication No. 21, International Commission on Radiological Protection; Pergamon Press, Oxford, U.K.

ICRP (1975). Report of the task group on reference man. Publication No. 23, International Commission on Radiological Protection; Pergamon Press, Oxford, U.K.

ICRU (1964). Physical aspects of irradiation. Recommendations of the International Commission on Radiological Units and Measurements. Handbook 85, Natl. Bur. of Standards.

ICRU (1970). Linear energy transfer. Report 16, International Commission on Radiation Units and Measurements, 7910 Woodmont Ave., Bethesda, MD 20814.

ICRU (1971). Radiation quantities and units. Report 19, International Commission on Radiation Units and Measurements, 7910 Woodmont Ave., Bethesda, MD, 20814.

ICRU (1972). Radiation dosimetry: Electrons with energies between 1 and 50 MeV. Report 35, International Commission on Radiation Units and Measurements, 7910 Woodmont Ave., Bethesdą, MD 20814.

ICRU (1977). Neutron dosimetry for biology and medicine. Report 26, International Commission on Radiological Units and Measurements, 7910 Woodmont Ave., Bethesda, MD 20814.

ICRU (1979a). Quantitative concepts and dosimetry in radiobiology. Report No. 30, International Commission on Radiation Units and Measurements, 7910 Woodmont Ave., Bethesda, MD 20814.

ICRU (1979b). Average energy required to produce an ion pair. Report 31, International Commission on Radiation Units and Measurements, 7910 Woodmont Ave., Bethesda, MD 20814.

ICRU (1980). Radiation quantities and units. Report 33, International Commission on Radiation Units and Measurements, 7910 Woodmont Ave., Bethesda, MD 20814.

ICRU (1983). Microdosimetry. Report 36, International Commission on Radiation Units and Measurements, 7910 Woodmont Ave., Bethesda, MD 20814.

ICRU (1984a). Stopping powers for electrons and positrons. Report 37, International Commission on Radiation Units and Measurements, 7910 Woodmont Ave., Bethesda, MD 20814.

ICRU (1984b). Radiation dosimetry: Electron beams with energies between 1 and 50 MeV. Report 35, International Commission on Radiation Units and Measurements, 7910 Woodmont Ave., Bethesda, MD 20814.

Janni, J. G. (1966). Calculation of energy loss, range, pathlength, straggling, multiple scattering, and the probability of inelastic nuclear collisions for 0.1 to 1000 MeV protons. Report AD 643837, Natl. Tech. Inform. Service, Springfield, VA 22151.

Janssens, A., Eggermont, G., Jacobs, R., and Thielens, G. (1974). Spectrum perturbation and energy deposition models for stopping-power ratio calculations in general cavity theory. *Phys. Med. Biol.* **19**, 619.

Janssens, A. (1981). Modified energy-deposition model for the computation of the stopping-power ratio for small cavity sizes. *Phys. Rev. A* **23**, 1164.

Janssens, A. (1983). A proposed modification of Burlin's general cavity theory for photons. *Phys. Med. Biol.* **28**, 745.

Janssens, A. (1984). The fundamental constraint of cavity theory. *Phys. Med. Biol.* **29**, 1157.

Jesse, W. P. and Sadauskis, J. (1952). Alpha-particle ionization in mixtures of the noble gases. *Phys. Rev.* **88**, 417.

Johansson, K., Mattson, L., Lindborg, L., and Svensson, H. (1977). Absorbed-dose determination with ionization chambers in electron and photon beams having energies between 1 and 50 MeV. Report IAEA-SM 222/35, International Atomic Energy Agency, Vienna.

Johns, H. E. and Cunningham, J. R. (1974). *The Physics of Radiology*, revised 3rd ed., Charles C Thomas, Springfield, IL.

Johns, H. E. and Cunningham, J. R. (1983). *The Physics of Radiology*, 4th ed., Charles C Thomas, Springfield, IL.

Johnson, T. R. (1970). The benzene-water dosimeter. In *Manual on Radiation Dosimetry* (N. W. Holm and R. J. Berry, eds.), Marcel Dekker, New York.

Johnson, T. L. and Luerson, R. B. (1980). Fading of unannealed ^{6}LiF (TLD-600) for thermal neutrons and gamma rays. *Health Phys.* **38**, 853.

Joyet, G. (1963). Standard free-air chamber with magnetic field for x- or γ-rays up to about 50 MeV. *J. Appl. Math. Physics (ZAMP)* **14**, 195.

Karlsson, B. G. (1964). Methoden zur Berechnung und Erzeilung Einiger für die Tiefentherapie mit Hochenergetichen Protonen gunstiger Dosisverteilungen. *Strahlentherapie* **124**, 481.

Kase, K. R. and Nelson, W. R. (1978). *Concepts of Radiation Dosimetry*, Pergamon Press, Oxford, U.K.

Katz, R., Sharma, S. C., and Homayoonfar, M. (1972). The structure of particle tracks. In *Topics in Radiation Dosimetry* (F. H. Attix, ed.), Chapter 6, Academic Press, New York.

Kearsley, E. E. (1984a). A comparison between the Burlin and the Horowitz–Burlin general cavity theories. *Phys. Med. Biol.* **29**, 57.

Kearsley, E. E. (1984b). A new general cavity theory. *Phys. Med. Biol.* **29**, 1179.

Keithley, J. F., Yeager, J. R., and Erdman, R. J. (1984). *Low Level Measurements*, Keithley Instruments, Cleveland, OH 44122.

Kellerer, A. M. and Chmelevsky, D. (1975). Criteria for the applicability of LET. *Radiat. Res.* **63**, 226.

Kellerer, A. (1985). Fundamentals of microdosimetry. In *The Dosimetry of Ionizing Radiation*, Vol. I (K. R. Kase, B. E. Bjarngard, and F. H. Attix, eds.), Chapter 2, Academic Press, New York.

Kessaris, N. D. (1970). Absorbed dose and cavity ionization for high-energy electron beams. *Rad. Res.* **43**, 288.

Kiefer, H., Maushart, R., and Mejdahl, V. (1969). Radiation protection dosimetry. In *Radiation Dosimetry*, Vol. III (F. H. Attix and E. Tochilin, eds.), Academic Press, New York.

Knoll, G. F. (1979). *Radiation Detection and Measurement*. Wiley, New York.

Kolbenstvedt, H. (1967). Simple theory for *K*-ionization by relativistic electrons. *J. Appl. Phys.* **38**, 4785.

Kramers, H. A. (1923). On the theory of x-ray absorption and of the continuous x-ray spectrum. *Phil. Mag.* **46**, 836.

Kutcher, G., Strubler, K., and Suntharalingam, N. (1977). High-energy-photon dose measurements using exposure-calibrated ionization chambers. *Med. Phys.* **4**, 414.

Laitano, R. F. and Toni, M. P. (1984). The primary exposure standard of ENEA for medium energy x rays: Characteristics and measurement procedures. Report RT/PROT(83)27,

Laboratorio di Metrologia della Radiazioni Ionizzanti ENEA, CRE Casaccia, c.p. 2400 Roma, Italia.

Larson, H. V., Myers, I. T., and Roesch, W. C. (1955). Wide-beam fluorescent x-ray source. *Nucleonics* **13**(11), 100.

Laughlin, J. S. and Genna, S. (1966). Calorimetry. In *Radiation Dosimetry*, Vol. II, (F. H. Attix and W. C. Roesch, eds.), Chapter 16, Academic Press, New York.

Lawson, R. C. and Watt, D. E. (1964). Neutron depth-dose measurements in a tissue-equivalent phantom for an incident Pu–Be spectrum. *Phys. Med. Biol.* **9**, 487.

Lea, D. E. (1946). *Actions of Radiation on Living Cells*, University Press, Cambridge.

Lederer, C. M. and Shirley, V. S. (1979). *Table of Isotopes*, 7th ed., Wiley-Interscience, New York.

Lempert, G. D., Nath, R., and Schulz, R. J. (1983). Fraction of ionization from electrons arising in the wall of an ionization chamber. *Med. Phys.* **10**, 1.

Lewis, E. E. and Miller, W. F., Jr. (1984). *Computational Methods of Neutron Transport*, Wiley, New York.

Liversage, W. E. (1952). The effects of x rays on the insulating properties of PTFE. *Brit. J. Radiol.* **25**, 434.

Loevinger, R., Japha, E. M., and Brownell, G. L. (1956). Discrete radioisotope sources. In *Radiation Dosimetry* 1st ed., (G. J. Hine and G. L. Brownell, eds.), Chapter 16, Academic Press, New York.

Loevinger, R. and Berman, M. (1968). A schema for absorbed-dose calculations for biologically-distributed radionuclides. MIRD Pamphlet 1, Society of Nuclear Medicine, 475 Park Ave. South, New York, NY 10016.

Loevinger, R. (1969). Distributed radionuclide sources. In *Radiation Dosimetry*, 2nd ed., Vol. III (F. H. Attix and E. Tochilin, eds.), Chapter 18, Academic Press, New York.

Loevinger, R. (1981). A formalism for calculation of absorbed dose to a medium from photon and electron beams. *Med. Phys.* **8**, 1.

Lubkin, G. B. (1981). Experiments set limits and a value for the neutrino mass. *Phys. Today*, July, p. 17.

Lucke, W. C. (1970). Intrinsic efficiency of thermoluminescent dosimetry phosphors. Report 7104, Naval Research Laboratory, Washington, DC.

Luo Zheng-Ming (1980). An electron transport theory of cavity ionization. *Rad. Res.* **84**, 1.

Malsky, S. J., Roswit, B., Reid, C. B., and Amato, C. G. (1970). Radioluminescent dosimetry system. In *Manual on Radiation Dosimetry* (N. W. Holm and R. J. Berry, eds.), Marcel Dekker, New York.

Mann, W. B. (1954). Use of Callendar's "Radio-Balance" for the measurement of the energy emission from radioactive sources. *J. Res. NBS* **52**, 177.

Martin, G. R., and Tuck, D. G. (1959). The specific activity of radium. *Int. J. Appl. Rad. and Isotopes* **5**, 141.

Mattsson, L. O., Johansson, K.-A., and Svensson, H. (1981). Calibration and use of plane-parallel ionization chambers for the determination of absorbed dose in electron beams. *Acta Radiol. Oncol.* **20**, 385.

Maushart, R. and Piesch, E. (1967). Phosphate glasses as routine personnel dosimeters. In Report CONF-650637, Symposium Series No. 8, p. 300, U.S. Atomic Energy Commission.

Mayneord, W. V. (1945). Energy absorption. IV: The mathematical theory of integral dose in radium therapy. *Brit. J. Radiol.* **18**, 12.

McCall, R. C., Jenkins, T. M., and Oliver, G. D., Jr. (1978). Photon and electron response of silicon-diode neutron detectors. *Med. Phys.* **5**, 37.

McConnell, W. J., Hubbell, Jr., H. H., and Birkhoff, R. D. (1964). Electron-slowing-down spectrum in Cu of beta rays from Cu-64. Report 3463, Oak Ridge National Laboratory.

McDonald, J. C., Laughlin, J. S., and Freeman, R. E. (1976). Portable tissue-equivalent calorimeter. *Med. Phys.* **3**, 80.

McGinley, P. H. (1972). Response of LiF to fast neutrons. *Health Phys.* **23**, 105.

McKinlay, A. F. (1981). *Thermoluminescence Dosimetry*, Adam Hilger, Bristol, England.

McLaughlin, W. L. (1970a). Films, dyes, and photographic systems. In *Manual on Radiation Dosimetry* (N. W. Holm and R. J. Berry, eds.), Marcel Dekker, New York.

McLaughlin, W. L. (1970b). Radiochromic dye-cyanide dosimeters. In *Manual on Radiation Dosimetry* (N. W. Holm and R. J. Berry, eds.), Marcel Dekker, New York.

McLaughlin, W. L. (1970c). Photographic film dosimeters. In *Manual on Radiation Dosimetry*, (N. W. Holm and R. J. Berry, eds.), Marcel Dekker, New York.

McMaster, W. H., Del Grande, N. K., Mallett, J. R., and Hubbell, J. H. (1969). Compilation of x-ray cross sections, Report UCRL-50174, Section 11, Rev. 1, Univ. of Calif., Livermore, CA 94550.

Merzbacher, E. and Lewis, H. W. (1958). X-ray production by heavy charged particles. In *Handbuch der Physik*, Vol. 34, (S. Flügge, ed.), p. 166, Springer-Verlag, Berlin.

Mijnheer, B. J., Guldbakke, S., Lewis, V. E., and Broerse, J. J. (1982). Comparison of the fast-neutron sensitivity of a Geiger–Müller counter using different techniques. *Phys. Med. Biol.* **27**, 91.

Mijnheer, B. J., van Wijk, P. C., Williams, J. R., and Bell, J. (1983). The influence of air humidity on gamma-ray calibration and neutron absorbed-dose measurements with different types of A-150 plastic tissue-equivalent ionisation chambers. *Phys. Med. Biol.* **28**, 277.

Mijnheer, B. J., Wootton, P., Williams, J. R., Eenmaa, J., and Parnell, C. J. (1986). Uniformity in dosimetry protocols for therapeutic applications of fast-neutron beams, supplement to the Protocol for Neutron Beam Dosimetry of the American Association of Physicists in Medicine and the European Protocol for Neutron Dosimetry for External Beam Therapy of the European Clinical Neutron Dosimetry Group (to be published).

Miller, G. L. (1961). The physics of semiconductor radiation detectors. Brookhaven Lecture Series No. 9, BNL 699, Brookhaven National Laboratory, Upton, NY 11973.

Mitacek, P., Jr. and Frigerio, N. A. (1965). Absolute neutron dosimetry by calorimetric means. Argonne National Laboratory Report ANL-6971, p. 112.

Møller, C. (1931). Über den Stoss zweier Teilchen unter Berücksichtigung der Retardation der Kräfte. *Z. Phys.* **70**, 786.

Moteff, J. (1969). Reactor neutron dosimetry in irradiation of materials. In *Radiation Do-*

simetry, 2nd ed., Vol. III (F. H. Attix and E. Tochilin, eds.), Chapter 21, Academic Press, New York.

Motz, J. W., Miller, W., and Wyckoff, H. O. (1953). Eleven-MeV thick target bremsstrahlung. *Phys. Rev.* **89**, 968.

Motz, J. W., Dick, C. E., Lucas, A. C., Placious, R. C., and Sparrow, J. H. (1971). Production of high-intensity K x-ray beams. *J. Appl. Phys.* **42**, 2131.

Murray, K. M. and Attix F. H. (1973). An adiabatic calorimeter for measuring x-ray dose in silicon. *Health Phys.* **25**, 169.

Myers, I. T. (1968). Ionization. In *Radiation Dosimetry*, Vol. I (F. H. Attix and W. C. Roesch eds.), Chapter 7, Academic Press, New York.

NACP (1980). Procedures in external radiation therapy dosimetry with electron and photon beams with maximum energies between 1 and 50 MeV. *Nordic Assoc. of Clinical Phys., Acta. Radiol. Oncol.* **19**, 55.

NACP (1981). Electron beams with mean energies at the phantom surface below 15 MeV. *Acta Radiol. Oncol.* **20**, 402.

NAS–NRC (1964). Studies in penetration of charged particles in matter. Publication 1133, Nuclear Science Series Report 39, National Academy of Sciences–National Research Council, Washington, DC.

NCRP (1961). Stopping powers for use with cavity chambers. Report 27, National Council on Radiation Protection and Measurements, or Handbook 79, National Bureau of Standards.

NCRP (1974). Specification of gamma-ray brachytherapy sources. Report 41, National Council on Radiation Protection and Measurements, 7910 Woodmont Ave., Bethesda, MD 20814.

NCRP (1976). Structural shielding design and evaluation for medical use of x rays and gamma rays of energies up to 10 MeV. Report 49, National Council on Radiation Protection and Measurements, 7910 Woodmont Ave., Bethesda, MD 20814.

NCRP (1977). Radiation protection design guidelines for 0.1–100 MeV particle accelerator facilities. NCRP Report 51, National Council on Radiation Protection and Measurements, 7910 Woodmont Ave., Bethesda, MD 20814.

Nachtigall, D. (1969). *Table of Specific Gamma-Ray Constants*, Karl Thiemig, Munich.

Nachtigall, D. and Burger, G. (1972). Dose equivalent determinations in neutron fields by means of moderator techniques. In *Topics in Radiation Dosimetry* (F. H. Attix, ed.,) Chapter 7, Academic Press, New York.

Nahum, A. E. and Greening, J. R. (1976). Inconsistency in derivation of C_λ and C_E. *Phys. Med. Biol.* **21**, 862.

Nahum, A. E. and Greening, J. R. (1978). A detailed re-evaluation of C_λ and C_E with application to ferrous sulphate G-values. *Phys. Med. Biol.* **23**, 894.

Nash, A. E. and Johnson, T. L. (1977). ^{6}LiF (TLD-600) thermoluminescence detectors for mixed thermal neutron and gamma dosimetry. In *Proceedings of Fifth International Conference on Luminescence Dosimetry, São Paulo, Brazil* (A. Scharmann, ed.), Physikalisches Institut, Justus-Liebig-Universität, Giessen, Germany.

Nelms, A. T. (1953). Graphs of the Compton energy–angle relationship and the Klein–Nishina formula from 10 keV to 500 MeV. Circular 542, U.S. National Bureau of Standards, Washington, DC.

Nelson, W. R. (1980). *Computer Techniques in Radiation Transport and Dosimetry* (W. R. Nelson and T. M. Jenkins, eds.), Plenum Press, New York.

Niatel, M.-T. (1969). Étude expérimentale de l'influence de la vapeur d'eau sur l'ionisation produite dans l'air. *Comptes Rendus Acad. Sci. Paris* **268**, 1650.

O'Brien, K. (1977). Monte Carlo calculations of the energy response of lithium fluoride dosimeters to high energy electrons (<30 MeV). *Phys. Med. Biol.* **22**, 836.

O. T. Ogunleye, F. H. Attix, and B. R. Paliwal (1980). Comparison of Burlin cavity theory with LiF TLD measurements for cobalt-60 gamma rays. *Phys. Med. Biol.* **25**, 203.

Ogunleye, O. T. (1982). Influence of electron path length on the evaluation of Burlin's cavity theory. *Brit. J. Radiol.* **55**, 588.

Orton, C. G. (1970). The clear PMMA dosimeter. In *Manual on Radiation Dosimetry* (N. W. Holm and R. J. Berry, eds.), Marcel Dekker, New York.

Paliwal, B. R. and Almond, P. R. (1976). Electron attenuation characteristics of LiF. *Health Phys.* **3**, 151.

Parker, H. M. and Roesch, W. C. (1962). Units, radiation: Historical development. In *Encyclopedia of X-Rays and Gamma Rays* (G. L. Clark, ed.), p. 1102, Reinhold, New York.

Patterson, H. W. and Thomas, R. H. (1973). *Accelerator Health Physics*, Academic Press, New York.

Pearson, D. W., Attix, F. H., DeLuca Jr., P. M., Goetsch, S. J., and Torti, R. P. (1980). Ionization error due to porosity in graphite ionization chambers. *Phys. Med. Biol.*, **25**, 333.

Perrin, F. (1933), *Compt. Rend.* **197**, 1100.

Platzman, R. (1961). Total ionization in gases by high-energy particles: An appraisal of our understanding. *Int. J. Appl. Rad. and Isot.* **10**, 116.

Podgorsak, E. B., Rawlinson, J. A., and Johns, H. E. (1975). X-ray depth doses from linear accelerators in the energy range from 10 to 32 MeV. *Am. J. Roent.* **123**, 182.

Proceedings of the First International Conference on Luminescence Dosimetry (1967). Report CONF-650637, U.S. Atomic Energy Commission, Washington, DC.

Proceedings of the Second International Conference on Luminescence Dosimetry (1968). Report CONF-680920, U.S. Atomic Energy Commission, Washington, DC.

Proceedings of the Third International Conference on Luminescence Dosimetry (1971). Report 249, Parts I, II, and III, Danish AEC Research Establishment, Risö, Denmark.

Proceedings of the Fourth International Conference on Luminescence Dosimetry (1974), Vols. 1, 2, and 3 (T. Niewiadomski, ed.), Institute of Nuclear Physics, Krakow, Poland.

Proceedings of the Fifth International Conference on Luminescence Dosimetry (1977) (A. Scharmann, ed.), Physikalisches Institut, Justus-Liebig-Universität, Giessen, Federal Republic of Germany.

Profio, A. E. (1979). *Radiation Shielding and Dosimetry*, Wiley, New York.

Pruitt, J. S., Domen, S. R., and Loevinger, R. (1981). The graphite calorimeter as a standard of absorbed dose for Co-60 gamma radiation. *J. Res. NBS* **86**, 495.

Radak, B. and Markovic, V. (1970). Calorimetry. In *Manual on Radiation Dosimetry* (N. W. Holm and R. J. Berry, eds.), Marcel Dekker, New York.

Rago, P. F., Goldstein, N., and Tochilin, E. (1970). Reactor neutron measurements with fission-foil Lexan detectors. *Nucl. Appl.* **8**, 302. (Journal now called *Nuclear Technology*.)

Raju, M. R., Lyman, J. T., Brustad, T., and Tobias, C. A. (1969). Heavy charged-particle beams. In *Radiation Dosimetry*, 2nd ed., Vol. III (F. H. Attix and E. Tochilin, eds.), Chapter 20, Academic Press, New York.

Raju, M. R., Lampo, E., Curtis, S. B., and Richman, C. (1971). Dosimetry of π^- mesons using silicon detectors and plastic scintillators. *Phys. Med. Biol.* **16**, 599.

Raju, M. R. and Richman, C. (1972). Negative pion radiotherapy: Physical and radiobiological aspects. *Current Topics Rad. Res. Quart.* **8**, 159.

Ramm, W. J. (1966). Scintillation detectors. In *Radiation Dosimetry*, Vol. II (F. H. Attix and W. C. Roesch, eds.), Chap. 11, Academic Press, New York.

Randall, J. T. and Wilkins, M. H. F. (1945). Phosphorescence and electron traps. *Proc. Roy. Soc.* **A184**, 366.

Richardson, J. E. (1954). Effect of chamber voltage on electron build-up measurements. *Radiology* **62**, 584.

Richman, C., Rodriguez, J. F., Jr., Malcom, J. E., and Stein, M. L. (1978). The three dose components of a negative pion beam and their role in pion radiotherapy. *Radiology* **128**, 757.

Roesch, W. C. (1958). Dose for nonelectronic equilibrium conditions. *Rad. Res.* **9**, 399.

Roesch, W. C., (1967), A correction for radiation non-equilibrium. *Health Phys.* **13**, 934 (abstract). Report BNWL-SA-1014, Pacific Northwest Laboratories, Battelle Memorial Institute, Richland, WA.

Roesch, W. C. (1968). Mathematical theory of radiation fields. In *Radiation Dosimetry*, Vol. I (F. H. Attix and W. C. Roesch, eds.), Chapter 5, Academic Press, New York.

Roesch, W. C. and Attix, F. H. (1968). Basic concepts of dosimetry. In *Radiation Dosimetry*, Vol. I (F. H. Attix and W. C. Roesch, eds.), Chapter 1, Academic Press, New York.

Rossi, H. H. and Rosenzweig, W. (1955). A device for the measurement of dose as a function of specific ionization. *Radiology* **64**, 404.

Rossi, H. H. (1959). Specification of radiation quality. *Rad. Res.* **10**, 522.

Rossi, H. H. and Roesch, W. C. (1962). Field equations in dosimetry. *Rad. Res.* **16**, 783.

Rossi, H. H. (1968). Microscopic energy distribution in irradiated matter. In *Radiation Dosimetry*, Vol. I (F. H. Attix and W. C. Roesch, eds.), Chapter 2, Academic Press, New York.

Schaeffer, N. M. (1973). Reactor shielding for nuclear engineers. Report TID-25951, U.S. Atomic Energy Commission, Natl. Tech. Inform. Service, Springfield, VA 22161.

Schiff, L. I. (1946). Energy–angle distribution of betatron target radiation. *Phys. Rev.* **70**, 87.

Schuler, R. H. (1958). Absolute dosimetry of irradiations with charged particles. In *Proceedings of the 2nd International Conference on Peaceful Uses of Atomic Energy*, Geneva, Vol. 21, p. 213.

Schwartz, R. B. and Grandl, J. A. (1978). NBS standard reference neutron fields for personnel dosimetry calibration. *National and International Standardization of Radiation Dosimetry*. International Atomic Energy Agency, Vienna.

Scott, P. B. and Greening, J. R. (1963). The determination of saturation currents in free-air ionization chambers by extrapolation methods. *Phys. Med. Biol.* **8**, 51.

Seagrave, J. D. (1958). D$(d,n)^3$He and T$(d,n)^4$He neutron source handbook. Report LAMS-2162, Los Alamos National Laboratory, Los Alamos, NM.

Seelentag, W. W., Panzer, W., Drexler, G., Platz, L., and Santner, F. (1979). Catalogue of spectra for the calibration of dosimeters. Report 560, Gesellschaft für Strahlen- und Umweltforschung mbH, Munich, Federal Republic of Germany.

Sehested, K. (1970). The Fricke dosimeter. In *Manual on Radiation Dosimetry* (N. W. Holm and R. J. Berry, eds.), Marcel Dekker, New York.

Seltzer, S. M. and Berger, M. J. (1985). Bremsstrahlung spectra from electron interactions with screened atomic nuclei and orbital electrons. *Nucl. Inst. and Meth. Phys. Res.* **B12**, 95.

Shalek, R. J., Sinclair, W. K., and Calkins, J. C. (1962). The relative biological effectiveness of 22 MeV x rays, cobalt-60 gamma rays, and 200 keV x rays. II. The use of the ferrous sulfate dosimeter for x-ray and gamma-ray beams. *Rad. Res.* **16**, 344.

Shalek, R. J. and Stovall, M. (1969). Dosimetry in implant therapy. In *Radiation Dosimetry*, Vol. III (F. H. Attix and E. Tochilin, eds.), Chapter 31, Academic Press, New York.

Sharp, J. (1964). *Nuclear Radiation Detectors*, Methuen, London.

Sheldon, R. (1970). The hydrogen pressure dosimeter. In *Manual on Radiation Dosimetry* (N. W. Holm and R. J. Berry, eds.), Marcel Dekker, New York.

Shiragai, A. (1984). A comment on a modification of Burlin's general cavity theory. *Phys. Med. Biol.* **29**, 427.

Shonka, F. R., Rose, J. E., and Failla, G. (1959). Conducting plastic equivalent to tissue, air and polystyrene. *Progr. Nucl. Energy Ser. 12* **1**, 160.

Sinclair, W. K. (1969). Radiobiological dosimetry. In *Radiation Dosimetry*, 2nd ed., Vol. III (F. H. Attix and E. Tochilin, eds.), Chapter 29, Academic Press, New York.

Singh, D. and Madvanath, U. (1981). Limitations of the ICRU standard tissue spherical phantom for organ dose estimation by highly degraded neutron spectra. *Health Phys.* **41**, 383.

Smathers, J. B., Otte, V. A., Smith, A. R., Almond, P. R., Attix, F. H., Spokas, J. J., Quam, W. M., and Goodman, L. J. (1977). Composition of A-150 tissue-equivalent plastic. *Med. Phys.* **4**, 74.

Snyder, W. S., Ford, M. R., Warner, G. G., and Watson, S. B. (1975). "*S*", absorbed dose per unit cumulated activity for selected radionuclides and organs. MIRD Pamphlet No. 11, Society of Nuclear Medicine, 475 Park Ave. South, New York, NY 10016.

Sondhaus, C. A. and Evans, R. D. (1969). Dosimetry of radiation in space flight. In *Radiation Dosimetry*, 2nd ed., Vol. III, (F. H. Attix and E. Tochilin, eds.), Chapter 26, Academic Press, New York.

Sparrow, J. H. and Dick, C. D. (1976). The development and application of monoenergetic x-ray sources. Report NBS SP456, National Bureau of Standards, Washington, DC.

Spencer, L. V. and F. H. Attix (1955). A theory of cavity ionization. *Rad. Res.* **3**, 239.

Spencer, L. V. (1959). Energy dissipation by fast electrons. NBS Monograph 1, National Bureau of Standards, Washington, DC.

Spencer, L. V. (1965). Note on the theory of cavity ionization chambers. *Rad. Res.* **25**, 352.

Spencer, L. V. (1971). Remarks on the theory of energy deposition in cavities. *Acta Radiol.* **10**, 1.

Spurny, F. and Tureck, K. (1977). Neutron dosimetry with solid state nuclear track detectors. *Nucl. Track Detection* **1**, 189.

Sternheimer, R. M. (1952). The density effect for the ionization loss in various materials. *Phys. Rev.* **88**, 95.

Sternheimer, R. M. and Peierls, R. F. (1971). General expression for the density effect for the ionization loss of charged particles, *Phys. Rev. B3*, 3681.

Sternheimer, R. M., Seltzer, S. M., and Berger, M. J. (1982). Density effect for the ionization loss of charged particles in various substances. *Phys. Rev. B* **26**, 6067.

Storm, E. and Israel, H. I. (1970). Photon cross sections from 1 keV to 100 MeV for elements from $Z = 1$ to $Z = 100$. In *Nuclear Data Tables*, Vol. A7, p. 565, Academic Press, New York.

Svensson, H. and Pettersson, S. (1967). Absorbed dose calibration of thimble chambers with high energy electrons at different phantom depth. *Ark. Fysik* **34**, 377.

Svensson, H. and Brahme, A. (1979). Ferrous sulphate dosimetry for electrons; a re-evaluation. *Acta Radiol. Oncol.* **18**, 326.

Swanson, W. P. (1979). Improved calculation of photoneutron yields released by incident electrons. *Health Phys.* **37**, 347.

Tabata, T. (1967). Backscattering of electrons from 3.2 to 14 MeV. *Phys. Rev.* **162**, 336.

Thoraeus, R. (1932). A study of the ionization method for measuring the intensity and absorption of roentgen rays and of the efficiency of different filters used in therapy. *Acta Radiol.* [Suppl., Stockholm] **15**.

Tochilin, E. and Kohler, G. D. (1958). Neutron beam characteristics from the University of California 60-in. cyclotron. *Health Phys.* **1**, 332.

Tochilin, E., Goldstein, N., and Lyman, J. T. (1968). The quality- and LET-dependence of three thermoluminescent dosimeters and their potential for use as secondary standards. In *Proceedings of 2nd International Conference on Luminescence Dosimetry*, CONF-680920, p. 424, U.S. Atomic Energy Commission, Washington, DC.

Tochilin, E. and Shumway, B. W. (1969). Dosimetry of neutrons and mixed $n + \gamma$ fields. In *Radiation Dosimetry*, Vol. III (F. H. Attix and E. Tochilin, eds.), Chapter 22, Academic Press, New York.

Todo, A. S., Hiromoto, G., Turner, J. E., Hamm, R. N., and Wright, H. A. (1982). Monte Carlo calculations of initial energies of electrons in water irradiated by photons with energies up to 1 GeV. *Health Phys.* **43**, 845.

Turner, J. E., Hamm, R. N., Wright, H. A., Módolo, J. T., and Sordi, G. M. A. A. (1980). Monte Carlo calculations of initial energies of Compton electrons and photoelectrons in water irradiated by photons with energies up to 2 MeV. *Health Phys.* **39**, 49.

Unger, L. M. and Trubey, D. K. (1982). Specific gamma-ray dose constants for nuclides important to dosimetry and radiological assessment. Report ORNL/RSIC-45/R1, Oak Ridge National Laboratory, Oak Ridge, TN.

Velkley, D. E., Manson, D. J., Purdy, J. A., and Oliver Jr., G. D. (1975). Buildup region of megavoltage photon radiation sources. *Med. Phys.* **2**, 14.

Wagner, E. B. and Hurst, G. S. (1959). Gamma response and energy losses in absolute fast-neutron dosimeters. *Health Phys.* **2,** 57.

Wagner, E. B. and Hurst, G. S. (1961). A Geiger–Müller gamma-ray dosimeter with low neutron sensitivity. *Health Phys.* **5,** 20.

Weaver, K., Bichsel, H., Eenmaa, J., and Wootton, P. (1977). Measurement of photon dose fraction in a neutron radiotherapy beam. *Med. Phys.* **4,** 379.

Whittaker, B. (1970). Red perspex dosimetry. In *Manual on Radiation Dosimetry* (N. W. Holm and R. J. Berry, eds.), Marcel Dekker, New York.

Whyte, G. N. (1959). *Principles of Radiation Dosimetry*, Wiley, New York.

Wilson, C. R. and Cameron, J. R. (1968). Dosimetric properties of $Li_2B_4O_7$:Mn (Harshaw). In *Proceedings of the 2nd International Conference on Luminscence Dosimetry*, CONF-680920, p. 161, U.S. Atomic Energy Commission, Washington, DC.

Wingate, C. L., Tochilin, E., and Goldstein, N. (1967). Response of lithium fluoride to neutrons and charged particles. In *Proceedings of International Conference on Luminescence Dosimetry, Stanford, CA*, CONF-650637, U.S. Atomic Energy Commission, Washington, DC.

Wright, K. A. and Trump, J. G. (1962). Backscattering of megavolt electrons from thick targets. *J. Appl. Phys.* **33,** 687.

Wright, A. E. and Gager, L. D. (1977). Silicon diode detectors used in radiological physics measurements. Part II: Measurement of dosimetry data for high energy photons. *Med. Phys.* **4,** 499.

Wyckoff, H. O. and Attix, F. H. (1957). *Design of Free-Air Ionization Chambers*, Handbook 64, National Bureau of Standards, Washington, DC.

Wyckoff, H. O. and Kirn, F. S. (1957). Standard ionization-chamber requirements for 250 to 500 kilovolt x rays. *J. Res. NBS* **58,** 111.

Wyckoff, H. O. (1960). Measurement of cobalt-60 and cesium-137 gamma rays with a free-air chamber. *J. Res. NBS* **64C,** 87.

Yang, C. N. (1951). Actual path length of electrons in foils. *Phys. Rev.* **84,** 599.

Yang Yin, DeLuca, P. M., Jr., Pearson, D. W., and Attix, F. H. (1984). Gamma-ray yield of a [239]Pu–Be source. Report WMP-170, DOE/EV/01105–310, Department of Medical Physics, Univ. of Wisconsin, Madison, WI 53706.

Zirkle, R. E., Marchbank, D. F., and Kuck, K. D. (1952). Exponential and sigmoid survival curves resulting from alpha and x-irradiation of Aspergillus spores. *J. Cell. Comp. Physiol.* **39,** Suppl. 1, 75.

APPENDIXES

APPENDIX A.1. **Physical Constants**

Quantity	Symbol	Value
Speed of light in vacuum	c	2.9979×10^8 m s^{-1}
Elementary charge	e	1.6022×10^{-19} C
		$= 4.8032 \times 10^{-10}$ esu
Planck constant	h	6.6262×10^{-34} J Hz^{-1}
Avogadro constant	N_A	6.0220×10^{23} mole^{-1}
Atomic mass unit	$1 \text{ u} = (10^{-3}$ kg mole$^{-1})/N_A$	1.6606×10^{-27} kg
Electron rest mass	m_0	0.91095×10^{-30} kg
Proton rest mass	$(M_0)_p$	1.6726×10^{-27} kg
Neutron rest mass	$(M_0)_n$	1.6750×10^{-27} kg
Ratio, proton mass to electron mass	$(M_0)_p/m_0$	1836
Classical electron radius	r_e	2.8179×10^{-15} m
Molar gas constant	R	8.3144 J mole^{-1} K^{-1}
Molar volume, ideal gas ($T_0 = 273.15$ K, $p_0 = 1$ atm)	$V_m = RT_0/P_0$	0.022414 m^3 mole^{-1}
Boltzmann constant	$k = R/N_A$	1.3807×10^{-23} J K^{-1}

$$1 \text{ kg} = 5.6095 \times 10^{29} \text{ MeV}$$
$$1 \text{ amu} = 931.50 \text{ MeV}$$
$$\text{Electron rest mass} = 0.51100 \text{ MeV}$$
$$\text{Proton rest mass} = 938.26 \text{ MeV}$$
$$\text{Neutron rest mass} = 939.55 \text{ MeV}$$
$$1 \text{ electron volt (eV)} = 1.6022 \times 10^{-19} \text{ J}$$
$$= 1.6022 \times 10^{-12} \text{ erg}$$
$$1 \text{ joule (J)} = 10^{7} \text{ erg}$$
$$1 \text{ coulomb (C)} = 2.9979 \times 10^{9} \text{ esu}$$
$$1 \text{ gray (Gy)} = 1 \text{ J/kg} = 10^{2} \text{ rad} = 10^{4} \text{ erg/g}$$
$$1 \text{ sievert (Sv)} = 1 \text{ J/kg}$$

Energy–wavelength conversion:

$$1.23985 \times 10^{-6} \text{ eV m}$$
$$12.3985 \text{ keV Å}$$

Exposure conversion:

$$1 \text{ roentgen (R)} = 2.58 \times 10^{-4} \text{ C/kg}$$
$$1 \text{ C/kg} = 3876 \text{ R}$$

Element	Symbol	At. No. Z	At. Wt. A	Z/A	$10^{-23}\,N_A Z/A^a$	Density^b (g/cm^3)	K-edge (keV)	L1-edge (keV)	I^c (eV)
Hydrogen	H	1	1.008	.9922	5.975	8.374×10^{-5}	0.014	—	19.2
Helium	He	2	4.003	.4997	3.009	1.663×10^{-4}	0.025	—	41.8
Lithium	Li	3	6.941	.4322	2.603	0.533	0.055	—	40.0
Beryllium	Be	4	9.012	.4438	2.673	1.848	0.111	—	63.7
Boron	B	5	10.81	.4625	2.785	2.34–2.37	0.188	—	—
Carbon (graphite)	C	6	12.01	.4995	3.008	1.9–2.3	0.284	—	78.0
Nitrogen	N	7	14.01	.4998	3.010	1.165×10^{-3}	0.402	—	82.0
Oxygen	O	8	16.00	.5000	3.011	1.331×10^{-3}	0.532	0.024	95.0
Fluorine	F	9	19.00	.4737	2.853	1.580×10^{-3}	0.685	0.031	—
Neon	Ne	10	20.18	.4956	2.984	8.385×10^{-4}	0.867	0.045	137
Sodium	Na	11	22.99	.4785	2.881	0.969	1.07	0.063	149
Magnesium	Mg	12	24.30	.4937	2.973	1.735	1.30	0.089	156
Aluminum	Al	13	26.98	.4818	2.901	2.69	1.56	0.118	166
Silicon	Si	14	28.09	.4985	3.002	2.32	1.84	0.149	173
Phosphorus	P	15	30.97	.4843	2.916	1.82–2.69	2.15	0.189	—
Sulfur	S	16	32.06	.4991	3.005	1.954, 2.07	2.47	0.229	—
Chlorine	Cl	17	35.45	.4795	2.888	2.995×10^{-3}	2.82	0.270	—
Argon	Ar	18	39.95	.4506	2.713	1.662×10^{-3}	3.20	0.320	188
Potassium	K	19	39.10	.4860	2.926	0.860	3.61	0.377	190
Calcium	Ca	20	40.08	.4990	3.005	1.55	4.04	0.438	191
Scandium	Sc	21	44.96	.4671	2.813	2.980	4.49	0.500	—
Titanium	Ti	22	47.90	.4593	2.766	4.54	4.97	0.564	233
Vanadium	V	23	50.94	.4515	2.719	6.10	5.47	0.628	245
Chromium	Cr	24	52.00	.4616	2.780	7.18	5.99	0.695	—
Manganese	Mn	25	54.94	.4551	2.740	7.21–7.44	6.54	0.769	272
Iron	Fe	26	55.85	.4656	2.804	7.86	7.11	0.846	286
Cobalt	Co	27	58.93	.4581	2.759	8.9	7.71	0.926	297
Nickel	Ni	28	58.71	.4769	2.872	8.88	8.33	1.01	311

APPENDIX B.1. (*Continued*)

Element	Symbol	At. No. Z	At. Wt. A	Z/A	$10^{-23} N_A Z/A$	Density[b] (g/cm^3)	K-edge (keV)	L1-edge (keV)	I^c (eV)
Copper	Cu	29	63.55	.4564	2.748	8.94	8.98	1.10	322
Zinc	Zn	30	65.38	.4589	2.763	7.11	9.66	1.19	330
Gallium	Ga	31	69.72	.4446	2.678	5.88	10.38	1.30	—
Germanium	Ge	32	72.59	.4408	2.655	5.31	11.10	1.41	350
Arsenic	As	33	74.92	.4405	2.652	5.73	11.87	1.53	—
Selenium	Se	34	78.96	.4306	2.593	4.28, 4.79	12.66	1.65	348
Bromine	Br	35	79.90	.4380	2.638	7.07×10^{-3}	13.47	1.78	—
Krypton	Kr	36	83.80	.4296	2.587	3.478×10^{-3}	14.33	1.92	352
Rubidium	Rb	37	85.47	.4329	2.607	1.529	15.20	2.07	363
Strontium	Sr	38	87.62	.4337	2.612	2.54	16.10	2.22	—
Yttrium	Y	39	88.91	.4387	2.642	4.46	17.04	2.37	—
Zirconium	Zr	40	91.22	.4385	2.641	6.49	18.00	2.53	—
Niobium	Nb	41	92.91	.4413	2.658	8.55	18.99	2.70	—
Molybdenum	Mo	42	95.94	.4378	2.636	10.20	20.00	2.87	—
Technetium	Tc	43	98.91	.4348	2.618	11.50	21.04	3.04	—
Ruthenium	Ru	44	101.1	.4353	2.622	12.41	22.12	3.22	—
Rhodium	Rh	45	102.9	.4373	2.633	12.41	23.22	3.41	—
Palladium	Pd	46	106.4	.4323	2.604	12.00	24.35	3.60	—
Silver	Ag	47	107.9	.4357	2.624	10.48	25.51	3.81	470
Cadmium	Cd	48	112.4	.4270	2.571	8.65	26.71	4.02	469
Indium	In	49	114.8	.4268	2.570	7.30	27.94	4.24	487
Tin (white)	Sn	50	118.7	.4213	2.537	7.31	29.20	4.46	488
Antimony	Sb	51	121.7	.4191	2.524	6.68	30.5	4.70	—
Tellurium	Te	52	127.6	.4075	2.454	6.23	31.8	4.94	—
Iodine	I	53	126.9	.4176	2.515	4.92	33.2	5.19	—
Xenon	Xe	54	131.3	.4113	2.477	5.485×10^{-3}	34.6	5.45	482
Cesium	Cs	55	132.9	.4138	2.492	1.870	36.0	5.71	488
Barium	Ba	56	137.3	.4078	2.456	3.5	37.4	5.99	—

APPENDIX B.1. (*Continued*)

Element	Symbol	At. No. Z	At. Wt. A	Z/A	$10^{-23} N_A Z/A$[a]	Density[b] (g/cm^3)	K-edge (keV)	L1-edge (keV)	I[c] (eV)
Lanthanum	La	57	138.9	.4104	2.471	6.13	38.9	6.27	—
Cerium	Ce	58	140.1	.4139	2.494	6.64	40.4	6.55	—
Praeseodymium	Pr	59	140.9	.4187	2.522	6.64, 6.77	42.0	6.83	—
Neodymium	Nd	60	144.2	.4160	2.505	6.80, 7.01	43.6	7.13	—
Promethium	Pm	61	(145)	.421	2.53	7.20	45.2	7.43	—
Samarium	Sm	62	150.4	.4122	2.482	7.40, 7.52	46.8	7.74	—
Europium	Eu	63	152.0	.4146	2.497	5.23	48.5	8.05	—
Gadolinium	Gd	64	157.2	.4070	2.451	7.88	50.2	8.38	591
Terbium	Tb	65	158.9	.4090	2.463	8.23	52.0	8.71	—
Dysprosium	Dy	66	162.5	.4062	2.446	8.52	53.8	9.05	—
Holmium	Ho	67	164.9	.4062	2.446	8.77	55.6	9.39	—
Erbium	Er	68	167.3	.4066	2.448	9.04	57.5	9.75	—
Thulium	Tm	69	168.9	.4084	2.460	9.29	59.4	10.1	—
Ytterbium	Yb	70	173.0	.4045	2.436	6.54, 6.96	61.3	10.5	718
Lutetium	Lu	71	175.0	.4058	2.444	9.81	63.3	10.9	727
Hafnium	Hf	72	178.5	.4034	2.429	13.29	65.4	11.3	—
Tantalum	Ta	73	180.9	.4034	2.429	16.65	67.4	11.7	—
Tungsten	W	74	183.8	.4025	2.424	19.3	69.5	12.1	—
Rhenium	Re	75	186.2	.4028	2.426	20.98	71.7	12.5	—
Osmium	Os	76	190.2	.3996	2.406	22.57	73.9	13.0	—
Iridium	Ir	77	192.2	.4006	2.412	22.39	76.1	13.4	—
Platinum	Pt	78	195.1	.3998	2.408	21.41	78.4	13.9	790
Gold	Au	79	197.0	.4011	2.415	19.29	80.7	14.4	790
Mercury	Hg	80	200.6	.3988	2.402	13.52	83.1	14.8	800
Thallium	Tl	81	204.4	.3963	2.387	11.83	85.5	15.3	—
Lead	Pb	82	207.2	.3958	2.383	11.33	88.0	15.9	823
Bismuth	Bi	83	209.0	.3972	2.392	9.73	90.5	16.4	—
Polonium	Po	84	(210)	.400	2.41	9.32	93.1	16.9	—

APPENDIX B.1. (Continued)

Element	Symbol	At. No. Z	At. Wt. A	Z/A	$10^{-23}\,N_A Z/A$[a]	Density[b] (g/cm^3)	K-edge (keV)	L1-edge (keV)	I[c] (eV)
Astatine	At	85	(210)	.405	2.44	—	95.7	17.5	—
Radon	Rn	86	(222)	.387	2.33	9.07×10^{-3}	98.4	18.0	794
Francium	Fr	87	(223)	.390	2.35	—	101.1	18.6	—
Radium	Ra	88	226.0	.3893	2.345	—	103.9	19.2	—
Actinium	Ac	89	(227)	.392	2.36	10.07	106.8	19.8	—
Thorium	Th	90	232.0	.3879	2.336	11.72	109.7	20.5	—
Protactinium	Pa	91	231.0	.3939	2.372	15.37	112.6	21.1	—
Uranium	U	92	238.0	.3865	2.328	18.95	115.6	21.8	890
Neptunium	Np	93	237.0	.3923	2.363	20.21	118.7	22.4	—
Plutonium	Pu	94	(244)	.385	2.32	19.78	121.8	23.1	—
Americium	Am	95	(243)	.391	2.35	13.65	125.0	23.8	—
Curium	Cm	96	(247)	.389	2.34	13.51	128.2	24.5	—
Berkelium	Bk	97	(247)	.393	2.36	$\cong 14$	131.6	25.3	—
Californium	Cf	98	(251)	.390	2.35	—	136.0	26.1	—
Einsteinium	Es	99	(254)	.390	2.35	—	139.5	26.9	—
Fermium	Fm	100	(257)	.389	2.34	—	143.1	27.7	—
Mendelevium	Md	101	(258)	.391	2.36	—	146.8	28.5	—
Nobelium	No	102	(259)	.394	2.37	—	150.5	29.4	—
Lawrencium	Lr	103	(260)	.396	2.39	—	154.4	30.2	—

[a] Number of electrons per gram of element (in units of 10^{23}).
[b] Assuming $T = 20°C$ and $P = 1$ atm, and Charles's law for gases. Multiply by 10^3 to convert to kg m^{-3}.
[c] From Berger and Seltzer (1983). I is the mean excitation potential for stopping power; see Chapter 8.

Appendix B.2.   Data Table for Compounds and Mixtures[a]

Material	Density (g/cm^3)[c]	Electron density $(10^{23}\ e/g)$	I (eV)[d]
A-150 plastic[b]	1.127	3.306	65.1
Adipose tissue			
(Fat, ICRP)[b]	0.92	3.363	63.2
Air[b]	1.205×10^{-3}	3.006	85.7
Bone, cortical (ICRP)[b]	1.85	3.139	106.4
Calcium fluoride, CaF_2	3.18	2.931	166
Carbon dioxide, CO_2	1.842×10^{-3}	3.010	85.0
Cesium iodide, CsI	4.51	2.503	553
Lithium fluoride, LiF	2.64	2.786	94.0
Lucite, $(C_5H_8O_2)_n$	1.19	3.248	74.0
Muscle, skeletal (ICRP)[b]	1.04	3.308	75.3
Mylar, $(C_{10}H_8O_4)_n$	1.40	3.134	78.7
Nylon, type 6			
$(C_6H_{11}NO)_n$	1.14	3.299	63.9
Polycarbonate			
$(C_{16}H_{14}O_3)_n$	1.20	3.173	73.1
Polyethylene $(C_2H_4)_n$	0.94	3.435	57.4
Polyimide $(C_{22}H_{10}N_2O_5)$	1.42	3.087	79.6
Polypropylene $(C_3H_5)_n$	0.90	3.372	59.2
Polystyrene $(C_8H_8)_n$	1.06	3.238	68.7
Polyvinyl Chloride			
$(C_2H_3Cl)_n$	1.30	3.083	108.2
Pyrex (borosilicate glass)[b]	2.23	2.993	134
Silicon dioxide, SiO_2	2.32	3.007	139.2
Silver bromide, AgBr	6.47	2.629	487
Sodium iodide, NaI	3.67	2.571	452
Teflon, $(C_2F_4)_n$	2.20	2.890	99.1
TE gas (methane-based)[b]	1.064×10^{-3}	3.312	61.2
TE gas (propane-based)[b]	1.826×10^{-3}	3.314	59.5
TE liquid (no sucrose)[b]	1.070	3.313	74.2
Water, H_2O	0.9982	3.343	75.0

[a] Data from Berger and Seltzer (1983)
[b] See compositions in Appendix B.3
[c] Assuming $T = 20°C.$, $P = 1$ atm., and Charles' Law for gases applies.
[d] I is the mean excitation potential for stopping power, see Chapter 8.

Appendix B.3 Compositions of Mixtures[a]

A-150 plastic: 10.13 H, 77.55 C, 3.51 N, 5.23 O, 1.74 F, 1.84 Ca

Muscle, skeletal (ICRP): 10.06 H, 10.78 C, 2.77 N, 75.48 O, 0.08 Na, 0.02 Mg, 0.18 P, 0.24 S, 0.08 Cl, 0.30 K, 0.01 (Ca + Fe + Zn)

Adipose tissue (ICRP): 11.95 H, 63.72 C, 0.80 N, 23.23 O, 0.05 Na, 0.02 P, 0.07 S, 0.12 Cl, 0.03 K, 0.01 (Mg + Ca + Fe + Zn)

Bone, cortical (ICRP): 4.72 H, 14.43 C, 4.20 N, 44.61 O, 0.22 Mg, 10.50 P, 0.32 S, 20.99 Ca, 0.01 Zn

Tissue-equivalent gas (methane-based): 10.19 H, 45.61 C, 3.52 N, 40.68 O

Tissue-equivalent gas (propane-based): 10.27 H, 56.89 C, 3.50 N, 29.34 O

Tissue-equivalent liquid (without sucrose): 10.20 H, 12.01 C, 3.54 N, 74.25 O

Air, dry: 0.0124 C, 75.5267 N, 23.1781 O, 1.2827 Ar

Borosilicate glass (Pyrex): 4.01 B, 53.96 O, 2.82 Na, 1.16 Al, 37.72 Si, 0.33 K

[a]After Berger and Seltzer (1983), Table 5.5. In percent by weight.

OUTPUT DATA

1 HYDROGEN 3   HALF LIFE = 12.3 YEARS

DECAY MODE- BETA MINUS

RADIATION	MEAN NUMBER/ DISINTE- GRATION n_i	MEAN ENERGY/ PAR- TICLE $\bar{E}_i$ (MeV)	EQUI- LIBRIUM DOSE CONSTANT Δ_i (g-rad/ μCi-h)
BETA MINUS 1	1.0000	0.0057	0.0121

OUTPUT DATA

8 OXYGEN 15   HALF LIFE = 124. SECONDS

DECAY MODE- BETA PLUS

RADIATION	MEAN NUMBER/ DISINTE- GRATION n_i	MEAN ENERGY/ PAR- TICLE $\bar{E}_i$ (MeV)	EQUI- LIBRIUM DOSE CONSTANT Δ_i (g-rad/ μCi-h)
BETA PLUS 1	1.0000	0.7206	1.5349
ANNIH. RADIATION	2.0000	0.5110	2.1768

OUTPUT DATA

6 CARBON 11   HALF LIFE = 20.3 MINUTES

DECAY MODE- BETA PLUS

RADIATION	MEAN NUMBER/ DISINTE- GRATION n_i	MEAN ENERGY/ PAR- TICLE $\bar{E}_i$ (MeV)	EQUI- LIBRIUM DOSE CONSTANT Δ_i (g-rad/ μCi-h)
BETA PLUS 1	0.9980	0.3942	0.8380
ANNIH. RADIATION	1.9960	0.5110	2.1725

OUTPUT DATA

9 FLUORINE 18   HALF LIFE = 109. MINUTES

DECAY MODES- ELECTRON CAPTURE AND BETA PLUS

RADIATION	MEAN NUMBER/ DISINTE- GRATION n_i	MEAN ENERGY/ PAR- TICLE $\bar{E}_i$ (MeV)	EQUI- LIBRIUM DOSE CONSTANT Δ_i (g-rad/ μCi-h)
BETA PLUS 1	0.9700	0.2496	0.5157
ANNIH. RADIATION	1.9400	0.5110	2.1115

OUTPUT DATA

6 CARBON 14   HALF LIFE = 5730. YEARS

DECAY MODE- BETA MINUS

RADIATION	MEAN NUMBER/ DISINTE- GRATION n_i	MEAN ENERGY/ PAR- TICLE $\bar{E}_i$ (MeV)	EQUI- LIBRIUM DOSE CONSTANT Δ_i (g-rad/ μCi-h)
BETA MINUS 1	1.0000	0.0493	0.1050

OUTPUT DATA

11 SODIUM 22   HALF LIFE = 2.60 YEARS

DECAY MODES- ELECTRON CAPTURE AND BETA PLUS

RADIATION	MEAN NUMBER/ DISINTE- GRATION n_i	MEAN ENERGY/ PAR- TICLE $\bar{E}_i$ (MeV)	EQUI- LIBRIUM DOSE CONSTANT Δ_i (g-rad/ μCi-h)
GAMMA 1	0.9999	1.2746	2.7148
KLL AUGER ELECT	0.0753	0.0008	0.0001
BETA PLUS 1	0.9060	0.2157	0.4163
BETA PLUS 2	0.0006	0.8356	0.0010
ANNIH. RADIATION	1.8132	0.5110	1.9735

OUTPUT DATA

7 NITROGEN 13   HALF LIFE = 10.0 MINUTES

DECAY MODE- BETA PLUS

RADIATION	MEAN NUMBER/ DISINTE- GRATION n_i	MEAN ENERGY/ PAR- TICLE $\bar{E}_i$ (MeV)	EQUI- LIBRIUM DOSE CONSTANT Δ_i (g-rad/ μCi-h)
BETA PLUS 1	1.0000	0.4880	1.0395
ANNIH. RADIATION	2.0000	0.5110	2.1768

OUTPUT DATA

11 SODIUM 24   HALF LIFE = 15.0 HOURS

DECAY MODE- BETA MINUS

RADIATION	MEAN NUMBER/ DISINTE- GRATION n_i	MEAN ENERGY/ PAR- TICLE $\bar{E}_i$ (MeV)	EQUI- LIBRIUM DOSE CONSTANT Δ_i (g-rad/ μCi-h)
BETA MINUS 2	0.9992	0.5547	1.1805
GAMMA 1	0.9999	1.3685	2.9149
GAMMA 2	0.9991	2.7539	5.8610
GAMMA 3	0.0008	3.8595	0.0065

533

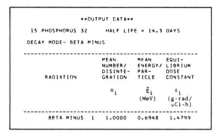

```
            ••OUTPUT DATA••

    15 PHOSPHORUS 32     HALF LIFE = 14.3 DAYS

    DECAY MODE- BETA MINUS

    ------------------------------------------
                      MEAN    MEAN    EQUI-
                      NUMBER/ ENERGY/ LIBRIUM
                      DISINTE- PAR-   DOSE
         RADIATION    GRATION TICLE   CONSTANT

                       n_i     Ē_i      Δ_i
                              (MeV)   (g-rad/
                                      µCi-h)
    ------------------------------------------
       BETA MINUS  1  1.0000  0.6948  1.4799
```

```
            ••OUTPUT DATA••

    20 CALCIUM 45      HALF LIFE = 163. DAYS

    DECAY MODE- BETA MINUS

    ------------------------------------------
                      MEAN    MEAN    EQUI-
                      NUMBER/ ENERGY/ LIBRIUM
                      DISINTE- PAR-   DOSE
         RADIATION    GRATION TICLE   CONSTANT

                       n_i     Ē_i      Δ_i
                              (MeV)   (g-rad/
                                      µCi-h)
    ------------------------------------------
       BETA MINUS  1  0.9999  0.0772  0.1645
```

```
            ••OUTPUT DATA••

    16 SULPHUR 35      HALF LIFE = 87.0 DAYS

    DECAY MODE- BETA MINUS

    ------------------------------------------
                      MEAN    MEAN    EQUI-
                      NUMBER/ ENERGY/ LIBRIUM
                      DISINTE- PAR-   DOSE
         RADIATION    GRATION TICLE   CONSTANT

                       n_i     Ē_i      Δ_i
                              (MeV)   (g-rad/
                                      µCi-h)
    ------------------------------------------
       BETA MINUS  1  1.0000  0.0488  0.1039
```

```
            ••OUTPUT DATA••

    24 CHROMIUM 51     HALF LIFE = 27.7 DAYS

    DECAY MODE- ELECTRON CAPTURE

    ------------------------------------------
                      MEAN    MEAN    EQUI-
                      NUMBER/ ENERGY/ LIBRIUM
                      DISINTE- PAR-   DOSE
         RADIATION    GRATION TICLE   CONSTANT

                       n_i     Ē_i      Δ_i
                              (MeV)   (g-rad/
                                      µCi-h)
    ------------------------------------------
              GAMMA  1  0.1018  0.3200  0.0694
    K ALPHA-1 X-RAY   0.1289  0.0049  0.0013
    K ALPHA-2 X-RAY   0.0659  0.0049  0.0006
      K BETA-1 X-RAY  0.0224  0.0054  0.0002
     KLL AUGER ELECT  0.5614  0.0044  0.0052
     KLX AUGER ELECT  0.1240  0.0048  0.0012
     LMM AUGER ELECT  1.5323  0.0004  0.0014
     MXY AUGER ELECT  3.2177  0.0000  0.0002
```

```
            ••OUTPUT DATA••

    18 ARGON 37       HALF LIFE = 34.8 DAYS

    DECAY MODE- ELECTRON CAPTURE

    ------------------------------------------
                      MEAN    MEAN    EQUI-
                      NUMBER/ ENERGY/ LIBRIUM
                      DISINTE- PAR-   DOSE
         RADIATION    GRATION TICLE   CONSTANT

                       n_i     Ē_i      Δ_i
                              (MeV)   (g-rad/
                                      µCi-h)
    ------------------------------------------
    K ALPHA-1 X-RAY   0.1044  0.0026  0.0005
     KLL AUGER ELECT  0.6865  0.0024  0.0035
     KLX AUGER ELECT  0.1174  0.0026  0.0006
     LMM AUGER ELECT  1.6837  0.0001  0.0006
```

```
            ••OUTPUT DATA••

    26 IRON 55        HALF LIFE = 2.70 YEARS

    DECAY MODE- ELECTRON CAPTURE

    ------------------------------------------
                      MEAN    MEAN    EQUI-
                      NUMBER/ ENERGY/ LIBRIUM
                      DISINTE- PAR-   DOSE
         RADIATION    GRATION TICLE   CONSTANT

                       n_i     Ē_i      Δ_i
                              (MeV)   (g-rad/
                                      µCi-h)
    ------------------------------------------
    K ALPHA-1 X-RAY   0.1553  0.0058  0.0019
    K ALPHA-2 X-RAY   0.0786  0.0058  0.0009
      K BETA-1 X-RAY  0.0257  0.0064  0.0003
     KLL AUGER ELECT  0.5151  0.0052  0.0057
     KLX AUGER ELECT  0.1220  0.0058  0.0015
     LMM AUGER ELECT  1.4807  0.0005  0.0017
     MXY AUGER ELECT  3.1174  0.0000  0.0003
```

```
            ••OUTPUT DATA••

    19 POTASSIUM 40      HALF LIFE = 1270. MEGAYEAR

    DECAY MODES- BETA MINUS AND ELECTRON CAPTURE

    ------------------------------------------
                      MEAN    MEAN    EQUI-
                      NUMBER/ ENERGY/ LIBRIUM
                      DISINTE- PAR-   DOSE
         RADIATION    GRATION TICLE   CONSTANT

                       n_i     Ē_i      Δ_i
                              (MeV)   (g-rad/
                                      µCi-h)
    ------------------------------------------
       BETA MINUS  1  0.8951  0.5555  1.0591
           GAMMA  1  0.1032  1.4609  0.3214
     KLL AUGER ELECT  0.0606  0.0026  0.0003
```

OUTPUT DATA

26 IRON 59   HALF LIFE = 45.0 DAYS

DECAY MODE- BETA MINUS

RADIATION		n_i MEAN NUMBER/ DISINTE- GRATION	$\bar{E}_i$ MEAN ENERGY/ PAR- TICLE (MeV)	Δ_i EQUI- LIBRIUM DOSE CONSTANT (g-rad/ μCi-h)
BETA MINUS	2	0.0122	0.0381	0.0009
BETA MINUS	3	0.4609	0.0808	0.0793
BETA MINUS	4	0.5228	0.1496	0.1666
BETA MINUS	5	0.0030	0.6396	0.0040
GAMMA	1	0.0096	0.1420	0.0029
GAMMA	2	0.0292	0.1922	0.0119
GAMMA	3	0.0023	0.3347	0.0017
GAMMA	4	0.0002	0.3810	0.0001
GAMMA	5	0.5548	1.0990	1.2987
K INT CON ELECT		0.0000	1.0912	0.0002
GAMMA	6	0.4411	1.2920	1.2140
K INT CON ELECT		0.0000	1.2842	0.0001
GAMMA	7	0.0009	1.4810	0.0028

OUTPUT DATA

27 COBALT 60   HALF LIFE = 5.26 YEARS

DECAY MODE- BETA MINUS

RADIATION		n_i MEAN NUMBER/ DISINTE- GRATION	$\bar{E}_i$ MEAN ENERGY/ PAR- TICLE (MeV)	Δ_i EQUI- LIBRIUM DOSE CONSTANT (g-rad/ μCi-h)
BETA MINUS	1	0.9980	0.0941	0.2000
BETA MINUS	2	0.0012	0.6243	0.0015
GAMMA	1	0.9978	1.1732	2.4935
K INT CON ELECT		0.0001	1.1648	0.0004
GAMMA	2	0.9998	1.3324	2.8378
K INT CON ELECT		0.0001	1.3241	0.0003

OUTPUT DATA

37 RUBIDIUM 86   HALF LIFE = 18.6 DAYS

DECAY MODE- BETA MINUS

RADIATION		n_i MEAN NUMBER/ DISINTE- GRATION	$\bar{E}_i$ MEAN ENERGY/ PAR- TICLE (MeV)	Δ_i EQUI- LIBRIUM DOSE CONSTANT (g-rad/ μCi-h)
BETA MINUS	1	0.0876	0.2304	0.0429
BETA MINUS	2	0.9124	0.7095	1.3789
GAMMA	1	0.0875	1.0766	0.2007

OUTPUT DATA

38 STRONTIUM 90   HALF LIFE = 28.1 YEARS

DECAY MODE- BETA MINUS

RADIATION		n_i MEAN NUMBER/ DISINTE- GRATION	$\bar{E}_i$ MEAN ENERGY/ PAR- TICLE (MeV)	Δ_i EQUI- LIBRIUM DOSE CONSTANT (g-rad/ μCi-h)
BETA MINUS	1	1.0000	0.1961	0.4177

DAUGHTER NUCLIDE, YTTRIUM 90 IS RADIOACTIVE
AND MAY CONTRIBUTE TO THE DOSE.

OUTPUT DATA

39 YTTRIUM 90   HALF LIFE = 64.0 HOURS

DECAY MODE- BETA MINUS

RADIATION		n_i MEAN NUMBER/ DISINTE- GRATION	$\bar{E}_i$ MEAN ENERGY/ PAR- TICLE (MeV)	Δ_i EQUI- LIBRIUM DOSE CONSTANT (g-rad/ μCi-h)
BETA MINUS	1	0.9998	0.9314	1.9836

OUTPUT DATA

43 TECHNETIUM 99M   HALF LIFE = 6.03 HOURS

DECAY MODE- ISOMERIC LEVEL

RADIATION		n_i MEAN NUMBER/ DISINTE- GRATION	$\bar{E}_i$ MEAN ENERGY/ PAR- TICLE (MeV)	Δ_i EQUI- LIBRIUM DOSE CONSTANT (g-rad/ μCi-h)
GAMMA	1	0.0000	0.0021	0.0000
M INT CON ELECT		0.9860	0.0016	0.0035
GAMMA	2	0.8787	0.1405	0.2630
K INT CON ELECT		0.0913	0.1194	0.0232
L INT CON ELECT		0.0118	0.1377	0.0034
M INT CON ELECT		0.0039	0.1400	0.0011
GAMMA	3	0.0003	0.1426	0.0001
K INT CON ELECT		0.0088	0.1215	0.0022
L INT CON ELECT		0.0035	0.1398	0.0010
M INT CON ELECT		0.0011	0.1422	0.0003
K ALPHA-1 X-RAY		0.0441	0.0183	0.0017
K ALPHA-2 X-RAY		0.0221	0.0182	0.0008
K BETA-1 X-RAY		0.0105	0.0206	0.0004
KLL AUGER ELECT		0.0152	0.0154	0.0005
KLX AUGER ELECT		0.0055	0.0178	0.0002
LMM AUGER ELECT		0.1093	0.0019	0.0004
MXY AUGER ELECT		1.2359	0.0004	0.0011

OUTPUT DATA

53 IODINE 125   HALF LIFE = 60.2 DAYS

DECAY MODE- ELECTRON CAPTURE

RADIATION	MEAN NUMBER/ DISINTE- GRATION n_i	MEAN ENERGY/ PAR- TICLE $\bar{E}_i$ (MeV)	EQUI- LIBRIUM DOSE CONSTANT Δ_i (g-rad/ μCi-h)
GAMMA 1	0.0666	0.0354	0.0050
K INT CON ELECT	0.8000	0.0036	0.0062
L INT CON ELECT	0.1142	0.0309	0.0075
M INT CON ELECT	0.0190	0.0346	0.0014
K ALPHA-1 X-RAY	0.7615	0.0274	0.0445
K ALPHA-2 X-RAY	0.3906	0.0272	0.0226
K BETA-1 X-RAY	0.2056	0.0309	0.0135
K BETA-2 X-RAY	0.0426	0.0318	0.0028
L X-RAYS	0.2226	0.0037	0.0017
KLL AUGER ELECT	0.1416	0.0226	0.0068
KLX AUGER ELECT	0.0597	0.0264	0.0033
KXY AUGER ELECT	0.0096	0.0301	0.0006
LMM AUGER ELECT	1.5442	0.0029	0.0096
MXY AUGER ELECT	3.6461	0.0008	0.0063

OUTPUT DATA

56 BARIUM 137M   HALF LIFE = 2.55 MINUTES

DECAY MODE- ISOMERIC LEVEL

RADIATION	MEAN NUMBER/ DISINTE- GRATION n_i	MEAN ENERGY/ PAR- TICLE $\bar{E}_i$ (MeV)	EQUI- LIBRIUM DOSE CONSTANT Δ_i (g-rad/ μCi-h)
GAMMA 1	0.8981	0.6616	1.2658
K INT CON ELECT	0.0820	0.6241	0.1091
L INT CON ELECT	0.0147	0.6560	0.0206
M INT CON ELECT	0.0049	0.6605	0.0069
K ALPHA-1 X-RAY	0.0392	0.0321	0.0026
K ALPHA-2 X-RAY	0.0203	0.0318	0.0013
K BETA-1 X-RAY	0.0110	0.0363	0.0008
K BETA-2 X-RAY	0.0023	0.0374	0.0001
L X-RAYS	0.0133	0.0044	0.0001
KLL AUGER ELECT	0.0059	0.0263	0.0003
KLX AUGER ELECT	0.0026	0.0308	0.0001
LMM AUGER ELECT	0.0756	0.0034	0.0005
MXY AUGER ELECT	0.1841	0.0010	0.0004

OUTPUT DATA

55 CESIUM 137   HALF LIFE = 30.0 YEARS

DECAY MODE- BETA MINUS

RADIATION	MEAN NUMBER/ DISINTE- GRATION n_i	MEAN ENERGY/ PAR- TICLE $\bar{E}_i$ (MeV)	EQUI- LIBRIUM DOSE CONSTANT Δ_i (g-rad/ μCi-h)
BETA MINUS 1	0.9460	0.1747	0.3520
BETA MINUS 2	0.0540	0.4269	0.0491

DAUGHTER NUCLIDE, BARIUM 137M IS RADIOACTIVE
AND MAY CONTRIBUTE TO THE DOSE.
BRANCHING TO 0.6616 MEV, 2.55 MINUTE HALF LIFE,
ISOMERIC LEVEL IN BARIUM-137 IS 0.946 PER
DISINTEGRATION OF CESIUM-137.

OUTPUT DATA

79 GOLD 198   HALF LIFE = 2.69 DAYS

DECAY MODE- BETA MINUS

RADIATION	MEAN NUMBER/ DISINTE- GRATION n_i	MEAN ENERGY/ PAR- TICLE $\bar{E}_i$ (MeV)	EQUI- LIBRIUM DOSE CONSTANT Δ_i (g-rad/ μCi-h)
BETA MINUS 1	0.0130	0.0811	0.0022
BETA MINUS 2	0.9860	0.3163	0.6643
BETA MINUS 3	0.0002	0.4648	0.0002
GAMMA 1	0.9555	0.4117	0.8380
K INT CON ELECT	0.0287	0.3286	0.0201
L INT CON ELECT	0.0095	0.3979	0.0081
M INT CON ELECT	0.0031	0.4089	0.0027
GAMMA 2	0.0107	0.6758	0.0154
K INT CON ELECT	0.0002	0.5927	0.0003
GAMMA 3	0.0022	1.0876	0.0053
K ALPHA-1 X-RAY	0.0139	0.0708	0.0021
K ALPHA-2 X-RAY	0.0076	0.0688	0.0011
K BETA-1 X-RAY	0.0048	0.0802	0.0008
K BETA-2 X-RAY	0.0013	0.0831	0.0002
L ALPHA X-RAYS	0.0060	0.0099	0.0001
L BETA X-RAYS	0.0056	0.0118	0.0001
LMM AUGER ELECT	0.0206	0.0081	0.0003
MXY AUGER ELECT	0.0622	0.0028	0.0003

[a] After Dillman and Von der Lage, 1975. Reproduced with permission from L. T. Dillman and the Society of Nuclear Medicine.

APPENDIX D.1 Klein–Nishina Interaction Cross Sections for Free Electrons[a]

$h\nu$ (keV)	${}_e\sigma$ (cm^2/e)	${}_e\sigma_{sc}$ (cm^2/e)	${}_e\sigma_{tr}$ (cm^2/e)
1.0	0.6627 −24	0.6614 −24	0.1291 −26
1.5	0.6614 −24	0.6594 −24	0.1929 −26
2.0	0.6601 −24	0.6575 −24	0.2561 −26
3.0	0.6576 −24	0.6537 −24	0.3811 −26
4.0	0.6550 −24	0.6500 −24	0.5041 −26
5.0	0.6525 −24	0.6463 −24	0.6251 −26
6.0	0.6501 −24	0.6426 −24	0.7441 −26
8.0	0.6452 −24	0.6355 −24	0.9766 −26
10.0	0.6405 −24	0.6285 −24	0.1202 −25
15.0	0.6290 −24	0.6116 −24	0.1735 −25
20.0	0.6180 −24	0.5957 −24	0.2228 −25
30.0	0.5975 −24	0.5664 −24	0.3109 −25
40.0	0.5787 −24	0.5400 −24	0.3871 −25
50.0	0.5615 −24	0.5162 −24	0.4532 −25
60.0	0.5456 −24	0.4945 −24	0.5109 −25
80.0	0.5173 −24	0.4567 −24	0.6059 −25
100.0	0.4927 −24	0.4247 −24	0.6800 −25
150.0	0.4436 −24	0.3631 −24	0.8054 −25
200.0	0.4065 −24	0.3185 −24	0.8794 −25
300.0	0.3535 −24	0.2581 −24	0.9531 −25
400.0	0.3167 −24	0.2186 −24	0.9805 −25
500.0	0.2892 −24	0.1905 −24	0.9871 −25
600.0	0.2675 −24	0.1692 −24	0.9831 −25
662.0	0.2561 −24	0.1584 −24	0.9775 −25
800.0	0.2350 −24	0.1389 −24	0.9602 −25
(MeV)			
1.0	0.2112 −24	0.1183 −24	0.9294 −25
1.25	0.1888 −24	0.9997 −25	0.8885 −25
1.5	0.1716 −24	0.8670 −25	0.8488 −25
2.0	0.1464 −24	0.6867 −25	0.7769 −25
3.0	0.1151 −24	0.4865 −25	0.6644 −25
4.0	0.9597 −25	0.3772 −25	0.5825 −25
5.0	0.8287 −25	0.3083 −25	0.5204 −25
6.0	0.7323 −25	0.2607 −25	0.4716 −25
8.0	0.5988 −25	0.1993 −25	0.3995 −25
10.0	0.5099 −25	0.1613 −25	0.3485 −25
15.0	0.3771 −25	0.1094 −25	0.2678 −25
20.0	0.3025 −25	0.8271 −26	0.2198 −25
30.0	0.2200 −25	0.5563 −26	0.1644 −25
40.0	0.1746 −25	0.4191 −26	0.1327 −25
50.0	0.1457 −25	0.3362 −26	0.1121 −25
60.0	0.1254 −25	0.2807 −26	0.9736 −26
80.0	0.9882 −26	0.2110 −26	0.7772 −26
100.0	0.8199 −26	0.1690 −26	0.6508 −26

[a]Table provided by Patrick D. Higgins, personal communication, 1986.

APPENDIX D.2. Photon Interaction Cross Sections in Units of 10^{-24} cm^2/atom^a

Hydrogen, Z = 1
Multiply data by 0.5975 to get cm^2/g
or by 0.05975 to get m^2/kg

Photon Energy (MeV)	Compton With and Without Coherent		Photoelectric	Nuclear and Electron Pair		Total With and Without Coherent	
	$_a\sigma + _a\sigma_R$	$_a\sigma$	$_a\tau$	$_a\kappa_{nuc}$	$_a\kappa_{elec}$	$_a\mu$	$_a\mu - _a\sigma_R$
1.00 −02	6.40 −01		4.57 −03	—	—	6.45 −01	
1.50 −02	6.29 −01		1.13 −03	—	—	6.30 −01	
2.00 −02	6.18 −01		4.19 −04	—	—	6.18 −01	
3.00 −02	5.97 −01		1.03 −04	—	—	5.98 −01	
4.00 −02	5.79 −01		3.84 −05	—	—	5.79 −01	
5.00 −02	5.61 −01		1.78 −05	—	—	5.61 −01	
6.00 −02	5.46 −01		9.51 −06	—	—	5.46 −01	
8.00 −02	5.17 −01		3.55 −06	—	—	5.17 −01	
1.00 −01	4.93 −01		1.66 −06	—	—	4.93 −01	
1.50 −01	4.44 −01		4.23 −07	—	—	4.44 −01	
2.00 −01	4.06 −01		1.64 −07	—	—	4.06 −01	
3.00 −01	3.53 −01		4.51 −08	—	—	3.53 −01	
4.00 −01	3.17 −01		1.91 −08	—	—	3.17 −01	
5.00 −01	2.89 −01		1.02 −08	—	—	2.89 −01	
6.00 −01	2.67 −01		6.35 −09	—	—	2.68 −01	
8.00 −01	2.35 −01		3.20 −09	—	—	2.35 −01	

1.00 +00	2.11 −01	1.99 −09	—	—	2.11 −01
1.50 +00	1.72 −01	9.25 −10	4.43 −05	—	1.72 −01
2.00 +00	1.46 −01	5.90 −10	1.77 −04	—	1.46 −01
3.00 +00	1.15 −01	3.32 −10	5.11 −04	4.02 −05	1.16 −01
4.00 +00	9.62 −02	2.28 −10	8.30 −04	1.65 −04	9.72 −02
5.00 +00	8.31 −02	1.75 −10	1.11 −03	3.25 −04	8.45 −02
6.00 +00	7.34 −02	1.40 −10	1.36 −03	4.99 −04	7.53 −02
8.00 +00	6.01 −02	1.00 −10	1.79 −03	8.54 −04	6.27 −02
1.00 +01	5.11 −02	7.89 −11	2.14 −03	1.17 −03	5.45 −02
1.50 +01	3.79 −02	—	2.79 −03	1.82 −03	4.25 −02
2.00 +01	3.04 −02	—	3.28 −03	2.33 −03	3.60 −02
3.00 +01	2.21 −02	—	3.97 −03	3.11 −03	2.92 −02
4.00 +01	1.76 −02	—	4.46 −03	3.68 −03	2.57 −02
5.00 +01	1.47 −02	—	4.85 −03	4.14 −03	2.37 −02
6.00 +01	1.26 −02	—	5.17 −03	4.51 −03	2.23 −02
8.00 +01	9.97 −03	—	5.66 −03	5.10 −03	2.07 −02
1.00 +02	8.28 −03	—	6.04 −03	5.56 −03	1.99 −02

[a] Data excerpted from tables by Hubbell, NSRDS-NBS 29, 1969. Reproduced with permission from J. H. Hubbell.

APPENDIX D.2. (*Continued*)

Carbon, Z = 6

Multiply data by 0.05014 to get cm²/g
or by 0.005014 to get m²/kg

Photon Energy (MeV)	Compton With and Without Coherent		Photoelectric	Nuclear and Electron Pair		Total With and Without Coherent	
	$_a\sigma + {_a\sigma_R}$	$_a\sigma$	$_a\tau$	$_a\kappa_{nuc}$	$_a\kappa_{elec}$	$_a\mu$	$_a\mu - {_a\sigma_R}$
1.00 −02	6.11 +00	3.84 +00	3.93 +01	—	—	4.54 +01	4.31 +01
1.50 −02	5.06 +00	3.77 +00	1.06 +01	—	—	1.57 +01	1.44 +01
2.00 −02	4.53 +00	3.71 +00	4.01 +00	—	—	8.54 +00	7.72 +00
3.00 −02	4.00 +00	3.58 +00	9.99 −01	—	—	5.00 +00	4.58 +00
4.00 −02	3.73 +00	3.47 +00	3.79 −01	—	—	4.10 +00	3.85 +00
5.00 −02	3.54 +00	3.37 +00	1.93 −01	—	—	3.73 +00	3.56 +00
6.00 −02	3.39 +00	3.27 +00	1.15 −01	—	—	3.51 +00	3.39 +00
8.00 −02	3.17 +00	3.10 +00	4.50 −02	—	—	3.21 +00	3.15 +00
1.00 −01	3.00 +00	2.96 +00	2.16 −02	—	—	3.02 +00	2.98 +00
1.50 −01	2.69 +00	2.66 +00	5.75 −03	—	—	2.69 +00	2.67 +00
2.00 −01	2.45 +00	2.44 +00	2.29 −03	—	—	2.45 +00	2.44 +00
3.00 −01	2.13 +00	2.12 +00	6.46 −04	—	—	2.13 +00	2.12 +00
4.00 −01	1.90 +00	1.90 +00	2.77 −04	—	—	1.91 +00	1.90 +00
5.00 −01	1.74 +00		1.49 −04	—	—	1.74 +00	
6.00 −01	1.61 +00		9.27 −05	—	—	1.61 +00	
8.00 −01	1.41 +00		4.68 −05	—	—	1.41 +00	

1.00 +00	1.27 +00	2.89 −05	—	—	1.27 +00
1.50 +00	1.03 +00	1.35 −05	1.60 −03	—	1.03 +00
2.00 +00	8.79 −01	8.61 −06	6.40 −03	—	8.86 −01
3.00 +00	6.92 −01	4.82 −06	1.84 −02	2.41 −04	7.11 −01
4.00 +00	5.77 −01	3.29 −06	2.98 −02	9.91 −04	6.08 −01
5.00 +00	4.98 −01	2.52 −06	4.00 −02	1.95 −03	5.40 −01
6.00 +00	4.40 −01	2.01 −06	4.90 −02	3.00 −03	4.93 −01
8.00 +00	3.60 −01	1.44 −06	6.42 −02	5.12 −03	4.30 −01
1.00 +01	3.07 −01	1.12 −06	7.66 −02	7.01 −03	3.90 −01
1.50 +01	2.27 −01	—	1.00 −01	1.09 −02	3.38 −01
2.00 +01	1.82 −01	—	1.17 −01	1.40 −02	3.14 −01
3.00 +01	1.33 −01	—	1.41 −01	1.87 −02	2.93 −01
4.00 +01	1.05 −01	—	1.58 −01	2.21 −02	2.86 −01
5.00 +01	8.80 −02	—	1.71 −01	2.48 −02	2.84 −01
6.00 +01	7.59 −02	—	1.81 −01	2.71 −02	2.84 −01
8.00 +01	5.98 −02	—	1.96 −01	3.06 −02	2.86 −01
1.00 +02	4.97 −02	—	2.07 −01	3.31 −02	2.90 −01

APPENDIX D.2.   (*Continued*)

Nitrogen, Z = 7

Multiply data by 0.04300 to get cm^2/g
or by 0.004300 to get m^2/kg

Photon Energy (MeV)	Compton With and Without Coherent		Photoelectric	Nuclear and Electron Pair		Total With and Without Coherent	
	$_a\sigma + _a\sigma_R$	$_a\sigma$	$_a\tau$	$_a\kappa_{nuc}$	$_a\kappa_{elec}$	$_a\mu$	$_a\mu - _a\sigma_R$
1.00 −02	8.03 +00	4.48 +00	7.86 +01	—	—	8.66 +01	8.31 +01
1.50 −02	6.38 +00	4.40 +00	2.10 +01	—	—	2.74 +01	2.54 +01
2.00 −02	5.60 +00	4.33 +00	8.26 +00	—	—	1.39 +01	1.26 +01
3.00 −02	4.83 +00	4.18 +00	2.23 +00	—	—	7.06 +00	6.41 +00
4.00 −02	4.44 +00	4.05 +00	8.78 −01	—	—	5.31 +00	4.93 +00
5.00 −02	4.18 +00	3.93 +00	4.25 −01	—	—	4.61 +00	4.35 +00
6.00 −02	4.00 +00	3.82 +00	2.38 −01	—	—	4.24 +00	4.06 +00
8.00 −02	3.73 +00	3.62 +00	9.40 −02	—	—	3.82 +00	3.72 +00
1.00 −01	3.52 +00	3.45 +00	4.54 −02	—	—	3.56 +00	3.49 +00
1.50 −01	3.13 +00	3.11 +00	1.22 −02	—	—	3.15 +00	3.12 +00
2.00 −01	2.86 +00	2.85 +00	4.85 −03	—	—	2.86 +00	2.85 +00
3.00 −01	2.48 +00	2.48 +00	1.38 −03	—	—	2.49 +00	2.48 +00
4.00 −01	2.22 +00		5.89 −04	—	—	2.22 +00	2.22 +00
5.00 −01	2.03 +00		3.16 −04	—	—	2.03 +00	2.03 +00
6.00 −01	1.87 +00		1.97 −04	—	—	1.87 +00	1.87 +00
8.00 −01	1.65 +00		9.94 −05	—	—	1.65 +00	1.65 +00

1.00 +00	1.48 +00	6.15 −05	—	—	1.48 +00
1.50 +00	1.20 +00	2.88 −05	2.19 −03	—	1.21 +00
2.00 +00	1.03 +00	1.84 −05	8.71 −03	—	1.03 +00
3.00 +00	8.07 −01	1.03 −05	2.50 −02	2.82 −04	8.33 −01
4.00 +00	6.73 −01	6.99 −06	4.06 −02	1.16 −03	7.15 −01
5.00 +00	5.81 −01	5.36 −06	5.44 −02	2.27 −03	6.38 −01
6.00 +00	5.14 −01	4.27 −06	6.67 −02	3.50 −03	5.84 −01
8.00 +00	4.20 −01	3.06 −06	8.73 −02	5.98 −03	5.14 −01
1.00 +01	3.58 −01	2.39 −06	1.04 −01	8.17 −03	4.70 −01
1.50 +01	2.65 −01	—	1.36 −01	1.27 −02	4.14 −01
2.00 +01	2.13 −01	—	1.59 −01	1.63 −02	3.88 −01
3.00 +01	1.55 −01	—	1.92 −01	2.18 −02	3.68 −01
4.00 +01	1.23 −01	—	2.14 −01	2.58 −02	3.63 −01
5.00 +01	1.03 −01	—	2.32 −01	2.90 −02	3.63 −01
6.00 +01	8.85 −02	—	2.45 −01	3.16 −02	3.65 −01
8.00 +01	6.98 −02	—	2.66 −01	3.56 −02	3.71 −01
1.00 +02	5.97 −02	—	2.81 −01	3.85 −02	3.79 −01

APPENDIX D.2. (Continued)

Oxygen, Z = 8
Multiply by 0.03764 to get cm²/g
or by 0.003764 to get m²/kg

Photon Energy (MeV)	Compton With and Without Coherent		Photoelectric	Nuclear and Electron Pair		Total With and Without Coherent	
	$_a\sigma + {}_a\sigma_R$	$_a\sigma$	$_a\tau$	$_a\kappa_{nuc}$	$_a\kappa_{elec}$	$_a\mu$	$_a\mu - {}_a\sigma_R$
1.00 −02	1.06 +01	5.12 +00	1.43 +02	—	—	1.54 +02	1.48 +02
1.50 −02	8.00 +00	5.03 +00	3.81 +01	—	—	4.61 +01	4.31 +01
2.00 −02	6.84 +00	4.94 +00	1.51 +01	—	—	2.19 +01	2.00 +01
3.00 −02	5.74 +00	4.78 +00	4.13 +00	—	—	9.87 +00	8.91 +00
4.00 −02	5.20 +00	4.63 +00	1.64 +00	—	—	6.84 +00	6.27 +00
5.00 −02	4.87 +00	4.49 +00	8.00 −01	—	—	5.67 +00	5.29 +00
6.00 −02	4.63 +00	4.36 +00	4.48 −01	—	—	5.08 +00	4.81 +00
8.00 −02	4.29 +00	4.14 +00	1.78 −01	—	—	4.47 +00	4.32 +00
1.00 −01	4.05 +00	3.94 +00	8.54 −02	—	—	4.13 +00	4.03 +00
1.50 −01	3.60 +00	3.55 +00	2.32 −02	—	—	3.62 +00	3.57 +00
2.00 −01	3.27 +00	3.25 +00	9.30 −03	—	—	3.28 +00	3.26 +00
3.00 −01	2.84 +00	2.83 +00	2.65 −03	—	—	2.84 +00	2.83 +00
4.00 −01	2.54 +00	2.53 +00	1.13 −03	—	—	2.54 +00	2.54 +00
5.00 −01	2.32 +00	2.31 +00	6.11 −04	—	—	2.32 +00	2.31 +00
6.00 −01	2.15 +00	2.14 +00	3.82 −04	—	—	2.15 +00	2.14 +00
8.00 −01	1.88 +00		1.92 −04	—	—		1.88 +00

1.00 +00	1.69 +00	1.19 −04	—	—	1.69 +00
1.50 +00	1.37 +00	5.57 −05	2.86 −03	—	1.38 +00
2.00 +00	1.17 +00	3.54 −05	1.14 −02	—	1.18 +00
3.00 +00	9.23 −01	1.98 −05	3.27 −02	3.22 −04	9.56 −01
4.00 +00	7.69 −01	1.35 −05	5.30 −02	1.32 −03	8.24 −01
5.00 +00	6.65 −01	1.03 −05	7.11 −02	2.60 −03	7.38 −01
6.00 +00	5.87 −01	8.22 −06	8.70 −02	3.99 −03	6.78 −01
8.00 +00	4.80 −01	5.88 −06	1.14 −01	6.83 −03	6.01 −01
1.00 +01	4.09 −01	4.61 −06	1.36 −01	9.34 −03	5.54 −01
1.50 +01	3.03 −01	—	1.77 −01	1.45 −02	4.95 −01
2.00 +01	2.43 −01	—	2.08 −01	1.87 −02	4.69 −01
3.00 +01	1.77 −01	—	2.50 −01	2.49 −02	4.52 −01
4.00 +01	1.41 −01	—	2.79 −01	2.95 −02	4.49 −01
5.00 +01	1.17 −01	—	3.01 −01	3.31 −02	4.52 −01
6.00 +01	1.01 −01	—	3.19 −01	3.61 −02	4.56 −01
8.00 +01	7.98 −02	—	3.46 −01	4.05 −02	4.66 −01
1.00 +02	6.62 −02	—	3.65 −01	4.39 −02	4.75 −01

APPENDIX D.2. *(Continued)*

Aluminum, Z = 13
Multiply by 0.02232 to get cm^2/g
or by 0.002232 to get m^2/kg

Photon Energy (MeV)	Compton With and Without Coherent		Photoelectric	Nuclear and Electron Pair		Total With and Without Coherent	
	$_a\sigma + _a\sigma_R$	$_a\sigma$	$_a\tau$	$_a\kappa_{nuc}$	$_a\kappa_{elec}$	$_a\mu$	$_a\mu - _a\sigma_R$
1.00 −02	3.04 +01	8.32 +00	1.15 +03	—	—	1.18 +03	1.16 +03
1.50 −02	2.03 +01	8.17 +00	3.35 +02	—	—	3.55 +02	3.43 +02
2.00 −02	1.57 +01	8.03 +00	1.37 +02	—	—	1.53 +02	1.45 +02
3.00 −02	1.17 +01	7.77 +00	3.85 +01	—	—	5.02 +01	4.63 +01
4.00 −02	9.89 +00	7.52 +00	1.55 +01	—	—	2.54 +01	2.30 +01
5.00 −02	8.88 +00	7.30 +00	7.65 +00	—	—	1.65 +01	1.49 +01
6.00 −02	8.22 +00	7.09 +00	4.33 +00	—	—	1.25 +01	1.14 +01
8.00 −02	7.38 +00	6.72 +00	1.73 +00	—	—	9.11 +00	8.45 +00
1.00 −01	6.83 +00	6.41 +00	8.45 −01	—	—	7.67 +00	7.25 +00
1.50 −01	5.96 +00	5.77 +00	2.33 −01	—	—	6.19 +00	6.00 +00
2.00 −01	5.39 +00	5.28 +00	9.53 −02	—	—	5.49 +00	5.38 +00
3.00 −01	4.64 +00	4.60 +00	2.76 −02	—	—	4.67 +00	4.62 +00
4.00 −01	4.14 +00	4.12 +00	1.19 −02	—	—	4.15 +00	4.13 +00
5.00 −01	3.78 +00	3.76 +00	6.43 −03	—	—	3.78 +00	3.77 +00
6.00 −01	3.49 +00	3.48 +00	4.02 −03	—	—	3.49 +00	3.48 +00
8.00 −01	3.06 +00	3.06 +00	2.04 −03	—	—	3.06 +00	3.06 +00

	2.75 +00	2.75 +00			2.75 +00
1.00 +00		1.26 −03	—	—	
1.50 +00	2.23 +00	5.89 −04	7.68 −03	—	2.24 +00
2.00 +00	1.91 +00	3.73 −04	3.03 −02	—	1.94 +00
3.00 +00	1.50 +00	2.07 −04	8.65 −02	5.23 −04	1.59 +00
4.00 +00	1.25 +00	1.41 −04	1.40 −01	2.15 −03	1.39 +00
5.00 +00	1.08 +00	1.07 −04	1.87 −01	4.22 −03	1.27 +00
6.00 +00	9.54 −01	8.53 −05	2.29 −01	6.49 −03	1.19 +00
8.00 +00	7.81 −01	6.09 −05	2.99 −01	1.11 −02	1.09 +00
1.00 +01	6.65 −01	4.76 −05	3.57 −01	1.52 −02	1.04 +00
1.50 +01	4.92 −01	—	4.65 −01	2.36 −02	9.80 −01
2.00 +01	3.95 −01	—	5.43 −01	3.03 −02	9.68 −01
3.00 +01	2.88 −01	—	6.52 −01	4.04 −02	9.81 −01
4.00 +01	2.29 −01	—	7.29 −01	4.79 −02	1.01 +00
5.00 +01	1.91 −01	—	7.86 −01	5.36 −02	1.03 +00
6.00 +01	1.64 −01	—	8.31 −01	5.81 −02	1.05 +00
8.00 +01	1.30 −01	—	8.98 −01	6.51 −02	1.09 +00
1.00 +02	1.08 −01	—	9.46 −01	7.03 −02	1.12 +00

APPENDIX D.2. (*Continued*)

Copper, Z = 29

Multiply by 0.009478 to get cm^2/g
or by 0.0009478 to get m^2/kg

Photon Energy (MeV)	Compton With and Without Coherent		Photoelectric	Nuclear and Electron Pair		Total With and Without Coherent	
	$_a\sigma + {}_a\sigma_R$	$_a\sigma$	$_a\tau$	$_a\kappa_{nuc}$	$_a\kappa_{elec}$	$_a\mu$	$_a\mu - {}_a\sigma_R$
1.00 −02	1.66 +02	1.86 +01	2.35 +04	—	—	2.37 +04	2.35 +04
1.50 −02	1.06 +02	1.82 +01	7.72 +03	—	—	7.83 +03	7.74 +03
2.00 −02	7.70 +01	1.79 +01	3.46 +03	—	—	3.54 +03	3.48 +03
3.00 −02	4.92 +01	1.73 +01	1.11 +03	—	—	1.15 +03	1.12 +03
4.00 −02	3.64 +01	1.68 +01	4.80 +02	—	—	5.16 +02	4.97 +02
5.00 −02	2.96 +01	1.63 +01	2.47 +02	—	—	2.77 +02	2.63 +02
6.00 −02	2.55 +01	1.58 +01	1.45 +02	—	—	1.71 +02	1.61 +02
8.00 −02	2.07 +01	1.50 +01	6.08 +01	—	—	8.14 +01	7.58 +01
1.00 −01	1.79 +01	1.43 +01	3.08 +01	—	—	4.87 +01	4.51 +01
1.50 −01	1.45 +01	1.29 +01	9.04 +00	—	—	2.36 +01	2.19 +01
2.00 −01	1.27 +01	1.18 +01	3.80 +00	—	—	1.65 +01	1.56 +01
3.00 −01	1.07 +01	1.02 +01	1.15 +00	—	—	1.18 +01	1.14 +01
4.00 −01	9.42 +00	9.19 +00	5.12 −01	—	—	9.93 +00	9.70 +00
5.00 −01	8.54 +00	8.39 +00	2.81 −01	—	—	8.82 +00	8.67 +00
6.00 −01	7.86 +00	7.76 +00	1.77 −01	—	—	8.04 +00	7.94 +00
8.00 −01	6.87 +00	6.82 +00	9.11 −02	—	—	6.96 +00	6.91 +00

1.00 +00	6.16 +00	6.13 +00	5.65 −02	—	—	6.22 +00	6.19 +00
1.50 +00	4.99 +00	4.98 +00	2.61 −02	4.23 −02	—	5.06 +00	5.05 +00
2.00 +00	4.25 +00	4.25 +00	1.63 −02	1.58 −01	—	4.43 +00	4.43 +00
3.00 +00	3.35 +00	3.34 +00	8.88 −03	4.38 −01	1.17 −03	3.79 +00	3.79 +00
4.00 +00	2.79 +00		5.96 −03	6.98 −01	4.79 −03	3.50 +00	
5.00 +00	2.41 +00		4.50 −03	9.28 −01	9.41 −03	3.35 +00	
6.00 +00	2.13 +00		3.56 −03	1.13 +00	1.45 −02	3.28 +00	
8.00 +00	1.74 +00		2.52 −03	1.46 +00	2.48 −02	3.23 +00	
1.00 +01	1.48 +00		1.95 −03	1.74 +00	3.39 −02	3.25 +00	
1.50 +01	1.10 +00		1.20 −03	2.25 +00	5.27 −02	3.41 +00	
2.00 +01	8.81 −01		9.00 −04	2.63 +00	6.77 −02	3.58 +00	
3.00 +01	6.41 −01		6.00 −04	3.15 +00	8.97 −02	3.89 +00	
4.00 +01	5.10 −01		4.00 −04	3.51 +00	1.05 −01	4.13 +00	
5.00 +01	4.25 −01		—	3.78 +00	1.17 −01	4.32 +00	
6.00 +01	3.67 −01		—	3.99 +00	1.26 −01	4.48 +00	
8.00 +01	2.89 −01		—	4.30 +00	1.41 −01	4.73 +00	
1.00 +02	2.40 −01		—	4.52 +00	1.51 −01	4.91 +00	

APPENDIX D.2. (*Continued*)

Tin, Z = 50

Multiply by 0.005074 to get cm²/g
or by 0.0005074 to get m²/kg

Photon Energy (MeV)	Compton With and Without Coherent		Photoelectric	Nuclear and Electron Pair		Total With and Without Coherent	
	$_a\sigma + _a\sigma_R$	$_a\sigma$	$_a\tau$	$_a\kappa_{nuc}$	$_a\kappa_{elec}$	$_a\mu$	$_a\mu - _a\sigma_R$
1.00 −02	5.38 +02	3.20 +01	2.73 +04	—	—	2.79 +04	2.74 +04
1.50 −02	3.60 +02	3.14 +01	8.91 +03	—	—	9.27 +03	8.94 +03
2.00 −02	2.59 +02	3.09 +01	3.95 +03	—	—	4.21 +03	3.98 +03
2.92 −02	1.61 +02	2.99 +01	1.33 +03	—	—	1.49 +03	1.36 +03
K 2.92 −02	1.61 +02	2.99 +01	8.57 +03	—	—	8.73 +03	8.60 +03
3.00 −02	1.56 +02	2.99 +01	7.98 +03	—	—	8.14 +03	8.01 +03
4.00 −02	1.10 +02	2.89 +01	3.70 +03	—	—	3.81 +03	3.73 +03
5.00 −02	8.44 +01	2.81 +01	2.02 +03	—	—	2.10 +03	2.04 +03
6.00 −02	6.85 +01	2.73 +01	1.22 +03	—	—	1.29 +03	1.25 +03
8.00 −02	5.02 +01	2.59 +01	5.45 +02	—	—	5.95 +02	5.71 +02
1.00 −01	4.05 +01	2.46 +01	2.90 +02	—	—	3.31 +02	3.15 +02
1.50 −01	2.96 +01	2.22 +01	9.15 +01	—	—	1.21 +02	1.14 +02
2.00 −01	2.45 +01	2.03 +01	4.02 +01	—	—	6.47 +01	6.06 +01
3.00 −01	1.96 +01	1.77 +01	1.28 +01	—	—	3.24 +01	3.05 +01

4.00 −01	1.69 +01	1.58 +01	5.93 +00	—	—	2.28 +01	2.18 +01
5.00 −01	1.51 +01	1.45 +01	3.50 +00	—	—	1.86 +01	1.80 +01
6.00 −01	1.39 +01	1.34 +01	2.20 +00	—	—	1.61 +01	1.56 +01
8.00 −01	1.20 +01	1.18 +01	1.15 +00	—	—	1.32 +01	1.29 +01
1.00 +00	1.07 +01	1.06 +01	6.90 −01	—	—	1.14 +01	1.13 +01
1.50 +00	8.65 +00	8.59 +00	3.13 −01	1.53 −01	—	9.12 +00	9.06 +00
2.00 +00	7.36 +00	7.33 +00	1.93 −01	5.23 −01	—	8.08 +00	8.04 +00
3.00 +00	5.77 +00	5.77 +00	1.05 −01	1.35 +00	2.01 −03	7.24 +00	7.23 +00
4.00 +00	4.82 +00	4.81 +00	6.93 −02	2.10 +00	8.26 −03	7.00 +00	6.98 +00
5.00 +00	4.16 +00	4.15 +00	5.18 −02	2.74 +00	1.62 −02	6.97 +00	6.96 +00
6.00 +00	3.68 +00	3.67 +00	4.05 −02	3.29 +00	2.50 −02	7.03 +00	7.03 +00
8.00 +00	3.00 +00		2.83 −02	4.21 +00	4.27 −02	7.28 +00	
1.00 +01	2.56 +00		2.18 −02	4.95 +00	5.84 −02	7.58 +00	
1.50 +01	1.89 +00		1.37 −02	6.38 +00	9.09 −02	8.37 +00	
2.00 +01	1.52 +00		9.94 −03	7.44 +00	1.16 −01	9.08 +00	
3.00 +01	1.11 +00		6.41 −03	8.92 +00	1.52 −01	1.02 +01	
4.00 +01	8.79 −01		4.73 −03	9.92 +00	1.77 −01	1.10 +01	
5.00 +01	7.34 −01		3.75 −03	1.07 +01	1.96 −01	1.16 +01	
6.00 +01	6.32 −01		3.10 −03	1.12 +01	2.11 −01	1.21 +01	
8.00 +01	4.98 −01		2.31 −03	1.21 +01	2.35 −01	1.28 +01	
1.00 +02	4.14 −01		1.84 −03	1.27 +01	2.52 −01	1.33 +01	

APPENDIX D.2. (*Continued*)

Lead, Z = 82

Multiply by 0.002907 to get cm^2/g
or by 0.0002907 to get m^2/kg

Photon Energy (MeV)	Compton With and Without Coherent		Photoelectric	Nuclear and Electron Pair		Total With and Without Coherent	
	$_a\sigma + {_a\sigma_R}$	$_a\sigma$	$_a\tau$	$_a\kappa_{nuc}$	$_a\kappa_{elec}$	$_a\mu$	$_a\mu - {_a\sigma_R}$
1.00 −02	1.73 +03	5.25 +01	4.40 +04	—	—	4.57 +04	4.41 +04
1.30 −02	1.34 +03	5.19 +01	2.20 +04	—	—	2.33 +04	2.20 +04
L_3 1.30 −02	1.34 +03	5.19 +01	5.58 +04	—	—	5.71 +04	5.59 +04
1.50 −02	1.15 +03	5.16 +01	3.84 +04	—	—	3.96 +04	3.85 +04
1.52 −02	1.13 +03	5.15 +01	3.75 +04	—	—	3.86 +04	3.76 +04
L_2 1.52 −02	1.13 +03	5.15 +01	4.90 +04	—	—	5.01 +04	4.91 +04
1.59 −02	1.08 +03	5.14 +01	4.35 +04	—	—	4.46 +04	4.36 +04
L_1 1.59 −02	1.08 +03	5.14 +01	5.29 +04	—	—	5.40 +04	5.29 +04
2.00 −02	8.17 +02	5.07 +01	2.86 +04	—	—	2.95 +04	2.87 +04
3.00 −02	4.91 +02	4.90 +01	9.71 +03	—	—	1.02 +04	9.76 +03
4.00 −02	3.36 +02	4.75 +01	4.47 +03	—	—	4.81 +03	4.52 +03
5.00 −02	2.48 +02	4.60 +01	2.44 +03	—	—	2.68 +03	2.48 +03
6.00 −02	1.94 +02	4.47 +01	1.48 +03	—	—	1.67 +03	1.52 +03
8.00 −02	1.32 +02	4.24 +01	6.70 +02	—	—	8.03 +02	7.13 +02
K 8.80 −02	1.16 +02	4.16 +01	5.15 +02	—	—	6.31 +02	5.56 +02
8.80 −02	1.16 +02	4.16 +01	2.45 +03	—	—	2.56 +03	2.49 +03
1.00 −01	9.93 +01	4.04 +01	1.76 +03	—	—	1.86 +03	1.80 +03

1.50 −01	6.39 +01	3.64 +01	6.14 +02	—	—	6.78 +02	6.51 +02
2.00 −01	4.92 +01	3.33 +01	2.92 +02	—	—	3.41 +02	3.25 +02
3.00 −01	3.61 +01	2.90 +01	1.03 +02	—	—	1.39 +02	1.32 +02
4.00 −01	3.00 +01	2.60 +01	4.96 +01	—	—	7.96 +01	7.56 +01
5.00 −01	2.63 +01	2.37 +01	2.92 +01	—	—	5.55 +01	5.29 +01
6.00 −01	2.37 +01	2.19 +01	1.92 +01	—	—	4.29 +01	4.11 +01
8.00 −01	2.03 +01	1.93 +01	1.02 +01	—	—	3.04 +01	2.95 +01
1.00 +00	1.79 +01	1.73 +01	6.39 +00	—	—	2.43 +01	2.37 +01
1.50 +00	1.43 +01	1.41 +01	2.89 +00	5.66 −01	—	1.78 +01	1.75 +01
2.00 +00	1.22 +01	1.20 +01	1.77 +00	1.70 +00	—	1.57 +01	1.55 +01
3.00 +00	9.51 +00	9.46 +00	9.14 −01	3.94 +00	3.30 −03	1.44 +01	1.43 +01
4.00 +00	7.94 +00	7.89 +00	5.89 −01	5.77 +00	1.35 −02	1.43 +01	1.43 +01
5.00 +00	6.84 +00	6.81 +00	4.34 −01	7.30 +00	2.66 −02	1.46 +01	1.46 +01
6.00 +00	6.04 +00	6.02 +00	3.36 −01	8.54 +00	4.09 −02	1.50 +01	1.49 +01
8.00 +00	4.93 +00	4.92 +00	2.31 −01	1.05 +01	7.00 −02	1.58 +01	1.58 +01
1.00 +01	4.20 +00	4.19 +00	1.78 −01	1.22 +01	9.57 −02	1.67 +01	1.67 +01
1.50 +01	3.10 +00		1.12 −01	1.55 +01	1.48 −01	1.89 +01	
2.00 +01	2.49 +00		8.10 −02	1.81 +01	1.86 −01	2.09 +01	
3.00 +01	1.81 +00		5.20 −02	2.18 +01	2.42 −01	2.39 +01	
4.00 +01	1.44 +00		3.80 −02	2.43 +01	2.81 −01	2.60 +01	
5.00 +01	1.20 +00		3.00 −02	2.61 +01	3.11 −01	2.77 +01	
6.00 +01	1.04 +00		2.50 −02	2.75 +01	3.35 −01	2.89 +01	
8.00 +01	8.18 −01		1.80 −02	2.96 +01	3.71 −01	3.06 +01	
1.00 +02	6.79 −01		1.41 −02	3.10 +01	3.97 −01	3.21 +01	

APPENDIX D.2. (Continued)

Uranium, Z = 92
Multiply by 0.002530 to get cm²/g
or by 0.0002530 to get m²/kg

Photon Energy (MeV)	Compton With and Without Coherent		Photoelectric	Nuclear and Electron Pair		Total With and Without Coherent	
	$_a\sigma + {_a}\sigma_R$	$_a\sigma$	$_a\tau$	$_a\kappa_{nuc}$	$_a\kappa_{elec}$	$_a\mu$	$_a\mu - {_a}\sigma_R$
1.00 −02	2.17 +03	5.89 +01	6.84 +04	—	—	7.05 +04	6.84 +04
1.50 −02	1.47 +03	5.79 +01	2.38 +04	—	—	2.53 +04	2.38 +04
1.72 −02	1.27 +03	5.74 +01	1.68 +01	—	—	1.81 +04	1.69 +04
L_3 1.72 −02	1.27 +03	5.74 +01	4.06 +04	—	—	4.19 +04	4.07 +04
2.00 −02	1.07 +03	5.68 +01	2.70 +04	—	—	2.81 +04	2.71 +04
2.09 −02	1.01 +03	5.67 +01	2.38 +04	—	—	2.48 +04	2.38 +04
L_2 2.09 −02	1.01 +03	5.67 +01	3.38 +04	—	—	3.48 +04	3.38 +04
2.18 −02	9.61 +02	5.65 +01	3.06 +04	—	—	3.15 +04	3.06 +04
L_1 2.18 −02	9.61 +02	5.65 +01	3.53 +04	—	—	3.63 +04	3.54 +04
3.00 −02	6.36 +02	5.50 +01	1.56 +04	—	—	1.62 +04	1.56 +04
4.00 −02	4.36 +02	5.32 +01	7.35 +03	—	—	7.79 +03	7.40 +03
5.00 −02	3.22 +02	5.16 +01	4.07 +03	—	—	4.39 +03	4.12 +03
6.00 −02	2.51 +02	5.02 +01	2.50 +03	—	—	2.75 +03	2.55 +03
8.00 −02	1.68 +02	4.76 +01	1.16 +03	—	—	1.32 +03	1.20 +03
1.00 −01	1.25 +02	4.53 +01	6.31 +02	—	—	7.56 +02	6.77 +02
1.16 −01	1.05 +02	4.38 +01	4.26 +02	—	—	5.31 +02	4.70 +02
K 1.16 −01	1.05 +02	4.38 +01	1.82 +03	—	—	1.92 +03	1.86 +03
1.50 −01	7.80 +01	4.08 +01	9.36 +02	—	—	1.01 +03	9.77 +02

2.00 −01	5.88 +01	3.74 +01	4.48 +02	—	—	5.07 +02	4.85 +02
3.00 −01	4.21 +01	3.25 +01	1.59 +02	—	—	2.01 +02	1.92 +02
4.00 −01	3.45 +01	2.91 +01	7.87 +01	—	—	1.13 +02	1.08 +02
5.00 −01	3.01 +01	2.66 +01	4.64 +01	—	—	7.65 +01	7.30 +01
6.00 −01	2.70 +01	2.46 +01	3.06 +01	—	—	5.76 +01	5.52 +01
8.00 −01	2.29 +01	2.16 −01	1.65 +01	—	—	3.94 +01	3.81 +01
1.00 +00	2.03 +01	1.94 +01	1.04 +01	—	—	3.07 +01	2.98 +01
1.50 +00	1.61 +01	1.58 +01	4.73 +00	7.77 −01	—	2.17 +01	2.13 +01
2.00 +00	1.37 +01	1.35 +01	2.84 +00	2.26 +00	—	1.88 +01	1.86 +01
3.00 +00	1.07 +01	1.06 +01	1.49 +00	5.09 +00	3.70 −03	1.73 +01	1.72 +01
4.00 +00	8.91 +00	8.85 +00	9.58 −01	7.32 +00	1.52 −02	1.72 +01	1.71 +01
5.00 +00	7.68 +00	7.64 +00	7.02 −01	9.16 +00	2.99 −02	1.76 +01	1.75 +01
6.00 +00	6.78 +00	6.75 +00	5.43 −01	1.06 +01	4.59 −02	1.80 +01	1.80 +01
8.00 +00	5.55 +00	5.52 +00	3.75 −01	1.30 +01	7.86 −02	1.90 +01	1.89 +01
1.00 +01	4.72 +00	4.71 +00	2.88 −01	1.49 +01	1.07 −01	2.00 +01	2.00 +01
1.50 +01	3.48 +00		1.80 −01	1.88 +01	1.65 −01	2.27 +01	
2.00 +01	2.80 +00		1.31 −01	2.20 +01	2.08 −01	2.51 +01	
3.00 +01	2.04 +00		8.50 −02	2.66 +01	2.69 −01	2.90 +01	
4.00 +01	1.62 +00		6.20 −02	2.96 +01	3.13 −01	3.16 +01	
5.00 +01	1.35 +00		5.00 −02	3.18 +01	3.46 −01	3.36 +01	
6.00 +01	1.16 +00		4.00 −02	3.36 +01	3.73 −01	3.51 +01	
8.00 +01	9.17 −01		3.00 −02	3.61 +01	4.12 −01	3.75 +01	
1.00 +02	7.62 −01		2.40 −02	3.77 +01	4.41 −01	3.89 +01	

APPENDIX D.3. Mass Attenuation Coefficients, Mass Energy-Transfer Coefficients, and Mass Energy-Absorption Coefficients for Photon Interactions in Various Media, in cm^2/g^a

Photon Energy (MeV)	Hydrogen μ/ρ	μ_{tr}/ρ	μ_{en}/ρ	Carbon μ/ρ	μ_{tr}/ρ	μ_{en}/ρ	Nitrogen μ/ρ	μ_{tr}/ρ	μ_{en}/ρ	Oxygen μ/ρ	μ_{tr}/ρ	μ_{en}/ρ
0.01	0.385	0.00986	0.00986	2.32	1.97	1.97	3.77	3.38	3.38	5.82	5.39	5.39
0.015	0.376	0.0110	0.0110	0.797	0.536	0.536	1.19	0.908	0.908	1.75	1.44	1.44
0.02	0.369	0.0135	0.0135	0.434	0.208	0.208	0.602	0.362	0.362	0.830	0.575	0.575
0.03	0.357	0.0185	0.0185	0.253	0.0594	0.0594	0.304	0.105	0.105	0.373	0.165	0.165
0.04	0.346	0.0231	0.0231	0.205	0.0306	0.0306	0.229	0.0493	0.0493	0.257	0.0733	0.0733
0.05	0.335	0.0271	0.0271	0.185	0.0233	0.0233	0.196	0.0319	0.0319	0.211	0.0437	0.0437
0.06	0.326	0.0306	0.0306	0.174	0.0211	0.0211	0.181	0.0256	0.0256	0.190	0.0322	0.0322
0.08	0.309	0.0362	0.0362	0.162	0.0205	0.0205	0.164	0.0223	0.0223	0.168	0.0249	0.0249
0.10	0.294	0.0406	0.0406	0.152	0.0215	0.0215	0.154	0.0224	0.0224	0.156	0.0237	0.0237
0.15	0.265	0.0481	0.0481	0.135	0.0245	0.0245	0.136	0.0247	0.0247	0.137	0.0251	0.0251
0.2	0.243	0.0525	0.0525	0.123	0.0265	0.0265	0.124	0.0267	0.0267	0.124	0.0268	0.0268
0.3	0.211	0.0569	0.0569	0.107	0.0287	0.0287	0.107	0.0287	0.0287	0.107	0.0288	0.0288
0.4	0.189	0.0586	0.0586	0.0953	0.0295	0.0295	0.0953	0.0295	0.0295	0.0957	0.0295	0.0295
0.5	0.173	0.0593	0.0593	0.0870	0.0297	0.0297	0.0870	0.0297	0.0296	0.0871	0.0297	0.0297
0.6	0.160	0.0587	0.0587	0.0805	0.0296	0.0295	0.0805	0.0296	0.0295	0.0805	0.0296	0.0296
0.8	0.140	0.0574	0.0574	0.0707	0.0289	0.0288	0.0707	0.0289	0.0289	0.0707	0.0289	0.0289
1.0	0.126	0.0555	0.0555	0.0637	0.0279	0.0279	0.0636	0.0280	0.0279	0.0637	0.0280	0.0278
1.5	0.103	0.0507	0.0507	0.0519	0.0256	0.0255	0.0518	0.0256	0.0255	0.0518	0.0256	0.0254
2	0.0875	0.0465	0.0464	0.0443	0.0235	0.0234	0.0444	0.0236	0.0234	0.0445	0.0236	0.0234
3	0.0691	0.0399	0.0398	0.0356	0.0206	0.0204	0.0357	0.0207	0.0205	0.0359	0.0208	0.0206
4	0.0581	0.0353	0.0352	0.0305	0.0187	0.0185	0.0308	0.0189	0.0186	0.0310	0.0191	0.0188
5	0.0505	0.0319	0.0317	0.0271	0.0174	0.0171	0.0274	0.0177	0.0173	0.0278	0.0179	0.0175
6	0.0450	0.0292	0.0290	0.0247	0.0164	0.0161	0.0251	0.0167	0.0163	0.0255	0.0171	0.0166
8	0.0375	0.0253	0.0252	0.0216	0.0151	0.0147	0.0221	0.0156	0.0151	0.0226	0.0160	0.0155
10	0.0325	0.0227	0.0225	0.0196	0.0143	0.0138	0.0203	0.0149	0.0143	0.0209	0.0154	0.0148

^{a}For m^2/kg multiply these data by 0.1. Data due to Hubbell, as given by Evans (1968). Reproduced with permission from J. H. Hubbell and Academic Press.

Photon Energy (MeV)	Aluminum μ/ρ	Aluminum μ_{tr}/ρ	Aluminum μ_{en}/ρ	Silicon μ/ρ	Silicon μ_{tr}/ρ	Silicon μ_{en}/ρ	Calcium μ/ρ	Calcium μ_{tr}/ρ	Calcium μ_{en}/ρ	Copper μ/ρ	Copper μ_{tr}/ρ	Copper μ_{en}/ρ
0.01	26.2	25.5	25.5	34.1	33.3	33.3	96.5	91.6	91.6	224.2	160.	160.
0.015	7.90	7.47	7.47	10.2	9.75	9.75	30.1	28.6	28.6	74.1	59.4	59.4
0.02	3.39	3.06	3.06	4.36	4.01	4.01	12.9	12.2	12.2	33.7	28.2	28.2
0.03	1.12	0.868	0.868	1.41	1.14	1.14	3.98	3.60	3.60	10.9	9.50	9.50
0.04	0.565	0.357	0.357	0.693	0.472	0.472	1.78	1.50	1.50	4.88	4.24	4.24
0.05	0.367	0.184	0.184	0.435	0.241	0.241	0.994	0.764	0.764	2.61	2.22	2.22
0.06	0.277	0.111	0.111	0.319	0.144	0.144	0.646	0.444	0.444	1.60	1.32	1.32
0.08	0.201	0.0562	0.0562	0.223	0.0700	0.0700	0.363	0.196	0.196	0.768	0.573	0.573
0.10	0.170	0.0386	0.0386	0.184	0.0459	0.0459	0.255	0.109	0.109	0.462	0.302	0.302
0.15	0.138	0.0285	0.0285	0.145	0.0312	0.0312	0.168	0.0497	0.0497	0.223	0.106	0.106
0.2	0.122	0.0276	0.0276	0.128	0.0292	0.0292	0.138	0.0371	0.0371	0.157	0.0597	0.0597
0.3	0.104	0.0282	0.0282	0.108	0.0294	0.0294	0.112	0.0318	0.0318	0.112	0.0370	0.0370
0.4	0.0926	0.0287	0.0287	0.0961	0.0298	0.0298	0.0980	0.0309	0.0309	0.0942	0.0318	0.0318
0.5	0.0844	0.0287	0.0286	0.0875	0.0298	0.0298	0.0886	0.0304	0.0304	0.0835	0.0298	0.0298
0.6	0.0779	0.0286	0.0286	0.0806	0.0296	0.0295	0.0813	0.0300	0.0299	0.0762	0.0287	0.0286
0.8	0.0682	0.0279	0.0277	0.0708	0.0289	0.0288	0.0712	0.0291	0.0289	0.0659	0.0272	0.0271
1.0	0.0613	0.0270	0.0269	0.0634	0.0279	0.0277	0.0639	0.0280	0.0278	0.0590	0.0261	0.0258
1.5	0.0500	0.0247	0.0245	0.0517	0.0255	0.0253	0.0519	0.0257	0.0254	0.0479	0.0237	0.0233
2	0.0431	0.0229	0.0226	0.0447	0.0237	0.0234	0.0452	0.0240	0.0236	0.0419	0.0222	0.0217
3	0.0353	0.0206	0.0202	0.0367	0.0214	0.0210	0.0377	0.0220	0.0214	0.0359	0.0211	0.0202
4	0.0311	0.0193	0.0188	0.0324	0.0202	0.0196	0.0340	0.0213	0.0205	0.0332	0.0211	0.0200
5	0.0284	0.0185	0.0179	0.0297	0.0194	0.0187	0.0317	0.0211	0.0200	0.0318	0.0214	0.0200
6	0.0266	0.0181	0.0172	0.0279	0.0191	0.0182	0.0304	0.0211	0.0198	0.0310	0.0220	0.0202
8	0.0244	0.0177	0.0168	0.0257	0.0187	0.0177	0.0289	0.0215	0.0198	0.0307	0.0234	0.0209
10	0.0232	0.0176	0.0165	0.0246	0.0188	0.0175	0.0284	0.0222	0.0201	0.0310	0.0248	0.0215

APPENDIX D.3. (*Continued*)

Photon Energy (MeV)	Tin			Photon Energy (MeV)	Lead		
	μ/ρ	μ_{tr}/ρ	μ_{en}/ρ		μ/ρ	μ_{tr}/ρ	μ_{en}/ρ
0.0010	11130	11110	11110	M$_1$ edge	—		
0.0015	3960	3950	3950	0.003854	1493	1454	1453
0.0020	1963	1954	1954	0.004	1333	1298	1297
0.0030	713	705	705	0.005	767	747	747
0.0039288	367	360	360	0.006	493	479	479
L$_3$ edge 0.0039288	1118	1067	1067	0.008	238	230	230
0.0040	1067	1019	1019	0.010	136.6	131.0	130.7
0.0041573	973	930	930	0.0130406	70.1	66.2	66.0
L$_2$ edge 0.0041573	1244	1187	1187	L$_3$ edge 0.0130406	165.7	128.8	128.8
0.0044648	1016	971	971	0.015	114.7	91.7	91.7
L$_1$ edge 0.0044648	1264	1207	1207	0.0152053	112.0	89.6	89.6
0.005	919	880	880	L$_2$ edge 0.0152053	145.4	113.0	113.0
0.006	561	540	539	0.015855	129.3	101.7	101.6
0.008	259	250	249	L$_1$ edge 0.015855	159.2	123.0	123.0
0.010	141.6	136.5	136.4	0.02	85.5	69.2	69.1
0.015	45.8	43.7	43.6	0.03	29.1	24.6	24.6
0.020	21.2	19.83	19.81				

Energy			
0.0291947	7.61	6.83	6.82
K edge			
0.0291947	45.4	16.70	16.69
0.030	42.1	16.18	16.17
0.04	18.77	9.97	9.96
0.05	10.20	6.25	6.24
0.06	6.34	4.20	4.19
0.08	3.07	2.19	2.18
0.10	1.720	1.257	1.250
0.15	0.634	0.446	0.442
0.20	0.333	0.211	0.209
0.30	0.1649	0.0853	0.0843
0.4	0.1163	0.0536	0.0530
0.5	0.0948	0.0423	0.0416
0.6	0.0811	0.0358	0.0353
0.8	0.0667	0.0301	0.0294
1.0	0.0578	0.0270	0.0264
1.5	0.0462	0.0233	0.0226
2.0	0.0410	0.0220	0.0210
3.0	0.0366	0.0219	0.0205
4	0.0355	0.0232	0.0212
5	0.0353	0.0247	0.0221
6	0.0357	0.0262	0.0230
8	0.0370	0.0292	0.0245
10	0.0387	0.0319	0.0258

Energy			
0.04	13.80	11.83	11.78
0.05	7.71	6.57	6.54
0.06	4.87	4.11	4.08
0.08	2.37	1.924	1.908
0.088005	1.865	1.494	1.481
K edge			
0.088005	7.30	2.47	2.47
0.10	5.78	2.28	2.28
0.15	2.07	1.164	1.154
0.2	1.014	0.637	0.629
0.3	0.406	0.265	0.259
0.4	0.233	0.1474	0.1432
0.5	0.1614	0.0984	0.0951
0.6	0.1249	0.0737	0.0710
0.8	0.0886	0.0503	0.0481
1.0	0.0708	0.0396	0.0377
1.5	0.0518	0.0288	0.0271
2	0.0455	0.0259	0.0240
3	0.0417	0.0260	0.0234
4	0.0415	0.0281	0.0245
5	0.0424	0.0306	0.0259
6	0.0436	0.0331	0.0272
8	0.0467	0.0378	0.0294
10	0.0496	0.0419	0.0310

APPENDIX D.3. (*Continued*)

Photon Energy (MeV)	Air			Water			ICRU Compact Bone			ICRU Striated Muscle		
	μ/ρ	μ_{tr}/ρ	μ_{en}/ρ	μ/ρ	μ_{tr}/ρ	μ_{en}/ρ	μ/ρ	μ_{tr}/ρ	μ_{en}/ρ	μ/ρ	μ_{tr}/ρ	μ_{en}/ρ
0.01	5.04	4.61	4.61	5.21	4.79	4.79	20.3	19.2	19.2	5.30	4.87	4.87
0.015	1.56	1.27	1.27	1.60	1.28	1.28	6.32	5.84	5.84	1.64	1.32	1.32
0.02	0.758	0.511	0.511	0.778	0.512	0.512	2.79	2.46	2.46	0.796	0.533	0.533
0.03	0.350	0.148	0.148	0.371	0.149	0.149	0.962	0.720	0.720	0.375	0.154	0.154
0.04	0.248	0.0668	0.0668	0.267	0.0677	0.0677	0.511	0.304	0.304	0.267	0.0701	0.0701
0.05	0.206	0.0406	0.0406	0.225	0.0418	0.0418	0.346	0.161	0.161	0.224	0.0431	0.0431
0.06	0.187	0.0305	0.0305	0.205	0.0320	0.0320	0.273	0.0998	0.0998	0.204	0.0328	0.0328
0.08	0.167	0.0243	0.0243	0.185	0.0262	0.0262	0.209	0.0537	0.0537	0.183	0.0264	0.0264
0.10	0.155	0.0234	0.0234	0.171	0.0256	0.0256	0.181	0.0387	0.0387	0.170	0.0256	0.0256
0.15	0.136	0.0250	0.0250	0.151	0.0277	0.0277	0.150	0.0305	0.0305	0.150	0.0275	0.0275
0.2	0.124	0.0268	0.0268	0.137	0.0297	0.0297	0.133	0.0301	0.0301	0.136	0.0294	0.0294
0.3	0.107	0.0287	0.0287	0.119	0.0319	0.0319	0.114	0.0310	0.0310	0.118	0.0317	0.0317
0.4	0.0954	0.0295	0.0295	0.106	0.0328	0.0328	0.102	0.0315	0.0315	0.105	0.0325	0.0325
0.5	0.0868	0.0297	0.0296	0.0966	0.0330	0.0330	0.0926	0.0317	0.0317	0.0958	0.0328	0.0328
0.6	0.0804	0.0296	0.0295	0.0894	0.0329	0.0329	0.0856	0.0315	0.0314	0.0886	0.0326	0.0325
0.8	0.0706	0.0289	0.0289	0.0785	0.0321	0.0321	0.0751	0.0307	0.0306	0.0778	0.0318	0.0318
1.0	0.0635	0.0280	0.0278	0.0706	0.0311	0.0309	0.0675	0.0297	0.0295	0.0699	0.0308	0.0306
1.5	0.0517	0.0256	0.0254	0.0575	0.0284	0.0282	0.0549	0.0272	0.0270	0.0570	0.0282	0.0280
2	0.0444	0.0236	0.0234	0.0493	0.0262	0.0260	0.0472	0.0251	0.0249	0.0489	0.0259	0.0257
3	0.0358	0.0207	0.0205	0.0396	0.0229	0.0227	0.0382	0.0221	0.0219	0.0392	0.0227	0.0225
4	0.0308	0.0189	0.0186	0.0340	0.0209	0.0206	0.0331	0.0204	0.0200	0.0337	0.0207	0.0204
5	0.0276	0.0178	0.0174	0.0303	0.0195	0.0191	0.0297	0.0192	0.0187	0.0300	0.0193	0.0189
6	0.0252	0.0168	0.0164	0.0277	0.0185	0.0180	0.0274	0.0184	0.0178	0.0274	0.0183	0.0178
8	0.0223	0.0157	0.0152	0.0243	0.0170	0.0166	0.0244	0.0173	0.0167	0.0240	0.0169	0.0164
10	0.0205	0.0151	0.0145	0.0222	0.0162	0.0157	0.0226	0.0168	0.0159	0.0219	0.0160	0.0155

Photon Energy (MeV)	Polystyrene			Methyl Methacrylate, Lucite, Plexiglas, Perspex			Polyethylene			Pyrex glass		
	μ/ρ	μ_{tr}/ρ	μ_{en}/ρ	μ/ρ	μ_{tr}/ρ	μ_{en}/ρ	μ/ρ	μ_{tr}/ρ	μ_{en}/ρ	μ/ρ	μ_{tr}/ρ	μ_{en}/ρ
0.01	2.17	1.82	1.82	3.31	2.91	2.91	2.04	1.69	1.69	17.1	16.5	16.5
0.015	0.764	0.495	0.495	1.07	0.783	0.783	0.737	0.461	0.461	5.11	4.75	4.75
0.02	0.429	0.193	0.193	0.555	0.310	0.310	0.425	0.180	0.180	2.24	1.94	1.94
0.03	0.261	0.0562	0.0562	0.300	0.0899	0.0899	0.268	0.0535	0.0535	0.785	0.554	0.554
0.04	0.216	0.0300	0.0300	0.233	0.0437	0.0437	0.225	0.0295	0.0295	0.430	0.232	0.232
0.05	0.197	0.0236	0.0236	0.205	0.0301	0.0301	0.207	0.0238	0.0238	0.299	0.122	0.122
0.06	0.186	0.0218	0.0218	0.191	0.0254	0.0254	0.196	0.0225	0.0225	0.241	0.0768	0.0768
0.08	0.173	0.0217	0.0217	0.176	0.0232	0.0232	0.183	0.0228	0.0228	0.190	0.0428	0.0428
0.10	0.164	0.0231	0.0231	0.165	0.0238	0.0238	0.173	0.0243	0.0243	0.166	0.0325	0.0325
0.15	0.145	0.0263	0.0263	0.146	0.0266	0.0266	0.154	0.0279	0.0279	0.139	0.0274	0.0274
0.2	0.132	0.0286	0.0286	0.133	0.0287	0.0287	0.140	0.0303	0.0303	0.125	0.0276	0.0276
0.3	0.115	0.0309	0.0309	0.115	0.0310	0.0310	0.122	0.0328	0.0328	0.107	0.0289	0.0289
0.4	0.103	0.0318	0.0318	0.103	0.0318	0.0318	0.109	0.0337	0.0337	0.0953	0.0295	0.0295
0.5	0.0937	0.0321	0.0321	0.0939	0.0322	0.0322	0.0994	0.0340	0.0340	0.0868	0.0297	0.0297
0.6	0.0867	0.0319	0.0318	0.0869	0.0319	0.0319	0.0919	0.0338	0.0337	0.0801	0.0295	0.0294
0.8	0.0761	0.0311	0.0310	0.0763	0.0312	0.0311	0.0807	0.0330	0.0329	0.0704	0.0288	0.0287
1.0	0.0683	0.0300	0.0300	0.0686	0.0302	0.0301	0.0725	0.0319	0.0319	0.0633	0.0279	0.0277
1.5	0.0557	0.0275	0.0275	0.0559	0.0276	0.0275	0.0591	0.0292	0.0291	0.0515	0.0254	0.0252
2	0.0476	0.0253	0.0252	0.0478	0.0254	0.0253	0.0505	0.0268	0.0267	0.0444	0.0235	0.0233
3	0.0381	0.0221	0.0219	0.0383	0.0222	0.0220	0.0403	0.0234	0.0232	0.0360	0.0209	0.0207
4	0.0326	0.0200	0.0198	0.0329	0.0202	0.0199	0.0345	0.0211	0.0209	0.0314	0.0194	0.0190
5	0.0289	0.0185	0.0182	0.0292	0.0187	0.0184	0.0305	0.0195	0.0192	0.0284	0.0184	0.0179
6	0.0263	0.0174	0.0171	0.0266	0.0177	0.0173	0.0276	0.0182	0.0180	0.0263	0.0178	0.0171
8	0.0227	0.0159	0.0155	0.0231	0.0162	0.0158	0.0238	0.0166	0.0162	0.0237	0.0170	0.0163
10	0.0206	0.0150	0.0145	0.0210	0.0153	0.0148	0.0215	0.0155	0.0151	0.0221	0.0166	0.0157

APPENDIX D.4. Mass Energy-Absorption Coefficients μ_{en}/ρ (cm^2/g) for Various Media[a]

γ-Ray Energy (MeV)	Li	F	LiF	Teflon $(CF_2)_n$	CaF_2	CaF_2:Mn[b]
0.01	0.150	7.61	5.61	6.26	50.7	51.7
0.015	0.0426	2.05	1.51	1.69	15.7	16.1
0.02	0.0205	0.821	0.607	0.674	6.66	6.86
0.03	0.0118	0.233	0.174	0.191	1.96	2.03
0.04	0.0115	0.100	0.0763	0.0833	0.818	0.850
0.05	0.0125	0.0566	0.0448	0.0486	0.419	0.436
0.06	0.0137	0.0391	0.0323	0.0348	0.247	0.256
0.08	0.0159	0.0270	0.0240	0.0254	0.114	0.118
0.10	0.0178	0.0241	0.0224	0.0235	0.0677	0.0697
0.15	0.0210	0.0243	0.0234	0.0243	0.0373	0.0379
0.2	0.0229	0.0256	0.0249	0.0258	0.0315	0.0317
0.3	0.0248	0.0273	0.0266	0.0276	0.0296	0.0296
0.4	0.0255	0.0281	0.0274	0.0284	0.0295	0.0295
0.5	0.0258	0.0282	0.0276	0.0286	0.0293	0.0293
0.6	0.0256	0.0281	0.0274	0.0284	0.0290	0.0290
0.8	0.0250	0.0273	0.0267	0.0277	0.0281	0.0281
1.0	0.0242	0.0264	0.0258	0.0268	0.0271	0.0270
1.5	0.0221	0.0241	0.0236	0.0244	0.0248	0.0247
2.0	0.0203	0.0222	0.0217	0.0225	0.0229	0.0229
3.0	0.0175	0.0196	0.0190	0.0198	0.0205	0.0205
4.0	0.0156	0.0179	0.0173	0.0180	0.0192	0.0192
5.0	0.0142	0.0168	0.0161	0.0169	0.0184	0.0184
6.0	0.0131	0.0160	0.0152	0.0160	0.0179	0.0179
8.0	0.0117	0.0150	0.0141	0.0149	0.0175	0.0175
10.0	0.0107	0.0144	0.0134	0.0143	0.0173	0.0173

[a]Data for Li, F, LiF, and Teflon are taken from Sinclair (1969); those for CaF_2 and CaF_2:Mn are from Attix (1970). Both references were derived from the data of J. H. Hubbell, as published in the review by Evans (1968).
[b]CaF_2:Mn (TLD phosphor) is 49.5% Ca, 48.4% F, and 2.1% Mn by weight.

APPENDIX E. Electron Mass Stopping Powers, Ranges, Radiation Yields, and Density Corrections[a]

				Hydrogen			

ENERGY	STOPPING POWER			CSDA	RADIATION	DENS.EFF.
	COLLISION	RADIATIVE	TOTAL	RANGE	YIELD	CORR.
						(DELTA)
MeV	MeV cm²/g	MeV cm²/g	MeV cm²/g	g/cm²		
0.0100	5.125E+01	9.702E-04	5.125E+01	1.076E-04	1.029E-05	0.0
0.0125	4.271E+01	9.793E-04	4.271E+01	1.613E-04	1.242E-05	0.0
0.0150	3.682E+01	9.881E-04	3.682E+01	2.245E-04	1.450E-05	0.0
0.0175	3.249E+01	9.964E-04	3.249E+01	2.970E-04	1.654E-05	0.0
0.0200	2.917E+01	1.004E-03	2.917E+01	3.783E-04	1.854E-05	0.0
0.0250	2.439E+01	1.019E-03	2.439E+01	5.667E-04	2.246E-05	0.0
0.0300	2.110E+01	1.034E-03	2.110E+01	7.878E-04	2.628E-05	0.0
0.0350	1.870E+01	1.048E-03	1.870E+01	1.040E-03	3.003E-05	0.0
0.0400	1.687E+01	1.061E-03	1.687E+01	1.322E-03	3.371E-05	0.0
0.0450	1.542E+01	1.074E-03	1.542E+01	1.632E-03	3.733E-05	0.0
0.0500	1.424E+01	1.088E-03	1.424E+01	1.970E-03	4.090E-05	0.0
0.0550	1.327E+01	1.101E-03	1.327E+01	2.334E-03	4.443E-05	0.0
0.0600	1.245E+01	1.113E-03	1.245E+01	2.724E-03	4.791E-05	0.0
0.0700	1.114E+01	1.138E-03	1.114E+01	3.575E-03	5.475E-05	0.0
0.0800	1.015E+01	1.164E-03	1.015E+01	4.517E-03	6.146E-05	0.0
0.0900	9.367E+00	1.190E-03	9.368E+00	5.543E-03	6.806E-05	0.0
0.1000	8.737E+00	1.216E-03	8.738E+00	6.650E-03	7.457E-05	0.0
0.1250	7.590E+00	1.285E-03	7.592E+00	9.732E-03	9.050E-05	0.0
0.1500	6.819E+00	1.357E-03	6.820E+00	1.322E-02	1.061E-04	0.0
0.1750	6.266E+00	1.433E-03	6.267E+00	1.705E-02	1.215E-04	0.0
0.2000	5.851E+00	1.511E-03	5.852E+00	2.118E-02	1.367E-04	0.0
0.2500	5.275E+00	1.677E-03	5.276E+00	3.021E-02	1.670E-04	0.0
0.3000	4.898E+00	1.852E-03	4.899E+00	4.007E-02	1.971E-04	0.0
0.3500	4.635E+00	2.038E-03	4.637E+00	5.057E-02	2.273E-04	0.0
0.4000	4.445E+00	2.232E-03	4.447E+00	6.159E-02	2.577E-04	0.0
0.4500	4.302E+00	2.436E-03	4.305E+00	7.303E-02	2.884E-04	0.0
0.5000	4.193E+00	2.648E-03	4.196E+00	8.480E-02	3.194E-04	0.0
0.5500	4.109E+00	2.869E-03	4.111E+00	9.684E-02	3.508E-04	0.0
0.6000	4.042E+00	3.096E-03	4.045E+00	1.091E-01	3.825E-04	0.0
0.7000	3.945E+00	3.573E-03	3.949E+00	1.341E-01	4.471E-04	0.0
0.8000	3.883E+00	4.076E-03	3.837E+00	1.597E-01	5.133E-04	0.0
0.9000	3.842E+00	4.603E-03	3.847E+00	1.856E-01	5.809E-04	0.0
1.0000	3.816E+00	5.152E-03	3.821E+00	2.117E-01	6.501E-04	0.0
1.2500	3.787E+00	6.614E-03	3.794E+00	2.774E-01	8.289E-04	0.0
1.5000	3.788E+00	8.190E-03	3.796E+00	3.433E-01	1.016E-03	0.0
1.7500	3.802E+00	9.862E-03	3.812E+00	4.090E-01	1.209E-03	0.0
2.0000	3.823E+00	1.162E-02	3.835E+00	4.744E-01	1.409E-03	0.0
2.5000	3.873E+00	1.534E-02	3.888E+00	6.039E-01	1.824E-03	0.0
3.0000	3.924E+00	1.931E-02	3.943E+00	7.316E-01	2.257E-03	0.0
3.5000	3.973E+00	2.348E-02	3.997E+00	8.575E-01	2.703E-03	0.0
4.0000	4.020E+00	2.782E-02	4.047E+00	9.818E-01	3.162E-03	0.0
4.5000	4.063E+00	3.230E-02	4.095E+00	1.105E+00	3.631E-03	0.0
5.0000	4.103E+00	3.693E-02	4.140E+00	1.226E+00	4.108E-03	0.0
5.5000	4.140E+00	4.166E-02	4.182E+00	1.346E+00	4.593E-03	0.0
6.0000	4.175E+00	4.651E-02	4.222E+00	1.465E+00	5.084E-03	.0.0
7.0000	4.239E+00	5.647E-02	4.295E+00	1.700E+00	6.083E-03	0.0
8.0000	4.295E+00	6.675E-02	4.361E+00	1.931E+00	7.101E-03	0.0
9.0000	4.345E+00	7.731E-02	4.422E+00	2.159E+00	8.133E-03	0.0
10.0000	4.391E+00	8.809E-02	4.479E+00	2.383E+00	9.177E-03	0.0
12.5000	4.488E+00	1.159E-01	4.604E+00	2.934E+00	1.183E-02	0.0
15.0000	4.569E+00	1.448E-01	4.714E+00	3.470E+00	1.451E-02	0.0
17.5000	4.638E+00	1.744E-01	4.813E+00	3.995E+00	1.722E-02	0.0
20.0000	4.698E+00	2.046E-01	4.903E+00	4.510E+00	1.994E-02	0.0
25.0000	4.799E+00	2.667E-01	5.065E+00	5.513E+00	2.540E-02	0.0
30.0000	4.881E+00	3.305E-01	5.212E+00	6.485E+00	3.084E-02	0.0
35.0000	4.951E+00	3.955E-01	5.347E+00	7.432E+00	3.625E-02	0.0
40.0000	5.010E+00	4.615E-01	5.471E+00	8.357E+00	4.161E-02	1.250E-02
45.0000	5.055E+00	5.283E-01	5.583E+00	9.261E+00	4.693E-02	6.872E-02
50.0000	5.091E+00	5.959E-01	5.686E+00	1.015E+01	5.221E-02	1.504E-01
55.0000	5.120E+00	6.640E-01	5.784E+00	1.102E+01	5.745E-02	2.452E-01
60.0000	5.144E+00	7.326E-01	5.876E+00	1.188E+01	6.264E-02	3.459E-01
70.0000	5.183E+00	8.713E-01	6.054E+00	1.355E+01	7.288E-02	5.514E-01
80.0000	5.213E+00	1.011E+00	6.225E+00	1.518E+01	8.293E-02	7.513E-01
90.0000	5.238E+00	1.153E+00	6.391E+00	1.677E+01	9.277E-02	9.405E-01

[a]Berger and Seltzer, 1983. Reproduced with permission from M. J. Berger.

Helium

ENERGY	STOPPING POWER COLLISION	STOPPING POWER RADIATIVE	TOTAL	CSDA RANGE	RADIATION YIELD	DENS.EFF. CORR. (DELTA)
MeV	MeV cm²/g	MeV cm²/g	MeV cm²/g	g/cm²		
0.0100	2.267E+01	9.885E-04	2.267E+01	2.467E-04	2.412E-05	0.0
0.0125	1.898E+01	9.941E-04	1.898E+01	3.678E-04	2.890E-05	0.0
0.0150	1.642E+01	9.995E-04	1.642E+01	5.098E-04	3.352E-05	0.0
0.0175	1.453E+01	1.005E-03	1.453E+01	6.720E-04	3.802E-05	0.0
0.0200	1.307E+01	1.010E-03	1.307E+01	8.537E-04	4.242E-05	0.0
0.0250	1.097E+01	1.020E-03	1.097E+01	1.273E-03	5.096E-05	0.0
0.0300	9.521E+00	1.029E-03	9.522E+00	1.764E-03	5.923E-05	0.0
0.0350	8.457E+00	1.039E-03	8.458E+00	2.322E-03	6.727E-05	0.0
0.0400	7.642E+00	1.048E-03	7.643E+00	2.945E-03	7.510E-05	0.0
0.0450	6.996E+00	1.057E-03	6.997E+00	3.630E-03	8.277E-05	0.0
0.0500	6.471E+00	1.066E-03	6.472E+00	4.374E-03	9.029E-05	0.0
0.0550	6.035E+00	1.075E-03	6.037E+00	5.174E-03	9.766E-05	0.0
0.0600	5.669E+00	1.084E-03	5.670E+00	6.029E-03	1.049E-04	0.0
0.0700	5.084E+00	1.101E-03	5.085E+00	7.896E-03	1.191E-04	0.0
0.0800	4.638E+00	1.119E-03	4.639E+00	9.958E-03	1.328E-04	0.0
0.0900	4.287E+00	1.138E-03	4.288E+00	1.220E-02	1.462E-04	0.0
0.1000	4.003E+00	1.157E-03	4.004E+00	1.462E-02	1.593E-04	0.0
0.1250	3.486E+00	1.207E-03	3.487E+00	2.134E-02	1.910E-04	0.0
0.1500	3.137E+00	1.260E-03	3.139E+00	2.891E-02	2.215E-04	0.0
0.1750	2.887E+00	1.316E-03	2.889E+00	3.723E-02	2.511E-04	0.0
0.2000	2.700E+00	1.375E-03	2.701E+00	4.619E-02	2.800E-04	0.0
0.2500	2.439E+00	1.499E-03	2.441E+00	6.573E-02	3.363E-04	0.0
0.3000	2.269E+00	1.632E-03	2.270E+00	8.702E-02	3.914E-04	0.0
0.3500	2.150E+00	1.774E-03	2.152E+00	1.097E-01	4.457E-04	0.0
0.4000	2.064E+00	1.924E-03	2.066E+00	1.334E-01	4.997E-04	0.0
0.4500	2.000E+00	2.081E-03	2.002E+00	1.580E-01	5.536E-04	0.0
0.5000	1.952E+00	2.245E-03	1.954E+00	1.833E-01	6.076E-04	0.0
0.5500	1.914E+00	2.416E-03	1.916E+00	2.092E-01	6.619E-04	0.0
0.6000	1.884E+00	2.592E-03	1.887E+00	2.355E-01	7.165E-04	0.0
0.7000	1.842E+00	2.961E-03	1.845E+00	2.891E-01	8.269E-04	0.0
0.8000	1.815E+00	3.350E-03	1.818E+00	3.437E-01	9.389E-04	0.0
0.9000	1.798E+00	3.757E-03	1.801E+00	3.990E-01	1.053E-03	0.0
1.0000	1.787E+00	4.180E-03	1.791E+00	4.547E-01	1.168E-03	0.0
1.2500	1.777E+00	5.306E-03	1.782E+00	5.947E-01	1.465E-03	0.0
1.5000	1.780E+00	6.515E-03	1.787E+00	7.349E-01	1.773E-03	0.0
1.7500	1.789E+00	7.793E-03	1.797E+00	8.744E-01	2.089E-03	0.0
2.0000	1.801E+00	9.132E-03	1.810E+00	1.013E+00	2.414E-03	0.0
2.5000	1.827E+00	1.196E-02	1.839E+00	1.287E+00	3.085E-03	0.0
3.0000	1.854E+00	1.495E-02	1.869E+00	1.557E+00	3.779E-03	0.0
3.5000	1.880E+00	1.809E-02	1.898E+00	1.822E+00	4.491E-03	0.0
4.0000	1.903E+00	2.134E-02	1.925E+00	2.084E+00	5.218E-03	0.0
4.5000	1.925E+00	2.469E-02	1.950E+00	2.342E+00	5.957E-03	0.0
5.0000	1.946E+00	2.813E-02	1.974E+00	2.597E+00	6.706E-03	0.0
5.5000	1.965E+00	3.165E-02	1.997E+00	2.848E+00	7.465E-03	0.0
6.0000	1.983E+00	3.523E-02	2.018E+00	3.098E+00	8.231E-03	0.0
7.0000	2.015E+00	4.260E-02	2.057E+00	3.588E+00	9.781E-03	0.0
8.0000	2.043E+00	5.018E-02	2.093E+00	4.070E+00	1.135E-02	0.0
9.0000	2.069E+00	5.793E-02	2.126E+00	4.544E+00	1.293E-02	0.0
10.0000	2.092E+00	6.584E-02	2.157E+00	5.011E+00	1.453E-02	0.0
12.5000	2.141E+00	8.617E-02	2.227E+00	6.151E+00	1.855E-02	0.0
15.0000	2.182E+00	1.071E-01	2.289E+00	7.258E+00	2.258E-02	0.0
17.5000	2.216E+00	1.286E-01	2.345E+00	8.337E+00	2.662E-02	0.0
20.0000	2.247E+00	1.505E-01	2.397E+00	9.391E+00	3.064E-02	0.0
25.0000	2.297E+00	1.952E-01	2.493E+00	1.144E+01	3.863E-02	0.0
30.0000	2.339E+00	2.410E-01	2.580E+00	1.341E+01	4.651E-02	0.0
35.0000	2.374E+00	2.875E-01	2.662E+00	1.531E+01	5.426E-02	0.0
40.0000	2.405E+00	3.346E-01	2.739E+00	1.717E+01	6.187E-02	0.0
45.0000	2.432E+00	3.822E-01	2.814E+00	1.897E+01	6.933E-02	0.0
50.0000	2.456E+00	4.303E-01	2.886E+00	2.072E+01	7.665E-02	0.0
55.0000	2.478E+00	4.786E-01	2.956E+00	2.243E+01	8.382E-02	0.0
60.0000	2.498E+00	5.272E-01	3.025E+00	2.410E+01	9.085E-02	0.0
70.0000	2.533E+00	6.252E-01	3.158E+00	2.734E+01	1.045E-01	0.0
80.0000	2.564E+00	7.239E-01	3.288E+00	3.044E+01	1.176E-01	0.0
90.0000	2.589E+00	8.231E-01	3.412E+00	3.343E+01	1.301E-01	2.142E-02

Carbon (Graphite)

ENERGY	STOPPING POWER COLLISION	RADIATIVE	TOTAL	CSDA RANGE	RADIATION YIELD	DENS.EFF. CORR.
MeV	MeV cm²/g	MeV cm²/g	MeV cm²/g	g/cm²		(DELTA)
0.0100	2.014E+01	3.150E-03	2.014E+01	2.820E-04	8.665E-05	1.920E-03
0.0125	1.694E+01	3.161E-03	1.695E+01	4.179E-04	1.036E-04	2.481E-03
0.0150	1.471E+01	3.168E-03	1.471E+01	5.767E-04	1.199E-04	3.073E-03
0.0175	1.305E+01	3.172E-03	1.305E+01	7.575E-04	1.355E-04	3.695E-03
0.0200	1.177E+01	3.176E-03	1.177E+01	9.595E-04	1.506E-04	4.347E-03
0.0250	9.913E+00	3.184E-03	9.916E+00	1.424E-03	1.796E-04	5.736E-03
0.0300	8.626E+00	3.194E-03	8.629E+00	1.966E-03	2.073E-04	7.236E-03
0.0350	7.679E+00	3.204E-03	7.682E+00	2.582E-03	2.340E-04	8.843E-03
0.0400	6.950E+00	3.215E-03	6.953E+00	3.267E-03	2.597E-04	1.055E-02
0.0450	6.372E+00	3.228E-03	6.375E+00	4.019E-03	2.847E-04	1.236E-02
0.0500	5.901E+00	3.241E-03	5.904E+00	4.835E-03	3.090E-04	1.425E-02
0.0550	5.510E+00	3.255E-03	5.513E+00	5.712E-03	3.327E-04	1.624E-02
0.0600	5.179E+00	3.270E-03	5.183E+00	6.648E-03	3.558E-04	1.832E-02
0.0700	4.652E+00	3.303E-03	4.655E+00	8.688E-03	4.008E-04	2.271E-02
0.0800	4.249E+00	3.337E-03	4.253E+00	1.094E-02	4.441E-04	2.740E-02
0.0900	3.931E+00	3.375E-03	3.935E+00	1.339E-02	4.860E-04	3.237E-02
0.1000	3.674E+00	3.414E-03	3.677E+00	1.602E-02	5.268E-04	3.760E-02
0.1250	3.204E+00	3.523E-03	3.207E+00	2.333E-02	6.243E-04	5.166E-02
0.1500	2.886E+00	3.640E-03	2.890E+00	3.156E-02	7.168E-04	6.694E-02
0.1750	2.657E+00	3.764E-03	2.661E+00	4.059E-02	8.055E-04	8.320E-02
0.2000	2.485E+00	3.896E-03	2.489E+00	5.032E-02	8.911E-04	1.003E-01
0.2500	2.245E+00	4.179E-03	2.249E+00	7.152E-02	1.055E-03	1.363E-01
0.3000	2.087E+00	4.489E-03	2.092E+00	9.462E-02	1.213E-03	1.740E-01
0.3500	1.977E+00	4.820E-03	1.981E+00	1.192E-01	1.367E-03	2.129E-01
0.4000	1.896E+00	5.173E-03	1.901E+00	1.450E-01	1.518E-03	2.524E-01
0.4500	1.835E+00	5.545E-03	1.841E+00	1.718E-01	1.668E-03	2.922E-01
0.5000	1.788E+00	5.935E-03	1.794E+00	1.993E-01	1.817E-03	3.321E-01
0.5500	1.752E+00	6.340E-03	1.758E+00	2.274E-01	1.966E-03	3.719E-01
0.6000	1.722E+00	6.759E-03	1.729E+00	2.561E-01	2.115E-03	4.114E-01
0.7000	1.679E+00	7.637E-03	1.687E+00	3.147E-01	2.416E-03	4.891E-01
0.8000	1.650E+00	8.559E-03	1.659E+00	3.745E-01	2.719E-03	5.648E-01
0.9000	1.631E+00	9.523E-03	1.640E+00	4.352E-01	3.026E-03	6.382E-01
1.0000	1.617E+00	1.053E-02	1.627E+00	4.964E-01	3.337E-03	7.091E-01
1.2500	1.599E+00	1.318E-02	1.612E+00	6.509E-01	4.133E-03	8.756E-01
1.5000	1.593E+00	1.602E-02	1.609E+00	8.062E-01	4.954E-03	1.028E+00
1.7500	1.594E+00	1.901E-02	1.613E+00	9.614E-01	5.799E-03	1.167E+00
2.0000	1.597E+00	2.213E-02	1.619E+00	1.116E+00	6.665E-03	1.295E+00
2.5000	1.608E+00	2.870E-02	1.637E+00	1.423E+00	8.450E-03	1.522E+00
3.0000	1.621E+00	3.561E-02	1.657E+00	1.727E+00	1.029E-02	1.720E+00
3.5000	1.634E+00	4.281E-02	1.677E+00	2.027E+00	1.218E-02	1.894E+00
4.0000	1.647E+00	5.026E-02	1.697E+00	2.323E+00	1.410E-02	2.051E+00
4.5000	1.658E+00	5.792E-02	1.716E+00	2.616E+00	1.606E-02	2.193E+00
5.0000	1.669E+00	6.576E-02	1.735E+00	2.906E+00	1.803E-02	2.323E+00
5.5000	1.679E+00	7.378E-02	1.753E+00	3.193E+00	2.003E-02	2.443E+00
6.0000	1.689E+00	8.193E-02	1.771E+00	3.476E+00	2.204E-02	2.555E+00
7.0000	1.706E+00	9.865E-02	1.804E+00	4.036E+00	2.610E-02	2.758E+00
8.0000	1.720E+00	1.158E-01	1.836E+00	4.585E+00	3.020E-02	2.939E+00
9.0000	1.733E+00	1.334E-01	1.867E+00	5.125E+00	3.432E-02	3.104E+00
10.0000	1.745E+00	1.513E-01	1.896E+00	5.657E+00	3.845E-02	3.256E+00
12.5000	1.769E+00	1.971E-01	1.966E+00	6.952E+00	4.877E-02	3.591E+00
15.0000	1.787E+00	2.444E-01	2.032E+00	8.202E+00	5.903E-02	3.879E+00
17.5000	1.803E+00	2.927E-01	2.095E+00	9.414E+00	6.918E-02	4.133E+00
20.0000	1.816E+00	3.417E-01	2.157E+00	1.059E+01	7.917E-02	4.361E+00
25.0000	1.836E+00	4.417E-01	2.278E+00	1.284E+01	9.861E-02	4.755E+00
30.0000	1.852E+00	5.435E-01	2.396E+00	1.498E+01	1.173E-01	5.088E+00
35.0000	1.865E+00	6.466E-01	2.512E+00	1.702E+01	1.351E-01	5.376E+00
40.0000	1.877E+00	7.508E-01	2.627E+00	1.897E+01	1.522E-01	5.628E+00
45.0000	1.886E+00	8.559E-01	2.742E+00	2.083E+01	1.685E-01	5.854E+00
50.0000	1.895E+00	9.617E-01	2.857E+00	2.262E+01	1.841E-01	6.057E+00
55.0000	1.903E+00	1.068E+00	2.971E+00	2.433E+01	1.991E-01	6.241E+00
60.0000	1.910E+00	1.175E+00	3.085E+00	2.598E+01	2.133E-01	6.411E+00
70.0000	1.922E+00	1.391E+00	3.313E+00	2.911E+01	2.401E-01	6.712E+00
80.0000	1.932E+00	1.608E+00	3.541E+00	3.203E+01	2.648E-01	6.974E+00
90.0000	1.942E+00	1.826E+00	3.768E+00	3.477E+01	2.875E-01	7.206E+00

Nitrogen

ENERGY	STOPPING POWER COLLISION	RADIATIVE	TOTAL	CSDA RANGE	RADIATION YIELD	DENS.EFF. CORR. (DELTA)
MeV	MeV cm²/g	MeV cm²/g	MeV cm²/g	g/cm²		
0.0100	1.995E+01	3.711E-03	1.996E+01	2.851E-04	1.023E-04	0.0
0.0125	1.679E+01	3.729E-03	1.680E+01	4.223E-04	1.227E-04	0.0
0.0150	1.458E+01	3.740E-03	1.459E+01	5.825E-04	1.421E-04	0.0
0.0175	1.294E+01	3.747E-03	1.295E+01	7.648E-04	1.608E-04	0.0
0.0200	1.168E+01	3.753E-03	1.168E+01	9.684E-04	1.789E-04	0.0
0.0250	9.838E+00	3.762E-03	9.842E+00	1.437E-03	2.135E-04	0.0
0.0300	8.564E+00	3.770E-03	8.568E+00	1.983E-03	2.465E-04	0.0
0.0350	7.626E+00	3.779E-03	7.629E+00	2.603E-03	2.781E-04	0.0
0.0400	6.904E+00	3.790E-03	6.908E+00	3.293E-03	3.086E-04	0.0
0.0450	6.331E+00	3.803E-03	6.335E+00	4.049E-03	3.382E-04	0.0
0.0500	5.865E+00	3.816E-03	5.868E+00	4.870E-03	3.669E-04	0.0
0.0550	5.477E+00	3.831E-03	5.481E+00	5.753E-03	3.949E-04	0.0
0.0600	5.150E+00	3.846E-03	5.154E+00	6.694E-03	4.222E-04	0.0
0.0700	4.628E+00	3.881E-03	4.632E+00	8.745E-03	4.751E-04	0.0
0.0800	4.229E+00	3.920E-03	4.233E+00	1.101E-02	5.260E-04	0.0
0.0900	3.914E+00	3.961E-03	3.918E+00	1.347E-02	5.752E-04	0.0
0.1000	3.660E+00	4.005E-03	3.664E+00	1.611E-02	6.229E-04	0.0
0.1250	3.195E+00	4.127E-03	3.199E+00	2.344E-02	7.368E-04	0.0
0.1500	2.881E+00	4.259E-03	2.885E+00	3.169E-02	8.447E-04	0.0
0.1750	2.655E+00	4.400E-03	2.660E+00	4.073E-02	9.477E-04	0.0
0.2000	2.486E+00	4.550E-03	2.491E+00	5.046E-02	1.047E-03	0.0
0.2500	2.251E+00	4.874E-03	2.256E+00	7.162E-02	1.236E-03	0.0
0.3000	2.097E+00	5.227E-03	2.103E+00	9.462E-02	1.418E-03	0.0
0.3500	1.991E+00	5.606E-03	1.996E+00	1.191E-01	1.593E-03	0.0
0.4000	1.914E+00	6.009E-03	1.920E+00	1.446E-01	1.765E-03	0.0
0.4500	1.857E+00	6.436E-03	1.863E+00	1.711E-01	1.935E-03	0.0
0.5000	1.813E+00	6.882E-03	1.820E+00	1.982E-01	2.103E-03	0.0
0.5500	1.779E+00	7.347E-03	1.787E+00	2.260E-01	2.271E-03	0.0
0.6000	1.753E+00	7.827E-03	1.761E+00	2.542E-01	2.438E-03	0.0
0.7000	1.716E+00	8.831E-03	1.725E+00	3.116E-01	2.773E-03	0.0
0.8000	1.693E+00	9.889E-03	1.703E+00	3.700E-01	3.109E-03	0.0
0.9000	1.679E+00	1.099E-02	1.690E+00	4.289E-01	3.447E-03	0.0
1.0000	1.670E+00	1.214E-02	1.683E+00	4.883E-01	3.788E-03	0.0
1.2500	1.665E+00	1.518E-02	1.680E+00	6.371E-01	4.655E-03	0.0
1.5000	1.670E+00	1.842E-02	1.688E+00	7.856E-01	5.541E-03	0.0
1.7500	1.681E+00	2.184E-02	1.702E+00	9.331E-01	6.444E-03	0.0
2.0000	1.693E+00	2.540E-02	1.719E+00	1.079E+00	7.364E-03	0.0
2.5000	1.721E+00	3.290E-02	1.754E+00	1.367E+00	9.243E-03	0.0
3.0000	1.749E+00	4.078E-02	1.790E+00	1.649E+00	1.116E-02	0.0
3.5000	1.775E+00	4.899E-02	1.824E+00	1.926E+00	1.311E-02	0.0
4.0000	1.799E+00	5.747E-02	1.857E+00	2.198E+00	1.509E-02	0.0
4.5000	1.821E+00	6.620E-02	1.888E+00	2.465E+00	1.708E-02	0.0
5.0000	1.842E+00	7.512E-02	1.917E+00	2.728E+00	1.909E-02	0.0
5.5000	1.861E+00	8.423E-02	1.945E+00	2.987E+00	2.110E-02	0.0
6.0000	1.879E+00	9.352E-02	1.972E+00	3.242E+00	2.312E-02	0.0
7.0000	1.911E+00	1.125E-01	2.024E+00	3.742E+00	2.718E-02	0.0
8.0000	1.940E+00	1.320E-01	2.072E+00	4.231E+00	3.124E-02	0.0
9.0000	1.965E+00	1.520E-01	2.117E+00	4.708E+00	3.530E-02	0.0
10.0000	1.988E+00	1.723E-01	2.161E+00	5.176E+00	3.934E-02	0.0
12.5000	2.038E+00	2.244E-01	2.262E+00	6.306E+00	4.938E-02	0.0
15.0000	2.079E+00	2.780E-01	2.356E+00	7.388E+00	5.926E-02	0.0
17.5000	2.113E+00	3.327E-01	2.446E+00	8.430E+00	6.894E-02	0.0
20.0000	2.144E+00	3.884E-01	2.532E+00	9.434E+00	7.842E-02	0.0
25.0000	2.194E+00	5.016E-01	2.696E+00	1.135E+01	9.672E-02	0.0
30.0000	2.235E+00	6.169E-01	2.852E+00	1.315E+01	1.142E-01	9.661E-03
35.0000	2.266E+00	7.336E-01	3.000E+00	1.486E+01	1.308E-01	6.591E-02
40.0000	2.290E+00	8.515E-01	3.142E+00	1.649E+01	1.467E-01	1.474E-01
45.0000	2.310E+00	9.704E-01	3.281E+00	1.804E+01	1.619E-01	2.393E-01
50.0000	2.327E+00	1.090E+00	3.417E+00	1.954E+01	1.765E-01	3.344E-01
55.0000	2.342E+00	1.211E+00	3.552E+00	2.097E+01	1.904E-01	4.291E-01
60.0000	2.355E+00	1.332E+00	3.686E+00	2.235E+01	2.038E-01	5.217E-01
70.0000	2.377E+00	1.575E+00	3.952E+00	2.497E+01	2.290E-01	6.973E-01
80.0000	2.395E+00	1.821E+00	4.216E+00	2.742E+01	2.523E-01	8.590E-01
90.0000	2.411E+00	2.067E+00	4.478E+00	2.972E+01	2.740E-01	1.008E+00

Oxygen

ENERGY	STOPPING POWER COLLISION	STOPPING POWER RADIATIVE	TOTAL	CSDA RANGE	RADIATION YIELD	DENS.EFF. CORR.
MeV	MeV cm²/g	MeV cm²/g	MeV cm²/g	g/cm²		(DELTA)
0.0100	1.937E+01	4.267E-03	1.937E+01	2.950E-04	1.207E-04	0.0
0.0125	1.632E+01	4.298E-03	1.633E+01	4.362E-04	1.449E-04	0.0
0.0150	1.419E+01	4.316E-03	1.419E+01	6.009E-04	1.681E-04	0.0
0.0175	1.260E+01	4.328E-03	1.261E+01	7.882E-04	1.903E-04	0.0
0.0200	1.138E+01	4.336E-03	1.138E+01	9.973E-04	2.118E-04	0.0
0.0250	9.595E+00	4.347E-03	9.600E+00	1.478E-03	2.529E-04	0.0
0.0300	8.359E+00	4.356E-03	8.363E+00	2.037E-03	2.919E-04	0.0
0.0350	7.447E+00	4.365E-03	7.452E+00	2.672E-03	3.293E-04	0.0
0.0400	6.746E+00	4.376E-03	6.750E+00	3.378E-03	3.653E-04	0.0
0.0450	6.189E+00	4.388E-03	6.193E+00	4.153E-03	4.001E-04	0.0
0.0500	5.735E+00	4.402E-03	5.739E+00	4.992E-03	4.339E-04	0.0
0.0550	5.358E+00	4.417E-03	5.362E+00	5.894E-03	4.668E-04	0.0
0.0600	5.039E+00	4.434E-03	5.044E+00	6.856E-03	4.988E-04	0.0
0.0700	4.530E+00	4.471E-03	4.535E+00	8.951E-03	5.608E-04	0.0
0.0800	4.142E+00	4.512E-03	4.146E+00	1.126E-02	6.204E-04	0.0
0.0900	3.835E+00	4.558E-03	3.839E+00	1.377E-02	6.779E-04	0.0
0.1000	3.586E+00	4.607E-03	3.591E+00	1.647E-02	7.337E-04	0.0
0.1250	3.133E+00	4.741E-03	3.137E+00	2.394E-02	8.666E-04	0.0
0.1500	2.826E+00	4.889E-03	2.831E+00	3.235E-02	9.921E-04	0.0
0.1750	2.606E+00	5.048E-03	2.611E+00	4.157E-02	1.112E-03	0.0
0.2000	2.441E+00	5.215E-03	2.446E+00	5.147E-02	1.227E-03	0.0
0.2500	2.211E+00	5.578E-03	2.217E+00	7.302E-02	1.447E-03	0.0
0.3000	2.061E+00	5.975E-03	2.067E+00	9.642E-02	1.656E-03	0.0
0.3500	1.957E+00	6.402E-03	1.963E+00	1.213E-01	1.859E-03	0.0
0.4000	1.882E+00	6.856E-03	1.889E+00	1.473E-01	2.057E-03	0.0
0.4500	1.826E+00	7.335E-03	1.833E+00	1.742E-01	2.253E-03	0.0
0.5000	1.784E+00	7.838E-03	1.791E+00	2.018E-01	2.446E-03	0.0
0.5500	1.751E+00	8.362E-03	1.759E+00	2.299E-01	2.639E-03	0.0
0.6000	1.725E+00	8.904E-03	1.734E+00	2.586E-01	2.831E-03	0.0
0.7000	1.690E+00	1.004E-02	1.700E+00	3.169E-01	3.215E-03	0.0
0.8000	1.667E+00	1.122E-02	1.679E+00	3.761E-01	3.600E-03	0.0
0.9000	1.654E+00	1.247E-02	1.666E+00	4.359E-01	3.987E-03	0.0
1.0000	1.646E+00	1.376E-02	1.659E+00	4.961E-01	4.377E-03	0.0
1.2500	1.641E+00	1.718E-02	1.658E+00	6.469E-01	5.366E-03	0.0
1.5000	1.647E+00	2.084E-02	1.667E+00	7.973E-01	6.376E-03	0.0
1.7500	1.658E+00	2.468E-02	1.682E+00	9.466E-01	7.405E-03	0.0
2.0000	1.671E+00	2.869E-02	1.699E+00	1.094E+00	8.452E-03	0.0
2.5000	1.699E+00	3.711E-02	1.736E+00	1.386E+00	1.059E-02	0.0
3.0000	1.727E+00	4.598E-02	1.773E+00	1.671E+00	1.276E-02	0.0
3.5000	1.753E+00	5.519E-02	1.808E+00	1.950E+00	1.497E-02	0.0
4.0000	1.777E+00	6.471E-02	1.842E+00	2.224E+00	1.720E-02	0.0
4.5000	1.799E+00	7.448E-02	1.874E+00	2.493E+00	1.945E-02	0.0
5.0000	1.820E+00	8.449E-02	1.905E+00	2.758E+00	2.171E-02	0.0
5.5000	1.839E+00	9.470E-02	1.934E+00	3.018E+00	2.398E-02	0.0
6.0000	1.857E+00	1.051E-01	1.962E+00	3.275E+00	2.626E-02	0.0
7.0000	1.889E+00	1.264E-01	2.016E+00	3.777E+00	3.081E-02	0.0
8.0000	1.918E+00	1.482E-01	2.066E+00	4.267E+00	3.536E-02	0.0
9.0000	1.944E+00	1.705E-01	2.114E+00	4.746E+00	3.990E-02	0.0
10.0000	1.967E+00	1.932E-01	2.160E+00	5.214E+00	4.441E-02	0.0
12.5000	2.016E+00	2.514E-01	2.268E+00	6.343E+00	5.558E-02	0.0
15.0000	2.057E+00	3.112E-01	2.368E+00	7.421E+00	6.652E-02	0.0
17.5000	2.092E+00	3.723E-01	2.464E+00	8.456E+00	7.720E-02	0.0
20.0000	2.122E+00	4.343E-01	2.556E+00	9.452E+00	8.762E-02	0.0
25.0000	2.173E+00	5.606E-01	2.733E+00	1.134E+01	1.076E-01	0.0
30.0000	2.214E+00	6.890E-01	2.903E+00	1.312E+01	1.266E-01	2.989E-03
35.0000	2.246E+00	8.189E-01	3.065E+00	1.479E+01	1.446E-01	4.425E-02
40.0000	2.272E+00	9.502E-01	3.222E+00	1.638E+01	1.617E-01	1.129E-01
45.0000	2.292E+00	1.083E+00	3.375E+00	1.790E+01	1.779E-01	1.940E-01
50.0000	2.310E+00	1.216E+00	3.526E+00	1.935E+01	1.934E-01	2.804E-01
55.0000	2.325E+00	1.350E+00	3.675E+00	2.074E+01	2.082E-01	3.682E-01
60.0000	2.338E+00	1.484E+00	3.823E+00	2.207E+01	2.224E-01	4.554E-01
70.0000	2.361E+00	1.755E+00	4.116E+00	2.459E+01	2.488E-01	6.239E-01
80.0000	2.379E+00	2.028E+00	4.407E+00	2.694E+01	2.732E-01	7.819E-01
90.0000	2.395E+00	2.302E+00	4.697E+00	2.914E+01	2.957E-01	9.288E-01

Aluminum

ENERGY	STOPPING POWER COLLISION	RADIATIVE	TOTAL	CSDA RANGE	RADIATION YIELD	DENS.EFF. CORR. (DELTA)
MeV	MeV cm²/g	MeV cm²/g	MeV cm²/g	g/cm²		
0.0100	1.649E+01	6.559E-03	1.650E+01	3.539E-04	2.132E-04	3.534E-04
0.0125	1.398E+01	6.700E-03	1.398E+01	5.192E-04	2.583E-04	4.937E-04
0.0150	1.220E+01	6.798E-03	1.221E+01	7.111E-04	3.016E-04	6.538E-04
0.0175	1.088E+01	6.871E-03	1.088E+01	9.284E-04	3.435E-04	8.332E-04
0.0200	9.844E+00	6.926E-03	9.851E+00	1.170E-03	3.840E-04	1.031E-03
0.0250	8.338E+00	7.004E-03	8.345E+00	1.724E-03	4.616E-04	1.483E-03
0.0300	7.287E+00	7.059E-03	7.294E+00	2.367E-03	5.353E-04	2.005E-03
0.0350	6.509E+00	7.100E-03	6.516E+00	3.093E-03	6.058E-04	2.593E-03
0.0400	5.909E+00	7.133E-03	5.916E+00	3.900E-03	6.736E-04	3.246E-03
0.0450	5.430E+00	7.162E-03	5.437E+00	4.783E-03	7.390E-04	3.960E-03
0.0500	5.039E+00	7.191E-03	5.046E+00	5.738E-03	8.022E-04	4.732E-03
0.0550	4.714E+00	7.217E-03	4.721E+00	6.763E-03	8.636E-04	5.560E-03
0.0600	4.439E+00	7.243E-03	4.446E+00	7.855E-03	9.232E-04	6.440E-03
0.0700	3.998E+00	7.295E-03	4.005E+00	1.023E-02	1.038E-03	8.351E-03
0.0800	3.661E+00	7.350E-03	3.668E+00	1.284E-02	1.147E-03	1.045E-02
0.0900	3.394E+00	7.411E-03	3.401E+00	1.568E-02	1.252E-03	1.271E-02
0.1000	3.177E+00	7.476E-03	3.185E+00	1.872E-02	1.353E-03	1.513E-02
0.1250	2.781E+00	7.659E-03	2.789E+00	2.714E-02	1.593E-03	2.175E-02
0.1500	2.513E+00	7.865E-03	2.521E+00	3.659E-02	1.816E-03	2.907E-02
0.1750	2.320E+00	8.096E-03	2.328E+00	4.693E-02	2.028E-03	3.694E-02
0.2000	2.174E+00	8.344E-03	2.183E+00	5.804E-02	2.231E-03	4.525E-02
0.2500	1.972E+00	8.888E-03	1.981E+00	8.217E-02	2.616E-03	6.280E-02
0.3000	1.839E+00	9.487E-03	1.849E+00	1.083E-01	2.982E-03	8.116E-02
0.3500	1.747E+00	1.013E-02	1.757E+00	1.361E-01	3.335E-03	9.997E-02
0.4000	1.680E+00	1.082E-02	1.691E+00	1.652E-01	3.678E-03	1.190E-01
0.4500	1.630E+00	1.154E-02	1.642E+00	1.952E-01	4.016E-03	1.380E-01
0.5000	1.592E+00	1.230E-02	1.604E+00	2.260E-01	4.349E-03	1.569E-01
0.5500	1.563E+00	1.309E-02	1.576E+00	2.575E-01	4.680E-03	1.757E-01
0.6000	1.540E+00	1.390E-02	1.554E+00	2.894E-01	5.009E-03	1.943E-01
0.7000	1.507E+00	1.560E-02	1.522E+00	3.545E-01	5.664E-03	2.307E-01
0.8000	1.486E+00	1.739E-02	1.503E+00	4.206E-01	6.319E-03	2.661E-01
0.9000	1.473E+00	1.925E-02	1.492E+00	4.874E-01	6.976E-03	3.005E-01
1.0000	1.465E+00	2.119E-02	1.486E+00	5.546E-01	7.636E-03	3.339E-01
1.2500	1.457E+00	2.630E-02	1.484E+00	7.231E-01	9.306E-03	4.138E-01
1.5000	1.460E+00	3.177E-02	1.491E+00	8.912E-01	1.101E-02	4.898E-01
1.7500	1.466E+00	3.752E-02	1.504E+00	1.058E+00	1.274E-02	5.632E-01
2.0000	1.475E+00	4.350E-02	1.518E+00	1.224E+00	1.449E-02	6.349E-01
2.5000	1.493E+00	5.605E-02	1.549E+00	1.550E+00	1.808E-02	7.757E-01
3.0000	1.510E+00	6.924E-02	1.580E+00	1.869E+00	2.173E-02	9.145E-01
3.5000	1.526E+00	8.292E-02	1.609E+00	2.183E+00	2.544E-02	1.051E+00
4.0000	1.540E+00	9.702E-02	1.637E+00	2.491E+00	2.918E-02	1.183E+00
4.5000	1.552E+00	1.115E-01	1.664E+00	2.794E+00	3.296E-02	1.311E+00
5.0000	1.564E+00	1.263E-01	1.690E+00	3.092E+00	3.675E-02	1.433E+00
5.5000	1.574E+00	1.413E-01	1.715E+00	3.386E+00	4.055E-02	1.550E+00
6.0000	1.583E+00	1.567E-01	1.739E+00	3.675E+00	4.436E-02	1.661E+00
7.0000	1.599E+00	1.879E-01	1.787E+00	4.242E+00	5.197E-02	1.868E+00
8.0000	1.613E+00	2.200E-01	1.833E+00	4.795E+00	5.955E-02	2.055E+00
9.0000	1.625E+00	2.526E-01	1.877E+00	5.334E+00	6.708E-02	2.226E+00
10.0000	1.636E+00	2.858E-01	1.921E+00	5.861E+00	7.454E-02	2.384E+00
12.5000	1.658E+00	3.706E-01	2.029E+00	7.127E+00	9.281E-02	2.727E+00
15.0000	1.676E+00	4.574E-01	2.134E+00	8.328E+00	1.105E-01	3.016E+00
17.5000	1.691E+00	5.459E-01	2.237E+00	9.472E+00	1.275E-01	3.265E+00
20.0000	1.704E+00	6.357E-01	2.340E+00	1.056E+01	1.438E-01	3.484E+00
25.0000	1.726E+00	8.180E-01	2.544E+00	1.261E+01	1.745E-01	3.857E+00
30.0000	1.743E+00	1.003E+00	2.746E+00	1.450E+01	2.027E-01	4.168E+00
35.0000	1.757E+00	1.190E+00	2.947E+00	1.626E+01	2.287E-01	4.435E+00
40.0000	1.769E+00	1.379E+00	3.148E+00	1.790E+01	2.528E-01	4.669E+00
45.0000	1.780E+00	1.569E+00	3.349E+00	1.944E+01	2.751E-01	4.878E+00
50.0000	1.789E+00	1.761E+00	3.550E+00	2.089E+01	2.959E-01	5.068E+00
55.0000	1.797E+00	1.953E+00	3.751E+00	2.226E+01	3.152E-01	5.241E+00
60.0000	1.805E+00	2.147E+00	3.951E+00	2.356E+01	3.333E-01	5.401E+00
70.0000	1.818E+00	2.535E+00	4.353E+00	2.597E+01	3.662E-01	5.687E+00
80.0000	1.829E+00	2.927E+00	4.755E+00	2.817E+01	3.953E-01	5.938E+00
90.0000	1.838E+00	3.320E+00	5.158E+00	3.019E+01	4.214E-01	6.161E+00

Silicon

ENERGY	STOPPING POWER COLLISION	STOPPING POWER RADIATIVE	TOTAL	CSDA RANGE	RADIATION YIELD	DENS.EFF. CORR.
MeV	MeV cm²/g	MeV cm²/g	MeV cm²/g	g/cm²		(DELTA)
0.0100	1.689E+01	7.255E-03	1.690E+01	3.461E-04	2.289E-04	1.037E-03
0.0125	1.432E+01	7.431E-03	1.433E+01	5.074E-04	2.780E-04	1.332E-03
0.0150	1.251E+01	7.555E-03	1.252E+01	6.946E-04	3.252E-04	1.641E-03
0.0175	1.115E+01	7.648E-03	1.116E+01	9.065E-04	3.709E-04	1.963E-03
0.0200	1.010E+01	7.720E-03	1.011E+01	1.142E-03	4.151E-04	2.298E-03
0.0250	8.556E+00	7.822E-03	8.564E+00	1.682E-03	5.000E-04	3.007E-03
0.0300	7.480E+00	7.892E-03	7.487E+00	2.308E-03	5.807E-04	3.766E-03
0.0350	6.682E+00	7.946E-03	6.690E+00	3.016E-03	6.579E-04	4.572E-03
0.0400	6.067E+00	7.988E-03	6.075E+00	3.802E-03	7.322E-04	5.424E-03
0.0450	5.576E+00	8.026E-03	5.584E+00	4.661E-03	8.038E-04	6.320E-03
0.0500	5.175E+00	8.061E-03	5.183E+00	5.591E-03	8.731E-04	7.257E-03
0.0550	4.842E+00	8.092E-03	4.850E+00	6.590E-03	9.402E-04	8.235E-03
0.0600	4.559E+00	8.123E-03	4.568E+00	7.653E-03	1.006E-03	9.251E-03
0.0700	4.107E+00	8.185E-03	4.116E+00	9.964E-03	1.131E-03	1.139E-02
0.0800	3.761E+00	8.248E-03	3.769E+00	1.251E-02	1.251E-03	1.368E-02
0.0900	3.487E+00	8.317E-03	3.496E+00	1.526E-02	1.366E-03	1.608E-02
0.1000	3.265E+00	8.389E-03	3.274E+00	1.822E-02	1.476E-03	1.861E-02
0.1250	2.859E+00	8.591E-03	2.867E+00	2.642E-02	1.737E-03	2.538E-02
0.1500	2.583E+00	8.821E-03	2.592E+00	3.561E-02	1.981E-03	3.271E-02
0.1750	2.385E+00	9.076E-03	2.394E+00	4.566E-02	2.212E-03	4.050E-02
0.2000	2.236E+00	9.349E-03	2.245E+00	5.646E-02	2.433E-03	4.868E-02
0.2500	2.028E+00	9.951E-03	2.038E+00	7.991E-02	2.852E-03	6.592E-02
0.3000	1.892E+00	1.062E-02	1.903E+00	1.054E-01	3.248E-03	8.402E-02
0.3500	1.797E+00	1.133E-02	1.809E+00	1.323E-01	3.631E-03	1.027E-01
0.4000	1.729E+00	1.209E-02	1.741E+00	1.606E-01	4.003E-03	1.216E-01
0.4500	1.677E+00	1.290E-02	1.690E+00	1.897E-01	4.368E-03	1.407E-01
0.5000	1.638E+00	1.374E-02	1.652E+00	2.197E-01	4.728E-03	1.599E-01
0.5500	1.608E+00	1.461E-02	1.623E+00	2.502E-01	5.085E-03	1.790E-01
0.6000	1.585E+00	1.551E-02	1.600E+00	2.812E-01	5.441E-03	1.980E-01
0.7000	1.551E+00	1.740E-02	1.568E+00	3.444E-01	6.148E-03	2.355E-01
0.8000	1.529E+00	1.938E-02	1.549E+00	4.086E-01	6.855E-03	2.721E-01
0.9000	1.516E+00	2.145E-02	1.537E+00	4.734E-01	7.564E-03	3.077E-01
1.0000	1.507E+00	2.360E-02	1.531E+00	5.386E-01	8.275E-03	3.424E-01
1.2500	1.500E+00	2.927E-02	1.529E+00	7.022E-01	1.007E-02	4.248E-01
1.5000	1.502E+00	3.533E-02	1.538E+00	8.652E-01	1.190E-02	5.020E-01
1.7500	1.509E+00	4.171E-02	1.551E+00	1.027E+00	1.376E-02	5.747E-01
2.0000	1.518E+00	4.833E-02	1.567E+00	1.188E+00	1.565E-02	6.439E-01
2.5000	1.538E+00	6.223E-02	1.600E+00	1.503E+00	1.949E-02	7.743E-01
3.0000	1.558E+00	7.682E-02	1.634E+00	1.812E+00	2.340E-02	8.976E-01
3.5000	1.575E+00	9.197E-02	1.667E+00	2.115E+00	2.736E-02	1.016E+00
4.0000	1.591E+00	1.076E-01	1.699E+00	2.412E+00	3.134E-02	1.131E+00
4.5000	1.605E+00	1.236E-01	1.729E+00	2.704E+00	3.535E-02	1.243E+00
5.0000	1.618E+00	1.399E-01	1.758E+00	2.991E+00	3.937E-02	1.351E+00
5.5000	1.629E+00	1.566E-01	1.786E+00	3.273E+00	4.340E-02	1.456E+00
6.0000	1.639E+00	1.735E-01	1.813E+00	3.551E+00	4.742E-02	1.557E+00
7.0000	1.657E+00	2.081E-01	1.865E+00	4.095E+00	5.546E-02	1.748E+00
8.0000	1.672E+00	2.435E-01	1.916E+00	4.624E+00	6.344E-02	1.925E+00
9.0000	1.685E+00	2.795E-01	1.965E+00	5.139E+00	7.136E-02	2.088E+00
10.0000	1.697E+00	3.161E-01	2.013E+00	5.642E+00	7.919E-02	2.239E+00
12.5000	1.721E+00	4.098E-01	2.130E+00	6.849E+00	9.833E-02	2.574E+00
15.0000	1.740E+00	5.057E-01	2.245E+00	7.992E+00	1.168E-01	2.858E+00
17.5000	1.756E+00	6.033E-01	2.359E+00	9.078E+00	1.345E-01	3.105E+00
20.0000	1.769E+00	7.023E-01	2.472E+00	1.011E+01	1.514E-01	3.323E+00
25.0000	1.791E+00	9.035E-01	2.695E+00	1.205E+01	1.832E-01	3.694E+00
30.0000	1.809E+00	1.108E+00	2.917E+00	1.383E+01	2.123E-01	4.003E+00
35.0000	1.824E+00	1.314E+00	3.139E+00	1.548E+01	2.391E-01	4.268E+00
40.0000	1.837E+00	1.523E+00	3.360E+00	1.702E+01	2.638E-01	4.501E+00
45.0000	1.848E+00	1.733E+00	3.581E+00	1.847E+01	2.865E-01	4.709E+00
50.0000	1.858E+00	1.944E+00	3.802E+00	1.982E+01	3.077E-01	4.897E+00
55.0000	1.866E+00	2.156E+00	4.023E+00	2.110E+01	3.273E-01	5.068E+00
60.0000	1.874E+00	2.369E+00	4.244E+00	2.231E+01	3.457E-01	5.226E+00
70.0000	1.888E+00	2.798E+00	4.686E+00	2.455E+01	3.789E-01	5.509E+00
80.0000	1.900E+00	3.230E+00	5.129E+00	2.659E+01	4.083E-01	5.757E+00
90.0000	1.910E+00	3.663E+00	5.573E+00	2.846E+01	4.344E-01	5.979E+00

				Copper			

ENERGY	STOPPING POWER			CSDA	RADIATION	DENS.EFF.
	COLLISION	RADIATIVE	TOTAL	RANGE	YIELD	CORR.
						(DELTA)
MeV	MeV cm²/g	MeV cm²/g	MeV cm²/g	g/cm²		
0.0100	1.318E+01	1.213E-02	1.319E+01	4.601E-04	4.701E-04	1.244E-03
0.0125	1.127E+01	1.277E-02	1.128E+01	6.658E-04	5.814E-04	1.585E-03
0.0150	9.904E+00	1.327E-02	9.917E+00	9.028E-04	6.904E-04	1.938E-03
0.0175	8.874E+00	1.366E-02	8.887E+00	1.170E-03	7.972E-04	2.304E-03
0.0200	8.066E+00	1.399E-02	8.080E+00	1.465E-03	9.019E-04	2.683E-03
0.0250	6.877E+00	1.449E-02	6.892E+00	2.138E-03	1.105E-03	3.481E-03
0.0300	6.040E+00	1.488E-02	6.055E+00	2.914E-03	1.301E-03	4.334E-03
0.0350	5.416E+00	1.518E-02	5.431E+00	3.788E-03	1.491E-03	5.247E-03
0.0400	4.931E+00	1.543E-02	4.947E+00	4.754E-03	1.674E-03	6.220E-03
0.0450	4.544E+00	1.564E-02	4.560E+00	5.808E-03	1.852E-03	7.259E-03
0.0500	4.226E+00	1.583E-02	4.242E+00	6.946E-03	2.025E-03	8.365E-03
0.0550	3.961E+00	1.600E-02	3.977E+00	8.164E-03	2.194E-03	9.542E-03
0.0600	3.736E+00	1.615E-02	3.753E+00	9.459E-03	2.358E-03	1.080E-02
0.0700	3.375E+00	1.641E-02	3.392E+00	1.227E-02	2.674E-03	1.354E-02
0.0800	3.098E+00	1.665E-02	3.114E+00	1.535E-02	2.977E-03	1.664E-02
0.0900	2.877E+00	1.688E-02	2.894E+00	1.868E-02	3.267E-03	2.013E-02
0.1000	2.698E+00	1.710E-02	2.715E+00	2.225E-02	3.547E-03	2.404E-02
0.1250	2.370E+00	1.763E-02	2.387E+00	3.211E-02	4.208E-03	3.583E-02
0.1500	2.146E+00	1.816E-02	2.164E+00	4.314E-02	4.822E-03	5.053E-02
0.1750	1.984E+00	1.870E-02	2.002E+00	5.517E-02	5.401E-03	6.758E-02
0.2000	1.861E+00	1.926E-02	1.881E+00	6.807E-02	5.950E-03	8.595E-02
0.2500	1.691E+00	2.045E-02	1.711E+00	9.603E-02	6.981E-03	1.236E-01
0.3000	1.579E+00	2.172E-02	1.601E+00	1.263E-01	7.945E-03	1.603E-01
0.3500	1.501E+00	2.307E-02	1.524E+00	1.584E-01	8.860E-03	1.958E-01
0.4000	1.444E+00	2.450E-02	1.469E+00	1.918E-01	9.741E-03	2.302E-01
0.4500	1.402E+00	2.600E-02	1.428E+00	2.263E-01	1.060E-02	2.635E-01
0.5000	1.370E+00	2.757E-02	1.398E+00	2.617E-01	1.143E-02	2.958E-01
0.5500	1.345E+00	2.919E-02	1.375E+00	2.978E-01	1.226E-02	3.273E-01
0.6000	1.326E+00	3.087E-02	1.357E+00	3.345E-01	1.307E-02	3.581E-01
0.7000	1.298E+00	3.437E-02	1.333E+00	4.089E-01	1.467E-02	4.173E-01
0.8000	1.281E+00	3.803E-02	1.319E+00	4.843E-01	1.625E-02	4.739E-01
0.9000	1.270E+00	4.185E-02	1.312E+00	5.604E-01	1.782E-02	5.280E-01
1.0000	1.263E+00	4.580E-02	1.309E+00	6.367E-01	1.938E-02	5.799E-01
1.2500	1.257E+00	5.623E-02	1.313E+00	8.276E-01	2.328E-02	7.011E-01
1.5000	1.259E+00	6.733E-02	1.327E+00	1.017E+00	2.720E-02	8.121E-01
1.7500	1.265E+00	7.896E-02	1.344E+00	1.204E+00	3.113E-02	9.149E-01
2.0000	1.273E+00	9.103E-02	1.364E+00	1.389E+00	3.509E-02	1.011E+00
2.5000	1.289E+00	1.162E-01	1.405E+00	1.750E+00	4.302E-02	1.186E+00
3.0000	1.305E+00	1.425E-01	1.448E+00	2.101E+00	5.095E-02	1.343E+00
3.5000	1.320E+00	1.697E-01	1.490E+00	2.441E+00	5.885E-02	1.486E+00
4.0000	1.334E+00	1.976E-01	1.531E+00	2.772E+00	6.668E-02	1.617E+00
4.5000	1.346E+00	2.261E-01	1.573E+00	3.094E+00	7.443E-02	1.738E+00
5.0000	1.358E+00	2.552E-01	1.613E+00	3.408E+00	8.209E-02	1.850E+00
5.5000	1.368E+00	2.847E-01	1.653E+00	3.715E+00	8.965E-02	1.954E+00
6.0000	1.378E+00	3.146E-01	1.693E+00	4.013E+00	9.710E-02	2.052E+00
7.0000	1.396E+00	3.756E-01	1.771E+00	4.591E+00	1.117E-01	2.229E+00
8.0000	1.411E+00	4.378E-01	1.849E+00	5.143E+00	1.258E-01	2.388E+00
9.0000	1.424E+00	5.009E-01	1.925E+00	5.673E+00	1.394E-01	2.532E+00
10.0000	1.436E+00	5.650E-01	2.001E+00	6.183E+00	1.526E-01	2.664E+00
12.5000	1.462E+00	7.282E-01	2.190E+00	7.376E+00	1.837E-01	2.951E+00
15.0000	1.482E+00	8.949E-01	2.377E+00	8.472E+00	2.122E-01	3.194E+00
17.5000	1.499E+00	1.064E+00	2.563E+00	9.484E+00	2.385E-01	3.407E+00
20.0000	1.513E+00	1.236E+00	2.749E+00	1.043E+01	2.628E-01	3.597E+00
25.0000	1.537E+00	1.583E+00	3.120E+00	1.213E+01	3.061E-01	3.927E+00
30.0000	1.555E+00	1.936E+00	3.491E+00	1.365E+01	3.437E-01	4.209E+00
35.0000	1.570E+00	2.291E+00	3.861E+00	1.501E+01	3.767E-01	4.456E+00
40.0000	1.582E+00	2.650E+00	4.233E+00	1.624E+01	4.059E-01	4.676E+00
45.0000	1.593E+00	3.012E+00	4.605E+00	1.738E+01	4.320E-01	4.874E+00
50.0000	1.603E+00	3.375E+00	4.978E+00	1.842E+01	4.554E-01	5.054E+00
55.0000	1.611E+00	3.740E+00	5.351E+00	1.939E+01	4.766E-01	5.219E+00
60.0000	1.619E+00	4.107E+00	5.725E+00	2.029E+01	4.959E-01	5.372E+00
70.0000	1.632E+00	4.844E+00	6.476E+00	2.193E+01	5.298E-01	5.646E+00
80.0000	1.643E+00	5.586E+00	7.229E+00	2.339E+01	5.587E-01	5.886E+00
90.0000	1.653E+00	6.330E+00	7.983E+00	2.471E+01	5.836E-01	6.100E+00

Tin

| ENERGY | STOPPING POWER | | | CSDA RANGE | RADIATION YIELD | DENS.EFF. CORR. |
| | COLLISION | RADIATIVE | TOTAL | | | (DELTA) |
MeV	MeV cm²/g	MeV cm²/g	MeV cm²/g	g/cm²		
0.0100	1.075E+01	1.645E-02	1.077E+01	5.861E-04	7.576E-04	6.966E-04
0.0125	9.263E+00	1.769E-02	9.281E+00	8.371E-04	9.496E-04	8.851E-04
0.0150	8.186E+00	1.869E-02	8.205E+00	1.124E-03	1.140E-03	1.079E-03
0.0175	7.366E+00	1.951E-02	7.386E+00	1.446E-03	1.329E-03	1.279E-03
0.0200	6.719E+00	2.021E-02	6.740E+00	1.801E-03	1.515E-03	1.484E-03
0.0250	5.759E+00	2.134E-02	5.781E+00	2.605E-03	1.882E-03	1.910E-03
0.0300	5.078E+00	2.224E-02	5.100E+00	3.528E-03	2.239E-03	2.358E-03
0.0350	4.567E+00	2.299E-02	4.590E+00	4.564E-03	2.589E-03	2.827E-03
0.0400	4.169E+00	2.364E-02	4.193E+00	5.705E-03	2.931E-03	3.316E-03
0.0450	3.850E+00	2.422E-02	3.874E+00	6.947E-03	3.266E-03	3.826E-03
0.0500	3.587E+00	2.473E-02	3.612E+00	8.285E-03	3.595E-03	4.355E-03
0.0550	3.367E+00	2.520E-02	3.393E+00	9.714E-03	3.917E-03	4.904E-03
0.0600	3.181E+00	2.564E-02	3.206E+00	1.123E-02	4.233E-03	5.473E-03
0.0700	2.880E+00	2.642E-02	2.907E+00	1.451E-02	4.849E-03	6.667E-03
0.0800	2.649E+00	2.713E-02	2.676E+00	1.810E-02	5.445E-03	7.935E-03
0.0900	2.465E+00	2.778E-02	2.492E+00	2.198E-02	6.023E-03	9.276E-03
0.1000	2.315E+00	2.838E-02	2.343E+00	2.612E-02	6.584E-03	1.069E-02
0.1250	2.039E+00	2.975E-02	2.069E+00	3.752E-02	7.920E-03	1.451E-02
0.1500	1.852E+00	3.100E-02	1.883E+00	5.021E-02	9.172E-03	1.875E-02
0.1750	1.717E+00	3.216E-02	1.749E+00	6.401E-02	1.035E-02	2.338E-02
0.2000	1.615E+00	3.328E-02	1.648E+00	7.876E-02	1.147E-02	2.838E-02
0.2500	1.473E+00	3.550E-02	1.508E+00	1.106E-01	1.356E-02	3.942E-02
0.3000	1.380E+00	3.776E-02	1.418E+00	1.448E-01	1.548E-02	5.166E-02
0.3500	1.316E+00	4.010E-02	1.356E+00	1.809E-01	1.729E-02	6.492E-02
0.4000	1.269E+00	4.252E-02	1.312E+00	2.185E-01	1.900E-02	7.898E-02
0.4500	1.235E+00	4.505E-02	1.280E+00	2.571E-01	2.065E-02	9.366E-02
0.5000	1.209E+00	4.766E-02	1.257E+00	2.965E-01	2.224E-02	1.088E-01
0.5500	1.189E+00	5.035E-02	1.239E+00	3.366E-01	2.379E-02	1.243E-01
0.6000	1.174E+00	5.311E-02	1.227E+00	3.772E-01	2.530E-02	1.399E-01
0.7000	1.152E+00	5.881E-02	1.211E+00	4.593E-01	2.825E-02	1.717E-01
0.8000	1.140E+00	6.472E-02	1.204E+00	5.421E-01	3.111E-02	2.036E-01
0.9000	1.132E+00	7.083E-02	1.203E+00	6.252E-01	3.391E-02	2.354E-01
1.0000	1.128E+00	7.712E-02	1.205E+00	7.083E-01	3.666E-02	2.669E-01
1.2500	1.127E+00	9.354E-02	1.220E+00	9.146E-01	4.340E-02	3.436E-01
1.5000	1.132E+00	1.108E-01	1.243E+00	1.118E+00	4.998E-02	4.168E-01
1.7500	1.140E+00	1.287E-01	1.269E+00	1.317E+00	5.646E-02	4.863E-01
2.0000	1.149E+00	1.472E-01	1.297E+00	1.512E+00	6.284E-02	5.525E-01
2.5000	1.168E+00	1.855E-01	1.354E+00	1.889E+00	7.534E-02	6.753E-01
3.0000	1.186E+00	2.251E-01	1.412E+00	2.251E+00	8.750E-02	7.874E-01
3.5000	1.203E+00	2.659E-01	1.469E+00	2.598E+00	9.933E-02	8.904E-01
4.0000	1.218E+00	3.075E-01	1.526E+00	2.932E+00	1.108E-01	9.857E-01
4.5000	1.232E+00	3.499E-01	1.582E+00	3.254E+00	1.220E-01	1.075E+00
5.0000	1.244E+00	3.930E-01	1.637E+00	3.564E+00	1.329E-01	1.158E+00
5.5000	1.256E+00	4.366E-01	1.692E+00	3.865E+00	1.434E-01	1.236E+00
6.0000	1.266E+00	4.808E-01	1.747E+00	4.155E+00	1.537E-01	1.311E+00
7.0000	1.285E+00	5.706E-01	1.856E+00	4.711E+00	1.734E-01	1.449E+00
8.0000	1.301E+00	6.620E-01	1.963E+00	5.234E+00	1.920E-01	1.576E+00
9.0000	1.315E+00	7.547E-01	2.070E+00	5.730E+00	2.097E-01	1.695E+00
10.0000	1.328E+00	8.486E-01	2.176E+00	6.202E+00	2.265E-01	1.805E+00
12.5000	1.353E+00	1.087E+00	2.441E+00	7.286E+00	2.649E-01	2.057E+00
15.0000	1.374E+00	1.331E+00	2.705E+00	8.258E+00	2.990E-01	2.279E+00
17.5000	1.390E+00	1.578E+00	2.969E+00	9.140E+00	3.295E-01	2.478E+00
20.0000	1.404E+00	1.829E+00	3.233E+00	9.947E+00	3.570E-01	2.658E+00
25.0000	1.426E+00	2.338E+00	3.764E+00	1.138E+01	4.045E-01	2.974E+00
30.0000	1.444E+00	2.854E+00	4.298E+00	1.262E+01	4.443E-01	3.244E+00
35.0000	1.459E+00	3.376E+00	4.834E+00	1.372E+01	4.782E-01	3.480E+00
40.0000	1.471E+00	3.902E+00	5.373E+00	1.470E+01	5.075E-01	3.689E+00
45.0000	1.481E+00	4.433E+00	5.914E+00	1.559E+01	5.332E-01	3.878E+00
50.0000	1.491E+00	4.966E+00	6.457E+00	1.639E+01	5.558E-01	4.049E+00
55.0000	1.499E+00	5.503E+00	7.002E+00	1.714E+01	5.760E-01	4.206E+00
60.0000	1.506E+00	6.041E+00	7.547E+00	1.783E+01	5.941E-01	4.351E+00
70.0000	1.519E+00	7.124E+00	8.643E+00	1.906E+01	6.253E-01	4.612E+00
80.0000	1.530E+00	8.213E+00	9.743E+00	2.015E+01	6.514E-01	4.843E+00
90.0000	1.540E+00	9.307E+00	1.085E+01	2.112E+01	6.736E-01	5.050E+00

Tungsten

| ENERGY | STOPPING POWER | | | CSDA | RADIATION | DENS.EFF. |
| | COLLISION | RADIATIVE | TOTAL | RANGE | YIELD | CORR. (DELTA) |
MeV	MeV cm²/g	MeV cm²/g	MeV cm²/g	g/cm²		
0.0100	8.974E+00	1.977E-02	8.993E+00	7.489E-04	1.076E-03	9.911E-04
0.0125	7.806E+00	2.165E-02	7.828E+00	1.048E-03	1.357E-03	1.263E-03
0.0150	6.945E+00	2.320E-02	6.968E+00	1.387E-03	1.639E-03	1.544E-03
0.0175	6.281E+00	2.450E-02	6.306E+00	1.765E-03	1.920E-03	1.834E-03
0.0200	5.753E+00	2.563E-02	5.779E+00	2.179E-03	2.200E-03	2.133E-03
0.0250	4.961E+00	2.752E-02	4.989E+00	3.114E-03	2.756E-03	2.758E-03
0.0300	4.394E+00	2.908E-02	4.423E+00	4.181E-03	3.304E-03	3.417E-03
0.0350	3.966E+00	3.042E-02	3.996E+00	5.372E-03	3.846E-03	4.109E-03
0.0400	3.631E+00	3.160E-02	3.662E+00	6.681E-03	4.381E-03	4.834E-03
0.0450	3.360E+00	3.267E-02	3.393E+00	8.101E-03	4.908E-03	5.591E-03
0.0500	3.137E+00	3.364E-02	3.171E+00	9.627E-03	5.430E-03	6.378E-03
0.0550	2.950E+00	3.454E-02	2.985E+00	1.125E-02	5.944E-03	7.195E-03
0.0600	2.791E+00	3.539E-02	2.826E+00	1.298E-02	6.453E-03	8.041E-03
0.0700	2.533E+00	3.694E-02	2.570E+00	1.669E-02	7.453E-03	9.817E-03
0.0800	2.335E+00	3.834E-02	2.373E+00	2.075E-02	8.430E-03	1.170E-02
0.0900	2.176E+00	3.964E-02	2.216E+00	2.511E-02	9.385E-03	1.369E-02
0.1000	2.047E+00	4.084E-02	2.088E+00	2.977E-02	1.032E-02	1.577E-02
0.1250	1.808E+00	4.355E-02	1.852E+00	4.253E-02	1.257E-02	2.139E-02
0.1500	1.646E+00	4.595E-02	1.692E+00	5.668E-02	1.470E-02	2.755E-02
0.1750	1.528E+00	4.814E-02	1.576E+00	7.202E-02	1.673E-02	3.420E-02
0.2000	1.439E+00	5.021E-02	1.490E+00	8.835E-02	1.865E-02	4.131E-02
0.2500	1.315E+00	5.414E-02	1.370E+00	1.235E-01	2.226E-02	5.677E-02
0.3000	1.234E+00	5.797E-02	1.292E+00	1.611E-01	2.558E-02	7.370E-02
0.3500	1.178E+00	6.179E-02	1.240E+00	2.007E-01	2.870E-02	9.188E-02
0.4000	1.138E+00	6.565E-02	1.203E+00	2.416E-01	3.164E-02	1.111E-01
0.4500	1.108E+00	6.956E-02	1.177E+00	2.836E-01	3.443E-02	1.310E-01
0.5000	1.085E+00	7.353E-02	1.159E+00	3.265E-01	3.712E-02	1.515E-01
0.5500	1.068E+00	7.755E-02	1.146E+00	3.699E-01	3.971E-02	1.723E-01
0.6000	1.055E+00	8.162E-02	1.136E+00	4.137E-01	4.221E-02	1.932E-01
0.7000	1.036E+00	8.993E-02	1.126E+00	5.022E-01	4.702E-02	2.352E-01
0.8000	1.025E+00	9.841E-02	1.124E+00	5.911E-01	5.161E-02	2.768E-01
0.9000	1.019E+00	1.071E-01	1.126E+00	6.800E-01	5.602E-02	3.176E-01
1.0000	1.016E+00	1.159E-01	1.132E+00	7.686E-01	6.030E-02	3.575E-01
1.2500	1.016E+00	1.387E-01	1.154E+00	9.875E-01	7.051E-02	4.528E-01
1.5000	1.021E+00	1.624E-01	1.183E+00	1.201E+00	8.022E-02	5.416E-01
1.7500	1.029E+00	1.868E-01	1.215E+00	1.410E+00	8.955E-02	6.242E-01
2.0000	1.037E+00	2.117E-01	1.249E+00	1.613E+00	9.856E-02	7.015E-01
2.5000	1.055E+00	2.630E-01	1.318E+00	2.003E+00	1.158E-01	8.423E-01
3.0000	1.072E+00	3.158E-01	1.388E+00	2.372E+00	1.321E-01	9.684E-01
3.5000	1.087E+00	3.698E-01	1.457E+00	2.724E+00	1.476E-01	1.083E+00
4.0000	1.101E+00	4.248E-01	1.526E+00	3.059E+00	1.625E-01	1.188E+00
4.5000	1.114E+00	4.806E-01	1.595E+00	3.380E+00	1.766E-01	1.286E+00
5.0000	1.126E+00	5.372E-01	1.663E+00	3.687E+00	1.902E-01	1.378E+00
5.5000	1.136E+00	5.945E-01	1.731E+00	3.981E+00	2.032E-01	1.463E+00
6.0000	1.146E+00	6.523E-01	1.798E+00	4.265E+00	2.157E-01	1.544E+00
7.0000	1.163E+00	7.697E-01	1.933E+00	4.801E+00	2.393E-01	1.694E+00
8.0000	1.178E+00	8.890E-01	2.067E+00	5.301E+00	2.612E-01	1.830E+00
9.0000	1.191E+00	1.010E+00	2.201E+00	5.770E+00	2.816E-01	1.955E+00
10.0000	1.203E+00	1.132E+00	2.335E+00	6.211E+00	3.006E-01	2.070E+00
12.5000	1.227E+00	1.443E+00	2.670E+00	7.212E+00	3.432E-01	2.324E+00
15.0000	1.247E+00	1.759E+00	3.006E+00	8.094E+00	3.800E-01	2.544E+00
17.5000	1.263E+00	2.081E+00	3.343E+00	8.882E+00	4.120E-01	2.737E+00
20.0000	1.277E+00	2.406E+00	3.682E+00	9.594E+00	4.403E-01	2.910E+00
25.0000	1.299E+00	3.065E+00	4.364E+00	1.084E+01	4.881E-01	3.212E+00
30.0000	1.316E+00	3.735E+00	5.051E+00	1.190E+01	5.270E-01	3.471E+00
35.0000	1.331E+00	4.412E+00	5.743E+00	1.283E+01	5.595E-01	3.698E+00
40.0000	1.343E+00	5.096E+00	6.439E+00	1.365E+01	5.871E-01	3.901E+00
45.0000	1.353E+00	5.784E+00	7.138E+00	1.439E+01	6.109E-01	4.084E+00
50.0000	1.362E+00	6.477E+00	7.840E+00	1.506E+01	6.316E-01	4.252E+00
55.0000	1.371E+00	7.174E+00	8.544E+00	1.567E+01	6.500E-01	4.405E+00
60.0000	1.378E+00	7.873E+00	9.251E+00	1.623E+01	6.662E-01	4.548E+00
70.0000	1.391E+00	9.280E+00	1.067E+01	1.724E+01	6.940E-01	4.804E+00
80.0000	1.401E+00	1.070E+01	1.210E+01	1.812E+01	7.169E-01	5.031E+00
90.0000	1.411E+00	1.212E+01	1.353E+01	1.890E+01	7.362E-01	5.233E+00

Lead

ENERGY	STOPPING POWER			CSDA RANGE	RADIATION YIELD	DENS.EFF. CORR. (DELTA)
	COLLISION	RADIATIVE	TOTAL			
MeV	MeV cm²/g	MeV cm²/g	MeV cm²/g	g/cm²		
0.0100	8.428E+00	2.045E-02	8.448E+00	8.253E-04	1.191E-03	4.841E-04
0.0125	7.357E+00	2.251E-02	7.379E+00	1.143E-03	1.500E-03	6.147E-04
0.0150	6.561E+00	2.421E-02	6.585E+00	1.502E-03	1.810E-03	7.491E-04
0.0175	5.946E+00	2.566E-02	5.971E+00	1.901E-03	2.121E-03	8.872E-04
0.0200	5.453E+00	2.693E-02	5.480E+00	2.339E-03	2.432E-03	1.029E-03
0.0250	4.714E+00	2.908E-02	4.743E+00	3.323E-03	3.051E-03	1.324E-03
0.0300	4.182E+00	3.086E-02	4.213E+00	4.444E-03	3.664E-03	1.633E-03
0.0350	3.779E+00	3.240E-02	3.812E+00	5.694E-03	4.271E-03	1.956E-03
0.0400	3.463E+00	3.376E-02	3.497E+00	7.066E-03	4.872E-03	2.294E-03
0.0450	3.208E+00	3.500E-02	3.243E+00	8.552E-03	5.467E-03	2.646E-03
0.0500	2.997E+00	3.613E-02	3.034E+00	1.015E-02	6.055E-03	3.011E-03
0.0550	2.821E+00	3.718E-02	2.858E+00	1.185E-02	6.638E-03	3.390E-03
0.0600	2.670E+00	3.817E-02	2.708E+00	1.365E-02	7.214E-03	3.783E-03
0.0700	2.426E+00	3.998E-02	2.466E+00	1.752E-02	8.349E-03	4.608E-03
0.0800	2.237E+00	4.162E-02	2.279E+00	2.175E-02	9.461E-03	5.485E-03
0.0900	2.087E+00	4.313E-02	2.130E+00	2.629E-02	1.055E-02	6.413E-03
0.1000	1.964E+00	4.454E-02	2.008E+00	3.113E-02	1.162E-02	7.392E-03
0.1250	1.738E+00	4.772E-02	1.785E+00	4.438E-02	1.419E-02	1.005E-02
0.1500	1.583E+00	5.054E-02	1.633E+00	5.905E-02	1.664E-02	1.300E-02
0.1750	1.471E+00	5.312E-02	1.524E+00	7.492E-02	1.896E-02	1.623E-02
0.2000	1.387E+00	5.555E-02	1.442E+00	9.180E-02	2.118E-02	1.971E-02
0.2500	1.269E+00	6.015E-02	1.329E+00	1.280E-01	2.533E-02	2.736E-02
0.3000	1.193E+00	6.460E-02	1.257E+00	1.668E-01	2.917E-02	3.579E-02
0.3500	1.140E+00	6.900E-02	1.209E+00	2.074E-01	3.276E-02	4.484E-02
0.4000	1.102E+00	7.340E-02	1.175E+00	2.494E-01	3.614E-02	5.437E-02
0.4500	1.074E+00	7.781E-02	1.152E+00	2.924E-01	3.935E-02	6.426E-02
0.5000	1.053E+00	8.228E-02	1.135E+00	3.361E-01	4.241E-02	7.442E-02
0.5500	1.037E+00	8.677E-02	1.124E+00	3.804E-01	4.536E-02	8.479E-02
0.6000	1.026E+00	9.132E-02	1.117E+00	4.250E-01	4.820E-02	9.529E-02
0.7000	1.009E+00	1.005E-01	1.110E+00	5.149E-01	5.363E-02	1.166E-01
0.8000	1.000E+00	1.098E-01	1.110E+00	6.050E-01	5.877E-02	1.380E-01
0.9000	9.957E-01	1.193E-01	1.115E+00	6.949E-01	6.369E-02	1.595E-01
1.0000	9.939E-01	1.290E-01	1.123E+00	7.843E-01	6.842E-02	1.809E-01
1.2500	9.966E-01	1.537E-01	1.150E+00	1.004E+00	7.960E-02	2.337E-01
1.5000	1.004E+00	1.792E-01	1.183E+00	1.219E+00	9.009E-02	2.854E-01
1.7500	1.014E+00	2.053E-01	1.219E+00	1.427E+00	1.001E-01	3.360E-01
2.0000	1.024E+00	2.319E-01	1.256E+00	1.629E+00	1.096E-01	3.855E-01
2.5000	1.044E+00	2.866E-01	1.331E+00	2.016E+00	1.277E-01	4.817E-01
3.0000	1.063E+00	3.427E-01	1.406E+00	2.381E+00	1.447E-01	5.743E-01
3.5000	1.080E+00	3.999E-01	1.480E+00	2.728E+00	1.608E-01	6.631E-01
4.0000	1.095E+00	4.582E-01	1.553E+00	3.057E+00	1.761E-01	7.479E-01
4.5000	1.108E+00	5.174E-01	1.626E+00	3.372E+00	1.906E-01	8.289E-01
5.0000	1.120E+00	5.773E-01	1.698E+00	3.673E+00	2.045E-01	9.061E-01
5.5000	1.132E+00	6.379E-01	1.769E+00	3.962E+00	2.177E-01	9.798E-01
6.0000	1.142E+00	6.991E-01	1.841E+00	4.239E+00	2.304E-01	1.050E+00
7.0000	1.160E+00	8.233E-01	1.983E+00	4.762E+00	2.543E-01	1.182E+00
8.0000	1.175E+00	9.495E-01	2.125E+00	5.249E+00	2.765E-01	1.304E+00
9.0000	1.189E+00	1.077E+00	2.266E+00	5.705E+00	2.970E-01	1.417E+00
10.0000	1.201E+00	1.206E+00	2.407E+00	6.133E+00	3.162E-01	1.523E+00
12.5000	1.226E+00	1.535E+00	2.761E+00	7.102E+00	3.589E-01	1.759E+00
15.0000	1.246E+00	1.870E+00	3.116E+00	7.954E+00	3.955E-01	1.964E+00
17.5000	1.262E+00	2.210E+00	3.472E+00	8.713E+00	4.274E-01	2.147E+00
20.0000	1.277E+00	2.554E+00	3.830E+00	9.399E+00	4.555E-01	2.310E+00
25.0000	1.299E+00	3.252E+00	4.551E+00	1.059E+01	5.028E-01	2.596E+00
30.0000	1.318E+00	3.961E+00	5.278E+00	1.161E+01	5.412E-01	2.841E+00
35.0000	1.332E+00	4.678E+00	6.011E+00	1.250E+01	5.731E-01	3.055E+00
40.0000	1.345E+00	5.402E+00	6.747E+00	1.329E+01	6.002E-01	3.247E+00
45.0000	1.356E+00	6.132E+00	7.488E+00	1.399E+01	6.235E-01	3.420E+00
50.0000	1.365E+00	6.865E+00	8.231E+00	1.463E+01	6.439E-01	3.579E+00
55.0000	1.374E+00	7.603E+00	8.977E+00	1.521E+01	6.618E-01	3.725E+00
60.0000	1.381E+00	8.345E+00	9.726E+00	1.574E+01	6.777E-01	3.861E+00
70.0000	1.395E+00	9.836E+00	1.123E+01	1.670E+01	7.048E-01	4.107E+00
80.0000	1.406E+00	1.134E+01	1.274E+01	1.753E+01	7.270E-01	4.326E+00
90.0000	1.415E+00	1.284E+01	1.426E+01	1.828E+01	7.457E-01	4.521E+00

Air (Dry)

ENERGY	STOPPING POWER COLLISION	RADIATIVE	TOTAL	CSDA RANGE	RADIATION YIELD	DENS.EFF. CORR. (DELTA)
MeV	MeV cm²/g	MeV cm²/g	MeV cm²/g	g/cm²		
0.0100	1.975E+01	3.897E-03	1.976E+01	2.883E-04	1.082E-04	0.0
0.0125	1.663E+01	3.921E-03	1.663E+01	4.269E-04	1.299E-04	0.0
0.0150	1.445E+01	3.937E-03	1.445E+01	5.886E-04	1.506E-04	0.0
0.0175	1.283E+01	3.946E-03	1.283E+01	7.726E-04	1.706E-04	0.0
0.0200	1.157E+01	3.954E-03	1.158E+01	9.781E-04	1.898E-04	0.0
0.0250	9.753E+00	3.966E-03	9.757E+00	1.451E-03	2.267E-04	0.0
0.0300	8.492E+00	3.976E-03	8.496E+00	2.001E-03	2.618E-04	0.0
0.0350	7.563E+00	3.986E-03	7.567E+00	2.626E-03	2.955E-04	0.0
0.0400	6.848E+00	3.998E-03	6.852E+00	3.322E-03	3.280E-04	0.0
0.0450	6.281E+00	4.011E-03	6.285E+00	4.085E-03	3.594E-04	0.0
0.0500	5.819E+00	4.025E-03	5.823E+00	4.912E-03	3.900E-04	0.0
0.0550	5.435E+00	4.040E-03	5.439E+00	5.801E-03	4.197E-04	0.0
0.0600	5.111E+00	4.057E-03	5.115E+00	6.750E-03	4.488E-04	0.0
0.0700	4.593E+00	4.093E-03	4.597E+00	8.817E-03	5.049E-04	0.0
0.0800	4.198E+00	4.133E-03	4.202E+00	1.110E-02	5.590E-04	0.0
0.0900	3.886E+00	4.175E-03	3.890E+00	1.357E-02	6.112E-04	0.0
0.1000	3.633E+00	4.222E-03	3.637E+00	1.623E-02	6.618E-04	0.0
0.1250	3.172E+00	4.348E-03	3.177E+00	2.362E-02	7.826E-04	0.0
0.1500	2.861E+00	4.485E-03	2.865E+00	3.193E-02	8.968E-04	0.0
0.1750	2.637E+00	4.633E-03	2.642E+00	4.103E-02	1.006E-03	0.0
0.2000	2.470E+00	4.789E-03	2.474E+00	5.082E-02	1.111E-03	0.0
0.2500	2.236E+00	5.126E-03	2.242E+00	7.212E-02	1.311E-03	0.0
0.3000	2.084E+00	5.495E-03	2.089E+00	9.527E-02	1.502E-03	0.0
0.3500	1.978E+00	5.890E-03	1.984E+00	1.199E-01	1.688E-03	0.0
0.4000	1.902E+00	6.311E-03	1.908E+00	1.456E-01	1.869E-03	0.0
0.4500	1.845E+00	6.757E-03	1.852E+00	1.722E-01	2.048E-03	0.0
0.5000	1.802E+00	7.223E-03	1.809E+00	1.995E-01	2.225E-03	0.0
0.5500	1.769E+00	7.708E-03	1.776E+00	2.274E-01	2.401E-03	0.0
0.6000	1.743E+00	8.210E-03	1.751E+00	2.558E-01	2.577E-03	0.0
0.7000	1.706E+00	9.258E-03	1.715E+00	3.135E-01	2.929E-03	0.0
0.8000	1.683E+00	1.036E-02	1.694E+00	3.722E-01	3.283E-03	0.0
0.9000	1.669E+00	1.151E-02	1.681E+00	4.315E-01	3.638E-03	0.0
1.0000	1.661E+00	1.271E-02	1.674E+00	4.912E-01	3.997E-03	0.0
1.2500	1.655E+00	1.588E-02	1.671E+00	6.408E-01	4.906E-03	0.0
1.5000	1.661E+00	1.927E-02	1.680E+00	7.900E-01	5.836E-03	0.0
1.7500	1.672E+00	2.284E-02	1.694E+00	9.382E-01	6.784E-03	0.0
2.0000	1.684E+00	2.656E-02	1.711E+00	1.085E+00	7.748E-03	0.0
2.5000	1.712E+00	3.437E-02	1.747E+00	1.374E+00	9.716E-03	0.0
3.0000	1.740E+00	4.260E-02	1.783E+00	1.658E+00	1.173E-02	0.0
3.5000	1.766E+00	5.115E-02	1.817E+00	1.935E+00	1.377E-02	0.0
4.0000	1.790E+00	5.999E-02	1.850E+00	2.208E+00	1.583E-02	0.0
4.5000	1.812E+00	6.908E-02	1.882E+00	2.476E+00	1.792E-02	0.0
5.0000	1.833E+00	7.838E-02	1.911E+00	2.740E+00	2.001E-02	0.0
5.5000	1.852E+00	8.787E-02	1.940E+00	2.999E+00	2.211E-02	0.0
6.0000	1.870E+00	9.754E-02	1.968E+00	3.255E+00	2.422E-02	0.0
7.0000	1.902E+00	1.173E-01	2.020E+00	3.757E+00	2.845E-02	0.0
8.0000	1.931E+00	1.376E-01	2.068E+00	4.246E+00	3.269E-02	0.0
9.0000	1.956E+00	1.584E-01	2.115E+00	4.724E+00	3.692E-02	0.0
10.0000	1.979E+00	1.795E-01	2.159E+00	5.192E+00	4.113E-02	0.0
12.5000	2.029E+00	2.337E-01	2.262E+00	6.323E+00	5.156E-02	0.0
15.0000	2.069E+00	2.895E-01	2.359E+00	7.405E+00	6.181E-02	0.0
17.5000	2.104E+00	3.464E-01	2.451E+00	8.444E+00	7.185E-02	0.0
20.0000	2.134E+00	4.042E-01	2.539E+00	9.446E+00	8.167E-02	0.0
25.0000	2.185E+00	5.219E-01	2.707E+00	1.135E+01	1.006E-01	7.636E-03
30.0000	2.226E+00	6.417E-01	2.868E+00	1.315E+01	1.186E-01	5.984E-02
35.0000	2.257E+00	7.630E-01	3.020E+00	1.485E+01	1.357E-01	
40.0000	2.282E+00	8.855E-01	3.167E+00	1.646E+01	1.520E-01	1.378E-01
45.0000	2.302E+00	1.009E+00	3.311E+00	1.801E+01	1.676E-01	2.266E-01
50.0000	2.319E+00	1.133E+00	3.452E+00	1.948E+01	1.825E-01	3.192E-01
55.0000	2.334E+00	1.258E+00	3.592E+00	2.090E+01	1.968E-01	4.120E-01
60.0000	2.347E+00	1.384E+00	3.731E+00	2.227E+01	2.104E-01	5.029E-01
70.0000	2.369E+00	1.637E+00	4.006E+00	2.486E+01	2.361E-01	6.762E-01
80.0000	2.387E+00	1.892E+00	4.279E+00	2.727E+01	2.598E-01	8.365E-01
90.0000	2.403E+00	2.148E+00	4.551E+00	2.954E+01	2.818E-01	9.842E-01

Water (Liquid)

ENERGY	STOPPING POWER			CSDA RANGE	RADIATION YIELD	DENS.EFF. CORR. (DELTA)
MeV	COLLISION MeV cm²/g	RADIATIVE MeV cm²/g	TOTAL MeV cm²/g	g/cm²		
0.0100	2.256E+01	3.898E-03	2.257E+01	2.515E-04	9.408E-05	0.0
0.0125	1.897E+01	3.927E-03	1.898E+01	3.728E-04	1.133E-04	0.0
0.0150	1.647E+01	3.944E-03	1.647E+01	5.147E-04	1.316E-04	0.0
0.0175	1.461E+01	3.955E-03	1.461E+01	6.761E-04	1.492E-04	0.0
0.0200	1.317E+01	3.963E-03	1.318E+01	8.566E-04	1.663E-04	0.0
0.0250	1.109E+01	3.974E-03	1.110E+01	1.272E-03	1.990E-04	0.0
0.0300	9.653E+00	3.984E-03	9.657E+00	1.756E-03	2.301E-04	0.0
0.0350	8.592E+00	3.994E-03	8.596E+00	2.306E-03	2.599E-04	0.0
0.0400	7.777E+00	4.005E-03	7.781E+00	2.919E-03	2.886E-04	0.0
0.0450	7.130E+00	4.018E-03	7.134E+00	3.591E-03	3.165E-04	0.0
0.0500	6.603E+00	4.031E-03	6.607E+00	4.320E-03	3.435E-04	0.0
0.0550	6.166E+00	4.046E-03	6.170E+00	5.103E-03	3.698E-04	0.0
0.0600	5.797E+00	4.062E-03	5.801E+00	5.940E-03	3.955E-04	0.0
0.0700	5.207E+00	4.098E-03	5.211E+00	7.762E-03	4.452E-04	0.0
0.0800	4.757E+00	4.138E-03	4.762E+00	9.773E-03	4.931E-04	0.0
0.0900	4.402E+00	4.181E-03	4.407E+00	1.196E-02	5.393E-04	0.0
0.1000	4.115E+00	4.228E-03	4.120E+00	1.431E-02	5.841E-04	0.0
0.1250	3.591E+00	4.355E-03	3.596E+00	2.083E-02	6.912E-04	0.0
0.1500	3.238E+00	4.494E-03	3.242E+00	2.817E-02	7.926E-04	0.0
0.1750	2.984E+00	4.643E-03	2.988E+00	3.622E-02	8.894E-04	0.0
0.2000	2.793E+00	4.801E-03	2.798E+00	4.487E-02	9.826E-04	0.0
0.2500	2.528E+00	5.141E-03	2.533E+00	6.372E-02	1.161E-03	0.0
0.3000	2.355E+00	5.514E-03	2.360E+00	8.421E-02	1.331E-03	0.0
0.3500	2.235E+00	5.913E-03	2.241E+00	1.060E-01	1.496E-03	0.0
0.4000	2.148E+00	6.339E-03	2.154E+00	1.288E-01	1.658E-03	0.0
0.4500	2.083E+00	6.787E-03	2.090E+00	1.523E-01	1.818E-03	0.0
0.5000	2.034E+00	7.257E-03	2.041E+00	1.766E-01	1.976E-03	0.0
0.5500	1.995E+00	7.747E-03	2.003E+00	2.013E-01	2.134E-03	1.103E-02
0.6000	1.963E+00	8.254E-03	1.972E+00	2.265E-01	2.292E-03	2.938E-02
0.7000	1.917E+00	9.312E-03	1.926E+00	2.778E-01	2.608E-03	7.435E-02
0.8000	1.886E+00	1.043E-02	1.896E+00	3.302E-01	2.928E-03	1.267E-01
0.9000	1.864E+00	1.159E-02	1.876E+00	3.832E-01	3.251E-03	1.835E-01
1.0000	1.849E+00	1.280E-02	1.862E+00	4.367E-01	3.579E-03	2.428E-01
1.2500	1.829E+00	1.600E-02	1.845E+00	5.717E-01	4.416E-03	3.944E-01
1.5000	1.822E+00	1.942E-02	1.841E+00	7.075E-01	5.281E-03	5.437E-01
1.7500	1.821E+00	2.303E-02	1.844E+00	8.432E-01	6.171E-03	6.866E-01
2.0000	1.824E+00	2.678E-02	1.850E+00	9.785E-01	7.085E-03	8.218E-01
2.5000	1.834E+00	3.468E-02	1.868E+00	1.247E+00	8.969E-03	1.069E+00
3.0000	1.846E+00	4.299E-02	1.889E+00	1.514E+00	1.092E-02	1.288E+00
3.5000	1.858E+00	5.164E-02	1.910E+00	1.777E+00	1.291E-02	1.484E+00
4.0000	1.870E+00	6.058E-02	1.931E+00	2.037E+00	1.495E-02	1.660E+00
4.5000	1.882E+00	6.976E-02	1.951E+00	2.295E+00	1.702E-02	1.821E+00
5.0000	1.892E+00	7.917E-02	1.971E+00	2.550E+00	1.911E-02	1.967E+00
5.5000	1.902E+00	8.876E-02	1.991E+00	2.802E+00	2.123E-02	2.102E+00
6.0000	1.911E+00	9.854E-02	2.010E+00	3.052E+00	2.336E-02	2.227E+00
7.0000	1.928E+00	1.185E-01	2.047E+00	3.545E+00	2.766E-02	2.453E+00
8.0000	1.943E+00	1.391E-01	2.082E+00	4.030E+00	3.200E-02	2.652E+00
9.0000	1.956E+00	1.601E-01	2.116E+00	4.506E+00	3.636E-02	2.831E+00
10.0000	1.968E+00	1.814E-01	2.149E+00	4.975E+00	4.072E-02	2.992E+00
12.5000	1.993E+00	2.362E-01	2.230E+00	6.117E+00	5.163E-02	3.341E+00
15.0000	2.014E+00	2.926E-01	2.306E+00	7.219E+00	6.243E-02	3.633E+00
17.5000	2.031E+00	3.501E-01	2.381E+00	8.286E+00	7.309E-02	3.885E+00
20.0000	2.046E+00	4.086E-01	2.454E+00	9.320E+00	8.355E-02	4.107E+00
25.0000	2.070E+00	5.277E-01	2.598E+00	1.130E+01	1.039E-01	4.487E+00
30.0000	2.089E+00	6.489E-01	2.738E+00	1.317E+01	1.233E-01	4.806E+00
35.0000	2.105E+00	7.716E-01	2.876E+00	1.496E+01	1.418E-01	5.082E+00
40.0000	2.118E+00	8.955E-01	3.013E+00	1.665E+01	1.594E-01	5.326E+00
45.0000	2.129E+00	1.021E+00	3.150E+00	1.828E+01	1.762E-01	5.544E+00
50.0000	2.139E+00	1.146E+00	3.286E+00	1.983E+01	1.923E-01	5.741E+00
55.0000	2.148E+00	1.273E+00	3.421E+00	2.132E+01	2.076E-01	5.921E+00
60.0000	2.156E+00	1.400E+00	3.556E+00	2.276E+01	2.222E-01	6.087E+00
70.0000	2.170E+00	1.656E+00	3.827E+00	2.547E+01	2.496E-01	6.383E+00
80.0000	2.182E+00	1.914E+00	4.096E+00	2.799E+01	2.747E-01	6.641E+00
90.0000	2.193E+00	2.173E+00	4.366E+00	3.035E+01	2.978E-01	6.871E+00

A-150 Tissue-Equivalent Plastic

| ENERGY | STOPPING POWER | | TOTAL | CSDA RANGE | RADIATION YIELD | DENS.EFF. CORR. (DELTA) |
| | COLLISION | RADIATIVE | | | | |
MeV	MeV cm²/g	MeV cm²/g	MeV cm²/g	g/cm²		
0.0100	2.294E+01	3.156E-03	2.295E+01	2.463E-04	7.529E-05	0.0
0.0125	1.927E+01	3.174E-03	1.927E+01	3.657E-04	9.048E-05	0.0
0.0150	1.671E+01	3.188E-03	1.671E+01	5.054E-04	1.050E-04	0.0
0.0175	1.482E+01	3.197E-03	1.482E+01	6.646E-04	1.191E-04	0.0
0.0200	1.335E+01	3.205E-03	1.336E+01	8.426E-04	1.327E-04	0.0
0.0250	1.124E+01	3.219E-03	1.124E+01	1.253E-03	1.588E-04	0.0
0.0300	9.769E+00	3.232E-03	9.772E+00	1.731E-03	1.838E-04	0.0
0.0350	8.691E+00	3.245E-03	8.694E+00	2.275E-03	2.079E-04	0.0
0.0400	7.863E+00	3.258E-03	7.866E+00	2.880E-03	2.311E-04	0.0
0.0450	7.206E+00	3.273E-03	7.209E+00	3.545E-03	2.537E-04	0.0
0.0500	6.671E+00	3.287E-03	6.675E+00	4.267E-03	2.756E-04	0.0
0.0550	6.228E+00	3.302E-03	6.231E+00	5.043E-03	2.971E-04	0.0
0.0600	5.853E+00	3.319E-03	5.857E+00	5.871E-03	3.180E-04	0.0
0.0700	5.256E+00	3.352E-03	5.259E+00	7.677E-03	3.586E-04	0.0
0.0800	4.800E+00	3.388E-03	4.803E+00	9.669E-03	3.977E-04	0.0
0.0900	4.441E+00	3.427E-03	4.444E+00	1.184E-02	4.356E-04	0.0
0.1000	4.150E+00	3.467E-03	4.153E+00	1.417E-02	4.723E-04	0.0
0.1250	3.620E+00	3.578E-03	3.623E+00	2.064E-02	5.602E-04	0.0
0.1500	3.262E+00	3.697E-03	3.265E+00	2.792E-02	6.436E-04	0.0
0.1750	3.005E+00	3.824E-03	3.009E+00	3.592E-02	7.234E-04	0.0
0.2000	2.812E+00	3.959E-03	2.816E+00	4.452E-02	8.003E-04	0.0
0.2500	2.544E+00	4.247E-03	2.548E+00	6.325E-02	9.476E-04	0.0
0.3000	2.369E+00	4.563E-03	2.373E+00	8.362E-02	1.089E-03	0.0
0.3500	2.247E+00	4.901E-03	2.252E+00	1.053E-01	1.226E-03	0.0
0.4000	2.156E+00	5.260E-03	2.161E+00	1.280E-01	1.361E-03	2.969E-02
0.4500	2.086E+00	5.639E-03	2.092E+00	1.515E-01	1.495E-03	6.264E-02
0.5000	2.033E+00	6.036E-03	2.039E+00	1.757E-01	1.628E-03	9.751E-02
0.5500	1.991E+00	6.448E-03	1.997E+00	2.005E-01	1.761E-03	1.337E-01
0.6000	1.957E+00	6.875E-03	1.964E+00	2.258E-01	1.895E-03	1.708E-01
0.7000	1.908E+00	7.768E-03	1.915E+00	2.774E-01	2.164E-03	2.464E-01
0.8000	1.874E+00	8.706E-03	1.883E+00	3.300E-01	2.436E-03	3.223E-01
0.9000	1.851E+00	9.687E-03	1.860E+00	3.835E-01	2.711E-03	3.975E-01
1.0000	1.834E+00	1.071E-02	1.845E+00	4.375E-01	2.990E-03	4.712E-01
1.2500	1.812E+00	1.341E-02	1.825E+00	5.739E-01	3.706E-03	6.472E-01
1.5000	1.803E+00	1.630E-02	1.819E+00	7.111E-01	4.447E-03	8.100E-01
1.7500	1.802E+00	1.934E-02	1.821E+00	8.485E-01	5.209E-03	9.601E-01
2.0000	1.804E+00	2.252E-02	1.827E+00	9.856E-01	5.992E-03	1.099E+00
2.5000	1.814E+00	2.920E-02	1.843E+00	1.258E+00	7.609E-03	1.346E+00
3.0000	1.827E+00	3.625E-02	1.863E+00	1.528E+00	9.281E-03	1.561E+00
3.5000	1.839E+00	4.358E-02	1.883E+00	1.795E+00	1.100E-02	1.751E+00
4.0000	1.852E+00	5.116E-02	1.903E+00	2.059E+00	1.275E-02	1.922E+00
4.5000	1.863E+00	5.896E-02	1.922E+00	2.320E+00	1.453E-02	2.077E+00
5.0000	1.874E+00	6.695E-02	1.941E+00	2.579E+00	1.633E-02	2.218E+00
5.5000	1.884E+00	7.511E-02	1.959E+00	2.836E+00	1.816E-02	2.349E+00
6.0000	1.894E+00	8.341E-02	1.977E+00	3.090E+00	2.000E-02	2.470E+00
7.0000	1.911E+00	1.004E-01	2.011E+00	3.591E+00	2.372E-02	2.691E+00
8.0000	1.926E+00	1.179E-01	2.044E+00	4.084E+00	2.748E-02	2.887E+00
9.0000	1.939E+00	1.358E-01	2.075E+00	4.570E+00	3.127E-02	3.064E+00
10.0000	1.951E+00	1.540E-01	2.105E+00	5.048E+00	3.508E-02	3.227E+00
12.5000	1.975E+00	2.007E-01	2.176E+00	6.216E+00	4.461E-02	3.582E+00
15.0000	1.995E+00	2.488E-01	2.243E+00	7.348E+00	5.411E-02	3.885E+00
17.5000	2.010E+00	2.979E-01	2.308E+00	8.446E+00	6.352E-02	4.150E+00
20.0000	2.024E+00	3.478E-01	2.372E+00	9.515E+00	7.282E-02	4.385E+00
25.0000	2.046E+00	4.496E-01	2.495E+00	1.157E+01	9.097E-02	4.788E+00
30.0000	2.063E+00	5.532E-01	2.616E+00	1.353E+01	1.085E-01	5.126E+00
35.0000	2.077E+00	6.582E-01	2.735E+00	1.540E+01	1.253E-01	5.417E+00
40.0000	2.089E+00	7.643E-01	2.854E+00	1.718E+01	1.414E-01	5.671E+00
45.0000	2.100E+00	8.714E-01	2.971E+00	1.890E+01	1.569E-01	5.897E+00
50.0000	2.109E+00	9.792E-01	3.089E+00	2.055E+01	1.717E-01	6.101E+00
55.0000	2.118E+00	1.088E+00	3.205E+00	2.214E+01	1.860E-01	6.286E+00
60.0000	2.125E+00	1.197E+00	3.322E+00	2.367E+01	1.996E-01	6.456E+00
70.0000	2.139E+00	1.416E+00	3.555E+00	2.658E+01	2.254E-01	6.758E+00
80.0000	2.151E+00	1.638E+00	3.788E+00	2.931E+01	2.491E-01	7.020E+00
90.0000	2.161E+00	1.860E+00	4.021E+00	3.187E+01	2.712E-01	7.253E+00

Skeletal Muscle (ICRP)

ENERGY	STOPPING POWER			CSDA	RADIATION	DENS.EFF.
	COLLISION	RADIATIVE	TOTAL	RANGE	YIELD	CORR.
						(DELTA)
MeV	MeV cm²/g	MeV cm²/g	MeV cm²/g	g/cm²		
0.0100	2.231E+01	3.835E-03	2.231E+01	2.543E-04	9.366E-05	0.0
0.0125	1.876E+01	3.863E-03	1.877E+01	3.771E-04	1.127E-04	0.0
0.0150	1.628E+01	3.880E-03	1.629E+01	5.205E-04	1.310E-04	0.0
0.0175	1.445E+01	3.892E-03	1.445E+01	6.838E-04	1.485E-04	0.0
0.0200	1.303E+01	3.901E-03	1.303E+01	8.662E-04	1.655E-04	0.0
0.0250	1.097E+01	3.913E-03	1.098E+01	1.286E-03	1.980E-04	0.0
0.0300	9.547E+00	3.924E-03	9.551E+00	1.776E-03	2.290E-04	0.0
0.0350	8.498E+00	3.934E-03	8.502E+00	2.332E-03	2.587E-04	0.0
0.0400	7.692E+00	3.946E-03	7.696E+00	2.951E-03	2.874E-04	0.0
0.0450	7.052E+00	3.959E-03	7.056E+00	3.631E-03	3.151E-04	0.0
0.0500	6.531E+00	3.973E-03	6.535E+00	4.368E-03	3.421E-04	0.0
0.0550	6.099E+00	3.988E-03	6.102E+00	5.160E-03	3.683E-04	0.0
0.0600	5.733E+00	4.004E-03	5.737E+00	6.006E-03	3.939E-04	0.0
0.0700	5.151E+00	4.040E-03	5.155E+00	7.848E-03	4.435E-04	0.0
0.0800	4.706E+00	4.079E-03	4.710E+00	9.881E-03	4.912E-04	0.0
0.0900	4.355E+00	4.122E-03	4.359E+00	1.209E-02	5.373E-04	0.0
0.1000	4.071E+00	4.168E-03	4.075E+00	1.447E-02	5.821E-04	0.0
0.1250	3.552E+00	4.294E-03	3.557E+00	2.106E-02	6.889E-04	0.0
0.1500	3.203E+00	4.431E-03	3.207E+00	2.848E-02	7.899E-04	0.0
0.1750	2.951E+00	4.579E-03	2.956E+00	3.662E-02	8.865E-04	0.0
0.2000	2.763E+00	4.734E-03	2.768E+00	4.537E-02	9.795E-04	0.0
0.2500	2.501E+00	5.070E-03	2.506E+00	6.442E-02	1.157E-03	0.0
0.3000	2.329E+00	5.438E-03	2.335E+00	8.513E-02	1.327E-03	0.0
0.3500	2.211E+00	5.832E-03	2.216E+00	1.071E-01	1.492E-03	0.0
0.4000	2.125E+00	6.252E-03	2.131E+00	1.302E-01	1.653E-03	0.0
0.4500	2.061E+00	6.694E-03	2.068E+00	1.540E-01	1.812E-03	0.0
0.5000	2.012E+00	7.158E-03	2.019E+00	1.785E-01	1.970E-03	2.181E-03
0.5500	1.972E+00	7.642E-03	1.980E+00	2.035E-01	2.128E-03	2.071E-02
0.6000	1.941E+00	8.141E-03	1.949E+00	2.290E-01	2.285E-03	4.241E-02
0.7000	1.895E+00	9.186E-03	1.904E+00	2.809E-01	2.602E-03	9.262E-02
0.8000	1.863E+00	1.028E-02	1.874E+00	3.339E-01	2.921E-03	1.488E-01
0.9000	1.842E+00	1.143E-02	1.853E+00	3.876E-01	3.244E-03	2.084E-01
1.0000	1.827E+00	1.262E-02	1.839E+00	4.418E-01	3.571E-03	2.697E-01
1.2500	1.806E+00	1.578E-02	1.822E+00	5.784E-01	4.408E-03	4.245E-01
1.5000	1.799E+00	1.916E-02	1.818E+00 —	7.158E-01	5.272E-03	5.750E-01
1.7500	1.799E+00	2.271E-02	1.821E+00	8.532E-01	6.162E-03	7.181E-01
2.0000	1.801E+00	2.642E-02	1.828E+00	9.903E-01	7.074E-03	8.529E-01
2.5000	1.812E+00	3.421E-02	1.846E+00	1.263E+00	8.956E-03	1.098E+00
3.0000	1.824E+00	4.241E-02	1.866E+00	1.532E+00	1.090E-02	1.316E+00
3.5000	1.836E+00	5.095E-02	1.887E+00	1.798E+00	1.289E-02	1.509E+00
4.0000	1.848E+00	5.977E-02	1.908E+00	2.062E+00	1.493E-02	1.683E+00
4.5000	1.860E+00	6.883E-02	1.928E+00	2.323E+00	1.699E-02	1.842E+00
5.0000	1.870E+00	7.811E-02	1.948E+00	2.580E+00	1.908E-02	1.986E+00
5.5000	1.880E+00	8.758E-02	1.968E+00	2.836E+00	2.119E-02	2.120E+00
6.0000	1.889E+00	9.722E-02	1.987E+00	3.089E+00	2.332E-02	2.243E+00
7.0000	1.906E+00	1.170E-01	2.023E+00	3.587E+00	2.761E-02	2.466E+00
8.0000	1.921E+00	1.372E-01	2.058E+00	4.077E+00	3.194E-02	2.664E+00
9.0000	1.934E+00	1.579E-01	2.092E+00	4.559E+00	3.629E-02	2.840E+00
10.0000	1.946E+00	1.790E-01	2.125E+00	5.033E+00	4.065E-02	3.001E+00
12.5000	1.971E+00	2.331E-01	2.205E+00	6.188E+00	5.152E-02	3.348E+00
15.0000	1.992E+00	2.887E-01	2.281E+00	7.303E+00	6.231E-02	3.640E+00
17.5000	2.009E+00	3.455E-01	2.354E+00	8.382E+00	7.294E-02	3.892E+00
20.0000	2.023E+00	4.032E-01	2.427E+00	9.428E+00	8.339E-02	4.115E+00
25.0000	2.047E+00	5.208E-01	2.568E+00	1.143E+01	1.037E-01	4.497E+00
30.0000	2.066E+00	6.403E-01	2.706E+00	1.333E+01	1.230E-01	4.818E+00
35.0000	2.081E+00	7.615E-01	2.842E+00	1.513E+01	1.415E-01	5.096E+00
40.0000	2.094E+00	8.838E-01	2.978E+00	1.685E+01	1.592E-01	5.341E+00
45.0000	2.105E+00	1.007E+00	3.112E+00	1.849E+01	1.760E-01	5.560E+00
50.0000	2.115E+00	1.131E+00	3.247E+00	2.006E+01	1.920E-01	5.758E+00
55.0000	2.124E+00	1.256E+00	3.380E+00	2.157E+01	2.073E-01	5.938E+00
60.0000	2.132E+00	1.382E+00	3.514E+00	2.302E+01	2.219E-01	6.105E+00
70.0000	2.146E+00	1.635E+00	3.780E+00	2.577E+01	2.492E-01	6.401E+00
80.0000	2.158E+00	1.889E+00	4.047E+00	2.832E+01	2.743E-01	6.660E+00
90.0000	2.168E+00	2.145E+00	4.313E+00	3.071E+01	2.974E-01	6.890E+00

Adipose Tissue (ICRP)

ENERGY	STOPPING POWER COLLISION	RADIATIVE	TOTAL	CSDA RANGE	RADIATION YIELD	DENS.EFF. CORR. (DELTA)
MeV	MeV cm²/g	MeV cm²/g	MeV cm²/g	g/cm²		
0.0100	2.347E+01	3.168E-03	2.347E+01	2.406E-04	7.396E-05	0.0
0.0125	1.971E+01	3.184E-03	1.971E+01	3.574E-04	8.884E-05	0.0
0.0150	1.709E+01	3.194E-03	1.709E+01	4.940E-04	1.031E-04	0.0
0.0175	1.515E+01	3.201E-03	1.515E+01	6.497E-04	1.168E-04	0.0
0.0200	1.365E+01	3.207E-03	1.365E+01	8.237E-04	1.301E-04	0.0
0.0250	1.148E+01	3.217E-03	1.149E+01	1.225E-03	1.556E-04	0.0
0.0300	9.984E+00	3.227E-03	9.987E+00	1.693E-03	1.800E-04	0.0
0.0350	8.881E+00	3.238E-03	8.884E+00	2.225E-03	2.034E-04	0.0
0.0400	8.034E+00	3.249E-03	8.037E+00	2.818E-03	2.260E-04	0.0
0.0450	7.362E+00	3.262E-03	7.365E+00	3.468E-03	2.480E-04	0.0
0.0500	6.816E+00	3.275E-03	6.819E+00	4.175E-03	2.693E-04	0.0
0.0550	6.362E+00	3.290E-03	6.365E+00	4.934E-03	2.902E-04	0.0
0.0600	5.979E+00	3.305E-03	5.983E+00	5.745E-03	3.106E-04	0.0
0.0700	5.369E+00	3.338E-03	5.372E+00	7.513E-03	3.501E-04	0.0
0.0800	4.903E+00	3.373E-03	4.906E+00	9.464E-03	3.881E-04	0.0
0.0900	4.535E+00	3.411E-03	4.539E+00	1.159E-02	4.250E-04	0.0
0.1000	4.238E+00	3.452E-03	4.241E+00	1.387E-02	4.608E-04	0.0
0.1250	3.696E+00	3.562E-03	3.700E+00	2.020E-02	5.464E-04	0.0
0.1500	3.330E+00	3.681E-03	3.334E+00	2.734E-02	6.277E-04	0.0
0.1750	3.068E+00	3.808E-03	3.071E+00	3.517E-02	7.055E-04	0.0
0.2000	2.871E+00	3.943E-03	2.875E+00	4.359E-02	7.806E-04	0.0
0.2500	2.597E+00	4.232E-03	2.601E+00	6.194E-02	9.244E-04	0.0
0.3000	2.418E+00	4.547E-03	2.422E+00	8.190E-02	1.062E-03	0.0
0.3500	2.294E+00	4.885E-03	2.299E+00	1.031E-01	1.196E-03	0.0
0.4000	2.204E+00	5.244E-03	2.209E+00	1.253E-01	1.328E-03	0.0
0.4500	2.135E+00	5.623E-03	2.141E+00	1.483E-01	1.458E-03	1.471E-02
0.5000	2.081E+00	6.020E-03	2.087E+00	1.720E-01	1.588E-03	4.184E-02
0.5500	2.039E+00	6.433E-03	2.045E+00	1.962E-01	1.718E-03	7.141E-02
0.6000	2.005E+00	6.860E-03	2.011E+00	2.209E-01	1.848E-03	1.028E-01
0.7000	1.954E+00	7.753E-03	1.962E+00	2.712E-01	2.109E-03	1.691E-01
0.8000	1.921E+00	8.692E-03	1.929E+00	3.227E-01	2.374E-03	2.381E-01
0.9000	1.897E+00	9.674E-03	1.907E+00	3.748E-01	2.642E-03	3.080E-01
1.0000	1.880E+00	1.070E-02	1.891E+00	4.275E-01	2.915E-03	3.776E-01
1.2500	1.858E+00	1.340E-02	1.871E+00	5.605E-01	3.612E-03	5.471E-01
1.5000	1.849E+00	1.629E-02	1.865E+00	6.944E-01	4.334E-03	7.067E-01
1.7500	1.848E+00	1.934E-02	1.867E+00	8.284E-01	5.078E-03	8.554E-01
2.0000	1.850E+00	2.252E-02	1.873E+00	9.621E-01	5.842E-03	9.936E-01
2.5000	1.860E+00	2.921E-02	1.889E+00	1.228E+00	7.421E-03	1.242E+00
3.0000	1.872E+00	3.626E-02	1.908E+00	1.491E+00	9.055E-03	1.459E+00
3.5000	1.885E+00	4.360E-02	1.928E+00	1.752E+00	1.073E-02	1.652E+00
4.0000	1.897E+00	5.120E-02	1.948E+00	2.010E+00	1.245E-02	1.825E+00
4.5000	1.909E+00	5.901E-02	1.968E+00	2.265E+00	1.419E-02	1.981E+00
5.0000	1.920E+00	6.701E-02	1.987E+00	2.518E+00	1.596E-02	2.125E+00
5.5000	1.930E+00	7.518E-02	2.005E+00	2.769E+00	1.774E-02	2.257E+00
6.0000	1.939E+00	8.350E-02	2.023E+00	3.017E+00	1.955E-02	2.379E+00
7.0000	1.956E+00	1.005E-01	2.057E+00	3.507E+00	2.319E-02	2.601E+00
8.0000	1.972E+00	1.181E-01	2.090E+00	3.990E+00	2.688E-02	2.798E+00
9.0000	1.985E+00	1.360E-01	2.121E+00	4.465E+00	3.059E-02	2.976E+00
10.0000	1.997E+00	1.542E-01	2.151E+00	4.933E+00	3.432E-02	3.137E+00
12.5000	2.022E+00	2.010E-01	2.223E+00	6.076E+00	4.368E-02	3.491E+00
15.0000	2.042E+00	2.492E-01	2.291E+00	7.183E+00	5.300E-02	3.790E+00
17.5000	2.059E+00	2.984E-01	2.357E+00	8.259E+00	6.225E-02	4.050E+00
20.0000	2.073E+00	3.485E-01	2.421E+00	9.305E+00	7.138E-02	4.282E+00
25.0000	2.095E+00	4.505E-01	2.546E+00	1.132E+01	8.923E-02	4.679E+00
30.0000	2.113E+00	5.544E-01	2.668E+00	1.324E+01	1.065E-01	5.012E+00
35.0000	2.128E+00	6.597E-01	2.788E+00	1.507E+01	1.230E-01	5.299E+00
40.0000	2.141E+00	7.661E-01	2.907E+00	1.683E+01	1.389E-01	5.551E+00
45.0000	2.152E+00	8.734E-01	3.025E+00	1.851E+01	1.542E-01	5.776E+00
50.0000	2.161E+00	9.815E-01	3.143E+00	2.013E+01	1.688E-01	5.979E+00
55.0000	2.170E+00	1.090E+00	3.260E+00	2.170E+01	1.829E-01	6.163E+00
60.0000	2.178E+00	1.200E+00	3.377E+00	2.320E+01	1.964E-01	6.332E+00
70.0000	2.192E+00	1.420E+00	3.611E+00	2.607E+01	2.218E-01	6.632E+00
80.0000	2.203E+00	1.642E+00	3.845E+00	2.875E+01	2.454E-01	6.894E+00
90.0000	2.214E+00	1.865E+00	4.079E+00	3.127E+01	2.673E-01	7.126E+00

Cortical Bone (ICRP)

ENERGY	STOPPING POWER COLLISION	RADIATIVE	TOTAL	CSDA RANGE	RADIATION YIELD	DENS.EFF. CORR. (DELTA)
MeV	MeV cm²/g	MeV cm²/g	MeV cm²/g	g/cm²		
0.0100	1.971E+01	5.461E-03	1.972E+01	2.909E-04	1.468E-04	0.0
0.0125	1.663E+01	5.579E-03	1.664E+01	4.295E-04	1.787E-04	0.0
0.0150	1.447E+01	5.664E-03	1.447E+01	5.911E-04	2.095E-04	0.0
0.0175	1.286E+01	5.728E-03	1.287E+01	7.747E-04	2.393E-04	0.0
0.0200	1.161E+01	5.778E-03	1.162E+01	9.795E-04	2.683E-04	0.0
0.0250	9.804E+00	5.853E-03	9.810E+00	1.450E-03	3.242E-04	0.0
0.0300	8.546E+00	5.907E-03	8.552E+00	1.997E-03	3.775E-04	0.0
0.0350	7.618E+00	5.951E-03	7.624E+00	2.618E-03	4.287E-04	0.0
0.0400	6.903E+00	5.989E-03	6.909E+00	3.308E-03	4.781E-04	0.0
0.0450	6.335E+00	6.022E-03	6.341E+00	4.064E-03	5.259E-04	0.0
0.0500	5.872E+00	6.054E-03	5.879E+00	4.884E-03	5.723E-04	0.0
0.0550	5.488E+00	6.084E-03	5.494E+00	5.764E-03	6.175E-04	0.0
0.0600	5.163E+00	6.113E-03	5.169E+00	6.703E-03	6.614E-04	0.0
0.0700	4.643E+00	6.171E-03	4.649E+00	8.748E-03	7.463E-04	0.0
0.0800	4.246E+00	6.230E-03	4.252E+00	1.100E-02	8.276E-04	0.0
0.0900	3.932E+00	6.292E-03	3.939E+00	1.345E-02	9.059E-04	0.0
0.1000	3.678E+00	6.356E-03	3.685E+00	1.607E-02	9.814E-04	0.0
0.1250	3.215E+00	6.530E-03	3.221E+00	2.336E-02	1.161E-03	0.0
0.1500	2.901E+00	6.719E-03	2.908E+00	3.155E-02	1.329E-03	0.0
0.1750	2.676E+00	6.923E-03	2.683E+00	4.051E-02	1.489E-03	0.0
0.2000	2.507E+00	7.140E-03	2.514E+00	5.015E-02	1.641E-03	0.0
0.2500	2.272E+00	7.612E-03	2.280E+00	7.111E-02	1.931E-03	0.0
0.3000	2.119E+00	8.129E-03	2.127E+00	9.386E-02	2.206E-03	0.0
0.3500	2.011E+00	8.685E-03	2.020E+00	1.180E-01	2.471E-03	8.920E-03
0.4000	1.931E+00	9.276E-03	1.941E+00	1.433E-01	2.730E-03	3.411E-02
0.4500	1.871E+00	9.901E-03	1.881E+00	1.695E-01	2.984E-03	6.200E-02
0.5000	1.825E+00	1.055E-02	1.836E+00	1.964E-01	3.236E-03	9.146E-02
0.5500	1.789E+00	1.124E-02	1.800E+00	2.239E-01	3.487E-03	1.219E-01
0.6000	1.760E+00	1.194E-02	1.772E+00	2.519E-01	3.737E-03	1.531E-01
0.7000	1.718E+00	1.341E-02	1.732E+00	3.090E-01	4.237E-03	2.166E-01
0.8000	1.690E+00	1.495E-02	1.705E+00	3.673E-01	4.749E-03	2.806E-01
0.9000	1.671E+00	1.657E-02	1.688E+00	4.262E-01	5.245E-03	3.442E-01
1.0000	1.658E+00	1.824E-02	1.677E+00	4.857E-01	5.755E-03	4.069E-01
1.2500	1.642E+00	2.267E-02	1.665E+00	6.354E-01	7.052E-03	5.580E-01
1.5000	1.637E+00	2.740E-02	1.665E+00	7.857E-01	8.382E-03	6.994E-01
1.7500	1.639E+00	3.237E-02	1.671E+00	9.356E-01	9.743E-03	8.310E-01
2.0000	1.643E+00	3.755E-02	1.681E+00	1.085E+00	1.113E-02	9.534E-01
2.5000	1.656E+00	4.840E-02	1.704E+00	1.380E+00	1.398E-02	1.174E+00
3.0000	1.670E+00	5.981E-02	1.730E+00	1.671E+00	1.689E-02	1.368E+00
3.5000	1.684E+00	7.165E-02	1.755E+00	1.958E+00	1.987E-02	1.541E+00
4.0000	1.697E+00	8.386E-02	1.781E+00	2.241E+00	2.288E-02	1.697E+00
4.5000	1.709E+00	9.638E-02	1.805E+00	2.520E+00	2.592E-02	1.839E+00
5.0000	1.720E+00	1.092E-01	1.829E+00	2.795E+00	2.898E-02	1.970E+00
5.5000	1.731E+00	1.222E-01	1.853E+00	3.067E+00	3.206E-02	2.091E+00
6.0000	1.740E+00	1.355E-01	1.876E+00	3.335E+00	3.514E-02	2.203E+00
7.0000	1.758E+00	1.626E-01	1.921E+00	3.862E+00	4.133E-02	2.408E+00
8.0000	1.773E+00	1.904E-01	1.964E+00	4.377E+00	4.752E-02	2.591E+00
9.0000	1.787E+00	2.188E-01	2.006E+00	4.880E+00	5.369E-02	2.757E+00
10.0000	1.799E+00	2.476E-01	2.046E+00	5.374E+00	5.983E-02	2.908E+00
12.5000	1.824E+00	3.214E-01	2.145E+00	6.567E+00	7.497E-02	3.241E+00
15.0000	1.844E+00	3.971E-01	2.241E+00	7.707E+00	8.974E-02	3.525E+00
17.5000	1.860E+00	4.742E-01	2.335E+00	8.800E+00	1.041E-01	3.773E+00
20.0000	1.874E+00	5.525E-01	2.427E+00	9.850E+00	1.180E-01	3.994E+00
25.0000	1.897E+00	7.117E-01	2.609E+00	1.184E+01	1.446E-01	4.375E+00
30.0000	1.915E+00	8.735E-01	2.788E+00	1.369E+01	1.694E-01	4.696E+00
35.0000	1.929E+00	1.037E+00	2.966E+00	1.543E+01	1.926E-01	4.973E+00
40.0000	1.942E+00	1.202E+00	3.144E+00	1.707E+01	2.143E-01	5.217E+00
45.0000	1.952E+00	1.369E+00	3.321E+00	1.861E+01	2.347E-01	5.434E+00
50.0000	1.962E+00	1.537E+00	3.498E+00	2.008E+01	2.538E-01	5.631E+00
55.0000	1.970E+00	1.705E+00	3.676E+00	2.147E+01	2.718E-01	5.810E+00
60.0000	1.978E+00	1.875E+00	3.853E+00	2.280E+01	2.888E-01	5.974E+00
70.0000	1.992E+00	2.215E+00	4.207E+00	2.529E+01	3.199E-01	6.267E+00
80.0000	2.003E+00	2.558E+00	4.561E+00	2.757E+01	3.480E-01	6.523E+00
90.0000	2.013E+00	2.903E+00	4.916E+00	2.968E+01	3.733E-01	6.749E+00

Polystyrene

ENERGY	STOPPING POWER		TOTAL	CSDA RANGE	RADIATION YIELD	DENS.EFF. CORR. (DELTA)
	COLLISION	RADIATIVE				
MeV	MeV cm²/g	MeV cm²/g	MeV cm²/g	g/cm²		
0.0100	2.223E+01	2.982E-03	2.224E+01	2.546E-04	7.406E-05	0.0
0.0125	1.868E+01	2.992E-03	1.869E+01	3.777E-04	8.869E-05	0.0
0.0150	1.621E+01	2.999E-03	1.621E+01	5.218E-04	1.027E-04	0.0
0.0175	1.437E+01	3.004E-03	1.438E+01	6.859E-04	1.162E-04	0.0
0.0200	1.296E+01	3.008E-03	1.296E+01	8.694E-04	1.292E-04	0.0
0.0250	1.091E+01	3.017E-03	1.091E+01	1.292E-03	1.543E-04	0.0
0.0300	9.485E+00	3.027E-03	9.488E+00	1.785E-03	1.782E-04	0.0
0.0350	8.440E+00	3.037E-03	8.443E+00	2.345E-03	2.013E-04	0.0
0.0400	7.637E+00	3.048E-03	7.640E+00	2.968E-03	2.235E-04	0.0
0.0450	7.000E+00	3.061E-03	7.003E+00	3.653E-03	2.452E-04	0.0
0.0500	6.481E+00	3.074E-03	6.484E+00	4.395E-03	2.662E-04	0.0
0.0550	6.051E+00	3.088E-03	6.054E+00	5.194E-03	2.867E-04	0.0
0.0600	5.688E+00	3.103E-03	5.691E+00	6.047E-03	3.068E-04	0.0
0.0700	5.108E+00	3.135E-03	5.111E+00	7.905E-03	3.458E-04	0.0
0.0800	4.666E+00	3.169E-03	4.669E+00	9.955E-03	3.834E-04	0.0
0.0900	4.317E+00	3.206E-03	4.320E+00	1.218E-02	4.197E-04	0.0
0.1000	4.034E+00	3.244E-03	4.038E+00	1.458E-02	4.550E-04	0.0
0.1250	3.520E+00	3.350E-03	3.523E+00	2.124E-02	5.396E-04	0.0
0.1500	3.172E+00	3.463E-03	3.176E+00	2.873E-02	6.199E-04	0.0
0.1750	2.923E+00	3.584E-03	2.926E+00	3.695E-02	6.967E-04	0.0
0.2000	2.735E+00	3.711E-03	2.739E+00	4.579E-02	7.709E-04	0.0
0.2500	2.475E+00	3.985E-03	2.479E+00	6.504E-02	9.131E-04	0.0
0.3000	2.305E+00	4.284E-03	2.309E+00	8.598E-02	1.050E-03	0.0
0.3500	2.187E+00	4.604E-03	2.192E+00	1.082E-01	1.182E-03	0.0
0.4000	2.101E+00	4.945E-03	2.106E+00	1.315E-01	1.312E-03	2.729E-03
0.4500	2.035E+00	5.304E-03	2.040E+00	1.557E-01	1.441E-03	2.688E-02
0.5000	1.984E+00	5.680E-03	1.990E+00	1.805E-01	1.570E-03	5.420E-02
0.5500	1.943E+00	6.071E-03	1.950E+00	2.059E-01	1.699E-03	8.383E-02
0.6000	1.911E+00	6.475E-03	1.918E+00	2.318E-01	1.827E-03	1.152E-01
0.7000	1.864E+00	7.322E-03	1.871E+00	2.846E-01	2.087E-03	1.810E-01
0.8000	1.832E+00	8.212E-03	1.840E+00	3.385E-01	2.349E-03	2.492E-01
0.9000	1.810E+00	9.142E-03	1.819E+00	3.932E-01	2.615E-03	3.179E-01
1.0000	1.794E+00	1.011E-02	1.804E+00	4.484E-01	2.885E-03	3.862E-01
1.2500	1.773E+00	1.267E-02	1.786E+00	5.878E-01	3.577E-03	5.515E-01
1.5000	1.766E+00	1.541E-02	1.781E+00	7.281E-01	4.293E-03	7.064E-01
1.7500	1.765E+00	1.830E-02	1.783E+00	8.684E-01	5.030E-03	8.501E-01
2.0000	1.768E+00	2.132E-02	1.789E+00	1.008E+00	5.788E-03	9.834E-01
2.5000	1.778E+00	2.766E-02	1.806E+00	1.287E+00	7.352E-03	1.222E+00
3.0000	1.791E+00	3.435E-02	1.825E+00	1.562E+00	8.970E-03	1.431E+00
3.5000	1.804E+00	4.132E-02	1.845E+00	1.835E+00	1.063E-02	1.616E+00
4.0000	1.816E+00	4.852E-02	1.865E+00	2.104E+00	1.233E-02	1.782E+00
4.5000	1.828E+00	5.593E-02	1.884E+00	2.371E+00	1.405E-02	1.932E+00
5.0000	1.839E+00	6.353E-02	1.902E+00	2.635E+00	1.580E-02	2.070E+00
5.5000	1.849E+00	7.129E-02	1.920E+00	2.897E+00	1.757E-02	2.197E+00
6.0000	1.859E+00	7.919E-02	1.938E+00	3.156E+00	1.936E-02	2.316E+00
7.0000	1.876E+00	9.539E-02	1.971E+00	3.667E+00	2.297E-02	2.531E+00
8.0000	1.891E+00	1.120E-01	2.003E+00	4.171E+00	2.662E-02	2.722E+00
9.0000	1.904E+00	1.290E-01	2.033E+00	4.666E+00	3.029E-02	2.896E+00
10.0000	1.916E+00	1.464E-01	2.062E+00	5.155E+00	3.399E-02	3.054E+00
12.5000	1.940E+00	1.909E-01	2.131E+00	6.347E+00	4.325E-02	3.403E+00
15.0000	1.960E+00	2.367E-01	2.196E+00	7.502E+00	5.249E-02	3.702E+00
17.5000	1.975E+00	2.835E-01	2.259E+00	8.625E+00	6.166E-02	3.963E+00
20.0000	1.989E+00	3.311E-01	2.320E+00	9.717E+00	7.072E-02	4.196E+00
25.0000	2.010E+00	4.282E-01	2.439E+00	1.182E+01	8.844E-02	4.596E+00
30.0000	2.027E+00	5.270E-01	2.554E+00	1.382E+01	1.056E-01	4.933E+00
35.0000	2.041E+00	6.271E-01	2.669E+00	1.574E+01	1.220E-01	5.223E+00
40.0000	2.053E+00	7.284E-01	2.782E+00	1.757E+01	1.378E-01	5.478E+00
45.0000	2.064E+00	8.306E-01	2.894E+00	1.933E+01	1.530E-01	5.704E+00
50.0000	2.073E+00	9.334E-01	3.006E+00	2.103E+01	1.676E-01	5.908E+00
55.0000	2.081E+00	1.037E+00	3.118E+00	2.266E+01	1.816E-01	6.093E+00
60.0000	2.089E+00	1.141E+00	3.230E+00	2.424E+01	1.951E-01	6.263E+00
70.0000	2.102E+00	1.351E+00	3.452E+00	2.723E+01	2.204E-01	6.565E+00
80.0000	2.113E+00	1.562E+00	3.675E+00	3.004E+01	2.439E-01	6.828E+00
90.0000	2.123E+00	1.774E+00	3.897E+00	3.268E+01	2.658E-01	7.060E+00

Polymethyl Methacrylate

ENERGY	STOPPING POWER COLLISION	RADIATIVE	TOTAL	CSDA RANGE	RADIATION YIELD	DENS.EFF. CORR. (DELTA)
MeV	MeV cm²/g	MeV cm²/g	MeV cm²/g	g/cm²		
0.0100	2.198E+01	3.332E-03	2.198E+01	2.580E-04	8.329E-05	0.0
0.0125	1.848E+01	3.349E-03	1.849E+01	3.826E-04	9.993E-05	0.0
0.0150	1.604E+01	3.359E-03	1.604E+01	5.282E-04	1.158E-04	0.0
0.0175	1.423E+01	3.366E-03	1.423E+01	6.940E-04	1.311E-04	0.0
0.0200	1.283E+01	3.372E-03	1.284E+01	8.792E-04	1.460E-04	0.0
0.0250	1.080E+01	3.382E-03	1.081E+01	1.306E-03	1.744E-04	0.0
0.0300	9.400E+00	3.391E-03	9.404E+00	1.803E-03	2.015E-04	0.0
0.0350	8.367E+00	3.401E-03	8.370E+00	2.368E-03	2.275E-04	0.0
0.0400	7.573E+00	3.413E-03	7.576E+00	2.997E-03	2.526E-04	0.0
0.0450	6.942E+00	3.425E-03	6.946E+00	3.687E-03	2.770E-04	0.0
0.0500	6.429E+00	3.438E-03	6.433E+00	4.436E-03	3.007E-04	0.0
0.0550	6.003E+00	3.453E-03	6.007E+00	5.241E-03	3.238E-04	0.0
0.0600	5.644E+00	3.468E-03	5.647E+00	6.100E-03	3.464E-04	0.0
0.0700	5.070E+00	3.502E-03	5.073E+00	7.972E-03	3.901E-04	0.0
0.0800	4.631E+00	3.538E-03	4.635E+00	1.004E-02	4.322E-04	0.0
0.0900	4.286E+00	3.577E-03	4.289E+00	1.228E-02	4.729E-04	0.0
0.1000	4.006E+00	3.619E-03	4.010E+00	1.470E-02	5.125E-04	0.0
0.1250	3.496E+00	3.732E-03	3.500E+00	2.140E-02	6.070E-04	0.0
0.1500	3.152E+00	3.855E-03	3.155E+00	2.894E-02	6.966E-04	0.0
0.1750	2.904E+00	3.987E-03	2.908E+00	3.721E-02	7.824E-04	0.0
0.2000	2.719E+00	4.126E-03	2.723E+00	4.610E-02	8.650E-04	0.0
0.2500	2.461E+00	4.425E-03	2.465E+00	6.547E-02	1.023E-03	0.0
0.3000	2.292E+00	4.751E-03	2.297E+00	8.653E-02	1.175E-03	0.0
0.3500	2.175E+00	5.101E-03	2.180E+00	1.089E-01	1.322E-03	0.0
0.4000	2.090E+00	5.474E-03	2.096E+00	1.323E-01	1.466E-03	0.0
0.4500	2.026E+00	5.867E-03	2.032E+00	1.566E-01	1.609E-03	1.466E-02
0.5000	1.975E+00	6.278E-03	1.981E+00	1.815E-01	1.751E-03	4.112E-02
0.5500	1.935E+00	6.707E-03	1.942E+00	2.070E-01	1.892E-03	6.992E-02
0.6000	1.903E+00	7.149E-03	1.910E+00	2.330E-01	2.035E-03	1.005E-01
0.7000	1.856E+00	8.076E-03	1.864E+00	2.860E-01	2.320E-03	1.650E-01
0.8000	1.825E+00	9.050E-03	1.834E+00	3.401E-01	2.609E-03	2.321E-01
0.9000	1.803E+00	1.007E-02	1.813E+00	3.950E-01	2.902E-03	3.001E-01
1.0000	1.788E+00	1.113E-02	1.799E+00	4.504E-01	3.199E-03	3.679E-01
1.2500	1.767E+00	1.393E-02	1.781E+00	5.902E-01	3.959E-03	5.330E-01
1.5000	1.760E+00	1.693E-02	1.776E+00	7.308E-01	4.744E-03	6.887E-01
1.7500	1.759E+00	2.009E-02	1.779E+00	8.715E-01	5.553E-03	8.339E-01
2.0000	1.762E+00	2.338E-02	1.785E+00	1.012E+00	6.383E-03	9.689E-01
2.5000	1.772E+00	3.031E-02	1.802E+00	1.291E+00	8.096E-03	1.212E+00
3.0000	1.784E+00	3.761E-02	1.822E+00	1.567E+00	9.868E-03	1.425E+00
3.5000	1.797E+00	4.521E-02	1.842E+00	1.839E+00	1.168E-02	1.613E+00
4.0000	1.809E+00	5.307E-02	1.862E+00	2.109E+00	1.354E-02	1.783E+00
4.5000	1.821E+00	6.115E-02	1.882E+00	2.376E+00	1.542E-02	1.936E+00
5.0000	1.832E+00	6.943E-02	1.901E+00	2.641E+00	1.733E-02	2.077E+00
5.5000	1.842E+00	7.788E-02	1.920E+00	2.903E+00	1.926E-02	2.207E+00
6.0000	1.851E+00	8.648E-02	1.938E+00	3.162E+00	2.120E-02	2.327E+00
7.0000	1.868E+00	1.041E-01	1.972E+00	3.673E+00	2.513E-02	2.545E+00
8.0000	1.883E+00	1.222E-01	2.005E+00	4.176E+00	2.910E-02	2.739E+00
9.0000	1.896E+00	1.407E-01	2.037E+00	4.671E+00	3.309E-02	2.914E+00
10.0000	1.908E+00	1.596E-01	2.067E+00	5.158E+00	3.710E-02	3.073E+00
12.5000	1.932E+00	2.079E-01	2.140E+00	6.346E+00	4.712E-02	3.421E+00
15.0000	1.952E+00	2.577E-01	2.210E+00	7.496E+00	5.709E-02	3.716E+00
17.5000	1.968E+00	3.086E-01	2.277E+00	8.610E+00	6.695E-02	3.974E+00
20.0000	1.982E+00	3.603E-01	2.342E+00	9.693E+00	7.667E-02	4.202E+00
25.0000	2.004E+00	4.656E-01	2.470E+00	1.177E+01	9.561E-02	4.596E+00
30.0000	2.022E+00	5.728E-01	2.595E+00	1.375E+01	1.138E-01	4.927E+00
35.0000	2.036E+00	6.815E-01	2.718E+00	1.563E+01	1.313E-01	5.212E+00
40.0000	2.049E+00	7.912E-01	2.840E+00	1.743E+01	1.480E-01	5.463E+00
45.0000	2.059E+00	9.020E-01	2.961E+00	1.915E+01	1.639E-01	5.687E+00
50.0000	2.069E+00	1.013E+00	3.082E+00	2.081E+01	1.792E-01	5.889E+00
55.0000	2.077E+00	1.126E+00	3.203E+00	2.240E+01	1.939E-01	6.072E+00
60.0000	2.085E+00	1.238E+00	3.323E+00	2.393E+01	2.079E-01	6.241E+00
70.0000	2.098E+00	1.465E+00	3.563E+00	2.684E+01	2.342E-01	6.541E+00
80.0000	2.109E+00	1.694E+00	3.804E+00	2.955E+01	2.585E-01	6.803E+00
90.0000	2.120E+00	1.924E+00	4.044E+00	3.210E+01	2.810E-01	7.034E+00

Polyethylene

ENERGY	STOPPING POWER COLLISION	RADIATIVE	TOTAL	CSDA RANGE	RADIATION YIELD	DENS.EFF. CORR. (DELTA)
MeV	MeV cm^2/g	MeV cm^2/g	MeV cm^2/g	g/cm^2		
0.0100	2.441E+01	2.837E-03	2.442E+01	2.308E-04	6.391E-05	0.0
0.0125	2.049E+01	2.847E-03	2.049E+01	3.430E-04	7.666E-05	0.0
0.0150	1.775E+01	2.854E-03	1.776E+01	4.745E-04	8.887E-05	0.0
0.0175	1.573E+01	2.860E-03	1.573E+01	6.244E-04	1.007E-04	0.0
0.0200	1.417E+01	2.864E-03	1.417E+01	7.921E-04	1.121E-04	0.0
0.0250	1.191E+01	2.873E-03	1.192E+01	1.179E-03	1.340E-04	0.0
0.0300	1.035E+01	2.883E-03	1.036E+01	1.630E-03	1.550E-04	0.0
0.0350	9.206E+00	2.894E-03	9.209E+00	2.143E-03	1.752E-04	0.0
0.0400	8.325E+00	2.905E-03	8.328E+00	2.715E-03	1.948E-04	0.0
0.0450	7.627E+00	2.918E-03	7.630E+00	3.343E-03	2.138E-04	0.0
0.0500	7.060E+00	2.931E-03	7.063E+00	4.025E-03	2.323E-04	0.0
0.0550	6.589E+00	2.945E-03	6.592E+00	4.758E-03	2.503E-04	0.0
0.0600	6.191E+00	2.960E-03	6.194E+00	5.541E-03	2.680E-04	0.0
0.0700	5.557E+00	2.992E-03	5.560E+00	7.249E-03	3.023E-04	0.0
0.0800	5.074E+00	3.025E-03	5.077E+00	9.134E-03	3.354E-04	0.0
0.0900	4.692E+00	3.061E-03	4.696E+00	1.118E-02	3.675E-04	0.0
0.1000	4.384E+00	3.099E-03	4.387E+00	1.339E-02	3.987E-04	0.0
0.1250	3.822E+00	3.201E-03	3.825E+00	1.952E-02	4.733E-04	0.0
0.1500	3.443E+00	3.312E-03	3.446E+00	2.642E-02	5.443E-04	0.0
0.1750	3.171E+00	3.429E-03	3.174E+00	3.399E-02	6.124E-04	0.0
0.2000	2.967E+00	3.553E-03	2.970E+00	4.215E-02	6.782E-04	0.0
0.2500	2.683E+00	3.820E-03	2.687E+00	5.991E-02	8.045E-04	0.0
0.3000	2.497E+00	4.110E-03	2.501E+00	7.923E-02	9.258E-04	0.0
0.3500	2.368E+00	4.420E-03	2.373E+00	9.979E-02	1.044E-03	0.0
0.4000	2.272E+00	4.750E-03	2.277E+00	1.213E-01	1.160E-03	2.626E-02
0.4500	2.199E+00	5.098E-03	2.204E+00	1.437E-01	1.276E-03	5.906E-02
0.5000	2.142E+00	5.462E-03	2.147E+00	1.667E-01	1.391E-03	9.409E-02
0.5500	2.097E+00	5.841E-03	2.103E+00	1.902E-01	1.506E-03	1.307E-01
0.6000	2.061E+00	6.233E-03	2.068E+00	2.142E-01	1.622E-03	1.683E-01
0.7000	2.008E+00	7.053E-03	2.016E+00	2.632E-01	1.856E-03	2.453E-01
0.8000	1.972E+00	7.915E-03	1.980E+00	3.133E-01	2.092E-03	3.231E-01
0.9000	1.947E+00	8.816E-03	1.956E+00	3.641E-01	2.332E-03	4.002E-01
1.0000	1.930E+00	9.754E-03	1.940E+00	4.155E-01	2.575E-03	4.759E-01
1.2500	1.905E+00	1.224E-02	1.917E+00	5.452E-01	3.200E-03	6.568E-01
1.5000	1.895E+00	1.490E-02	1.910E+00	6.759E-01	3.848E-03	8.243E-01
1.7500	1.893E+00	1.770E-02	1.911E+00	8.068E-01	4.516E-03	9.785E-01
2.0000	1.895E+00	2.062E-02	1.916E+00	9.375E-01	5.203E-03	1.121E+00
2.5000	1.905E+00	2.678E-02	1.932E+00	1.197E+00	6.623E-03	1.375E+00
3.0000	1.917E+00	3.327E-02	1.950E+00	1.455E+00	8.095E-03	1.596E+00
3.5000	1.930E+00	4.004E-02	1.970E+00	1.710E+00	9.608E-03	1.791E+00
4.0000	1.942E+00	4.704E-02	1.989E+00	1.963E+00	1.116E-02	1.966E+00
4.5000	1.954E+00	5.424E-02	2.008E+00	2.213E+00	1.273E-02	2.124E+00
5.0000	1.965E+00	6.162E-02	2.026E+00	2.461E+00	1.433E-02	2.269E+00
5.5000	1.975E+00	6.916E-02	2.044E+00	2.706E+00	1.594E-02	2.402E+00
6.0000	1.984E+00	7.684E-02	2.061E+00	2.950E+00	1.758E-02	2.527E+00
7.0000	2.002E+00	9.259E-02	2.094E+00	3.431E+00	2.089E-02	2.751E+00
8.0000	2.017E+00	1.088E-01	2.126E+00	3.905E+00	2.424E-02	2.952E+00
9.0000	2.030E+00	1.253E-01	2.156E+00	4.372E+00	2.762E-02	3.132E+00
10.0000	2.042E+00	1.422E-01	2.184E+00	4.833E+00	3.102E-02	3.298E+00
12.5000	2.067E+00	1.855E-01	2.253E+00	5.960E+00	3.956E-02	3.660E+00
15.0000	2.087E+00	2.301E-01	2.317E+00	7.054E+00	4.811E-02	3.967E+00
17.5000	2.103E+00	2.757E-01	2.379E+00	8.119E+00	5.661E-02	4.235E+00
20.0000	2.117E+00	3.220E-01	2.439E+00	9.157E+00	6.503E-02	4.473E+00
25.0000	2.139E+00	4.166E-01	2.556E+00	1.116E+01	8.156E-02	4.880E+00
30.0000	2.157E+00	5.129E-01	2.670E+00	1.307E+01	9.759E-02	5.221E+00
35.0000	2.171E+00	6.105E-01	2.782E+00	1.491E+01	1.131E-01	5.514E+00
40.0000	2.184E+00	7.092E-01	2.893E+00	1.667E+01	1.280E-01	5.770E+00
45.0000	2.195E+00	8.088E-01	3.004E+00	1.837E+01	1.424E-01	5.997E+00
50.0000	2.204E+00	9.092E-01	3.114E+00	2.000E+01	1.562E-01	6.202E+00
55.0000	2.213E+00	1.010E+00	3.223E+00	2.158E+01	1.695E-01	6.388E+00
60.0000	2.221E+00	1.112E+00	3.333E+00	2.310E+01	1.824E-01	6.558E+00
70.0000	2.235E+00	1.316E+00	3.551E+00	2.601E+01	2.067E-01	6.861E+00
80.0000	2.247E+00	1.522E+00	3.769E+00	2.874E+01	2.293E-01	7.125E+00
90.0000	2.257E+00	1.730E+00	3.987E+00	3.132E+01	2.504E-01	7.357E+00

Teflon

ENERGY	STOPPING POWER COLLISION	STOPPING POWER RADIATIVE	TOTAL	CSDA RANGE	RADIATION YIELD	DENS.EFF. CORR. (DELTA)
MeV	MeV cm²/g	MeV cm²/g	MeV cm²/g	g/cm²		
0.0100	1.843E+01	4.211E-03	1.843E+01	3.105E-04	1.249E-04	0.0
0.0125	1.553E+01	4.247E-03	1.554E+01	4.589E-04	1.502E-04	0.0
0.0150	1.351E+01	4.271E-03	1.351E+01	6.320E-04	1.743E-04	0.0
0.0175	1.200E+01	4.287E-03	1.201E+01	8.287E-04	1.975E-04	0.0
0.0200	1.084E+01	4.300E-03	1.084E+01	1.048E-03	2.199E-04	0.0
0.0250	9.141E+00	4.316E-03	9.146E+00	1.553E-03	2.629E-04	0.0
0.0300	7.965E+00	4.329E-03	7.970E+00	2.140E-03	3.037E-04	0.0
0.0350	7.098E+00	4.341E-03	7.102E+00	2.806E-03	3.428E-04	0.0
0.0400	6.430E+00	4.353E-03	6.435E+00	3.547E-03	3.805E-04	0.0
0.0450	5.900E+00	4.366E-03	5.904E+00	4.359E-03	4.169E-04	0.0
0.0500	5.468E+00	4.380E-03	5.472E+00	5.239E-03	4.522E-04	0.0
0.0550	5.109E+00	4.395E-03	5.113E+00	6.185E-03	4.865E-04	0.0
0.0600	4.806E+00	4.410E-03	4.810E+00	7.194E-03	5.200E-04	0.0
0.0700	4.321E+00	4.444E-03	4.325E+00	9.391E-03	5.847E-04	0.0
0.0800	3.951E+00	4.483E-03	3.955E+00	1.181E-02	6.467E-04	0.0
0.0900	3.658E+00	4.525E-03	3.663E+00	1.444E-02	7.065E-04	0.0
0.1000	3.421E+00	4.571E-03	3.426E+00	1.727E-02	7.643E-04	0.0
0.1250	2.989E+00	4.700E-03	2.994E+00	2.511E-02	9.021E-04	0.0
0.1500	2.697E+00	4.844E-03	2.702E+00	3.392E-02	1.032E-03	0.0
0.1750	2.487E+00	5.000E-03	2.492E+00	4.357E-02	1.156E-03	0.0
0.2000	2.330E+00	5.167E-03	2.335E+00	5.395E-02	1.275E-03	0.0
0.2500	2.111E+00	5.530E-03	2.117E+00	7.651E-02	1.503E-03	0.0
0.3000	1.968E+00	5.928E-03	1.974E+00	1.010E-01	1.721E-03	0.0
0.3500	1.869E+00	6.353E-03	1.875E+00	1.271E-01	1.931E-03	0.0
0.4000	1.797E+00	6.805E-03	1.804E+00	1.543E-01	2.137E-03	2.294E-03
0.4500	1.742E+00	7.279E-03	1.749E+00	1.824E-01	2.341E-03	2.338E-02
0.5000	1.699E+00	7.775E-03	1.707E+00	2.114E-01	2.543E-03	4.753E-02
0.5500	1.665E+00	8.291E-03	1.674E+00	2.410E-01	2.744E-03	7.398E-02
0.6000	1.639E+00	8.823E-03	1.647E+00	2.711E-01	2.945E-03	1.022E-01
0.7000	1.600E+00	9.937E-03	1.610E+00	3.326E-01	3.347E-03	1.623E-01
0.8000	1.573E+00	1.111E-02	1.585E+00	3.952E-01	3.753E-03	2.253E-01
0.9000	1.555E+00	1.233E-02	1.568E+00	4.587E-01	4.162E-03	2.896E-01
1.0000	1.543E+00	1.360E-02	1.557E+00	5.227E-01	4.575E-03	3.541E-01
1.2500	1.527E+00	1.697E-02	1.544E+00	6.841E-01	5.631E-03	5.127E-01
1.5000	1.522E+00	2.057E-02	1.542E+00	8.462E-01	6.719E-03	6.637E-01
1.7500	1.522E+00	2.437E-02	1.546E+00	1.008E+00	7.837E-03	8.056E-01
2.0000	1.525E+00	2.834E-02	1.553E+00	1.169E+00	8.983E-03	9.382E-01
2.5000	1.535E+00	3.667E-02	1.572E+00	1.490E+00	1.134E-02	1.178E+00
3.0000	1.546E+00	4.544E-02	1.592E+00	1.806E+00	1.377E-02	1.390E+00
3.5000	1.558E+00	5.456E-02	1.612E+00	2.118E+00	1.626E-02	1.578E+00
4.0000	1.569E+00	6.399E-02	1.633E+00	2.426E+00	1.879E-02	1.748E+00
4.5000	1.579E+00	7.367E-02	1.653E+00	2.730E+00	2.136E-02	1.902E+00
5.0000	1.589E+00	8.357E-02	1.672E+00	3.031E+00	2.395E-02	2.043E+00
5.5000	1.598E+00	9.367E-02	1.692E+00	3.328E+00	2.656E-02	2.173E+00
6.0000	1.606E+00	1.040E-01	1.710E+00	3.622E+00	2.919E-02	2.294E+00
7.0000	1.621E+00	1.250E-01	1.746E+00	4.201E+00	3.447E-02	2.512E+00
8.0000	1.635E+00	1.466E-01	1.781E+00	4.768E+00	3.978E-02	2.706E+00
9.0000	1.646E+00	1.686E-01	1.815E+00	5.324E+00	4.509E-02	2.880E+00
10.0000	1.657E+00	1.910E-01	1.848E+00	5.870E+00	5.040E-02	3.039E+00
12.5000	1.679E+00	2.483E-01	1.927E+00	7.194E+00	6.355E-02	3.385E+00
15.0000	1.697E+00	3.071E-01	2.004E+00	8.466E+00	7.643E-02	3.677E+00
17.5000	1.712E+00	3.672E-01	2.079E+00	9.691E+00	8.913E-02	3.930E+00
20.0000	1.724E+00	4.281E-01	2.152E+00	1.087E+01	1.015E-01	4.155E+00
25.0000	1.745E+00	5.521E-01	2.297E+00	1.312E+01	1.252E-01	4.541E+00
30.0000	1.761E+00	6.781E-01	2.439E+00	1.523E+01	1.476E-01	4.866E+00
35.0000	1.774E+00	8.056E-01	2.579E+00	1.723E+01	1.687E-01	5.146E+00
40.0000	1.785E+00	9.344E-01	2.719E+00	1.911E+01	1.886E-01	5.394E+00
45.0000	1.795E+00	1.064E+00	2.859E+00	2.091E+01	2.075E-01	5.614E+00
50.0000	1.803E+00	1.195E+00	2.998E+00	2.262E+01	2.253E-01	5.814E+00
55.0000	1.811E+00	1.326E+00	3.137E+00	2.425E+01	2.421E-01	5.996E+00
60.0000	1.818E+00	1.458E+00	3.276E+00	2.580E+01	2.581E-01	6.163E+00
70.0000	1.830E+00	1.724E+00	3.554E+00	2.874E+01	2.878E-01	6.461E+00
80.0000	1.840E+00	1.991E+00	3.831E+00	3.144E+01	3.147E-01	6.721E+00
90.0000	1.849E+00	2.260E+00	4.109E+00	3.396E+01	3.392E-01	6.952E+00

Borosilicate Glass

ENERGY	STOPPING POWER			CSDA RANGE	RADIATION YIELD	DENS.EFF. CORR. (DELTA)
	COLLISION	RADIATIVE	TOTAL			
MeV	MeV cm²/g	MeV cm²/g	MeV cm²/g	g/cm²		
0.0100	1.787E+01	5.400E-03	1.788E+01	3.237E-04	1.632E-04	0.0
0.0125	1.511E+01	5.488E-03	1.512E+01	4.764E-04	1.971E-04	0.0
0.0150	1.317E+01	5.548E-03	1.317E+01	6.540E-04	2.296E-04	0.0
0.0175	1.172E+01	5.593E-03	1.173E+01	8.556E-04	2.610E-04	0.0
0.0200	1.060E+01	5.626E-03	1.060E+01	1.080E-03	2.914E-04	0.0
0.0250	8.962E+00	5.674E-03	8.968E+00	1.595E-03	3.495E-04	0.0
0.0300	7.822E+00	5.707E-03	7.828E+00	2.194E-03	4.048E-04	0.0
0.0350	6.980E+00	5.735E-03	6.986E+00	2.871E-03	4.578E-04	0.0
0.0400	6.331E+00	5.759E-03	6.336E+00	3.624E-03	5.087E-04	0.0
0.0450	5.814E+00	5.781E-03	5.820E+00	4.448E-03	5.579E-04	0.0
0.0500	5.393E+00	5.803E-03	5.398E+00	5.341E-03	6.055E-04	0.0
0.0550	5.042E+00	5.824E-03	5.048E+00	6.300E-03	6.518E-04	0.0
0.0600	4.746E+00	5.847E-03	4.752E+00	7.321E-03	6.968E-04	0.0
0.0700	4.272E+00	5.893E-03	4.278E+00	9.544E-03	7.837E-04	0.0
0.0800	3.909E+00	5.943E-03	3.915E+00	1.199E-02	8.668E-04	0.0
0.0900	3.622E+00	5.997E-03	3.628E+00	1.465E-02	9.467E-04	0.0
0.1000	3.390E+00	6.055E-03	3.396E+00	1.750E-02	1.024E-03	0.0
0.1250	2.966E+00	6.215E-03	2.972E+00	2.540E-02	1.207E-03	0.0
0.1500	2.679E+00	6.393E-03	2.685E+00	3.427E-02	1.379E-03	0.0
0.1750	2.473E+00	6.588E-03	2.479E+00	4.398E-02	1.542E-03	0.0
0.2000	2.318E+00	6.796E-03	2.325E+00	5.440E-02	1.698E-03	0.0
0.2500	2.102E+00	7.250E-03	2.110E+00	7.706E-02	1.995E-03	0.0
0.3000	1.962E+00	7.749E-03	1.970E+00	1.016E-01	2.277E-03	0.0
0.3500	1.864E+00	8.286E-03	1.873E+00	1.277E-01	2.549E-03	0.0
0.4000	1.793E+00	8.857E-03	1.802E+00	1.549E-01	2.814E-03	8.985E-03
0.4500	1.739E+00	9.461E-03	1.749E+00	1.831E-01	3.075E-03	2.665E-02
0.5000	1.698E+00	1.009E-02	1.708E+00	2.121E-01	3.333E-03	4.637E-02
0.5500	1.665E+00	1.075E-02	1.676E+00	2.416E-01	3.590E-03	6.760E-02
0.6000	1.640E+00	1.143E-02	1.651E+00	2.717E-01	3.846E-03	8.997E-02
0.7000	1.603E+00	1.285E-02	1.616E+00	3.330E-01	4.359E-03	1.371E-01
0.8000	1.579E+00	1.434E-02	1.593E+00	3.953E-01	4.873E-03	1.860E-01
0.9000	1.563E+00	1.590E-02	1.579E+00	4.584E-01	5.391E-03	2.359E-01
1.0000	1.552E+00	1.751E-02	1.570E+00	5.220E-01	5.913E-03	2.859E-01
1.2500	1.540E+00	2.179E-02	1.561E+00	6.818E-01	7.240E-03	4.090E-01
1.5000	1.538E+00	2.636E-02	1.564E+00	8.418E-01	8.599E-03	5.271E-01
1.7500	1.541E+00	3.117E-02	1.572E+00	1.001E+00	9.990E-03	6.390E-01
2.0000	1.547E+00	3.617E-02	1.583E+00	1.160E+00	1.141E-02	7.448E-01
2.5000	1.561E+00	4.668E-02	1.608E+00	1.473E+00	1.431E-02	9.392E-01
3.0000	1.576E+00	5.771E-02	1.634E+00	1.782E+00	1.729E-02	1.114E+00
3.5000	1.590E+00	6.918E-02	1.660E+00	2.085E+00	2.032E-02	1.273E+00
4.0000	1.604E+00	8.102E-02	1.685E+00	2.384E+00	2.339E-02	1.419E+00
4.5000	1.616E+00	9.315E-02	1.709E+00	2.679E+00	2.649E-02	1.554E+00
5.0000	1.627E+00	1.056E-01	1.733E+00	2.970E+00	2.961E-02	1.679E+00
5.5000	1.637E+00	1.182E-01	1.756E+00	3.256E+00	3.275E-02	1.797E+00
6.0000	1.647E+00	1.311E-01	1.778E+00	3.539E+00	3.590E-02	1.907E+00
7.0000	1.664E+00	1.574E-01	1.821E+00	4.095E+00	4.222E-02	2.110E+00
8.0000	1.678E+00	1.844E-01	1.863E+00	4.638E+00	4.853E-02	2.292E+00
9.0000	1.691E+00	2.119E-01	1.903E+00	5.169E+00	5.483E-02	2.458E+00
10.0000	1.703E+00	2.399E-01	1.943E+00	5.689E+00	6.109E-02	2.611E+00
12.5000	1.726E+00	3.115E-01	2.038E+00	6.945E+00	7.653E-02	2.945E+00
15.0000	1.746E+00	3.850E-01	2.131E+00	8.145E+00	9.159E-02	3.229E+00
17.5000	1.761E+00	4.599E-01	2.221E+00	9.294E+00	1.062E-01	3.476E+00
20.0000	1.775E+00	5.360E-01	2.311E+00	1.040E+01	1.204E-01	3.695E+00
25.0000	1.797E+00	6.906E-01	2.487E+00	1.248E+01	1.474E-01	4.071E+00
30.0000	1.814E+00	8.477E-01	2.662E+00	1.442E+01	1.725E-01	4.388E+00
35.0000	1.828E+00	1.007E+00	2.835E+00	1.624E+01	1.961E-01	4.661E+00
40.0000	1.840E+00	1.167E+00	3.007E+00	1.796E+01	2.180E-01	4.901E+00
45.0000	1.851E+00	1.329E+00	3.179E+00	1.957E+01	2.386E-01	5.115E+00
50.0000	1.860E+00	1.491E+00	3.351E+00	2.111E+01	2.579E-01	5.309E+00
55.0000	1.868E+00	1.655E+00	3.523E+00	2.256E+01	2.761E-01	5.486E+00
60.0000	1.876E+00	1.819E+00	3.695E+00	2.395E+01	2.932E-01	5.649E+00
70.0000	1.889E+00	2.150E+00	4.039E+00	2.653E+01	3.246E-01	5.940E+00
80.0000	1.900E+00	2.483E+00	4.383E+00	2.891E+01	3.527E-01	6.194E+00
90.0000	1.909E+00	2.817E+00	4.727E+00	3.111E+01	3.782E-01	6.420E+00

Lithium Fluoride

ENERGY	STOPPING POWER COLLISION	RADIATIVE	TOTAL	CSDA RANGE	RADIATION YIELD	DENS.EFF. CORR.
MeV	MeV cm²/g	MeV cm²/g	MeV cm²/g	g/cm²		(DELTA)
0.0100	1.796E+01	3.678E-03	1.796E+01	3.181E-04	1.117E-04	0.0
0.0125	1.513E+01	3.712E-03	1.514E+01	4.704E-04	1.344E-04	0.0
0.0150	1.315E+01	3.735E-03	1.316E+01	6.480E-04	1.561E-04	0.0
0.0175	1.168E+01	3.750E-03	1.169E+01	8.501E-04	1.770E-04	0.0
0.0200	1.055E+01	3.762E-03	1.055E+01	1.076E-03	1.973E-04	0.0
0.0250	8.894E+00	3.779E-03	8.898E+00	1.594E-03	2.360E-04	0.0
0.0300	7.748E+00	3.792E-03	7.751E+00	2.198E-03	2.729E-04	0.0
0.0350	6.902E+00	3.804E-03	6.906E+00	2.883E-03	3.082E-04	0.0
0.0400	6.252E+00	3.815E-03	6.256E+00	3.645E-03	3.423E-04	0.0
0.0450	5.736E+00	3.827E-03	5.739E+00	4.480E-03	3.752E-04	0.0
0.0500	5.315E+00	3.840E-03	5.319E+00	5.386E-03	4.071E-04	0.0
0.0550	4.965E+00	3.853E-03	4.969E+00	6.359E-03	4.382E-04	0.0
0.0600	4.670E+00	3.867E-03	4.674E+00	7.397E-03	4.684E-04	0.0
0.0700	4.198E+00	3.898E-03	4.202E+00	9.659E-03	5.269E-04	0.0
0.0800	3.838E+00	3.932E-03	3.842E+00	1.215E-02	5.831E-04	0.0
0.0900	3.553E+00	3.970E-03	3.557E+00	1.486E-02	6.372E-04	0.0
0.1000	3.323E+00	4.011E-03	3.327E+00	1.777E-02	6.896E-04	0.0
0.1250	2.903E+00	4.125E-03	2.907E+00	2.584E-02	8.143E-04	0.0
0.1500	2.619E+00	4.253E-03	2.623E+00	3.492E-02	9.321E-04	0.0
0.1750	2.415E+00	4.392E-03	2.419E+00	4.486E-02	1.045E-03	0.0
0.2000	2.261E+00	4.540E-03	2.266E+00	5.555E-02	1.153E-03	0.0
0.2500	2.048E+00	4.863E-03	2.053E+00	7.881E-02	1.360E-03	6.058E-03
0.3000	1.907E+00	5.215E-03	1.912E+00	1.041E-01	1.558E-03	2.136E-02
0.3500	1.809E+00	5.592E-03	1.814E+00	1.310E-01	1.750E-03	3.978E-02
0.4000	1.737E+00	5.992E-03	1.743E+00	1.591E-01	1.939E-03	6.095E-02
0.4500	1.683E+00	6.412E-03	1.690E+00	1.883E-01	2.125E-03	8.445E-02
0.5000	1.642E+00	6.852E-03	1.649E+00	2.183E-01	2.310E-03	1.098E-01
0.5500	1.609E+00	7.308E-03	1.617E+00	2.489E-01	2.495E-03	1.367E-01
0.6000	1.583E+00	7.779E-03	1.591E+00	2.801E-01	2.679E-03	1.648E-01
0.7000	1.546E+00	8.765E-03	1.555E+00	3.437E-01	3.048E-03	2.236E-01
0.8000	1.521E+00	9.800E-03	1.530E+00	4.086E-01	3.419E-03	2.846E-01
0.9000	1.503E+00	1.088E-02	1.514E+00	4.743E-01	3.794E-03	3.467E-01
1.0000	1.491E+00	1.200E-02	1.504E+00	5.406E-01	4.173E-03	4.093E-01
1.2500	1.476E+00	1.499E-02	1.491E+00	7.077E-01	5.141E-03	5.644E-01
1.5000	1.471E+00	1.818E-02	1.489E+00	8.756E-01	6.138E-03	7.142E-01
1.7500	1.471E+00	2.154E-02	1.493E+00	1.043E+00	7.163E-03	8.568E-01
2.0000	1.474E+00	2.505E-02	1.499E+00	1.210E+00	8.214E-03	9.917E-01
2.5000	1.483E+00	3.244E-02	1.515E+00	1.542E+00	1.038E-02	1.240E+00
3.0000	1.493E+00	4.021E-02	1.533E+00	1.870E+00	1.262E-02	1.461E+00
3.5000	1.503E+00	4.830E-02	1.552E+00	2.194E+00	1.491E-02	1.660E+00
4.0000	1.513E+00	5.666E-02	1.570E+00	2.515E+00	1.725E-02	1.839E+00
4.5000	1.523E+00	6.524E-02	1.588E+00	2.832E+00	1.962E-02	2.003E+00
5.0000	1.531E+00	7.402E-02	1.605E+00	3.145E+00	2.202E-02	2.154E+00
5.5000	1.539E+00	8.298E-02	1.622E+00	3.455E+00	2.444E-02	2.293E+00
6.0000	1.547E+00	9.211E-02	1.639E+00	3.761E+00	2.687E-02	2.422E+00
7.0000	1.560E+00	1.108E-01	1.671E+00	4.365E+00	3.178E-02	2.655E+00
8.0000	1.572E+00	1.299E-01	1.702E+00	4.958E+00	3.672E-02	2.861E+00
9.0000	1.583E+00	1.494E-01	1.732E+00	5.541E+00	4.168E-02	3.046E+00
10.0000	1.592E+00	1.693E-01	1.761E+00	6.113E+00	4.663E-02	3.214E+00
12.5000	1.612E+00	2.201E-01	1.832E+00	7.504E+00	5.894E-02	3.577E+00
15.0000	1.629E+00	2.723E-01	1.901E+00	8.844E+00	7.108E-02	3.881E+00
17.5000	1.642E+00	3.256E-01	1.968E+00	1.014E+01	8.299E-02	4.143E+00
20.0000	1.654E+00	3.797E-01	2.034E+00	1.139E+01	9.463E-02	4.374E+00
25.0000	1.673E+00	4.896E-01	2.163E+00	1.377E+01	1.171E-01	4.769E+00
30.0000	1.688E+00	6.014E-01	2.289E+00	1.602E+01	1.384E-01	5.099E+00
35.0000	1.700E+00	7.146E-01	2.415E+00	1.814E+01	1.585E-01	5.383E+00
40.0000	1.711E+00	8.289E-01	2.540E+00	2.016E+01	1.776E-01	5.633E+00
45.0000	1.720E+00	9.441E-01	2.664E+00	2.208E+01	1.957E-01	5.856E+00
50.0000	1.728E+00	1.060E+00	2.788E+00	2.392E+01	2.129E-01	6.057E+00
55.0000	1.736E+00	1.177E+00	2.912E+00	2.567E+01	2.292E-01	6.240E+00
60.0000	1.742E+00	1.294E+00	3.036E+00	2.735E+01	2.447E-01	6.408E+00
70.0000	1.754E+00	1.530E+00	3.283E+00	3.052E+01	2.735E-01	6.707E+00
80.0000	1.764E+00	1.767E+00	3.531E+00	3.346E+01	2.998E-01	6.968E+00
90.0000	1.772E+00	2.006E+00	3.778E+00	3.619E+01	3.238E-01	7.199E+00

Calcium Fluoride

ENERGY	STOPPING POWER COLLISION	RADIATIVE	TOTAL	CSDA RANGE	RADIATION YIELD	DENS.EFF. CORR. (DELTA)
MeV	MeV cm²/g	MeV cm²/g	MeV cm²/g	g/cm²		
0.0100	1.666E+01	7.284E-03	1.667E+01	3.503E-04	2.300E-04	0.0
0.0125	1.412E+01	7.499E-03	1.413E+01	5.139E-04	2.809E-04	0.0
0.0150	1.233E+01	7.657E-03	1.233E+01	7.039E-04	3.301E-04	0.0
0.0175	1.099E+01	7.778E-03	1.099E+01	9.190E-04	3.778E-04	0.0
0.0200	9.945E+00	7.874E-03	9.953E+00	1.158E-03	4.243E-04	0.0
0.0250	8.424E+00	8.016E-03	8.432E+00	1.706E-03	5.138E-04	0.0
0.0300	7.363E+00	8.118E-03	7.371E+00	2.343E-03	5.993E-04	0.0
0.0350	6.577E+00	8.197E-03	6.585E+00	3.062E-03	6.813E-04	0.0
0.0400	5.970E+00	8.263E-03	5.979E+00	3.860E-03	7.604E-04	0.0
0.0450	5.487E+00	8.319E-03	5.495E+00	4.733E-03	8.368E-04	0.0
0.0500	5.093E+00	8.370E-03	5.101E+00	5.678E-03	9.109E-04	0.0
0.0550	4.764E+00	8.416E-03	4.773E+00	6.693E-03	9.829E-04	0.0
0.0600	4.486E+00	8.458E-03	4.495E+00	7.773E-03	1.053E-03	0.0
0.0700	4.041E+00	8.541E-03	4.050E+00	1.012E-02	1.188E-03	0.0
0.0800	3.701E+00	8.621E-03	3.709E+00	1.271E-02	1.316E-03	0.0
0.0900	3.432E+00	8.704E-03	3.440E+00	1.551E-02	1.440E-03	0.0
0.1000	3.213E+00	8.788E-03	3.222E+00	1.851E-02	1.559E-03	0.0
0.1250	2.814E+00	9.016E-03	2.823E+00	2.684E-02	1.840E-03	0.0
0.1500	2.544E+00	9.265E-03	2.553E+00	3.617E-02	2.102E-03	0.0
0.1750	2.349E+00	9.534E-03	2.359E+00	4.638E-02	2.350E-03	0.0
0.2000	2.203E+00	9.821E-03	2.213E+00	5.733E-02	2.586E-03	0.0
0.2500	2.000E+00	1.045E-02	2.011E+00	8.111E-02	3.033E-03	0.0
0.3000	1.867E+00	1.113E-02	1.878E+00	1.069E-01	3.455E-03	5.037E-03
0.3500	1.774E+00	1.187E-02	1.786E+00	1.342E-01	3.859E-03	1.737E-02
0.4000	1.706E+00	1.266E-02	1.719E+00	1.628E-01	4.252E-03	3.256E-02
0.4500	1.656E+00	1.348E-02	1.669E+00	1.923E-01	4.638E-03	5.026E-02
0.5000	1.617E+00	1.435E-02	1.631E+00	2.226E-01	5.017E-03	7.003E-02
0.5500	1.587E+00	1.525E-02	1.602E+00	2.536E-01	5.394E-03	9.144E-02
0.6000	1.563E+00	1.618E-02	1.579E+00	2.850E-01	5.768E-03	1.141E-01
0.7000	1.528E+00	1.812E-02	1.547E+00	3.491E-01	6.512E-03	1.623E-01
0.8000	1.506E+00	2.016E-02	1.526E+00	4.142E-01	7.256E-03	2.128E-01
0.9000	1.491E+00	2.229E-02	1.513E+00	4.800E-01	8.002E-03	2.645E-01
1.0000	1.481E+00	2.450E-02	1.505E+00	5.463E-01	8.752E-03	3.167E-01
1.2500	1.470E+00	3.034E-02	1.500E+00	7.128E-01	1.065E-02	4.459E-01
1.5000	1.468E+00	3.658E-02	1.505E+00	8.793E-01	1.258E-02	5.700E-01
1.7500	1.471E+00	4.313E-02	1.515E+00	1.045E+00	1.456E-02	6.875E-01
2.0000	1.477E+00	4.995E-02	1.527E+00	1.209E+00	1.656E-02	7.980E-01
2.5000	1.491E+00	6.423E-02	1.555E+00	1.534E+00	2.065E-02	9.994E-01
3.0000	1.506E+00	7.922E-02	1.585E+00	1.852E+00	2.481E-02	1.178E+00
3.5000	1.520E+00	9.476E-02	1.615E+00	2.165E+00	2.903E-02	1.338E+00
4.0000	1.533E+00	1.108E-01	1.644E+00	2.472E+00	3.328E-02	1.482E+00
4.5000	1.545E+00	1.272E-01	1.673E+00	2.773E+00	3.755E-02	1.614E+00
5.0000	1.557E+00	1.439E-01	1.701E+00	3.070E+00	4.183E-02	1.735E+00
5.5000	1.567E+00	1.610E-01	1.728E+00	3.361E+00	4.611E-02	1.848E+00
6.0000	1.577E+00	1.783E-01	1.755E+00	3.649E+00	5.038E-02	1.953E+00
7.0000	1.594E+00	2.137E-01	1.808E+00	4.210E+00	5.889E-02	2.144E+00
8.0000	1.610E+00	2.499E-01	1.859E+00	4.755E+00	6.732E-02	2.316E+00
9.0000	1.623E+00	2.868E-01	1.910E+00	5.286E+00	7.566E-02	2.472E+00
10.0000	1.635E+00	3.243E-01	1.959E+00	5.803E+00	8.388E-02	2.615E+00
12.5000	1.660E+00	4.199E-01	2.079E+00	7.041E+00	1.039E-01	2.931E+00
15.0000	1.679E+00	5.180E-01	2.197E+00	8.210E+00	1.231E-01	3.203E+00
17.5000	1.695E+00	6.177E-01	2.313E+00	9.319E+00	1.415E-01	3.442E+00
20.0000	1.709E+00	7.189E-01	2.428E+00	1.037E+01	1.590E-01	3.656E+00
25.0000	1.731E+00	9.243E-01	2.655E+00	1.234E+01	1.917E-01	4.026E+00
30.0000	1.748E+00	1.133E+00	2.881E+00	1.415E+01	2.217E-01	4.338E+00
35.0000	1.762E+00	1.344E+00	3.106E+00	1.582E+01	2.491E-01	4.609E+00
40.0000	1.774E+00	1.557E+00	3.331E+00	1.738E+01	2.742E-01	4.848E+00
45.0000	1.784E+00	1.771E+00	3.555E+00	1.883E+01	2.974E-01	5.061E+00
50.0000	1.793E+00	1.987E+00	3.780E+00	2.019E+01	3.189E-01	5.253E+00
55.0000	1.802E+00	2.204E+00	4.005E+00	2.148E+01	3.388E-01	5.429E+00
60.0000	1.809E+00	2.422E+00	4.231E+00	2.269E+01	3.574E-01	5.590E+00
70.0000	1.822E+00	2.860E+00	4.682E+00	2.494E+01	3.909E-01	5.878E+00
80.0000	1.833E+00	3.301E+00	5.134E+00	2.698E+01	4.205E-01	6.130E+00
90.0000	1.843E+00	3.744E+00	5.587E+00	2.884E+01	4.468E-01	6.353E+00

APPENDIX F. Neutron Kerma Factors F_n, rad (or cGy) per n/cm^2 [a,b]

En/MeV	ΔEn/MeV	H	Li-6	Li-7	B	C	N	O
.253-07	.000	.420-11	.722-05	.130-13	.159-05	.241-14	.785-09	.356-16
.360-07	.200-07	.355-11	.611-05	.110-13	.135-05	.206-14	.665-09	.337-16
.630-07	.340-07	.269-11	.462-05	.837-14	.102-05	.158-14	.502-09	.345-16
.110-06	.660-07	.204-11	.349-05	.637-14	.770-06	.123-14	.380-09	.418-16
.200-06	.120-06	.153-11	.260-05	.478-14	.572-06	.981-15	.282-09	.610-16
.360-06	.200-06	.116-11	.193-05	.363-14	.426-06	.846-15	.210-09	.986-16
.630-06	.340-06	.909-12	.145-05	.286-14	.321-06	.834-15	.159-09	.165-15
.110-05	.600-06	.749-12	.110-05	.237-14	.243-06	.971-15	.120-09	.282-15
.200-05	.120-05	.672-12	.821-06	.213-14	.181-06	.137-14	.894-10	.508-15
.360-05	.200-05	.707-12	.611-06	.225-14	.135-06	.217-14	.665-10	.911-15
.630-05	.340-05	.885-12	.462-06	.283-14	.102-06	.359-14	.502-10	.159-14
.110-04	.600-05	.128-11	.349-06	.412-14	.768-07	.611-14	.380-10	.278-14
.200-04	.120-04	.211-11	.260-06	.682-14	.570-07	.110-13	.283-10	.505-14
.360-04	.200-04	.364-11	.193-06	.118-13	.424-07	.197-13	.211-10	.909-14
.630-04	.340-04	.625-11	.146-06	.203-13	.320-07	.344-13	.159-10	.159-13
.110-03	.600-04	.108-10	.110-06	.351-13	.242-07	.600-13	.121-10	.278-13
.200-03	.120-03	.196-10	.820-07	.636-13	.179-07	.109-12	.910-11	.505-13
.360-03	.200-03	.352-10	.610-07	.114-12	.133-07	.196-12	.694-11	.909-13
.630-03	.340-03	.614-10	.461-07	.200-12	.100-07	.343-12	.552-11	.159-12
.110-02	.600-03	.107-09	.349-07	.349-12	.756-08	.599-12	.464-11	.278-12
.200-02	.120-02	.193-09	.259-07	.635-12	.559-08	.109-11	.429-11	.505-12
.360-02	.200-02	.345-09	.193-07	.114-11	.415-08	.195-11	.462-11	.909-12
.630-02	.340-02	.593-09	.147-07	.200-11	.313-08	.341-11	.582-11	.159-11
.110-01	.600-02	.100-08	.112-07	.344-11	.237-08	.593-11	.826-11	.278-11
.200-01	.120-01	.174-08	.849-08	.578-11	.178-08	.107-10	.128-10	.506-11
.360-01	.200-01	.287-08	.660-08	.944-11	.136-08	.190-10	.197-10	.912-11
.630-01	.340-01	.444-08	.555-08	.148-10	.108-08	.325-10	.289-10	.160-10
.820-01	.400-02	.535-08	.532-08	.179-10	.968-09	.416-10	.342-10	.209-10
.860-01	.400-02	.553-08	.533-08	.186-10	.952-09	.435-10	.353-10	.220-10
.900-01	.400-02	.570-08	.534-08	.192-10	.938-09	.454-10	.364-10	.230-10
.940-01	.400-02	.587-08	.538-08	.198-10	.924-09	.473-10	.374-10	.240-10
.980-01	.400-02	.603-08	.543-08	.204-10	.911-09	.491-10	.384-10	.251-10
.105+00	.100-01	.631-08	.554-08	.217-10	.891-09	.523-10	.403-10	.269-10
.115+00	.100-01	.669-08	.575-08	.237-10	.865-09	.569-10	.430-10	.296-10
.125+00	.100-01	.705-08	.614-08	.257-10	.842-09	.613-10	.456-10	.322-10
.135+00	.100-01	.739-08	.664-08	.281-10	.822-09	.657-10	.482-10	.350-10
.145+00	.100-01	.772-08	.731-08	.312-10	.804-09	.700-10	.507-10	.377-10
.155+00	.100-01	.803-08	.821-08	.350-10	.787-09	.743-10	.531-10	.404-10
.165+00	.100-01	.832-08	.942-08	.394-10	.772-09	.784-10	.555-10	.432-10
.175+00	.100-01	.861-08	.110-07	.448-10	.758-09	.825-10	.579-10	.461-10
.185+00	.100-01	.867-08	.131-07	.519-10	.745-09	.865-10	.602-10	.489-10
.195+00	.100-01	.913-08	.159-07	.620-10	.733-09	.905-10	.624-10	.518-10
.210+00	.200-01	.951-08	.210-07	.869-10	.717-09	.963-10	.657-10	.562-10
.230+00	.200-01	.999-08	.275-07	.220-09	.697-09	.104-09	.700-10	.623-10
.250+00	.200-01	.104-07	.277-07	.627-09	.678-09	.111-09	.742-10	.688-10
.270+00	.200-01	.109-07	.218-07	.614-09	.659-09	.118-09	.778-10	.758-10
.290+00	.200-01	.113-07	.159-07	.349-09	.642-09	.125-09	.814-10	.836-10
.310+00	.200-01	.117-07	.117-07	.238-09	.627-09	.132-09	.848-10	.926-10
.330+00	.200-01	.120-07	.918-08	.199-09	.616-09	.138-09	.882-10	.104-09
.350+00	.200-01	.124-07	.746-08	.173-09	.608-09	.145-09	.915-10	.118-09
.370+00	.200-01	.127-07	.631-08	.166-09	.606-09	.151-09	.950-10	.139-09
.390+00	.200-01	.131-07	.551-08	.166-09	.618-09	.157-09	.998-10	.174-09
.420+00	.400-01	.135-07	.471-08	.171-09	.708-09	.165-09	.129-09	.298-09
.460+00	.400-01	.141-07	.403-08	.177-09	.693-09	.176-09	.102-09	.239-09
.500+00	.400-01	.147-07	.361-08	.185-09	.625-09	.186-09	.159-09	.991-10
.540+00	.400-01	.153-07	.334-08	.197-09	.585-09	.196-09	.102-09	.908-10
.580+00	.400-01	.158-07	.314-08	.211-09	.546-09	.205-09	.102-09	.975-10
.620+00	.400-01	.163-07	.300-08	.228-09	.511-09	.214-09	.171-09	.106-09

[a]The notation in Appendix F: for example .253-07, means 0.253×10^{-7}.
[b]From Caswell, Coyne, and Randolph, *Rad. Res.* **83**, 217 (1980).
Reproduced with permission from R. S. Caswell and Academic Press.

En/MeV	ΔEn/MeV	H	Li-6	Li-7	B	C	N	O
.660+00	.400-01	.168-07	.290-08	.246-09	.482-09	.222-09	.269-09	.114-09
.700+00	.400-01	.173-07	.283-08	.267-09	.461-09	.230-09	.182-09	.123-09
.740+00	.400-01	.177-07	.278-08	.289-09	.447-09	.237-09	.155-09	.131-09
.780+00	.400-01	.182-07	.274-08	.313-09	.438-09	.244-09	.142-09	.140-09
.820+00	.400-01	.186-07	.271-08	.340-09	.433-09	.251-09	.133-09	.152-09
.860+00	.400-01	.190-07	.269-08	.371-09	.429-09	.257-09	.124-09	.169-09
.900+00	.400-01	.194-07	.268-08	.404-09	.427-09	.263-09	.114-09	.202-09
.940+00	.400-01	.198-07	.268-08	.441-09	.428-09	.269-09	.984-10	.287-09
.980+00	.400-01	.202-07	.268-08	.480-09	.426-09	.275-09	.122-09	.479-09
.105+01	.100+00	.209-07	.270-08	.542-09	.434-09	.284-09	.202-09	.422-09
.115+01	.100+00	.218-07	.274-08	.614-09	.482-09	.296-09	.176-09	.259-09
.125+01	.100+00	.227-07	.281-08	.672-09	.658-09	.306-09	.172-09	.273-09
.135+01	.100+00	.235-07	.289-08	.714-09	.662-09	.316-09	.417-09	.269-09
.145+01	.100+00	.243-07	.301-08	.748-09	.616-09	.325-09	.405-09	.216-09
.155+01	.100+00	.250-07	.314-08	.789-09	.645-09	.334-09	.313-09	.218-09
.165+01	.100+00	.257-07	.328-08	.831-09	.720-09	.343-09	.294-09	.268-09
.175+01	.100+00	.264-07	.338-08	.876-09	.866-09	.352-09	.443-09	.214-09
.185+01	.100+00	.271-07	.343-08	.928-09	.908-09	.361-09	.364-09	.284-09
.195+01	.100+00	.277-07	.345-08	.982-09	.870-09	.371-09	.328-09	.220-09
.210+01	.200+00	.286-07	.347-08	.107-08	.821-09	.458-09	.371-09	.203-09
.230+01	.200+00	.297-07	.348-08	.120-08	.745-09	.420-09	.484-09	.113-09
.250+01	.200+00	.307-07	.347-08	.134-08	.897-09	.471-09	.495-09	.137-09
.270+01	.200+00	.317-07	.350-08	.147-08	.934-09	.569-09	.717-09	.175-09
.290+01	.200+00	.326-07	.358-08	.159-08	.923-09	.800-09	.838-09	.188-09
.310+01	.200+00	.335-07	.374-08	.170-08	.876-09	.585-09	.104-08	.279-09
.330+01	.200+00	.343-07	.395-08	.181-08	.861-09	.907-09	.112-08	.561-09
.350+01	.200+00	.350-07	.413-08	.198-08	.939-09	.105-08	.137-08	.542-09
.370+01	.200+00	.357-07	.428-08	.221-08	.986-09	.101-08	.127-08	.591-09
.390+01	.200+00	.364-07	.441-08	.247-08	.101-08	.908-09	.154-08	.407-09
.420+01	.400+00	.373-07	.453-08	.274-08	.106-08	.742-09	.172-08	.479-09
.460+01	.400+00	.384-07	.468-08	.290-08	.124-08	.555-09	.135-08	.378-09
.500+01	.400+00	.394-07	.480-08	.289-08	.131-08	.520-09	.113-08	.584-09
.540+01	.400+00	.402-07	.493-08	.286-08	.131-08	.534-09	.104-08	.315-09
.580+01	.400+00	.410-07	.504-08	.304-08	.136-08	.558-09	.976-09	.486-09
.620+01	.400+00	.417-07	.521-08	.303-08	.138-08	.782-09	.115-08	.456-09
.660+01	.400+00	.423-07	.537-08	.299-08	.131-08	.462-09	.884-09	.653-09
.700+01	.400+00	.428-07	.550-08	.298-08	.130-08	.450-09	.983-09	.866-09
.740+01	.400+00	.433-07	.562-08	.299-08	.127-08	.794-09	.125-08	.110-08
.780+01	.400+00	.438-07	.575-08	.304-08	.135-08	.132-08	.121-08	.838-09
.820+01	.400+00	.442-07	.587-08	.315-08	.128-08	.914-09	.113-08	.800-09
.860+01	.400+00	.445-07	.597-08	.327-08	.129-08	.751-09	.112-08	.101-08
.900+01	.400+00	.448-07	.606-08	.339-08	.130-08	.119-08	.118-08	.102-08
.940+01	.400+00	.452-07	.611-08	.350-08	.132-08	.151-08	.127-08	.963-09
.980+01	.400+00	.454-07	.615-08	.361-08	.141-08	.125-08	.138-08	.115-08
.105+02	.100+01	.459-07	.625-08	.379-08	.146-08	.121-08	.156-08	.127-08
.115+02	.100+01	.463-07	.634-08	.401-08	.157-08	.144-08	.177-08	.173-08
.125+02	.100+01	.467-07	.637-08	.419-08	.171-08	.181-08	.211-08	.157-08
.135+02	.100+01	.469-07	.641-08	.434-08	.186-08	.201-08	.234-08	.182-08
.145+02	.100+01	.471-07	.645-08	.448-08	.200-08	.239-08	.253-08	.206-08
.155+02	.100+01	.471-07	.649-08	.467-08	.209-08	.294-08	.269-08	.218-08
.165+02	.100+01	.472-07	.658-08	.488-08	.217-08	.327-08	.282-08	.223-08
.175+02	.100+01	.471-07	.669-08	.506-08	.223-08	.337-08	.296-08	.234-08
.185+02	.100+01	.470-07	.679-08	.523-08	.228-08	.355-08	.313-08	.246-08
.195+02	.100+01	.469-07	.688-08	.537-08	.231-08	.367-08	.329-08	.262-08
.210+02	.200+01	.467-07	.704-08	.556-08	.245-08	.403-08	.349-08	.277-08
.230+02	.200+01	.463-07	.723-08	.578-08	.255-08	.427-08	.366-08	.275-08
.250+02	.200+01	.458-07	.741-08	.595-08	.265-08	.452-08	.378-08	.270-08
.270+02	.200+01	.453-07	.757-08	.607-08	.273-08	.466-08	.386-08	.278-08
.290+02	.200+01	.447-07	.771-08	.617-08	.285-08	.490-08	.394-08	.264-08

En/MeV	ΔEn/MeV	F	Na	Mg	Al	Si	P	S-32
.253-07	.000	.364-14	.941-13	.176-13	.499-13	.436-13	.371-13	.145-11
.360-07	.200-07	.309-14	.797-13	.149-13	.423-13	.370-13	.321-13	.323-11
.630-07	.340-07	.234-14	.602-13	.113-13	.320-13	.279-13	.240-13	.330-11
.110-06	.600-07	.178-14	.456-13	.853-14	.242-13	.212-13	.184-13	.186-11
.200-06	.120-06	.135-14	.339-13	.636-14	.180-13	.158-13	.141-13	.185-11
.360-06	.200-06	.104-14	.253-13	.476-14	.134-13	.117-13	.113-13	.151-11
.630-06	.340-06	.858-15	.191-13	.364-14	.101-13	.890-14	.757-14	.154-11
.110-05	.600-06	.771-15	.145-13	.282-14	.768-14	.676-14	.581-14	.141-11
.200-05	.120-05	.803-15	.109-13	.222-14	.575-14	.508-14	.471-14	.142-11
.360-05	.200-05	.101-14	.836-14	.188-14	.435-14	.388-14	.346-14	.142-11
.630-05	.340-05	.146-14	.669-14	.178-14	.341-14	.310-14	.284-14	.141-11
.110-04	.600-05	.231-14	.573-14	.199-14	.279-14	.267-14	.278-14	.140-11
.200-04	.120-04	.402-14	.552-14	.270-14	.247-14	.257-14	.345-14	.140-11
.360-04	.200-04	.710-14	.636-14	.418-14	.255-14	.295-14	.467-14	.140-11
.630-04	.340-04	.123-13	.870-14	.686-14	.312-14	.400-14	.678-14	.140-11
.110-03	.600-04	.214-13	.134-13	.116-13	.447-14	.611-14	.104-13	.140-11
.200-03	.120-03	.380-13	.229-13	.208-13	.735-14	.104-13	.175-13	.140-11
.360-03	.200-03	.659-13	.405-13	.373-13	.126-13	.182-13	.300-13	.140-11
.630-03	.340-03	.108-12	.721-13	.651-13	.216-13	.314-13	.511-13	.141-11
.110-02	.600-03	.186-12	.150-12	.113-12	.373-13	.546-13	.878-13	.142-11
.200-02	.120-02	.337-12	.186-11	.205-12	.675-13	.990-13	.158-12	.143-11
.360-02	.200-02	.608-12	.121-10	.368-12	.120-12	.178-12	.283-12	.146-11
.630-02	.340-02	.107-11	.172-11	.638-12	.305-12	.309-12	.541-12	.152-11
.110-01	.600-02	.186-11	.184-11	.112-11	.347-12	.480-12	.105-11	.164-11
.200-01	.120-01	.344-11	.280-11	.286-11	.401-12	.713-12	.155-11	.174-11
.360-01	.200-01	.106-10	.467-11	.381-11	.821-11	.118-11	.301-11	.190-11
.630-01	.340-01	.195-10	.114-10	.117-10	.368-11	.269-11	.528-11	.228-11
.820-01	.400-02	.186-10	.592-11	.893-10	.199-10	.300-11	.664-11	.421-11
.860-01	.400-02	.270-10	.104-10	.107-09	.376-10	.287-11	.692-11	.522-11
.900-01	.400-02	.418-10	.108-10	.698-10	.382-10	.272-11	.710-11	.655-11
.940-01	.400-02	.732-10	.112-10	.401-10	.230-10	.262-11	.666-11	.831-11
.980-01	.400-02	.107-09	.117-10	.294-10	.149-10	.257-11	.605-11	.105-10
.105+00	.100-01	.759-10	.125-10	.222-10	.920-11	.253-11	.564-11	.246-10
.115+00	.100-01	.376-10	.136-10	.180-10	.112-10	.237-11	.540-11	.324-10
.125+00	.100-01	.303-10	.147-10	.160-10	.945-11	.200-11	.489-11	.224-10
.135+00	.100-01	.278-10	.153-10	.156-10	.129-10	.159-11	.358-11	.172-10
.145+00	.100-01	.275-10	.169-10	.174-10	.371-10	.123-11	.664-11	.145-10
.155+00	.100-01	.284-10	.179-10	.203-10	.389-10	.190-11	.123-10	.127-10
.165+00	.100-01	.285-10	.185-10	.203-10	.265-10	.608-11	.771-11	.118-10
.175+00	.100-01	.293-10	.195-10	.205-10	.175-10	.201-10	.738-11	.112-10
.185+00	.100-01	.305-10	.204-10	.222-10	.147-10	.438-10	.122-10	.104-10
.195+00	.100-01	.315-10	.224-10	.251-10	.173-10	.567-10	.796-11	.108-10
.210+00	.200-01	.381-10	.356-10	.314-10	.282-10	.479-10	.118-10	.155-10
.230+00	.200-01	.504-10	.321-10	.448-10	.207-10	.367-10	.809-11	.118-10
.250+00	.200-01	.646-10	.423-10	.635-10	.154-10	.316-10	.135-10	.105-10
.270+00	.200-01	.104-09	.285-10	.703-10	.130-10	.293-10	.128-10	.150-10
.290+00	.200-01	.106-09	.261-10	.604-10	.371-10	.281-10	.134-10	.176-10
.310+00	.200-01	.103-09	.366-10	.581-10	.325-10	.276-10	.106-10	.136-10
.330+00	.200-01	.108-09	.338-10	.518-10	.240-10	.275-10	.114-10	.118-10
.350+00	.200-01	.112-09	.361-10	.445-10	.199-10	.276-10	.168-10	.976-11
.370+00	.200-01	.116-09	.405-10	.413-10	.403-10	.279-10	.301-10	.124-10
.390+00	.200-01	.126-09	.553-10	.428-10	.226-10	.284-10	.188-10	.250-10
.420+00	.400-01	.130-09	.453-10	.934-10	.420-10	.293-10	.213-10	.179-10
.460+00	.400-01	.946-10	.502-10	.756-10	.424-10	.306-10	.302-10	.170-10
.500+00	.400-01	.108-09	.363-10	.506-10	.368-10	.322-10	.218-10	.170-10
.540+00	.400-01	.986-10	.594-10	.495-10	.473-10	.441-10	.217-10	.182-10
.580+00	.400-01	.102-09	.794-10	.492-10	.475-10	.529-10	.307-10	.279-10
.620+00	.400-01	.111-09	.865-10	.364-10	.414-10	.303-10	.246-10	.159-10

En/MeV	ΔEn/MeV	F	Na	Mg	Al	Si	P	S-32
.660+00	.400-01	.817-10	.108-09	.592-10	.534-10	.331-10	.249-10	.158-10
.700+00	.400-01	.833-10	.148-09	.600-10	.422-10	.350-10	.250-10	.228-10
.740+00	.400-01	.111-09	.101-09	.533-10	.451-10	.395-10	.250-10	.293-10
.780+00	.400-01	.119-09	.106-09	.519-10	.751-10	.479-10	.249-10	.241-10
.820+00	.400-01	.124-09	.868-10	.651-10	.640-10	.881-10	.247-10	.247-10
.860+00	.400-01	.131-09	.758-10	.843-10	.675-10	.490-10	.362-10	.212-10
.900+00	.400-01	.125-09	.106-09	.536-10	.484-10	.551-10	.346-10	.214-10
.940+00	.400-01	.140-09	.710-10	.515-10	.504-10	.653-10	.569-10	.306-10
.980+00	.400-01	.119-09	.866-10	.517-10	.468-10	.681-10	.422-10	.278-10
.105+01	.100+00	.134-09	.945-10	.515-10	.520-10	.479-10	.372-10	.303-10
.115+01	.100+00	.155-09	.884-10	.650-10	.757-10	.344-10	.530-10	.274-10
.125+01	.100+00	.189-09	.962-10	.744-10	.658-10	.512-10	.515-10	.365-10
.135+01	.100+00	.172-09	.980-10	.816-10	.636-10	.553-10	.535-10	.463-10
.145+01	.100+00	.161-09	.897-10	.729-10	.756-10	.714-10	.566-10	.453-10
.155+01	.100+00	.193-09	.916-10	.625-10	.801-10	.767-10	.606-10	.472-10
.165+01	.100+00	.214-09	.106-09	.850-10	.770-10	.126-09	.650-10	.531-10
.175+01	.100+00	.193-09	.124-09	.114-09	.911-10	.574-10	.697-10	.726-10
.185+01	.100+00	.191-09	.101-09	.909-10	.771-10	.120-09	.739-10	.916-10
.195+01	.100+00	.223-09	.123-09	.105-09	.980-10	.103-09	.779-10	.134-09
.210+01	.200+00	.217-09	.142-09	.819-10	.106-09	.794-10	.814-10	.149-09
.230+01	.200+00	.227-09	.145-09	.115-09	.958-10	.826-10	.887-10	.173-09
.250+01	.200+00	.284-09	.152-09	.118-09	.106-09	.103-09	.105-09	.184-09
.270+01	.200+00	.282-09	.137-09	.159-09	.110-09	.966-10	.130-09	.271-09
.290+01	.200+00	.260-09	.145-09	.142-09	.110-09	.103-09	.153-09	.321-09
.310+01	.200+00	.265-09	.124-09	.138-09	.118-09	.110-09	.170-09	.351-09
.330+01	.200+00	.260-09	.154-09	.134-09	.125-09	.102-09	.175-09	.411-09
.350+01	.200+00	.278-09	.171-09	.169-09	.128-09	.105-09	.178-09	.478-09
.370+01	.200+00	.280-09	.181-09	.153-09	.134-09	.884-10	.194-09	.518-09
.390+01	.200+00	.288-09	.170-09	.146-09	.132-09	.117-09	.206-09	.622-09
.420+01	.400+00	.364-09	.188-09	.201-09	.141-09	.133-09	.223-09	.520-09
.460+01	.400+00	.460-09	.185-09	.219-09	.154-09	.163-09	.229-09	.499-09
.500+01	.400+00	.495-09	.197-09	.236-09	.173-09	.175-09	.245-09	.500-09
.540+01	.400+00	.625-09	.221-09	.220-09	.189-09	.163-09	.273-09	.525-09
.580+01	.400+00	.773-09	.239-09	.232-09	.216-09	.229-09	.284-09	.596-09
.620+01	.400+00	.772-09	.268-09	.213-09	.238-09	.279-09	.302-09	.652-09
.660+01	.400+00	.786-09	.275-09	.277-09	.268-09	.374-09	.333-09	.676-09
.700+01	.400+00	.879-09	.279-09	.313-09	.292-09	.473-09	.358-09	.695-09
.740+01	.400+00	.916-09	.314-09	.333-09	.316-09	.598-09	.381-09	.718-09
.780+01	.400+00	.915-09	.343-09	.395-09	.349-09	.748-09	.407-09	.742-09
.820+01	.400+00	.974-09	.382-09	.465-09	.375-09	.713-09	.436-09	.764-09
.860+01	.400+00	.106-08	.415-09	.458-09	.411-09	.791-09	.470-09	.782-09
.900+01	.400+00	.109-08	.453-09	.534-09	.437-09	.786-09	.507-09	.802-09
.940+01	.400+00	.116-08	.497-09	.592-09	.476-09	.847-09	.534-09	.826-09
.980+01	.400+00	.124-08	.537-09	.663-09	.517-09	.912-09	.562-09	.854-09
.105+02	.100+01	.140-08	.621-09	.810-09	.608-09	.100-08	.611-09	.914-09
.115+02	.100+01	.162-08	.696-09	.979-09	.810-09	.110-08	.684-09	.992-09
.125+02	.100+01	.184-08	.753-09	.116-08	.102-08	.116-08	.747-09	.105-08
.135+02	.100+01	.199-08	.783-09	.131-08	.121-08	.118-08	.802-09	.111-08
.145+02	.100+01	.213-08	.812-09	.143-08	.132-08	.125-08	.827-09	.115-08
.155+02	.100+01	.228-08	.880-09	.144-08	.135-08	.134-08	.846-09	.121-08
.165+02	.100+01	.241-08	.983-09	.147-08	.134-08	.140-08	.846-09	.126-08
.175+02	.100+01	.245-08	.109-08	.152-08	.133-08	.148-08	.852-09	.130-08
.185+02	.100+01	.254-08	.119-08	.153-08	.130-08	.157-08	.855-09	.132-08
.195+02	.100+01	.234-08	.130-08	.150-08	.126-08	.161-08	.848-09	.130-08
.210+02	.200+01	.220-08	.142-08	.153-08	.124-08	.165-08	.884-09	.136-08
.230+02	.200+01	.208-08	.154-08	.152-08	.119-08	.166-08	.936-09	.136-08
.250+02	.200+01	.209-08	.164-08	.151-08	.115-08	.167-08	.101-08	.139-08
.270+02	.200+01	.215-08	.175-08	.153-08	.112-08	.161-08	.110-08	.142-08
.290+02	.200+01	.230-08	.184-08	.157-08	.111-08	.163-08	.118-08	.149-08

APPENDIX F. (*Continued*)

En/MeV	ΔEn/MeV	Cl	Ar	K	Ca	Fe
.253-07	.000	.653-10	.483-13	.441-11	.110-11	.214-12
.360-07	.200-07	.553-10	.423-13	.374-11	.242-11	.181-12
.630-07	.340-07	.418-10	.312-13	.282-11	.172-11	.137-12
.110-06	.600-07	.316-10	.227-13	.214-11	.118-11	.104-12
.200-06	.120-06	.235-10	.175-13	.159-11	.143-11	.770-13
.360-06	.200-06	.175-10	.129-13	.118-11	.114-11	.573-13
.630-06	.340-06	.133-10	.969-14	.893-12	.120-11	.433-13
.110-05	.600-06	.994-11	.761-14	.676-12	.113-11	.328-13
.200-05	.120-05	.679-11	.569-14	.502-12	.109-11	.245-13
.360-05	.200-05	.440-11	.436-14	.374-12	.108-11	.184-13
.630-05	.340-05	.294-11	.354-14	.282-12	.106-11	.141-13
.110-04	.600-05	.197-11	.254-14	.214-12	.106-11	.111-13
.200-04	.120-04	.128-11	.241-14	.159-12	.106-11	.908-14
.360-04	.200-04	.837-12	.235-14	.119-12	.106-11	.821-14
.630-04	.340-04	.550-12	.224-14	.906-13	.106-11	.866-14
.110-03	.600-04	.356-12	.206-14	.698-13	.106-11	.108-13
.200-03	.120-03	.319-12	.231-14	.539-13	.106-11	.160-13
.360-03	.200-03	.182-10	.359-14	.436-13	.106-11	.254-13
.630-03	.340-03	.702-11	.582-14	.385-13	.107-11	.397-13
.110-02	.600-03	.979-12	.937-14	.380-13	.109-11	.989-13
.200-02	.120-02	.416-12	.182-13	.431-13	.111-11	.954-13
.360-02	.200-02	.783-12	.351-13	.327-12	.116-11	.145-12
.630-02	.340-02	.640-12	.692-13	.129-12	.123-11	.404-12
.110-01	.600-02	.631-12	.149-12	.501-12	.136-11	.395-12
.200-01	.120-01	.118-11	.368-12	.482-12	.158-11	.183-12
.360-01	.200-01	.152-11	.683-12	.119-11	.179-11	.350-11
.630-01	.340-01	.243-11	.116-11	.235-11	.211-11	.179-11
.820-01	.400-02	.268-11	.147-11	.174-11	.252-11	.357-11
.860-01	.400-02	.245-11	.153-11	.210-11	.331-11	.627-11
.900-01	.400-02	.256-11	.159-11	.220-11	.415-11	.316-11
.940-01	.400-02	.270-11	.166-11	.190-11	.219-11	.256-11
.980-01	.400-02	.276-11	.172-11	.346-11	.269-11	.257-11
.105+00	.100-01	.304-11	.183-11	.374-11	.309-11	.224-11
.115+00	.100-01	.327-11	.199-11	.291-11	.232-11	.188-11
.125+00	.100-01	.261-11	.217-11	.251-11	.252-11	.193-11
.135+00	.100-01	.481-11	.235-11	.322-11	.127-11	.232-11
.145+00	.100-01	.508-11	.253-11	.361-11	.614-11	.767-11
.155+00	.100-01	.394-11	.272-11	.476-11	.412-11	.311-11
.165+00	.100-01	.392-11	.290-11	.350-11	.536-11	.277-11
.175+00	.100-01	.302-11	.309-11	.252-11	.128-10	.355-11
.185+00	.100-01	.707-11	.328-11	.262-11	.259-11	.526-11
.195+00	.100-01	.759-11	.346-11	.412-11	.217-11	.786-11
.210+00	.200-01	.489-11	.375-11	.289-11	.746-11	.383-11
.230+00	.200-01	.584-11	.413-11	.350-11	.599-11	.511-11
.250+00	.200-01	.561-11	.451-11	.457-11	.203-10	.403-11
.270+00	.200-01	.585-11	.490-11	.524-11	.103-10	.442-11
.290+00	.200-01	.858-11	.528-11	.106-10	.783-11	.457-11
.310+00	.200-01	.751-11	.559-11	.741-11	.404-11	.330-11
.330+00	.200-01	.740-11	.536-11	.590-11	.166-10	.709-11
.350+00	.200-01	.125-10	.497-11	.862-11	.111-10	.357-11
.370+00	.200-01	.829-11	.451-11	.825-11	.884-11	.703-11
.390+00	.200-01	.114-10	.398-11	.811-11	.638-11	.121-10
.420+00	.400-01	.120-10	.424-11	.107-10	.587-11	.106-10
.460+00	.400-01	.128-10	.541-11	.979-11	.102-10	.842-11
.500+00	.400-01	.131-10	.603-11	.106-10	.889-11	.848-11
.540+00	.400-01	.143-10	.525-11	.992-11	.580-11	.665-11
.580+00	.400-01	.139-10	.101-10	.116-10	.132-10	.702-11
.620+00	.400-01	.153-10	.153-10	.122-10	.242-10	.465-11

En/MeV	ΔEn/MeV	Cl	Ar	K	Ca	Fe
.660+00	.400-01	.161-10	.136-10	.131-10	.150-10	.666-11
.700+00	.400-01	.176-10	.113-10	.139-10	.109-10	.919-11
.740+00	.400-01	.177-10	.103-10	.148-10	.112-10	.150-10
.780+00	.400-01	.196-10	.937-11	.156-10	.156-10	.156-10
.820+00	.400-01	.200-10	.967-11	.166-10	.119-10	.102-10
.860+00	.400-01	.221-10	.104-10	.176-10	.187-10	.984-11
.900+00	.400-01	.239-10	.129-10	.185-10	.335-10	.795-11
.940+00	.400-01	.240-10	.144-10	.190-10	.232-10	.616-11
.980+00	.400-01	.237-10	.143-10	.205-10	.196-10	.116-10
.105+01	.100+00	.272-10	.219-10	.234-10	.227-10	.127-10
.115+01	.100+00	.308-10	.271-10	.274-10	.263-10	.111-10
.125+01	.100+00	.347-10	.267-10	.289-10	.306-10	.180-10
.135+01	.100+00	.385-10	.376-10	.352-10	.245-10	.167-10
.145+01	.100+00	.433-10	.369-10	.415-10	.309-10	.204-10
.155+01	.100+00	.481-10	.399-10	.472-10	.462-10	.244-10
.165+01	.100+00	.529-10	.342-10	.574-10	.478-10	.221-10
.175+01	.100+00	.580-10	.485-10	.592-10	.567-10	.209-10
.185+01	.100+00	.620-10	.531-10	.712-10	.577-10	.222-10
.195+01	.100+00	.680-10	.553-10	.873-10	.665-10	.271-10
.210+01	.200+00	.780-10	.612-10	.998-10	.836-10	.292-10
.230+01	.200+00	.906-10	.644-10	.121-09	.108-09	.301-10
.250+01	.200+00	.104-09	.669-10	.133-09	.150-09	.377-10
.270+01	.200+00	.116-09	.726-10	.164-09	.198-09	.367-10
.290+01	.200+00	.123-09	.739-10	.185-09	.259-09	.390-10
.310+01	.200+00	.140-09	.739-10	.216-09	.331-09	.432-10
.330+01	.200+00	.153-09	.748-10	.271-09	.395-09	.437-10
.350+01	.200+00	.165-09	.775-10	.311-09	.467-09	.453-10
.370+01	.200+00	.186-09	.800-10	.354-09	.341-09	.493-10
.390+01	.200+00	.205-09	.811-10	.393-09	.612-09	.523-10
.420+01	.400+00	.230-09	.823-10	.439-09	.697-09	.571-10
.460+01	.400+00	.260-09	.828-10	.462-09	.773-09	.615-10
.500+01	.400+00	.284-09	.821-10	.491-09	.821-09	.683-10
.540+01	.400+00	.305-09	.810-10	.517-09	.860-09	.751-10
.580+01	.400+00	.328-09	.763-10	.548-09	.894-09	.835-10
.620+01	.400+00	.354-09	.772-10	.586-09	.923-09	.925-10
.660+01	.400+00	.375-09	.829-10	.621-09	.976-09	.103-09
.700+01	.400+00	.392-09	.886-10	.654-09	.102-08	.113-09
.740+01	.400+00	.407-09	.943-10	.668-09	.107-08	.125-09
.780+01	.400+00	.423-09	.998-10	.722-09	.111-08	.137-09
.820+01	.400+00	.437-09	.105-09	.759-09	.115-08	.149-09
.860+01	.400+00	.450-09	.111-09	.801-09	.119-08	.161-09
.900+01	.400+00	.464-09	.116-09	.849-09	.123-08	.174-09
.940+01	.400+00	.481-09	.123-09	.904-09	.126-08	.188-09
.980+01	.400+00	.497-09	.129-09	.964-09	.130-08	.202-09
.105+02	.100+01	.532-09	.139-09	.108-08	.137-08	.228-09
.115+02	.100+01	.589-09	.152-09	.126-08	.149-08	.270-09
.125+02	.100+01	.649-09	.166-09	.142-08	.160-08	.317-09
.135+02	.100+01	.708-09	.181-09	.152-08	.164-08	.360-09
.145+02	.100+01	.758-09	.200-09	.158-08	.164-08	.402-09
.155+02	.100+01	.790-09	.214-09	.157-08	.166-08	.441-09
.165+02	.100+01	.822-09	.227-09	.152-08	.157-08	.474-09
.175+02	.100+01	.843-09	.241-09	.143-08	.151-08	.499-09
.185+02	.100+01	.861-09	.255-09	.132-08	.146-08	.534-09
.195+02	.100+01	.879-09	.269-09	.119-08	.147-08	.575-09
.210+02	.200+01	.919-09	.291-09	.117-08	.162-08	.668-09
.230+02	.200+01	.982-09	.320-09	.111-08	.195-08	.807-09
.250+02	.200+01	.105-08	.350-09	.109-08	.232-08	.999-09
.270+02	.200+01	.112-08	.382-09	.105-08	.270-08	.120-08
.290+02	.200+01	.118-08	.414-09	.103-08	.305-08	.144-08

En/MeV	ΔEn/MeV	Tissue Appx	Bone (Femur)	Muscle ICRU	Std Man	A-150 Plast
.110−04	.600−05	.145−11	.127−11	.147−11	.129−11	.149−11
.200−04	.120−04	.120−11	.106−11	.122−11	.109−11	.124−11
.360−04	.200−04	.111−11	.969−12	.112−11	.103−11	.115−11
.630−04	.340−04	.120−11	.101−11	.122−11	.114−11	.124−11
.110−03	.600−04	.154−11	.121−11	.156−11	.150−11	.159−11
.200−03	.120−03	.233−11	.171−11	.237−11	.230−11	.242−11
.360−03	.200−03	.386−11	.269−11	.393−11	.387−11	.399−11
.630−03	.340−03	.651−11	.440−11	.662−11	.650−11	.672−11
.110−02	.600−03	.112−10	.742−11	.114−10	.112−10	.115−10
.200−02	.120−02	.200−10	.132−10	.204−10	.200−10	.207−10
.360−02	.200−02	.356−10	.233−10	.362−10	.356−10	.367−10
.630−02	.340−02	.612−10	.359−10	.622−10	.611−10	.631−10
.110−01	.600−02	.104−09	.676−10	.106−09	.104−09	.107−09
.200−01	.120−01	.180−09	.117−09	.183−09	.179−09	.185−09
.360−01	.200−01	.298−09	.194−09	.303−09	.297−09	.308−09
.630−01	.340−01	.463−09	.302−09	.470−09	.462−09	.479−09
.820−01	.400−02	.558−09	.365−09	.567−09	.557−09	.578−09
.860−01	.400−02	.577−09	.377−09	.587−09	.576−09	.598−09
.900−01	.400−02	.596−09	.389−09	.605−09	.594−09	.617−09
.940−01	.400−02	.614−09	.401−09	.624−09	.613−09	.637−09
.980−01	.400−02	.631−09	.412−09	.641−09	.630−09	.655−09
.105+00	.100−01	.661−09	.432−09	.672−09	.660−09	.686−09
.115+00	.100−01	.701−09	.458−09	.713−09	.700−09	.727−09
.125+00	.100−01	.740−09	.483−09	.752−09	.738−09	.767−09
.135+00	.100−01	.777−09	.509−09	.789−09	.776−09	.806−09
.145+00	.100−01	.813−09	.532−09	.825−09	.811−09	.842−09
.155+00	.100−01	.846−09	.554−09	.860−09	.844−09	.877−09
.165+00	.100−01	.878−09	.575−09	.892−09	.876−09	.910−09
.175+00	.100−01	.910−09	.597−09	.924−09	.907−09	.943−09
.185+00	.100−01	.939−09	.615−09	.954−09	.937−09	.973−09
.195+00	.100−01	.968−09	.634−09	.983−09	.965−09	.100−08
.210+00	.200−01	.101−08	.662−09	.103−08	.101−08	.105−08
.230+00	.200−01	.106−08	.697−09	.108−08	.106−08	.110−08
.250+00	.200−01	.111−08	.733−09	.113−08	.111−08	.115−08
.270+00	.200−01	.116−08	.764−09	.113−08	.116−08	.120−08
.290+00	.200−01	.121−08	.795−09	.123−08	.121−08	.125−08
.310+00	.200−01	.126−08	.825−09	.128−08	.125−08	.130−08
.330+00	.200−01	.130−08	.857−09	.132−08	.130−08	.134−08
.350+00	.200−01	.135−08	.887−09	.137−08	.135−08	.138−08
.370+00	.200−01	.140−08	.920−09	.142−08	.139−08	.142−08
.390+00	.200−01	.146−08	.956−09	.148−08	.145−08	.146−08
.420+00	.400−01	.160−08	.104−08	.162−08	.158−08	.152−08
.460+00	.400−01	.162−08	.106−08	.164−08	.160−08	.159−08
.500+00	.400−01	.158−08	.104−08	.160−08	.158−08	.165−08
.540+00	.400−01	.163−08	.107−08	.165−08	.162−08	.171−08
.580+00	.400−01	.169−08	.112−08	.171−08	.168−08	.177−08
.620+00	.400−01	.175−08	.116−08	.177−08	.174−08	.184−08
.660+00	.400−01	.181−08	.119−08	.183−08	.180−08	.189−08
.700+00	.400−01	.186−08	.123−08	.189−08	.185−08	.195−08
.740+00	.400−01	.191−08	.126−08	.194−08	.191−08	.200−08
.780+00	.400−01	.196−08	.130−08	.199−08	.196−08	.205−08

En/MeV	ΔEn/MeV	Tissue Appx	Bone (Femur)	Muscle ICRU	Std Man	A-150 Plast
.820+00	.400−01	.202−08	.133−08	.204−08	.201−08	.210−08
.860+00	.400−01	.207−08	.137−08	.210−08	.206−08	.215−08
.900+00	.400−01	.214−08	.141−08	.217−08	.213−08	.219−08
.940+00	.400−01	.224−08	.147−08	.227−08	.222−08	.224−08
.980+00	.400−01	.241−08	.158−08	.245−08	.239−08	.230−08
.105+01	.100+00	.245−08	.160−08	.248−08	.242−08	.237−08
.115+01	.100+00	.242−08	.160−08	.246−08	.241−08	.247−08
.125+01	.100+00	.252−08	.166−08	.256−08	.251−08	.256−08
.135+01	.100+00	.261−08	.172−08	.265−08	.260−08	.266−08
.145+01	.100+00	.265−08	.175−08	.269−08	.264−08	.275−08
.155+01	.100+00	.273−08	.180−08	.277−08	.272−08	.283−08
.165+01	.100+00	.283−08	.187−08	.287−08	.282−08	.291−08
.175+01	.100+00	.287−08	.190−08	.291−08	.286−08	.299−08
.185+01	.100+00	.298−08	.197−08	.303−08	.297−08	.306−08
.195+01	.100+00	.300−08	.199−08	.304−08	.299−08	.313−08
.210+01	.200+00	.309−08	.207−08	.313−08	.309−08	.328−08
.230+01	.200+00	.314−08	.210−08	.318−08	.314−08	.337−08
.250+01	.200+00	.326−08	.220−08	.331−08	.327−08	.352−08
.270+01	.200+00	.341−08	.232−08	.346−08	.341−08	.370−08
.290+01	.200+00	.355−08	.246−08	.360−08	.356−08	.398−08
.310+01	.200+00	.368−08	.251−08	.373−08	.367−08	.391−08
.330+01	.200+00	.401−08	.278−08	.406−08	.400−08	.426−08
.350+01	.200+00	.410−08	.287−08	.415−08	.409−08	.446−08
.370+01	.200+00	.420−08	.294−08	.425−08	.419−08	.450−08
.390+01	.200+00	.413−08	.290−08	.418−08	.413−08	.449−08
.420+01	.400+00	.425−08	.296−08	.431−08	.424−08	.447−08
.460+01	.400+00	.425−08	.293−08	.431−08	.424−08	.442−08
.500+01	.400+00	.448−08	.307−08	.455−08	.446−08	.449−08
.540+01	.400+00	.437−08	.303−08	.444−08	.437−08	.458−08
.580+01	.400+00	.457−08	.316−08	.464−08	.456−08	.468−08
.620+01	.400+00	.469−08	.328−08	.475−08	.469−08	.493−08
.660+01	.400+00	.481−08	.330−08	.489−08	.479−08	.475−08
.700+01	.400+00	.501−08	.342−08	.510−08	.498−08	.481−08
.740+01	.400+00	.529−08	.367−08	.537−08	.526−08	.515−08
.780+01	.400+00	.522−08	.374−08	.529−08	.522−08	.559−08
.820+01	.400+00	.517−08	.364−08	.525−08	.516−08	.531−08
.860+01	.400+00	.534−08	.371−08	.542−08	.531−08	.523−08
.900+01	.400+00	.544−08	.387−08	.551−08	.542−08	.561−08
.940+01	.400+00	.548−08	.397−08	.555−08	.548−08	.589−08
.980+01	.400+00	.561−08	.400−08	.566−08	.559−08	.573−08
.105+02	.100+01	.574−08	.408−08	.582−08	.571−08	.577−08
.115+02	.100+01	.616−08	.439−08	.624−08	.611−08	.602−08
.125+02	.100+01	.614−08	.448−08	.621−08	.612−08	.636−08
.135+02	.100+01	.638−08	.467−08	.645−08	.635−08	.656−08
.145+02	.100+01	.663−08	.489−08	.670−08	.659−08	.689−08
.155+02	.100+01	.682−08	.511−08	.687−08	.679−08	.734−08
.165+02	.100+01	.691−08	.521−08	.695−08	.688−08	.761−08
.175+02	.100+01	.701−08	.528−08	.705−08	.698−08	.769−08
.185+02	.100+01	.711−08	.537−08	.715−08	.708−08	.784−08
.195+02	.100+01	.724−08	.547−08	.727−08	.720−08	.793−08
.210+02	.200+01	.739−08	.565−08	.742−08	.735−08	.820−08
.230+02	.200+01	.737−08	.574−08	.739−08	.735−08	.836−08
.250+02	.200+01	.733−08	.581−08	.734−08	.732−08	.851−08
.270+02	.200+01	.735−08	.591−08	.736−08	.736−08	.858−08
.290+02	.200+01	.723−08	.595−08	.724−08	.726−08	.871−08

594

En/MeV	ΔEn/MeV	Nylon 6.6/6	Lucite	Liq.Musc Eq	Water	Acetylene
.110−04	.600−05	.484−11	.108−12	.148−11	.146−12	.105−12
.200−04	.120−04	.371−11	.178−12	.122−11	.241−12	.173−12
.360−04	.200−04	.298−11	.308−12	.113−11	.415−12	.300−12
.630−04	.340−04	.261−11	.529−12	.122−11	.714−12	.516−12
.110−03	.600−04	.260−11	.917−12	.156−11	.124−11	.894−12
.200−03	.120−03	.312−11	.166−11	.237−11	.224−11	.162−11
.360−03	.200−03	.444−11	.298−11	.392−11	.402−11	.290−11
.630−03	.340−03	.694−11	.520−11	.662−11	.701−11	.507−11
.110−02	.600−03	.115−10	.906−11	.114−10	.122−10	.883−11
.200−02	.120−02	.202−10	.164−10	.204−10	.221−10	.160−10
.360−02	.200−02	.357−10	.292−10	.362−10	.394−10	.285−10
.630−02	.340−02	.612−10	.503−10	.622−10	.677−10	.490−10
.110−01	.600−02	.104−09	.853−10	.106−09	.115−09	.833−10
.200−01	.120−01	.179−09	.148−09	.183−09	.199−09	.144−09
.360−01	.200−01	.297−09	.246−09	.303−09	.330−09	.240−09
.630−01	.340−01	.462−09	.382−09	.470−09	.512−09	.374−09
.820−01	.400−02	.558−09	.462−09	.567−09	.617−09	.453−09
.860−01	.400−02	.577−09	.478−09	.587−09	.638−09	.468−09
.900−01	.400−02	.595−09	.493−09	.605−09	.658−09	.483−09
.940−01	.400−02	.614−09	.509−09	.624−09	.678−09	.498−09
.980−01	.400−02	.631−09	.523−09	.641−09	.697−09	.512−09
.105+00	.100−01	.661−09	.548−09	.672−09	.730−09	.537−09
.115+00	.100−01	.701−09	.582−09	.713−09	.775−09	.570−09
.125+00	.100−01	.740−09	.615−09	.752−09	.817−09	.602−09
.135+00	.100−01	.777−09	.646−09	.790−09	.858−09	.633−09
.145+00	.100−01	.813−09	.675−09	.826−09	.897−09	.662−09
.155+00	.100−01	.846−09	.704−09	.860−09	.934−09	.690−09
.165+00	.100−01	.878−09	.730−09	.892−09	.969−09	.716−09
.175+00	.100−01	.910−09	.757−09	.924−09	.100−08	.742−09
.185+00	.100−01	.939−09	.782−09	.954−09	.104−08	.767−09
.195+00	.100−01	.968−09	.806−09	.983−09	.107−08	.790−09
.210+00	.200−01	.101−08	.841−09	.103−08	.111−08	.825−09
.230+00	.200−01	.106−08	.886−09	.108−08	.117−08	.869−09
.250+00	.200−01	.111−08	.929−09	.113−08	.123−08	.911−09
.270+00	.200−01	.116−08	.970−09	.118−08	.128−08	.951−09
.290+00	.200−01	.121−08	.101−08	.123−08	.134−08	.989−09
.310+00	.200−01	.125−08	.105−08	.128−08	.139−08	.103−08
.330+00	.200−01	.129−08	.109−08	.132−08	.144−08	.106−08
.350+00	.200−01	.133−08	.112−08	.137−08	.149−08	.109−08
.370+00	.200−01	.137−08	.116−08	.142−08	.155−08	.112−08
.390+00	.200−01	.142−08	.120−08	.148−08	.162−08	.116−08
.420+00	.400−01	.149−08	.128−08	.163−08	.178−08	.120−08
.460+00	.400−01	.154−08	.132−08	.164−08	.179−08	.126−08
.500+00	.400−01	.160−08	.133−08	.160−08	.174−08	.131−08
.540+00	.400−01	.165−08	.133−08	.165−08	.179−08	.136−08
.580+00	.400−01	.171−08	.143−08	.171−08	.185−08	.141−08
.620+00	.400−01	.177−08	.148−08	.177−08	.192−08	.146−08
.660+00	.400−01	.184−08	.152−08	.183−08	.198−08	.151−08
.700+00	.400−01	.188−08	.157−08	.189−08	.204−08	.155−08
.740+00	.400−01	.193−08	.161−08	.194−08	.210−08	.159−08
.780+00	.400−01	.197−08	.165−08	.199−08	.216−08	.163−08

En/MeV	ΔEn/MeV	Nylon 6.6/6	Lucite	Liq.Musc Eq	Water	Acetylene
.820+00	.400-01	.202-08	.170-08	.205-08	.222-08	.167-08
.860+00	.400-01	.207-08	.174-08	.210-08	.228-08	.171-08
.900+00	.400-01	.212-08	.179-08	.217-08	.235-08	.175-08
.940+00	.400-01	.217-08	.185-08	.227-08	.247-08	.178-08
.980+00	.400-01	.224-08	.195-08	.240-08	.269-08	.182-08
.105+01	.100+00	.231-08	.199-08	.249-08	.271-08	.188-08
.115+01	.100+00	.239-08	.202-08	.246-08	.267-08	.196-08
.125+01	.100+00	.248-08	.210-08	.250-08	.278-08	.204-08
.135+01	.100+00	.260-08	.217-08	.265-08	.287-08	.211-08
.145+01	.100+00	.267-08	.222-08	.269-08	.291-08	.213-08
.155+01	.100+00	.274-08	.229-08	.277-08	.300-08	.225-08
.165+01	.100+00	.282-08	.236-08	.288-08	.312-08	.231-08
.175+01	.100+00	.290-08	.241-08	.291-08	.315-08	.237-08
.185+01	.100+00	.297-08	.249-08	.303-08	.328-08	.243-08
.195+01	.100+00	.302-08	.252-08	.304-08	.329-08	.248-08
.210+01	.200+00	.317-08	.264-08	.313-08	.338-08	.263-08
.230+01	.200+00	.325-08	.268-08	.318-08	.342-08	.269-08
.250+01	.200+00	.339-08	.280-08	.331-08	.356-08	.281-08
.270+01	.200+00	.358-08	.295-08	.346-08	.370-08	.298-08
.290+01	.200+00	.384-08	.317-08	.359-08	.382-08	.326-08
.310+01	.200+00	.382-08	.313-08	.373-08	.399-08	.313-08
.330+01	.200+00	.415-08	.348-08	.406-08	.433-08	.349-08
.350+01	.200+00	.434-08	.362-08	.415-08	.440-08	.368-08
.370+01	.200+00	.438-08	.367-08	.425-08	.452-08	.370-08
.390+01	.200+00	.435-08	.360-08	.418-08	.443-08	.365-08
.420+01	.400+00	.441-08	.360-08	.431-08	.460-08	.357-08
.460+01	.400+00	.433-08	.354-08	.431-08	.463-08	.348-08
.500+01	.400+00	.441-08	.367-08	.455-08	.492-08	.353-08
.540+01	.400+00	.446-08	.366-08	.444-08	.478-08	.361-08
.580+01	.400+00	.456-08	.379-08	.464-08	.502-08	.369-08
.620+01	.400+00	.479-08	.393-08	.475-08	.510-08	.395-08
.660+01	.400+00	.464-08	.385-08	.489-08	.531-08	.370-08
.700+01	.400+00	.473-08	.399-08	.510-08	.556-08	.373-08
.740+01	.400+00	.506-08	.432-08	.538-08	.583-08	.409-08
.780+01	.400+00	.540-08	.458-08	.529-08	.564-08	.460-08
.820+01	.400+00	.516-08	.436-08	.525-08	.565-08	.426-08
.860+01	.400+00	.512-08	.436-08	.542-08	.588-08	.414-08
.900+01	.400+00	.544-08	.465-08	.551-08	.592-08	.457-08
.940+01	.400+00	.568-08	.485-08	.555-08	.591-08	.489-08
.980+01	.400+00	.558-08	.477-08	.568-08	.610-08	.467-08
.105+02	.100+01	.564-08	.483-08	.582-08	.626-08	.467-08
.115+02	.100+01	.592-08	.514-08	.625-08	.672-08	.491-08
.125+02	.100+01	.621-08	.534-08	.622-08	.661-08	.528-08
.135+02	.100+01	.642-08	.556-08	.646-08	.686-08	.548-08
.145+02	.100+01	.674-08	.588-08	.670-08	.709-08	.585-08
.155+02	.100+01	.713-08	.626-08	.688-08	.721-08	.636-08
.165+02	.100+01	.737-08	.647-08	.696-08	.726-08	.667-08
.175+02	.100+01	.746-08	.656-08	.706-08	.736-08	.676-08
.185+02	.100+01	.761-08	.671-08	.716-08	.745-08	.692-08
.195+02	.100+01	.771-08	.681-08	.729-08	.757-08	.701-08
.210+02	.200+01	.797-08	.706-08	.743-08	.769-08	.733-08
.230+02	.200+01	.810-08	.717-08	.741-08	.762-08	.752-08
.250+02	.200+01	.822-08	.726-08	.735-08	.752-08	.772-08
.270+02	.200+01	.827-08	.733-08	.738-08	.753-08	.780-08
.290+02	.200+01	.836-08	.738-08	.724-08	.734-08	.798-08

APPENDIX F. (*Continued*)

En/MeV	ΔEn/MeV	Air-Dry	Air H$_2$O Sat	CO$_2$	Ethylene	Gas,TE,wCH$_4$
.110-04	.600-05	.287-10	.283-10	.369-14	.189-12	.147-11
.200-04	.120-04	.214-10	.210-10	.667-14	.313-12	.122-11
.360-04	.200-04	.159-10	.157-10	.120-13	.540-12	.112-11
.630-04	.340-04	.120-10	.119-10	.209-13	.928-12	.122-11
.110-03	.600-04	.916-11	.904-11	.366-13	.161-11	.157-11
.200-03	.120-03	.689-11	.682-11	.564-13	.291-11	.239-11
.360-03	.200-03	.526-11	.524-11	.120-12	.522-11	.395-11
.630-03	.340-03	.421-11	.425-11	.209-12	.912-11	.667-11
.110-02	.600-03	.357-11	.370-11	.365-12	.159-10	.115-10
.200-02	.120-02	.336-11	.363-11	.664-12	.287-10	.206-10
.360-02	.200-02	.370-11	.421-11	.119-11	.512-10	.365-10
.630-02	.340-02	.476-11	.566-11	.209-11	.881-10	.628-10
.110-01	.600-02	.688-11	.843-11	.364-11	.149-09	.107-09
.200-01	.120-01	.108-10	.135-10	.660-11	.259-09	.184-09
.360-01	.200-01	.170-10	.215-10	.118-10	.429-09	.306-09
.630-01	.340-01	.256-10	.325-10	.205-10	.667-09	.475-09
.820-01	.400-02	.307-10	.391-10	.266-10	.804-09	.574-09
.860-01	.400-02	.318-10	.404-10	.279-10	.832-09	.593-09
.900-01	.400-02	.328-10	.418-10	.291-10	.858-09	.612-09
.940-01	.400-02	.338-10	.431-10	.304-10	.884-09	.631-09
.980-01	.400-02	.349-10	.443-10	.316-10	.905-09	.649-09
.105+00	.100-01	.367-10	.466-10	.338-10	.952-09	.680-09
.115+00	.100-01	.394-10	.499-10	.370-10	.101-08	.721-09
.125+00	.100-01	.420-10	.530-10	.402-10	.107-08	.761-09
.135+00	.100-01	.445-10	.561-10	.433-10	.112-08	.799-09
.145+00	.100-01	.470-10	.592-10	.465-10	.117-08	.836-09
.155+00	.100-01	.495-10	.622-10	.497-10	.122-08	.870-09
.165+00	.100-01	.520-10	.651-10	.528-10	.126-08	.903-09
.175+00	.100-01	.544-10	.680-10	.560-10	.131-08	.935-09
.185+00	.100-01	.568-10	.708-10	.592-10	.135-08	.966-09
.195+00	.100-01	.592-10	.736-10	.623-10	.139-08	.995-09
.210+00	.200-01	.627-10	.777-10	.672-10	.145-08	.104-08
.230+00	.200-01	.674-10	.832-10	.737-10	.152-08	.109-08
.250+00	.200-01	.720-10	.886-10	.804-10	.160-08	.115-08
.270+00	.200-01	.764-10	.937-10	.874-10	.166-08	.120-08
.290+00	.200-01	.809-10	.989-10	.949-10	.173-08	.124-08
.310+00	.200-01	.856-10	.104-09	.103-09	.179-08	.129-08
.330+00	.200-01	.907-10	.110-09	.113-09	.185-08	.134-08
.350+00	.200-01	.965-10	.116-09	.125-09	.190-08	.138-08
.370+00	.200-01	.104-09	.125-09	.142-09	.196-08	.143-08
.390+00	.200-01	.116-09	.137-09	.169-09	.201-08	.148-08
.420+00	.400-01	.166-09	.189-09	.262-09	.209-08	.153-08
.460+00	.400-01	.133-09	.157-09	.222-09	.218-08	.162-08
.500+00	.400-01	.143-09	.166-09	.123-09	.227-08	.163-08
.540+00	.400-01	.979-10	.122-09	.120-09	.236-08	.169-08
.580+00	.400-01	.100-09	.125-09	.127-09	.245-08	.175-08
.620+00	.400-01	.154-09	.179-09	.135-09	.253-08	.181-08
.660+00	.400-01	.230-09	.255-09	.143-09	.260-08	.187-08
.700+00	.400-01	.167-09	.193-09	.152-09	.268-08	.192-08
.740+00	.400-01	.148-09	.176-09	.160-09	.275-08	.197-08
.780+00	.400-01	.140-09	.169-09	.169-09	.282-08	.203-08

En/MeV	ΔEn/MeV	Air-Dry	Air H_2O Sat	CO_2	Ethylene	Gas,TE,wCH_4
.820+00	.400−01	.136−09	.166−09	.179−09	.239−08	.208−08
.860+00	.400−01	.133−09	.164−09	.193−09	.296−08	.213−08
.900+00	.400−01	.133−09	.165−09	.219−09	.302−08	.219−08
.940+00	.400−01	.141−09	.174−09	.282−09	.308−08	.226−08
.980+00	.400−01	.203−09	.239−09	.423−09	.314−08	.239−08
.105+01	.100+00	.251−09	.286−09	.385−09	.325−08	.244−08
.115+01	.100+00	.194−09	.229−09	.269−09	.339−08	.247−08
.125+01	.100+00	.193−09	.230−09	.282−09	.352−08	.257−08
.135+01	.100+00	.378−09	.413−09	.282−09	.365−08	.267−08
.145+01	.100+00	.357−09	.393−09	.246−09	.377−08	.273−08
.155+01	.100+00	.291−09	.330−09	.253−09	.388−08	.280−08
.165+01	.100+00	.285−09	.325−09	.288−09	.399−08	.290−08
.175+01	.100+00	.385−09	.424−09	.252−09	.410−08	.296−08
.185+01	.100+00	.341−09	.383−09	.305−09	.420−08	.305−08
.195+01	.100+00	.300−09	.342−09	.261−09	.430−08	.309−08
.210+01	.200+00	.328−09	.372−09	.273−09	.450−08	.322−08
.230+01	.200+00	.393−09	.436−09	.196−09	.463−08	.328−08
.250+01	.200+00	.406−09	.451−09	.228−09	.482−08	.342−08
.270+01	.200+00	.583−09	.628−09	.283−09	.504−08	.359−08
.290+01	.200+00	.678−09	.723−09	.355−09	.537−08	.380−08
.310+01	.200+00	.848−09	.893−09	.363−09	.531−08	.383−08
.330+01	.200+00	.976−09	.102−08	.656−09	.570−08	.417−08
.350+01	.200+00	.116−08	.121−08	.680−09	.593−08	.431−08
.370+01	.200+00	.110−08	.115−08	.705−09	.600−08	.438−08
.390+01	.200+00	.126−08	.130−08	.544−09	.601−08	.434−08
.420+01	.400+00	.141−08	.146−08	.551−09	.599−08	.439−08
.460+01	.400+00	.110−08	.115−08	.426−09	.599−08	.437−08
.500+01	.400+00	.991−09	.105−08	.567−09	.610−08	.452−08
.540+01	.400+00	.860−09	.916−09	.375−09	.624−08	.451−08
.580+01	.400+00	.851−09	.910−09	.506−09	.637−08	.466−08
.620+01	.400+00	.988−09	.105−08	.574−09	.666−08	.485−08
.660+01	.400+00	.820−09	.884−09	.601−09	.648−08	.482−08
.700+01	.400+00	.944−09	.101−08	.753−09	.654−08	.496−08
.740+01	.400+00	.120−08	.127−08	.102−08	.691−08	.527−08
.780+01	.400+00	.111−08	.118−08	.969−09	.742−08	.544−08
.820+01	.400+00	.104−08	.111−08	.831−09	.713−08	.528−08
.860+01	.400+00	.108−08	.115−08	.942−09	.704−08	.533−08
.900+01	.400+00	.113−08	.120−08	.106−08	.747−08	.557−08
.940+01	.400+00	.118−08	.125−08	.111−08	.778−08	.573−08
.980+01	.400+00	.131−08	.138−08	.117−08	.760−08	.571−08
.105+02	.100+01	.147−08	.154−08	.125−08	.763−08	.580−08
.115+02	.100+01	.174−08	.181−08	.165−08	.789−08	.614−08
.125+02	.100+01	.196−08	.202−08	.163−08	.826−08	.625−08
.135+02	.100+01	.219−08	.226−08	.187−08	.846−08	.652−08
.145+02	.100+01	.239−08	.245−08	.215−08	.881−08	.681−08
.155+02	.100+01	.254−08	.261−08	.239−08	.929−08	.713−08
.165+02	.100+01	.265−08	.272−08	.251−08	.958−08	.730−08
.175+02	.100+01	.278−08	.285−08	.262−08	.966−08	.740−08
.185+02	.100+01	.294−08	.300−08	.276−08	.980−08	.753−08
.195+02	.100+01	.310−08	.316−08	.290−08	.988−08	.763−08
.210+02	.200+01	.328−08	.334−08	.312−08	.102−07	.785−08
.230+02	.200+01	.341−08	.347−08	.315−08	.103−07	.791−08
.250+02	.200+01	.348−08	.354−08	.320−08	.105−07	.796−08
.270+02	.200+01	.357−08	.362−08	.329−08	.105−07	.800−08
.290+02	.200+01	.359−08	.365−08	.325−08	.106−07	.800−08

Index